Evidence-Based Physical Diagnosis

Evidence-Based Physical Diagnosis

Steven McGee, MD
Associate Professor, Internal Medicine
University of Washington

W.B. SAUNDERS COMPANY
A Harcourt Health Sciences Company
Philadelphia   London   New York   St. Louis   Sydney   Toronto

W.B. Saunders Company
A Harcourt Health Sciences Company

The Curtis Center
Independence Square West
Philadelphia, PA 19106

Library of Congress Cataloging-in-Publication Data

McGee, Steven R.
 Evidence-based physical diagnosis/Steven McGee.
  p. cm.
  Includes bibliographical references and index.
  ISBN 0-7216-8693-1
  1. Physical diagnosis. 2. Evidence-based medicine.
RC76 .M347 2001
616.07′54—dc21

00-052252

Publishing Director: Richard Zorab
Editor: Liz Fathman
Editorial Assistant: Paige Mosher Wilke
Project Manager: Linda McKinley
Senior Production Editor: Julie Eddy
Designer: Julia Ramirez

EVIDENCE-BASED PHYSICAL DIAGNOSIS

Printed in the United States of America

Last digit is the print number: 9 8 7 6 5 4 3 2 1

To Rosalie, Connor, and Matthew

ACKNOWLEDGMENT

I am very grateful to several colleagues, Drs. Eric Kraus, Brad Anawalt, and Ed Boyko, who looked over sections of the manuscript and provided many helpful suggestions, and to Dr. Jan Hirschmann, who not only had the patience and kindness to review the entire manuscript but also taught me the importance of precise observation and critical thinking at the bedside.

Contents

Part Nine
Abdomen

Part Ten
Extremities

Part Eleven
Neurologic Examination

Part Twelve
Likelihood Ratios and their Confidence Intervals

INTRODUCTION

The purpose of this book is to explore the origins, pathophysiology, and diagnostic accuracy of many of the physical signs used today in adult patients. We have a wonderfully rich tradition of physical diagnosis, and my hope is that this book will help square this tradition, now almost two centuries old, with the realities of modern diagnosis, which often rely more on technologic tests such as clinical imaging and laboratory testing. The tension between physical diagnosis and technologic tests has never been greater. Having taught physical diagnosis for 20 years, I frequently observe medical students purchasing textbooks of physical diagnosis during their preclinical years to study and master traditional physical signs but then neglecting or even discarding this knowledge during their clinical years, after observing that modern diagnosis often takes place at a distance from the bedside. One can hardly fault a student who, caring for a patient with pneumonia, does not talk seriously about crackles and diminished breath sounds when all of the teachers are focused on the subtleties of the patient's chest radiograph. Disregard for physical diagnosis also pervades our residency programs, most of which have formal x-ray rounds, pathology rounds, microbiology rounds, and clinical conferences addressing the nuances of laboratory tests. Very few have formal physical diagnosis rounds.

Reconciling traditional physical diagnosis with contemporary diagnostic standards has been a continuous process throughout the history of physical diagnosis. In the 1830s, the inventor of topographic percussion, Professor Pierre Adolphe Piorry, taught that there were nine distinct percussion sounds, which he used to outline the patient's liver, heart, lungs, stomach, and even individual heart chambers or lung cavities. Piorry's methods flourished for over a century and once filled 200-page manuals,[1] although today, thanks to the introduction of clinical imaging in the early 1900s, the only vestige of his methods is percussion of the liver span. In his 1819 *A Treatise on Diseases of the Chest*,[2] Laennec wrote that lung auscultation could detect "every possible case" of pneumonia. It was only a matter of 20 years before other careful physical diagnosticians tempered Laennec's enthusiasm and pointed out that the stethoscope had diagnostic limitations.[3] And for most of the twentieth century, expert clinicians believed that all late systolic murmurs were benign until Barlow in 1963 showed they often represented mitral regurgitation, sometimes of significant severity.[4]

There are two contemporary polar opinions of physical diagnosis. Holding the less common position are clinicians who believe that all traditional physical signs remain accurate today, and these clinicians continue to quiz students about Krönig's isthmus and splenic percussion signs. A more common position is that physical diagnosis has little to offer the modern clinician and that traditional signs, although interesting, cannot compete with the accuracy of our more technologic diagnostic tools. Neither position, of course, is completely correct. I hope this book, by examining the best evidence comparing physical signs to current diagnostic standards, will bring clinicians to a more appropriate middle ground: that physical diagnosis is a reliable diagnostic tool that can still help clinicians with many but not all clinical problems.

Although some regard evidence-based medicine as "cookbook medicine," this is incorrect because there are immeasurable subtleties in our interaction with patients that clinical studies cannot address (at least, not as yet) and because the diagnostic power of any physical sign (or any test for that matter) depends in part on our ideas about disease prevalence, which in turn depend on our own personal interviewing skills and clinical experience.[a] Instead, evidence-based physical diagnosis

---

[a]These subjects are discussed fully in Chapters 1 and 3.

simply summarizes the best evidence available whether a physical sign is accurate or not. The clinician who understands this evidence can then approach patients with the confidence and wisdom that would have developed had the clinician personally examined and learned from the thousands of patients reviewed in the studies of this book.

Sometimes, comparing physical signs with modern diagnostic standards reveals that the physical sign is outdated and perhaps best discarded (e.g., capillary refill time, topographic percussion of diaphragm excursion). Other times the comparison reveals that physical signs are extremely accurate and probably underused (e.g., early diastolic murmur at the left lower sternal area for aortic regurgitation, conjunctival rim pallor for anemia, a palpable gallbladder for extrahepatic obstruction of the biliary ducts). And still other times the comparison reveals that the physical sign *is* the diagnostic standard, just as most of physical examination was a century ago (e.g., systolic murmur and click of mitral valve prolapse, hemiparesis for stroke, neovascularization for proliferative diabetic retinopathy). For some diagnoses, a tension remains between physical signs and technologic tests, making it still unclear which should be the diagnostic standard (e.g., the diagnoses of cardiac tamponade or carpal tunnel syndrome). And for still others, the comparison is impossible because clinical studies comparing physical signs to traditional diagnostic standards do not exist.

My hope is that the material in this book will allow clinicians of all levels—students, house officers, and seasoned clinicians alike—to examine patients more confidently and accurately, thus restoring physical diagnosis to its appropriate and often pivotal diagnostic role. Once well-versed in evidence-based physical diagnosis, clinicians can then settle many important clinical questions at the time and place they should be first addressed—the patient's bedside.

Steven McGee, MD
July 31, 2000

REFERENCES

1. Weil A. *Handbuch und Atlas der topographischen Perkussion,* Leipzig 1880, FCW Vogel.
2. Laennec RTH. *A treatise on the diseases of the chest* (facsimile edition by Classics of Medicine library), London, 1821, T & G Underwood.
3. Addison T. The difficulties and fallacies attending physical diagnosis of diseases of the chest. In Wilks, Daldy, editors. *A collection of the published writings of the late Thomas Addison* (facsimile edition by Classics of Medicine library), London, 1846, The New Sydenham Society.
4. Barlow JB and others. The significance of late systolic murmurs, *Am Heart J* 66:443-452, 1963.

PART ONE

Understanding the Evidence

CHAPTER 1

Diagnostic Accuracy of Physical Findings

I. INTRODUCTION. If a physical sign characteristic of a suspected diagnosis is present (i.e., **positive** finding), that diagnosis becomes more likely; if the finding is absent (i.e., **negative** finding), the suspected diagnosis becomes less likely. How much these positive and negative results modify probability, however, is distinct for each physical sign. Some findings, when positive, shift probability upward greatly, but they change it little when negative. Other signs are more useful if they are absent because the negative finding practically excludes disease, although the positive one changes it little.

Much of this book consists of tables that specifically describe how positive or negative findings change the probability of disease, a property called "diagnostic accuracy." Understanding these tables first requires review of four concepts: pretest probability, sensitivity, specificity, and likelihood ratios.

II. PRETEST PROBABILITY. Pretest probability is the probability of disease (i.e., prevalence) before application of the results of a physical finding. Pretest probability is the starting point for all clinical decisions. For example, the clinician may know that a certain physical finding shifts the probability of disease upward 40%, but this information alone is unhelpful unless the clinician also knows the starting point: if the pretest probability for the particular diagnosis was 50%, the finding is diagnostic (i.e., posttest probability = 50% + 40% = 90%); if the pretest probability was only 10%, the finding is less helpful because the probability of disease is still the flip of a coin (i.e., posttest probability = 10% + 40% = 50%).

Published estimates of disease prevalence, given a particular clinical setting, are available for many clinical problems (Table 1-1), although the clinician must adjust these estimates with information from his or her own practice. For example, large studies based in emergency departments show that 12% to 30% of patients presenting with cough and fever have pneumonia (see Table 1-1). The probability of pneumonia, however, is certainly lower in patients presenting with cough and fever to an office-based practice in the community, and it may be higher if cough and fever develops in patients with cancer or human immunodeficiency virus (HIV) infection. In fact, because the best estimate of pretest probability incorporates information from the clinician's own practice—how specific underlying diseases, risks, and exposures make disease more or less likely— the practice of evidence-based medicine is never "cookbook" medicine, but instead consists of decisions based on the unique characteristics of the patients the clinician sees.

III. SENSITIVITY AND SPECIFICITY

   A. Definitions. Sensitivity and specificity describe the discriminatory power of physical signs. **Sensitivity** is the proportion of patients *with* the diagnosis who *have* the physical sign (i.e., have the *positive* result). **Specificity** is the proportion of patients *without* the diagnosis who *lack* the physical sign (i.e., have the *negative* result).

TABLE 1-1 Pretest probability

Setting (ref)	Diagnosis	Probability (%)
Acute abdominal pain[1-3]	Small bowel obstruction	4
Aortic flow murmur[4]	Severe aortic stenosis	5
Acute calf pain or swelling[5,6]	Proximal deep vein thrombosis	18
Cough and fever[7]	Pneumonia	12-30
Pleuritic chest pain, dyspnea, or hemoptysis[8,9]	Pulmonary embolism	26
Murmur of mitral regurgitation, referred for echocardiography[10]	Moderate-to-severe mitral regurgitation	33
Murmur of aortic regurgitation, referred for echocardiography or angiography[10-12]	Moderate-to-severe aortic regurgitation	49

Calculation of sensitivity and specificity requires construction of a 2×2 table (Figure 1-1) that has 2 columns (one for "diagnosis present" and another for "diagnosis absent") and 2 rows (one for "physical sign present" and another for "physical sign absent"). These rows and columns create 4 boxes: one for the "true positives"

Significant tricuspid regurgitation:

	Present	Absent	
Holosystolic murmur:			
Present	22 (a)	3 (b)	25
Absent	20 (c)	55 (d)	75
	42 (n_1)	58 (n_2)	

FIGURE 1-1 2×2 Table. The total number of patients with disease (tricuspid regurgitation in this example) is the sum of the first column, or $n_1 = a + c$. The total number of patients without disease is the sum of the second column, or $n_2 = b + d$. The *sensitivity* of a physical finding (holosystolic murmur at the left lower sternal edge, in this example) is the proportion of patients with disease who have the finding (i.e., $a/(a + c)$ or a/n_1). The *specificity* of a physical finding is the proportion of patients without disease who lack the finding (i.e., $d/(b + d)$ or d/n_2). The *positive likelihood ratio (LR)* is proportion of patients with disease who have a positive finding (a/n_1) divided by the proportion of patients without disease who have a positive finding (b/n_2), or sensitivity/ (1 − specificity). The *negative LR* is the proportion of patients with disease who lack the finding (c/n_1) divided by the proportion of patients without disease who lack the finding (d/n_2), or (1 − sensitivity)/specificity.

In this example, the sensitivity is 0.52 (22/42), the specificity is 0.95 (55/58), the positive LR is 10.1 [(22/42)/(3/58)], and the negative LR is 0.5 [(20/42)/(55/58)].

(cell a, sign and diagnosis present), one for "false positives" (cell b, sign present but disease absent), one for the "false negatives" (cell c, sign absent but disease present), and one for the "true negatives" (cell d, sign and disease absent).

Figure 1-1 presents data from a hypothetical study of 100 patients presenting with pulmonary hypertension. The clinician knows that tricuspid regurgitation is a complication of pulmonary hypertension and wonders how accurately a single physical sign—the presence of a holosystolic murmur at the left lower sternal border—detects this complication.[a] In this study, 42 patients have significant tricuspid regurgitation (the sum of column 1) and 58 patients do not (the sum of column 2). The **sensitivity** of the holosystolic murmur is the proportion of patients with disease (i.e., tricuspid regurgitation, 42 patients) who have the characteristic murmur (i.e., the *positive* result, 22 patients), which is 22/42 = 0.52 or 52%. The **specificity** of the holosystolic murmur is the proportion of patients *without* disease (i.e., no tricuspid regurgitation, 58 patients) who *lack* the murmur (i.e., the *negative* result, 55 patients), which is 55/58 = 0.95 or 95%.

To recall how to calculate sensitivity and specificity, Sackett and others have suggested helpful mnemonics: sensitivity is "pelvic inflammatory disease" (or "PID," meaning "positivity in disease") and specificity is "National Institutes of Health" (or "NIH," meaning "negativity in health").[14,15]

B. Using sensitivity and specificity to determine probability of disease. The completed 2 × 2 table can be used to determine the accu-

---

[a] The numbers used in this example are very close to those in reference 13. See also Chapter 41.

racy of the holosystolic murmur, which is how well its presence or absence discriminates between those with tricuspid regurgitation and those without it. In Figure 1-1, the first row includes all 25 patients with the murmur (i.e. the positive results). Of these 25 patients, 22 have tricuspid regurgitation; therefore the probability of tricuspid regurgitation, if the murmur is present (*positive* finding), is 22/25 or 88% (i.e., the "posttest probability" if the murmur is present). The second row includes all 75 patients without the murmur. Of these 75 patients, 20 have tricuspid regurgitation; therefore, the posttest probability of tricuspid regurgitation, if the murmur is absent (i.e., *negative* finding) is 20/75 or 27%.

In this example, the pretest probability of tricuspid regurgitation is 42%. The presence of the murmur (positive result) shifts the probability of disease upward considerably more (i.e., 46%, from 42% to 88%) than the absence of the murmur (negative result) shifts it downward (i.e., 15%, from 42% to 27%). This illustrates an important property of physical signs with a high specificity: when *present*, physical signs with a *high specificity* greatly *increase* the probability of disease. A corollary to this applies to findings with high sensitivity: when *absent*, physical signs with a high *sensitivity*, greatly *decrease* the probability of disease. The holosystolic murmur has a high specificity (95%) but only a meager sensitivity (52%), meaning that, at the bedside, a positive result (the presence of a murmur) has greater diagnostic importance than the negative result (the absence of the murmur). The presence of the characteristic murmur argues compellingly for tricuspid regurgitation, but its absence is less helpful, simply because many patients with significant regurgitation lack the characteristic murmur.

Sackett and others have suggested mnemonics for these characteristics as well: "SpPin" (i.e., a *Sp*ecific test, when *P*ositive, rules *in* disease) and "SnNout" (i.e., a *Sn*sitive test, when *N*egative, rules *out* disease).[15]

IV. LIKELIHOOD RATIOS.

Likelihood ratios, like sensitivity and specificity, describe the discriminatory power of physical signs. Although they have many advantages, the most important is how simply and quickly they can be used to estimate posttest probability.

A. Definition.

The likelihood ratio ("LR") of a physical sign is the proportion of patients *with* disease who have a particular finding divided by the proportion of patients *without* disease who also have the same finding.[b] The adjectives "positive" or "negative" indicate whether that LR refers to the presence of the physical sign (i.e. "positive" result) or to the absence of the physical sign (i.e., the "negative" result).

A **positive LR**, therefore, is the proportion of patients *with* disease who *have* a physical sign divided by the proportion of patients *without* disease who also *have* the same sign. The numerator of this equation—proportion of patients with disease who have the physical sign—is the sign's sensitivity. The denominator—proportion of patients without disease who have the sign—is the complement of specificity, or (1 – specificity). Therefore,

$$Positive\ LR = \frac{(sens)}{(1 - spec)}$$

In our hypothetical study (Figure 1-1), the proportion of patients with tricuspid regurgita-

---

[b] The usual definition of LR is the *odds* that a given finding would occur in a patient with disease as opposed to a patient without disease.

tion who have the murmur 22/42 or 52.4% (i.e., the finding's sensitivity) and the proportion of patients without tricuspid regurgitation who also have the murmur is 3/58 or 5.2% (i.e., 1 – specificity). The ratio of these proportions (i.e., [sensitivity]/[1 – specificity]) is 10.1, which is the positive LR for a holosystolic murmur at the lower sternal border. This number means that patients *with* tricuspid regurgitation are 10.1 times more likely to have the holosystolic murmur than those *without* tricuspid regurgitation.

Similarly, the **negative LR** is the proportion of patients *with* disease *lacking* a physical sign divided by the proportion of patients *without* disease also *lacking* the sign. The numerator of this equation—proportion of patients with disease *lacking* the finding—is the complement of sensitivity, or (1 – sensitivity). The denominator of the equation—proportion of patients without disease *lacking* the finding—is the specificity. Therefore,

$$Negative\ LR = \frac{(1 - sens)}{(spec)}$$

In our hypothetical study, the proportion of patients with tricuspid regurgitation lacking the murmur is 20/42 or 47.6% (i.e., 1 – sensitivity) and the proportion of patients without tricuspid regurgitation lacking the fluid wave is 55/58 or 94.8% (i.e., the specificity). The ratio of these proportions (i.e., [1 – sensitivity]/[specificity]) is 0.5, which is the negative LR for the holosystolic murmur. This number means that patients *with* tricuspid regurgitation are 0.5 times less likely to lack the murmur than those *without* tricuspid regurgitation (the inverse statement is less confusing: patients *without* tricuspid regurgitation are 2 times more likely to lack a murmur than those *with* tricuspid regurgitation).

Although these formulae are difficult to recall, the interpretation of LRs is straightforward. Physical signs with LRs greater than 1 increase the probability of disease; the greater the LR, the more compelling the argument *for* disease. Physical signs that have LRs between 1 and 0 decrease the probability of disease; the closer the LR is to zero, the more convincing the finding argues *against* disease. "Positive LR" describes how probability changes when the finding is *present.* "Negative LR" describes how probability changes when the finding is *absent.*

B. Using LRs to determine probability. The clinician can use the LR of a physical finding to estimate probability of disease in three ways: (1) using graphs or other easy-to-use nomograms,[16] (2) using bedside approximations, or (3) using formulas.

    1. Using graphs

        a. Parts of the graph. Figure 1-2 displays an easy-to-use graph that illustrates the relationship between pretest probability (x-axis) and posttest probability (y-axis), given the finding's LR. The straight line bisecting the graph into an upper left half and lower right half describes the LR of 1, which has no discriminatory value because for findings with this LR, posttest probability always equals pretest probability. Physical findings that argue *for* disease (i.e., LRs >1) appear in the upper left half of the graph; the larger the LR the more the curve approaches the upper left corner. Physical findings that argue *against* disease (i.e., LRs <1) appear in the lower right half of the graph: the closer the LR is to zero the more the curve approaches the lower right corner.

        In Figure 1-2, the 3 depicted curves with LRs greater than 1 (i.e., LR = 2, 5, and 10) are mirror images of the 3 curves

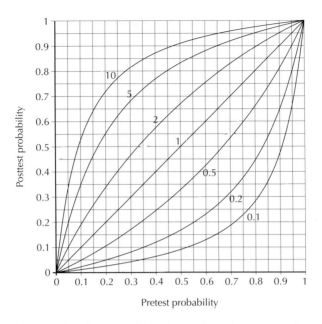

FIGURE 1-2 Probability and Likelihood Ratios. The curves describe how pretest probability (x-axis) relates to posttest probability (y-axis), given the likelihood ratio (LR) for the physical finding. Only the curves for 7 likelihood ratios are depicted (from LR = 0.1 to LR = 10). See text.

with LRs less than 1 (i.e., LR = 0.5, 0.2, and 0.1) (This assumes the "mirror" is the line LR = 1). This symmetry indicates that findings with an LR of 10 argue as much *for* disease as those with an LR = 0.1 argue *against* disease (though this is true only for the intermediate pretest probabilities). Similarly, LR = 5 argues as much for disease as LR = 0.2 argues against it, and LR = 2 mirrors LR = 0.5. Keeping these companion curves in mind will help the clinician interpret the LRs throughout this book.[c]

If a finding has an LR other than one of these depicted 7 curves, its position can be estimated with little loss in accuracy. For example, the curve for LR = 4 lies between LR = 5 and LR = 2, though closer to LR = 5 than to LR = 2.

b. **Using the graph to determine probability.** To use this graph, the clinician identifies on the x-axis the patient's pretest probability, derived from published estimates and clinical experience, and extends a line upward from that point to meet the LR curve for the physical finding. The clinician then extends a horizontal line from this point to the y-axis to identify posttest probability.

Figure 1-3 depicts this process for the lower sternal holosystolic murmur and tricuspid regurgitation. The pretest probability of tricuspid regurgitation is 42%. If the characteristic murmur is present (positive LR = 10), a line is drawn upward from 0.42 on the x-axis to the LR = 10 curve; from this point, a horizontal line is drawn to the y-axis to find the posttest probability (88%). If the murmur is absent (negative LR = 0.5), the posttest probability is the y-value where the vertical line intersects the LR = 0.5 curve (i.e., posttest probability of 27%).

These curves illustrate an additional important point: Physical signs are diagnostically most useful when they are applied to patients who have pretest prob-

---

[c] These companion pairs are easy to recall because they are the inverse of each other: the inverse of 10 is $1/10 = 0.1$; the inverse of 5 is $1/5 = 0.2$; the inverse of 2 is $1/2 = 0.5$.

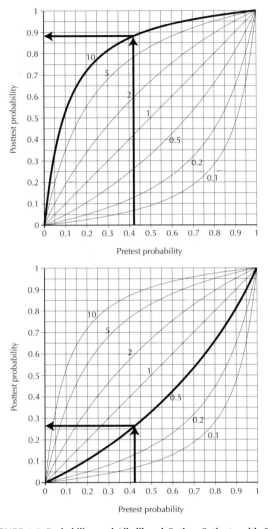

FIGURE 1-3 Probability and Likelihood Ratios: Patients with Pulmonary Hypertension. In our hypothetical clinician's practice, 42% of patients with pulmonary hypertension have the complication of tricuspid regurgitation (i.e., pretest probability is 42%). To use the curves, the clinician finds 0.42 on the x-axis and extends a line upward. The posttest probability of tricuspid regurgitation is read off the y-axis where the vertical line intersects the curve of the appropriate LR. The probability of tricuspid regurgitation if a holosystolic murmur is present at the left lower sternal edge is 88%; the probability if the finding is absent is 27%.

abilities in the intermediate range (i.e., 20% to 80%) because in this range, the different LR curves diverge the most from the LR = 1 curve (thus, shifting probability up or down a large amount). If instead the pretest probability is already very low or very high, all the LR curves cluster close to the line LR = 1 curve in either the bottom left or upper right corners, thus changing probability relatively little.

2. **Approximating probability.** The clinician can avoid using graphs and instead approximate posttest probability by remembering the following two points: (1) The companion LR curves in Figure 1-2 are LR = 2 and LR = 0.5, LR = 5 and LR = 0.2, and LR = 10 and LR = 0.1. (2) The first 3 multiples of 15 are 15, 30, and 45. Using this rule, the LRs of 2, 5, and 10 increase probability about 15%, 30%, and 45%, respectively. The LRs of 0.5, 0.2, and 0.1 decrease probability about 15%, 30%, and 45%, respectively. These estimates are accurate to within 5% to 10% of the actual value, as long as the clinician rounds posttest probability estimates over 100 to an even 100% and those below 0 to an even 0%.

Therefore, in our hypothetical patient with pulmonary hypertension, the finding of a holosystolic murmur (LR = 10) increases the probability of tricuspid regurgitation from 42% to 87% (i.e., 42% + 45%, which is only 1% lower from the actual value). The absence of the murmur (LR = 0.5) decreases the probability of tricuspid regurgitation from 42% to 27% (i.e., 42% − 15%, which is identical to the actual value).

3. **Calculating probability.** The posttest probability also can be calculated by first

converting pretest probability (P_{pre}) into pretest odds (O_{pre}):

$$O_{pre} = \frac{P_{pre}}{(1 - P_{pre})}$$

The pretest odds (O_{pre}) is multiplied by the LR for the physical sign to determine the posttest odds (O_{post}):

$$O_{post} = O_{pre} \times LR$$

The posttest odds (O_{post}) converts back to posttest probability (P_{post}), using:

$$P_{post} = \frac{O_{post}}{(1 + O_{post})}$$

Therefore, in our hypothetical example of the patients with pulmonary hypertension, the pretest odds for tricuspid regurgitation is [(0.42)/(1 − 0.42)] or 0.72. If the murmur is present (LR = 10), the posttest odds is [0.72 × 10] or 7.2, which translates to a posttest probability of [(7.2)/(1 + 7.2)] or 0.88 (i.e., 88%). If the murmur wave is absent (LR = 0.5), the posttest odds is [0.72 × 0.5] or 0.36, which translates to a posttest probability of [(0.36)/(1 + 0.36)] or 0.27 (i.e., 27%).

Clinical medicine, however, is rarely as precise as these calculations suggest, and for most decisions at the bedside, the approximations described in the preceding Section 2 are more than adequate.

C. Advantages of likelihood ratios

    1. Simplicity. In a single number, the LR conveys to clinicians how convincingly a physical sign argues for or against disease. If the LR of a finding is large, disease is likely; and if the LR of a finding is close to zero, disease is doubtful. "Positive LR" refers to the presence of the finding; "negative LR" to its absence. By comparing LRs of various findings, the clinician can easily assess which findings best rule in or rule out disease.

2. **Accuracy.** Using LRs to describe diagnostic accuracy is superior to sensitivity and specificity because the earlier described mnemonics, "SpPin" and "SnNout," are sometimes misleading. For example, according to the mnemonic "SpPin," a finding with a specificity of 95% should argue conclusively for disease, but it does so only if the positive LR for the finding is a high number. If the finding's sensitivity is 60%, the positive LR is 12.0 and the finding does argue convincingly for disease (i.e., consistent with the "SpPin" mnemonic); if the finding's sensitivity is only 5%, however, the positive LR is 1.0 and posttest probability does not change at all (i.e., inconsistent with "SpPin" mnemonic). Similarly, a highly sensitive finding argues convincingly against disease (i.e., "SnNout") only when its calculated negative LR is a number close to zero.

3. **Levels of findings.** Another advantage of LRs is that a physical sign measured on an ordinal scale (e.g., 0, 1+, 2+, 3+) or continuous scale (e.g., blood pressure) can be categorized into different levels to determine the LR for each level, thereby increasing the accuracy of the finding. Other examples include continuous findings such as heart rate, respiratory rate, temperature, and percussed span of the liver, and ordinal findings such as intensity of murmurs and degree of edema.

For example, in patients with chronic obstructive lung disease (i.e., emphysema, chronic bronchitis), breath sounds are typically faint. If the clinician grades the intensity of breath sounds on a scale from 0 (absent) to 24 (very loud), based on the methods discussed in Chapter 26, he can classify the patient's breath sounds into 1 of

4 groups: scores of 9 or less (very faint), 10 to 12, 13 to 15, or greater than 15 (loud). Each category then has its own LR (Table 1-2): scores of 9 or less argue strongly for obstructive disease (LR = 10.2), whereas scores greater than 15 argue convincingly against it (LR = 0.1). Scores from 10 to 12 argue somewhat for disease (LR = 3.6), and scores from 13 to 15 provide no diagnostic information (LR not significantly different from 1.0). If the clinician had instead identified breath sounds as simply "faint" or "normal/increased" (i.e., the traditional positive or negative finding), the finding may still discriminate between patients with and without obstructive disease, but it misses the point that the discriminatory power of the sign resides mostly with scores less than 10 and greater than 15.

When findings are categorized into levels, the term "specificity" becomes meaningless. For example, the "specificity" of a breath sound score of 13 to 15 is 80%, which means that 80% of patients without chronic airflow limitation have values other than 13 to 15, though the "80%" does not convey whether most of these other values are greater than 15 or less than 13. Similarly, when findings are put in more than 2 categories, the LR de-

TABLE 1-2 Breath sound intensity and chronic airflow limitation

Breath Sound Score	Likelihood Ratio
9 or less	10.2
10-12	3.6
13-15	NS
> 15	0.1

From references 17 and 18.

NS, Not significant.

scriptor "negative" is no longer necessary because all LRs are "positive" ones for their respective category.

4. **Combining findings.** A final advantage of LRs is that clinicians can use them to combine findings, which is particularly important for those physical signs with positive LRs around 2.0 or negative LRs around 0.5, signs that by themselves change probability little but when combined change probability a greater amount. Individual LRs can be combined, however, only if the findings are "independent."

   a. **Independence of findings.** "Independence" means that the LR for the second finding does not change once the clinician determines whether the first finding is present or absent. For a few diagnostic problems, investigators have identified which findings are independent of each other. These findings appear as components of "diagnostic scoring schemes" in the tables throughout this book. For most physical findings, however, very little information is available about independence, and the clinician must judge whether combining findings is appropriate.

   One important clue is that most independent findings have unique pathophysiology. For example, when considering pneumonia in patients with cough and fever, the clinician could combine the findings of abnormal mental status and diminished breath sounds, using the individual LRs of each finding because abnormal mental status and diminished breath sounds probably have separate pathophysiology. Similarly, when considering heart failure in patients with dyspnea, the clinician could combine the findings of elevated neck veins and third heart sound because these findings also have different pathophysiology.

Examples of findings whose individual LRs should *not* be combined (because the findings share the same pathophysiology) are flank dullness and shifting dullness in the diagnosis of ascites (both depend on intraabdominal contents dampening the vibrations of the abdominal wall during percussion), neck stiffness and Kernig's sign in the diagnosis of meningitis (both are caused by meningeal irritation), and edema and elevated neck veins in the diagnosis of heart failure (both depend on elevated right atrial pressure).

Until more information is available, the safest policy for the clinician to follow, when combining LRs of individual findings, is to combine no more than 3 findings, all of which have distinct pathophysiology.

b. How to combine findings. The clinician can use any of the methods previously described to combine findings, simply by making the posttest probability from the first finding the pretest probability for the second finding. For example, a hypothetical patient with acute fever and cough has 2 positive findings that we believe have separate pathophysiology and therefore are independent: abnormal mental status (LR = 2.2 for pneumonia) and diminished breath sounds (LR = 2.0 for pneumonia). The pretest probability of pneumonia, derived from published estimates and clinical experience is estimated to be 20%. Using the graph, the finding of abnormal mental status increases the probability form 20% to 36%; this posttest probability then becomes the pretest probability for the second finding, diminished breath sounds, which increases probability from 36% to 52%—the overall probability after application of the 2 findings. Using the approximating rules, both findings (LRs ≈ 2.0) increase the probability about 15%; the posttest probability is thus 20% + 15% + 15% = 50% (an error of only 2%). Using formulas to calculate probability, the LRs of the separate findings are multiplied together and the product is used to convert pretest into posttest odds. The product of the 2 LRs is 4.4 (2.2 × 2.0); the pretest odds is 0.2/0.8 = 0.25; the posttest odds is 0.25 × 4.4 = 1.1, which equals a probability of 1.1/2.1 = 52%.

REFERENCES

1. Eskelinen M, Ikonen J, and Lipponen P. Contributions of history-taking, physical examination, and computer assistance to diagnosis of acute small-bowel obstruction: A prospective study of 1333 patients with acute abdominal pain, *Scand J Gastroenterol* 29:715-721, 1994.
2. Brewer RJ and others. Abdominal pain: an analysis of 1000 consecutive cases in a University hospital emergency room, *Am J Surg* 131:219-223, 1976.
3. Bohner H and others. Simple data from history and physical examination help to exclude bowel obstruction and to avoid radiographic studies in patients with acute abdominal pain, *Eur J Surg* 164:777-784, 1998.
4. Aronow WS and Kronzon I. Correlation of prevalence and severity of valvular aortic stenosis determined by continuous-wave doppler echocardiography with physical signs of aortic stenosis in patients aged 62 to 100 years with aortic systolic ejection murmurs, *Am J Cardiol* 60:399-401, 1987.
5. Wells PS and others. Value of assessment of pretest probability of deep-vein thrombosis in clinical management, *Lancet* 350:1795-1798, 1997.

6. Miron MJ, Perrier A, and Bounameaux H. Clinical assessment of suspected deep vein thrombosis: comparison between a score and empirical assessment, *J Intern Med* 247:249-254, 2000.

7. Heckerling PS and others. Clinical prediction rule for pulmonary infiltrates, *Ann Intern Med* 113:664-670, 1990.

8. Hull RD and others. Pulmonary embolism in outpatients with pleuritic chest pain, *Arch Intern Med* 148:838-844, 1988.

9. Hoellerich VL and Wigton RS. Diagnosing pulmonary embolism using clinical findings, *Arch Intern Med* 146:1699-1704, 1986.

10. Desjardins VA and others. Intensity of murmurs correlates with severity of valvular regurgitation, *Am J Med* 100:149-156, 1996.

11. Frank MJ and others. The clinical evaluation of aortic regurgitation, *Arch Intern Med* 116:357-365, 1965.

12. Linhart JW. Aortic regurgitation: clinical, hemodynamic, surgical, and angiographic correlations, *Ann Thorac Surg* 11:27-37, 1971.

13. Rahko PS. Prevalence of regurgitant murmurs in patients with valvular regurgitation detected by Doppler echocardiography, *Ann Intern Med* 111:466-472, 1989.

14. Sackett DL and others. *Evidence-based medicine: how to practice and teach EBM,* New York, 1997, Churchill Livingstone.

15. Sackett DL, Haynes RB, and Tugwell P. *Clinical epidemiology: a basic science for clinical medicine,* ed 1, Boston, 1985 Little, Brown and Co.

16. Fagan TJ. Nomogram for Bayes' theorem, *N Engl J Med* 293:257, 1975.

17. Bohadana AB, Peslin R, and Uffholtz H. Breath sounds in the clinical assessment of airflow obstruction, *Thorax* 33:345-351, 1978.

18. Pardee NE, Martin CJ, and Morgan EH. A test of the practical value of estimating breath sound intensity: breath sounds related to measured ventilatory function, *Chest* 70:341-344, 1976.

CHAPTER 2

Using the Tables
in This Book

I. INTRODUCTION. Information about the diagnostic accuracy of physical findings is presented in two types of tables in this book: (1) "Frequency of Findings" tables, which display only the sensitivity of physical signs and (2) "Diagnostic Accuracy" tables, which present the sensitivity, specificity, and likelihood ratios of various physical signs.

II. FREQUENCY OF FINDINGS TABLES
  A. Definition. Frequency of Findings tables summarize multiple studies of patients with a specific diagnosis and present the sensitivity of physical signs found in that disorder. These tables provide no information about a sign's specificity. An example is Table 2-1, listing the frequency of findings in constrictive pericarditis, a disorder in which a diseased and unyielding pericardium interferes with diastolic filling of the heart.
  B. Parts of the table
    1. Finding. The first column lists the various physical signs, organized by organ system, with the findings of each organ system listed from most to least frequent.
    2. Frequency. The second column lists the sensitivity (or frequency) of the physical

TABLE 2-1 Constrictive pericarditis*

Physical Finding	Frequency (%)†
Neck Veins	
Elevated neck veins	98
Prominent Y descent (Friedrich's sign)	57-94
Kussmaul's sign	50
Arterial Pulse	
Irregularly irregular (atrial fibrillation)	36-70
Blood Pressure	
Pulsus paradoxus >10 mm Hg	17-43
Auscultation of Heart	
Pericardial knock	28-94
Pericardial rub	4
Other	
Hepatomegaly	87-100
Edema	63
Ascites	53-89

From references 1 to 8 (181 patients).

*Diagnostic standard: For constrictive pericarditis, surgical and postmortem findings,[1,2,5,6] sometimes in combination with hemodynamic findings.[3,4,7,8]

†Results are overall mean frequency or, if statistically heterogeneous, the range of values.

signs. If the sensitivity from all the studies is statistically similar, the overall mean frequency is presented (e.g., in Table 2-1, 98% of patients with constrictive pericarditis have elevated neck veins). If the sensitivities from the different studies are statistically diverse ($p <.05$ by the χ^2 test), the range of values instead is presented (e.g., in Table 2-1, 28% to 94% have a pericardial knock—a loud heart sound heard near the apex during early diastole).

3. **Footnotes.** The footnotes to these tables present the source of the information and the diagnostic standards used. For example, the

information in Table 2-1 is based on 181 patients from 8 different studies, which based the diagnosis of constrictive pericarditis on surgical, postmortem, or hemodynamic findings.

C. Interpretation. Because the Frequency of Findings tables provide just information about a sign's sensitivity, they can only be used to support a statement that a physical sign, when *absent*, probably argues *against* disease. The absence of any finding whose sensitivity (or frequency) is greater than 95% is a compelling argument against that diagnosis (i.e., the LR is 0.1 or less, even if the specificity of the finding, which is unknown, is as low as 50%). In Table 2-1, elevated venous pressure is such a finding (sensitivity 98%): if the clinician is considering the diagnosis of constrictive pericarditis, but the patient's bedside estimate of venous pressure is normal, the diagnosis becomes very unlikely.

Similarly, the absence of 2 or 3 independent findings having sensitivities greater than 80% is also a compelling argument against disease[a] (Chapter 1 defines "independent findings").

III. DIAGNOSTIC ACCURACY TABLES

A. Definition. Diagnostic Accuracy tables summarize information from large numbers of patients who present with similar symptoms but different diagnoses. The tables present the physical sign's sensitivity, specificity, and positive and negative LRs, which then indicate how well that physical sign discriminates between pa-

---

[a] This statement assumes that the product of the LRs being combined is less than 0.1. Therefore, $LR^n = \left[\dfrac{(1 - sens)}{(spec)} \right]^n \leq 0.1$, where n = number of findings being combined. If the specificity of the findings is as low as 50%, each of 2 findings being combined must have a sensitivity greater than 84%, and each of 3 findings being combined must have a sensitivity greater than 77%.

tients with a particular diagnosis of interest and those without it. The criteria for selecting these studies appear in Section IV below.

Table 2-2 presents an example that summarizes the diagnostic accuracy of physical signs for pneumonia, as applied to a large number of patients with cough and fever (see Chapter 28 for complete table). In these studies, only about 20% of patients had pneumonia; the remainder had other causes of cough and fever such as sinusitis, bronchitis, or rhinitis.

B. Parts of the table

1. **Finding.** The first column presents the physical signs, organized by organ system and the source of the information. Validated scoring schemes that combine findings appear in the bottom rows of these tables.

2. **Sensitivity and specificity.** The second and third columns present the range of a physical sign's sensitivity and specificity observed in these studies.

3. **Likelihood ratios.** The third and fourth columns present the physical sign's positive and negative LR. In contrast to sensitivity and specificity, which are presented as a range of values, LRs are described by a single number, derived by using a statistical technique called the random effects model (see Section V below).[16] Only statistically significant LRs are presented in these tables. If the 95% confidence intervals for an LR, positive or negative, include the value of 1.0, that result of the physical finding does not statistically discriminate between patients with disease and those without it, and the notation "NS" for "not significant" is recorded in the table.[b]

---

[b] For interested readers, the point estimates and 95% confidence intervals for all LRs are presented in Chapter 60.

TABLE 2-2 Pneumonia*

Finding (ref)†	Sensitivity (%)	Specificity (%)	Positive LR	Negative LR
General Appearance				
Cachexia[9]	10	97	4.0	NS
Abnormal mental status[10,11]	13-14	92-95	2.2	NS
Lung Findings				
Percussion dullness[9-13]	4-26	82-99	3.0	NS
Diminished breath sounds[10-13]	15-49	73-95	2.3	0.8
Bronchial breath sounds[10]	14	96	3.3	NS
Egophony[9-11]	4-16	96-99	4.1	NS
Crackles[9-14]	19-64	48-94	2.0	0.8
Wheezing[10-14]	15-36	50-85	NS	NS
Diagnostic Score (Heckerling and Others)[10,15]				
0 or 1 findings	7-29	33-65	0.3	—
2 or 3 findings	48-55	—	NS	—
4 or 5 findings	38-41	92-97	8.2	—

NS, Not significant.

**Diagnostic standard*: For *pneumonia*, infiltrate on chest radiograph.

†*Definition of findings*: For Heckerling's diagnostic score, the clinician scores 1 point for each of the following 5 findings that are present: temperature >37.8° C, heart rate >100 beats/min, crackles, diminished breath sounds, and *absence* of asthma.

    4. Footnote. The footnotes to these tables describe the diagnostic standards used in the studies and, if necessary, definitions of findings that appear in the table. The footnote for Table 2-2, for example, indicates that the diagnostic standard for pneumonia was the chest radiograph; it also describes the components of Heckerling's diagnostic scoring scheme presented at the bottom of the table.

C. Interpretation. To use these tables, the clinician needs only to glance at the LR columns to appreciate the discriminatory power of different findings. Positive LRs with the highest value argue the most *for* disease when that sign is *present*; negative LRs with the value closest to zero argue the most *against* disease when that sign is *absent*.

    In patients with cough and fever (Table 2-2), the findings that argue the most convincingly for pneumonia are egophony (LR = 4.1), cachexia (LR = 4.0), bronchial breath sounds (LR = 3.3), and percussion dullness (LR = 3.0). In contrast, the absence of *individual* findings never argues *against* the diagnosis of pneumonia (all negative LRs are either close to 1.0 or not significant), primarily because all of these findings have low sensitivity (i.e., the highest is 26% for percussion dullness) and thus, frequently are absent in proven cases of pneumonia.

    Table 2-2 also shows that 4 or more points using Heckerling's diagnostic scheme argues strongly *for* pneumonia (LR = 8.2), whereas the presence of 0 or 1 point argues *against* the diagnosis (LR = 0.3).

IV. CRITERIA FOR SELECTING STUDIES USED IN DIAGNOSTIC ACCURACY TABLES. All studies of adult patients that met the following four criteria were included in the tables of this book.

A. Patients were symptomatic. The study had to enroll patients presenting to clinicians with symptoms or other problems suggestive of a particular diagnosis. Therefore, studies using asymptomatic controls, which tend to inflate the specificity of a physical sign, were excluded. Clinicians do not need a physical sign to help them distinguish patients with pneumonia from healthy persons (who would not be consulting the doctor); instead, they are interested in those physical signs distinguishing pneumonia from other causes of cough and fever.

B. Definition of physical sign. The physical sign in the study had to be clearly defined.

C. Independent comparison to a diagnostic standard. There had to be an independent comparison to an acceptable diagnostic standard. "Independent comparison" means that the physical sign was not used to select patients for testing with the diagnostic standard. Acceptable diagnostic standards include laboratory testing, clinical imaging, surgical findings, or postmortem analysis.

D. 2 × 2 table could be constructed. The studies had to provide figures or tables from which numbers could be extracted to construct 2 × 2 tables and calculate sensitivity, specificity, and likelihood ratios. If any cell of the 2 × 2 table contained the value of zero, 0.5 was added to all cells to avoid creating the unlikely LRs of 0 or infinity.

V. SUMMARIZING LIKELIHOOD RATIOS. The random effects model by Dersimonian and Laird,[16] which considers both within-study and between-study variance to calculate a pooled LR, was used to summarize the LRs from the various studies. Table 2-3 illustrates how this model works. In the top rows of this table are the individual data from all studies of egophony that appeared in Table 2-2, including the finding's sensitivity, specificity, the positive and negative LRs, and the LRs' 95% confidence intervals (CIs). The bottom row of Table 2-3 shows how all of this information is summarized throughout the book.

TABLE 2-3 Egophony and pneumonia—individual studies

Reference	Sensitivity (%)	Specificity (%)	Positive LR (95% CI)	Negative LR (95% CI)
Heckerling and others[10]	16	97	4.91 (2.88, 8.37)	0.87 (0.81, 0.94)
Gennis and others[11]	8	96	2.07 (0.79, 5.41)	0.96 (0.90, 1.02)
Diehr and others[9]	4	99	7.97 (1.77, 35.91)	0.96 (0.91, 1.02)
Pooled result			4.08 (2.14, 7.79)	0.93 (0.88, 1.01)
Notation used in book	4-16	96-99	4.1	NS

NS, Not significant.

In each of the studies, egophony was very specific (96% to 99%) but insensitive (4% to 16%), and the positive LRs were all greater than 1, indicating that the finding of egophony argues for pneumonia. For 1 of the 3 studies (i.e., Gennis and others[11]), the positive LR was not significant because the 95% CI includes the value of 1 (i.e., the LR value of 1 has no discriminatory value). For the other 2 studies, the 95% confidence interval of the positive LR excluded the value of 1, thus making them statistically significant. The summary measure for the positive LR (fourth row of this table) is both clinically significant (4.08, a large positive number) and statistically significant (its 95% CI excludes 1.0). All of this information is summarized, in the notation used in this book (last row), by simply presenting the pooled LR of 4.1. (Interested readers may consult Chapter 60 for the 95% CIs for all LRs in this book.)

In contrast, the negative LRs from each study have both meager clinical significance (i.e., 0.87 to 0.96, values close to 1) and, for 2 of the 3 studies, no statistical significance (i.e., the 95% CI includes 1). The pooled negative LR also lacks clinical and statistical significance. Because statistically it is no different from 1.0 (i.e., the 95% CI of the pooled value, 0.88 to 1.01, includes 1), it is summarized using the notation "NS" for "not significant."

Presenting the single pooled result for statistically significant LRs and "NS" for the statistically insignificant ones simplifies the table and makes it much simpler to grasp the point that the finding of egophony in patients with cough and fever argues for pneumonia (LR 4.1), but the absence of egophony changes probability very little or not at all.

REFERENCES

1. Paul O, Castleman B, and White PD. Chronic constrictive pericarditis: a study of 53 cases. *Am J Med Sci* 216:361-377, 1948.

2. Mounsey P. The early diastolic sound of constrictive pericarditis, *Br Heart J* 17:143-152, 1955.

3. Tyberg TI, Goodyer AVN, and Langou RA. Genesis of pericardial knock in constrictive pericarditis, *Am J Cardiol* 46:570-575, 1980.

4. Schiavone WA. The changing etiology of constrictive pericarditis in a large referral center, *Am J Cardiol* 58:373-375, 1986.

5. Lange RL and others. Diagnostic signs in compressive cardiac disorders: constrictive pericarditis, pericardial effusion, and tamponade, *Circulation* 33:763-777, 1966.

6. Evans W and Jackson F. Constrictive pericarditis, *Br Heart J* 14:53-69, 1952.

7. Wood P. Chronic constrictive pericarditis, *Am J Cardiol* 7:48-61, 1961.

8. El-Sherif A and El-Said G. Jugular, hepatic, and praecordial pulsations in constrictive pericarditis, *Br Heart J* 33: 305-312, 1971.

9. Diehr P and others. Prediction of pneumonia in outpatients with acute cough—a statistical approach, *J Chron Dis* 37:215-225, 1984.

10. Heckerling PS and others. Clinical prediction rule for pulmonary infiltrates, *Ann Intern Med* 113:664-670, 1990.

11. Gennis P and others. Clinical criteria for the detection of pneumonia in adults: guidelines for ordering chest roentgenograms in the emergency department *J Emerg Med* 7:263-268, 1989.

12. Melbye H and others. Diagnosis of pneumonia in adults in general practice, *Scand J Prim Health Care* 10:226-233, 1992.

13. Melbye H and others. The diagnosis of adult pneumonia in general practice, *Scand J Prim Health Care* 6:111-117, 1988.

14. Singal BM, Hedges JR, and Radack KL. Decision rules and clinical prediction of pneumonia: evaluation of low-yield criteria *Ann Emerg Med* 18:13-20, 1989.

15. Emerman CL and others. Comparison of physician judgment and decision aids for ordering chest radiographs for pneumonia in outpatients, *Ann Emerg Med* 20:1215-1219, 1991.

16. DerSimonian R and Laird N. Meta analysis in clinical trials, *Control Clin Trials* 7:177-188, 1986.

CHAPTER 3

Reliability of Physical Findings

"Reliability" refers to how often multiple clinicians, examining the same patients, agree that a particular physical sign is present or absent. As characteristics of a physical sign, reliability and accuracy are distinct qualities, although significant interobserver disagreement tends to undermine the finding's accuracy and prevents clinicians from applying it confidently to their own practice. Disagreement about physical signs also contributes to the growing sense among clinicians, not necessarily justified, that physical examination is less scientific than more technologic tests, such as clinical imaging and laboratory testing, and that physical examination lacks their diagnostic authority.

The most straightforward way to express reliability, or interobserver agreement, is "simple agreement," which is the proportion of total observations in which clinicians agree about the finding. For example, if 2 clinicians examining 100 patients with dyspnea agree that a third heart sound is present in 5 patients and is absent in 75 patients, simple agreement would be 80% (i.e., $(5 + 75)/100 = 0.80$; in the remaining 20 patients, only 1 of the 2 clinicians heard a third heart sound). Simple agreement has advantages, including being easy to calculate and understand, but a significant disadvantage is that agreement may be quite high by chance alone. For example, if one of the clinicians in our hypothetical study heard a third heart sound in 10 of the 100 dyspneic patients and the other heard it in 20 of the patients (even though they agreed about the presence of the heart sound in only 5 patients), simple agreement *by chance alone* would be 74%.[a] With chance agreement this high, the observed 80% agreement no longer seems so impressive.

To address this problem, most clinical studies now express interobserver agreement using the kappa (κ)–statistic, which usually has values between 0 and 1 (Appendix 1 at the end of this chapter shows how to calculate the κ-statistic). A κ-value of 0 indicates that observed agreement is the same as that expected by chance, and a κ-value of 1 indicates perfect agreement. According to convention, a kappa value of 0 to 0.2 indicates *slight* agreement; 0.2 to 0.4, *fair* agreement; 0.4 to 0.6, *moderate* agreement; 0.6 to 0.8, *substantial* agreement; and 0.8 to 1.0 almost *perfect* agreement.[b] Rarely, physical signs have κ-values less than 0 (theoretically as low as –1), indicating the observed agreement was worse than chance agreement.

Table 3-1 presents the κ-statistic for most of the physical signs discussed in this book, demonstrating that, with rare exceptions, observed agreement is better than chance agreement (i.e., κ-statistic >0). About 60% of findings have a κ-statistic of 0.4 or more, indicating that observed agreement is moderate or better.

Clinical disagreement occurs for many reasons—some causes clinicians can control, but others are inextricably linked to the very nature of clinical medicine and human observation in general. The most prominent reasons include the following: (1) The physical sign's

Text continued on p. 40

---

[a] Agreement by chance approaches 100% as the percentage of positive observations for both clinicians approaches 0% or 100% (i.e., both clinicians agree that a finding is very uncommon or very common). Appendix 1 shows how to calculate chance agreement.

[b] No measure of reliability is perfect, especially for findings whose prevalence clinicians agree approaches 0% or 100%. For these findings, simple agreement tends to overestimate reliability, and the κ-statistic tends to underestimate the reliability.

TABLE 3-1 Interobserver agreement and physical signs

FINDING (REF)	κ-STATISTIC*
General Appearance	
Mental Status Examination	
Mini-Mental Status examination[1]	0.28-0.80
Clock-drawing test (Wolf-Klein method)[2]	0.73
Confusion Assessment Method for delirium[3]	0.81
Stance and Gait	
Abnormal gait[4]	0.11-0.52
Skin	
Patient appears anemic[5,6]	0.23-0.48
Nail bed pallor[7]	0.19-0.34
Conjunctival pallor (rim method)[8]	0.54-0.75
Cyanosis[5,9]	0.36-0.70
Jaundice[10]	0.65
Vascular spiders[10,11]	0.64-0.73
Palmar erythema[10,11]	0.37-0.49
Hydration Status	
Patient appears dehydrated[5]	0.44-0.53
Axillary dryness[12]	0.5
Increased moisture on skin[5]	0.31-0.53
Nutritional Assessment	
Abnormal nutritional state[5]	0.27-0.36
Other	
Consciousness impaired[5]	0.65-0.88
Patient appears older than age[5]	0.38-0.42
Patient appears in pain[5]	0.43-0.75
Generally unwell in appearance[5]	0.52-0.64
Vital Signs	
Hypotension, systolic blood pressure <90 mm Hg[13]	> 0.90
Osler's sign[14-16]	0.26-0.72
Elevated body temperature, palpating the skin[5]	0.09-0.23
Tachypnea[9]	0.25

Continued

TABLE 3-1 Interobserver agreement and physical signs—cont'd

Finding (ref)	κ-Statistic*
Head and Neck	
Diabetic Retinopathy	
Microaneurysms[17,18]	0.58-0.66
Intraretinal hemorrhages[17,18]	0.89
Hard exudates[17,18]	0.66-0.74
Cotton wool spots[17,18]	0.56-0.67
Intraretinal microvascular abnormalities (IRMA)[17,18]	0.46
Neovascularization near disc[17,18]	0.21-0.48
Macular edema[17,18]	0.21-0.67
Overall grade[17,18]	0.65
Hearing	
Whispered voice test[19]	0.16-1.0
Thyroid	
Thyroid gland diffuse, multinodular, or solitary nodule[20]	0.25-0.70
Goiter present or absent[21]	0.38-0.77
Meninges	
Nuchal rigidity, present or absent[22]	0.76
Lungs	
Inspection	
Clubbing[9,23]	0.33-0.45
Breathing difficulties[5]	0.54-0.69
Reduced chest movement[9,24]	0.14-0.38
Scalene or sternocleidomastoid muscle contraction[25]	0.52
Kyphosis[23]	0.37
Displaced trachea[9]	0.01
Palpation	
Tracheal descent during inspiration[25]	0.62
Impalpable apex beat[9,23]	0.33-0.44
Decreased tactile fremitus[9]	0.24
Increased tactile fremitus[9]	0.01
Subxiphoid point of maximal cardiac impulse[26]	0.30
Paradoxical costal margin movement[25]	0.56

TABLE 3-1 Interobserver agreement and physical signs—cont'd

FINDING (REF)	κ-STATISTIC*
Lungs—cont'd	
Percussion	
Hyperresonant percussion note[9,24,26]	0.26-0.50
Dull percussion note[9,24,27]	0.16-0.52
Diaphragm excursion more or less than 2 cm, by percussion[26]	−0.04
Diminished cardiac dullness[26]	0.49
Auscultatory percussion abnormal[28]	0.18-0.39
Auscultation	
Reduced breath sound intensity[9,24,26,27,29]	0.16-0.47
Bronchial breathing[9,24]	0.19-0.32
Whispering pectoriloquy[9]	0.11
Crackles[9,27,29,30]	0.21-0.63
Wheezes[9,26,27,29]	0.43-0.93
Rhonchi[24]	0.55
Pleural rub[9]	0.51
Special Tests	
Snider test <10 cm[26]	0.39
Forced expiratory time[26,31,32]	0.27-0.70
Wells system for clinical probability for pulmonary embolus[33]	0.86
Heart	
Neck Veins	
Neck veins, elevated or normal[30,34]	0.38-0.69
Abdominojugular test[34]	0.92
Palpation	
Palpable apical impulse present[35-37]	0.68-0.82
Palpable apical impulse measurable[38]	0.56
Palpable apical impulse displaced lateral to midclavicular line[30,35,36]	0.43-0.64
Percussion	
Cardiac dullness >10.5 cm from midsternal line[39,40]	0.57

Continued

TABLE 3-1 Interobserver agreement and physical signs—cont'd

Finding (ref)	κ-Statistic*
Heart–cont'd	
Auscultation	
S_2 diminished or absent vs. normal[41]	0.54
Third heart sound[30,34,42,43]	−0.17-0.69
Fourth heart sound[43]	0.15-0.52
Presence of systolic murmur[41]	0.19
Systolic murmur radiates to right carotid[41]	0.33
Systolic murmur, long systolic or early systolic[44]	0.78
Carotid Pulsation	
Delayed carotid upstroke[41]	0.26
Reduced carotid volume[41]	0.24
Abdomen	
Inspection	
Abdominal distension[45]	0.35
Abdominal wall collateral veins, present vs. absent[10]	0.47
Palpation and Percussion	
Ascites[10,11]	0.63-0.75
Abdominal tenderness[45,46]	0.31-0.68
Rebound tenderness[45]	0.25
Guarding[45]	0.36
Rigidity[45]	0.14
Palpable spleen[10,11]	0.33-0.75
Liver consistency, normal or abnormal[10]	0.4
Liver, nodular or not[10]	0.29
Liver, tender or not[11]	0.49
Liver, span >9 cm by percussion[30]	0.11
Spleen palpable or not[47]	0.56-0.70
Spleen percussion sign (Traube's), positive or not[48]	0.19-0.41
Abdominal aortic aneurysm, present vs. absent[49]	0.53

TABLE 3-1 Interobserver agreement and physical signs—cont'd

FINDING (REF)	κ-STATISTIC*
Extremities	
Peripheral pulse, present vs. absent[50,51]	0.52-0.92
Peripheral pulse, normal or diminished[50]	0.01-0.15
Monofilament sensation, normal or abnormal[52]	0.72-0.83
Dependent edema[30]	0.39
Well's pretest probability for DVT[53]	0.75
Neurologic Examination	
Cranial Nerves	
Pharyngeal sensation, present or absent[54]	1.0
Facial palsy, present or absent[55]	0.48-0.68
Motor Examination	
Muscle strength, MRC scale[56-58]	0.69-0.93
Muscle atrophy[59]	0.32-0.81
Spasticity, 6-point scale[60]	0.21-0.61
Rigidity, 4-point scale[61]	0.64
Asterixis, present or absent[10]	0.42
Sensory Examination	
Light touch sensation, normal, diminished, or increased[59]	0.63
Pain sensation, normal, diminished, or increased[57,59]	0.41-0.57
Vibratory sensation, normal or diminished[59]	0.45-0.54
Reflex Examination	
Reflex amplitude, NINDS scale[62]	0.51-0.61
Ankle jerk, present or absent[63]	0.34-0.94
Asymmetric leg reflexes[57]	0.52
Primitive reflexes, amplitude and persistence[64]	0.46-1.0
Babinski response[55,65]	0.17-0.61
Coordination	
Finger-nose test[55]	0.55-0.79
Dysmetria, finger-to-nose test, rated 0-3[66]	0.36-0.40

Continued

TABLE 3-1 Interobserver agreement and physical signs—cont'd

FINDING (REF)	κ-STATISTIC*
Neurologic Examination—cont'd	
Peripheral Nerve	
Positive straight-leg raising test[57,67,68]	0.33-0.68

DVT, Deep vein thrombosis; *MRC,* Medical Research Council; *NINDS,* National Institute of Neurological Disorders.

*Interpretation of the κ-statistic: 0-0.2 slight agreement, 0.2-0.4 fair agreement, 0.4-0.6 moderate agreement, 0.6-0.8 substantial agreement, 0.8-1.0 almost perfect agreement.

definition is vague or ambiguous. For example, experts recommend about a dozen different ways to perform auscultatory percussion of the liver, thus making the sign so nebulous that significant interobserver agreement is guaranteed. Ambiguity also results if signs are defined with terms that are not easily measurable. For example, clinicians assessing whether a peripheral pulse is present or absent demonstrate moderate-to-almost perfect agreement (κ = 0.52 to 0.92, Table 3-1), but when the same clinicians are asked to record whether the palpable pulse is normal or diminished, they have great difficulty agreeing about the sign (κ = 0.01 to 0.15) simply because they have no idea what the next clinician means by "diminished." (2) The clinician's technique is flawed. For example, common mistakes are using the diaphragm instead of the bell of the stethoscope to detect the third heart sound or stating a muscle stretch reflex is absent without first trying to elicit it using a reinforcing maneuver (e.g., Jendrassik maneuver). (3) Biologic variation of the physical sign. The pericardial friction rub, pulsus alternans, cannon A waves, Cheyne-Stokes respirations, and many other signs are notoriously evanescent, tending to come and go over time. (4) The clinician is careless or inattentive. The bustle of an active practice may lead clinicians to listen to the lungs while conducting the patient interview or to search for a subtle murmur in a noisy emergency room. Reliable observations require undistracted attention and an alert mind. (5) The clinician's biases influence the observation. When findings are equivocal, expectations influence perceptions. For example, in a patient who just started blood pressure medications, borderline hypertension may become normal blood pressure; in a patient with increasing bilateral edema, borderline distended neck veins may become clearly elevated venous pressure, or in a patient with new weakness, the equivocal Babinski sign may become clearly positive. Sometimes, biases actually create the finding: if the clinician holds a flashlight too long over an eye with suspected optic nerve disease, he may temporarily bleach the retina of that eye and produce the Marcus Gunn pupil, thus confirming the original suspicion.

The lack of perfect reliability with physical diagnosis is sometimes regarded as a significant weakness, a reason that physical diagnosis is less reliable and scientific than clinical imaging and laboratory testing. Nonetheless, Table 3-2 shows that, for most of our *diagnostic standards*—chest radiography, computed tomography, angiography, magnetic resonance imaging, ultrasonography, endoscopy, and pathology—interobserver agreement is also less than perfect, with κ-statistics similar to those for physical signs. Even with laboratory tests, which present the clinician with a single, indisputable number, interobserver disagreement is still possible and even common, simply because the clinician has to interpret the laboratory test's *significance*. For example, in one study of 3 endocrinologists reviewing the same thyroid function tests and other clinical data of 55 consecutive outpatients with suspected thyroid disease, the endocrinologists disagreed about the final diagnosis 40% of the time.[20] Computerized interpretation of test results performs no better: in a study of pairs of electrocardiograms taken only 1 minute apart from 92 patients, the computer interpretation was significantly different 40% of the time, even though the tracings showed no change.[82]

By defining abnormal findings precisely, by studying and mastering examination technique, and by observ-

TABLE 3-2 Interobserver agreement—diagnostic standards

FINDING (REF)	κ-STATISTIC*
Chest Radiography	
Cardiomegaly[34]	0.48
Interstitial edema[34]	0.83
Pulmonary vascular redistribution[34]	0.50
Grading pulmonary fibrosis, 4-point scale[69]	0.45
Contrast Venography	
DVT in leg[70]	0.53
Digital Subtraction Angiography	
Renal artery stenosis[71]	0.65
Coronary Arteriography	
Classification of coronary artery lesions[72]	0.33
Computed Tomography of Head	
Normal or abnormal, patient with stroke[73]	0.60
Lesion on right or left side, patient with stroke[73]	0.65
Mass effect, present or absent[73]	0.52
Computed Tomography of the Chest	
Lung cancer staging[74]	0.40-0.60
Magnetic Resonance Imaging of Head	
Compatible with multiple sclerosis[75]	0.57-0.87
Magnetic Resonance Imaging of Lumbar Spine	
Intervertebral disc extrusion, protrusion, bulge, or normal[76]	0.59
Ultrasonography	
Calf DVT, present or absent[77]	0.69
Thyroid nodule, present or absent[78,79]	0.57-0.66
Endoscopy	
Grade of reflux esophagitis[80]	0.55
Pathologic Examination of Liver Biopsy	
Cholestasis[81]	0.40
Alcoholic liver disease[81]	0.49
Cirrhosis[81]	0.59

*Interpretation of the κ-statistic: 0-0.2 slight agreement, 0.2-0.4 fair agreement, 0.4-0.6 moderate agreement, 0.6-0.8 substantial agreement, 0.8-1.0 almost perfect agreement.

ing every detail at the bedside attentively and without bias or distraction, we can minimize interobserver disagreement and make physical diagnosis more precise. But, it is simply impossible to abstract every detail of our observations of patients into exact physical signs, and in this way physical diagnosis is no different than any of the other tools we use to categorize disease. So long as both the material and the observers of clinical medicine are human beings, a certain amount of subjectivity always will be with us.

APPENDIX 1: CALCULATION OF THE κ-STATISTIC

The observations of 2 observers who are examining the same N patients independently are customarily displayed in a 2×2 table, similar to that in Figure 3-1. Observer A finds the sign to be present in w_1 patients and absent in w_2 patients; observer B finds the sign to be present in y_1 patients and absent in y_2 patients. The 2 observers agree the sign is present in a patients and absent in d patients. Therefore, the observed agreement (P_O) is:

$$P_O = (a + d)/N$$

Calculation of the κ-statistic first requires calculation of the agreement that would have occurred by chance alone. Among all the patients, observer A found the fraction w_1/N to have the sign; therefore, by chance alone, among the y_1 patients with the sign according to observer B, observer A would find the sign in (w_1/N) times y_1 or ($w_1 y_1/N$) patients (i.e., this is the *number* of patients in which both observers agree the sign is present, by chance alone). Similarly, both observers would agree the sign is absent by chance alone in ($w_2 y_2/N$) patients. Therefore, the expected chance agreement (P_E) is their sum, divided by N:

$$P_E = (w_1 y_1 + w_2 y_2)/N^2$$

This equation shows that agreement by chance alone (P_E) approaches 100% as both w_1 and y_1 approach 0 or

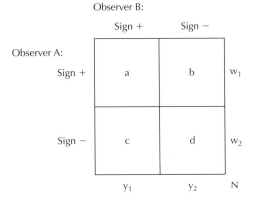

Observer B:

	Sign +	Sign −	
Observer A:			
Sign +	a	b	w_1
Sign −	c	d	w_2
	y_1	y_2	N

Sample problem:

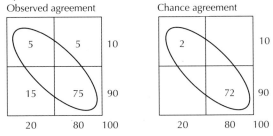

Observed agreement

5	5	10
15	75	90
20	80	100

Chance agreement

2		10
	72	90
20	80	100

FIGURE 3-1 Interobserver Agreement and the κ-Statistic. *Top half:* Conventional 2 × 2 table displaying data for calculation of κ-statistic. *Bottom half:* A sample case, in which observed agreement is 80%, chance agreement is 74%, and the κ-statistic is 0.23 (see Appendix 1 for discussion).

N (i.e., both clinicians agree that a finding is rare or that it is very common).

The κ-statistic is the increment in observed agreement beyond that expected by chance ($P_O–P_E$), divided by the maximal increment that could have been observed had the observed agreement been perfect ($1–P_E$):

$$\kappa = \frac{(P_O - P_E)}{(1 - P_E)}$$

For example, Figure 3-1 depicts the observations of 2 observers in a study of 100 patients with dyspnea. Both agree the third heart sound is present in 5 patients and absent in 75 patients; therefore simple agreement is $(5 + 75)/100$ or 0.80. By chance alone, they would have agreed about the sound being present in $(10 \times 20)/100$ patients (i.e., 2 patients) and absent in $(90 \times 80)/100$ patients (i.e., 72 patients); therefore, chance agreement is $(2 + 72)/100$ patients or 0.74. The κ-statistic for this finding becomes $(0.80 - 0.74)/(1 - 0.74) = (0.06)/(0.26) = 0.23$.

REFERENCES

1. O'Connor DW and others. The reliability and validity of the mini-mental state in a British community survey, *J Psychiatr Res* 23:87-96, 1989.
2. Ainslie NK and Murden RA. Effect of education on the clock-drawing dementia screen in non-demented elderly persons, *J Am Geriatr Soc* 41:249-252, 1993.
3. Inouye SK and others. Clarifying confusion: the confusion assessment method. A new method for detection of delirium, *Ann Intern Med* 113:941-948, 1990.
4. Eastlack ME and others. Interrater reliability of video-taped observational gait-analysis assessments, *Phys Ther* 71:465-472, 1991.
5. Gjorup T and others. Global assessment of patients—a bedside study. II. Interobserver variation and frequency of clinical findings, *J Intern Med* 228:147-150, 1990.
6. Gjorup T and others. A critical evaluation of the clinical diagnosis of anemia, *Am J Epidemiol* 124:657-665, 1986.
7. Nardone DA and others. Usefulness of physical examination in detecting the presence or absence of anemia, *Arch Intern Med* 150:201-204, 1990.
8. Sheth TN and others. The relation of conjunctival pallor to the presence of anemia, *J Gen Intern Med* 12:102-106, 1997.
9. Spiteri MA, Cook DG, and Clarke SW. Reliability of eliciting physical signs in examination of the chest, *Lancet* 2:873-875, 1988.
10. Espinoza P and others. Interobserver agreement in the physical diagnosis of alcoholic liver disease, *Dig Dis Sci* 32:244-247, 1987.

11. Theodossi A and others. Inter-observer variation of symptoms and signs in jaundice, *Liver* 1:21-32, 1981.

12. Eaton D and others. Axillary sweating in clinical assessment of dehydration in ill elderly patients, *Br Med J* 308:1271, 1994.

13. Lemeshow S and others. Mortality probability models (MPM II) based on an international cohort of intensive care unit patients, *JAMA* 270:2478-2486, 1993.

14. Hla KM and others. Observer variability of Osler's maneuver in detection of pseudohypertension, *J Clin Epidemiol* 44:513-518, 1991.

15. Belmin J and others. Osler's maneuver: absence of usefulness for the detection of pseudohypertension in an elderly population, *Am J Med* 98:42-49, 1995.

16. Tsapatasaris NP, Napolitana BT, and Rothchild J. Osler's maneuver in an outpatient clinic setting, *Arch Intern Med* 151:2209-2211, 1991.

17. Milton RC, Ganley JP, and Lynk RH. Variability in grading diabetic retinopathy from stereo fundus photographs: comparison of physician and lay readers, *Br J Ophthalmol* 61:192-201, 1977.

18. Early Treatment Diabetic Retinopathy Study Research Group. Grading diabetic retinopathy from stereoscopic color fundus photographs: an extension of the modified Airlie House Classification. ETDRS report number 10. *Ophthalmology* 98:786-806, 1991.

19. Eekhof JAH and others. The whispered voice: the best test for screening for hearing impairment in general practice? *Br J Gen Pract* 46:473-474, 1996.

20. Jarlov AE and others. Observer variation in the clinical and laboratory evaluation of patients with thyroid dysfunction and goiter, *Thyroid* 8:393-398, 1998.

21. Siminoski K. The rational clinical examination: does this patient have a goiter? *JAMA* 273:813-817, 1995.

22. Lindsay KW, Teasdale GM, and Knill-Jones RP. Observer variability in assessing the clinical features of subarachnoid hemorrhage, *J Neurosurg* 58:57-62, 1983.

23. Schilling RSF, Hughes JPW, and Dingwall-Fordyce I. Disagreement between observers in an epidemiological study of respiratory disease, *Br Med J* 1:65-68, 1955.

24. Gjorup T, Bugge PM, and Jensen AM. Interobserver variation in assessment of respiratory signs: physicians' guesses as to interobserver variation, *Acta Med Scand* 216:61-66, 1984.

25. Stubbing DG and others. Some physical signs in patients with chronic airflow obstruction, *Am Rev Respir Dis* 125: 549-552, 1982.

26. Badgett RG and others. Can moderate chronic obstructive pulmonary disease be diagnosed by historical and physical findings alone? *Am J Med* 94:188-196, 1993.

27. Mulrow CD and others. Observer variation in the pulmonary examination, *J Gen Intern Med* 1:364-367, 1986.

28. Nelson RS and others. Rapid clinical diagnosis of pulmonary abnormalities in HIV-seropositive patients by auscultatory percussion, *Chest* 105:402-407, 1994.

29. Holleman DR, Simel DL, and Goldberg JS. Diagnosis of obstructive airways disease from the clinical examination, *J Gen Intern Med* 8:63-68, 1993.

30. Gadsboll N and others. Symptoms and signs of heart failure in patients with myocardial infarction: Reproducibility and relationship to chest X-ray, radionuclide ventriculography and right heart catheterization, *Eur Heart J* 10:1017-1028, 1989.

31. Schapira RM and others. The value of the forced expiratory time in the physical diagnosis of obstructive airways disease, *JAMA* 270:731-736, 1993.

32. Badgett R and Tanaka D. The diagnostic value of the forced expiratory time, *JAMA* 271:25, 1994.

33. Wells PS and others. Use of a clinical model for safe management of patients with suspected pulmonary embolism, *Ann Intern Med* 129:997-1005, 1998.

34. Butman SM and others. Bedside cardiovascular examination in patients with severe chronic heart failure: Importance of rest or inducible jugular venous distension, *J Am Coll Cardiol* 22:968-974, 1993.

35. O'Neill TW and others. Diagnostic value of the apex beat, *Lancet* 1:410-411, 1989.

36. O'Neill TW and others. Diagnostic value of the apex beat, *Lancet* 2:499, 1989.

37. Mulkerrin E and others. The apex cardiac beat: not a reliable clinical sign in elderly patients, *Age Ageing* 20: 304-306, 1991.

38. Dans AL and others. Evaluation of the reproducibility and accuracy of apex beat measurement in the detection of echocardiographic left ventricular dilation, *Can J Cardiol* 11:493-497, 1995.

39. Heckerling PS and others. Accuracy of precordial percussion in detecting cardiomegaly, *Am J Med* 91:328-334, 1991.

40. Heckerling PS and others. Accuracy and reproducibility of precordial percussion and palpation for detecting increased left ventricular end-diastolic volume and mass: a comparison of physical findings and ultrafast computed tomography of the heart, *JAMA* 270:1943-1948, 1993.

41. Etchells E and others. A bedside clinical prediction rule for detecting moderate or severe aortic stenosis, *J Gen Intern Med* 13:699-704, 1998.

42. Ishmail AA and others. Interobserver agreement by auscultation in the presence of a third heart sound in patients with congestive heart failure, *Chest* 91:870-873, 1987.

43. Lok CE, Morgan CD, and Ranganathan N. The accuracy and interobserver agreement in detecting the "gallop sounds" by cardiac auscultation, *Chest* 114:1283-1288, 1998.

44. Forssell G, Jonasson R, and Orinius E. Identifying severe aortic valvular stenosis by bedside examination, *Acta Med Scand* 218:397-400, 1985.

45. Bjerregaard B and others. The reliability of medical history and physical examination in patients with acute abdominal pain, *Meth Inform Med* 22:15-18, 1983.

46. Priebe WM, DaCosta LR, and Beck IT. Is epigastric tenderness a sign of peptic ulcer disease? *Gastroenterology* 82:16-19, 1982.

47. Barkun AN and others. The bedside assessment of splenic enlargement, *Am J Med* 91:512-518, 1991.

48. Barkun AN and others. Splenic enlargement and Traube's space: how useful is percussion? *Am J Med* 87:562-566, 1989.

49. Fink HA and others. The accuracy of physical examination to detect abdominal aortic aneurysm, *Arch Intern Med* 160:833-836, 2000.

50. Myers KA and others. Palpation of the femoral and popliteal pulses: a study of the accuracy as assessed by agreement between multiple observers, *Eur J Vasc Surg* 1:245-249, 1987.

51. Brearley S, Shearman CP, and Simms MH. Peripheral pulse palpation: an unreliable physical sign, *Ann Roy Coll Surg Eng* 74:169-171, 1992.

52. Diamond JE and others. Reliability of diabetic foot evaluation, *Physical Ther* 69:797-802, 1989.

53. Wells PS and others. Value of assessment of pretest probability of deep-vein thrombosis in clinical management, *Lancet* 350:1795-1798, 1997.

54. Davies AE and others. Pharyngeal sensation and gag reflex in healthy subjects, *Lancet* 345:487-488, 1995.

55. Hansen M and others. Inter-observer variation in the evaluation of neurological signs: patient-related factors, *J Neurol* 241:492-496, 1994.

56. Segatore M. Determining the interrater reliability of motor power assessments using a spinal cord testing record, *J Neurosci Nurs* 23:220-223, 1991.

57. Vroomen PCAJ, De Krom MCTFM, and Knottnerus JA. Consistency of history taking and physical examination in patients with suspected lumbar nerve root involvement, *Spine* 25:91-97, 2000.

58. Brandsma JW and others. Manual muscle strength testing: intraobserver and interobserver reliabilities for the intrinsic muscles of the hand, *J Hand Ther* 8:185-190, 1995.

59. Viikari-Juntura E. Interexaminer reliability of observations in physical examinations of the neck, *Phys Ther* 67:1526-1532, 1987.

60. Haas BM and others. The inter-rater reliability of the original and of the modified Ashworth scale for the assessment of spasticity in patients with spinal cord injury, *Spin Cord* 34:560-564, 1996.

61. van Dillen L and Roach KE. Interrater reliability of a clinical scale of rigidity, *Phys Ther* 68:1679-1681, 1988.

62. Litvan I and others. Reliability of the NINDS myotatic reflex scale, *Neurology* 47:969-972, 1996.

63. O'Keeffe STO and others. A comparison of two techniques for ankle jerk assessment in elderly subjects, *Lancet* 344: 1619-1620, 1994.

64. Vreeling FW and others. Primitive reflexes in healthy, adult volunteers and neurological patients: Methodological issues, *J Neurol* 240:495-504, 1993.

65. Maher J and others. Plantar power: reproducibility of the plantar response, *Br Med J* 304:482, 1992.

66. Swaine BR and Sullivan SJ. Reliability of the scores for the finger-to-nose test in adults with traumatic brain injury, *Phys Ther* 73:71-78, 1993.

67. McCombe PF and others. Reproducibility of physical signs in low-back pain, *Spine* 14:909-918, 1989.

68. Van den Hoogen HJM and others. The inter-observer reproducibility of Lasegue's sign in patients with low back pain in general practice, *Br J Gen Pract* 46:727-730, 1996.

69. Baughman RP and others. Crackles in interstitial lung disease: comparison of sarcoidosis and fibrosing alveolitis, *Chest* 100:96-101, 1991.

70. Illescas FF and others. Interobserver variability in the interpretation of contrast venography, technetium-99m red blood cell venography and impedance plethysmography for deep vein thrombosis, *J Can Assoc Radiol* 41:264-269, 1990.

71. DeVries AR and others. Interobserver variability in assessing renal artery stenosis by digital subtraction angiography, *Diagn Imag Clin Med* 53:277-281, 1984.

72. Herrman JPR and others. Inter- and intra-observer variability in the qualitative categorization of coronary angiograms, *Int J Card Imag* 12:21-30, 1996.

73. Shinar D and others. Interobserver reliability in the interpretation of computed tomographic scans of stroke patients, *Arch Neurol* 44:149-155, 1987.

74. Webb WR and others. Interobserver variability in CT and MR staging of lung cancer, *J Comput Assist Tomogr* 17:841-846, 1993.

75. Barkhof F and others. Interobserver agreement for diagnostic MRI criteria in suspected multiple sclerosis, *Neuroradiology* 41:347-350, 1999.

76. Jensen MC and others. Magnetic resonance imaging of the lumbar spine in people without back pain, *N Engl J Med* 331:69-73, 1994.

77. Atri M and others. Accuracy of sonography in the evaluation of calf deep vein thrombosis in both postoperative surveillance and symptomatic patients, *Am J Radiol* 166:1361-1367, 1996.

78. Jarlov AE and others. Observer variation in ultrasound assessment of the thyroid gland, *Br J Radiol* 66:625-627, 1993.

79. Schneider AB and others. Thyroid nodules in the follow-up of irradiated individuals: Comparison of thyroid ultrasound with scanning and palpation, *J Clin Endocrinol Metab* 82:4020-4027, 1997.

80. Bytzer P, Havelund T, and Moeller Hansen J. Interobserver variation in the endoscopic diagnosis of reflux esophagitis, *Scand J Gastroenterol* 28:119-125, 1993.

81. Theodossi A and others. Observer variation in assessment of liver biopsies including analysis by kappa statistics, *Gastroenterology* 79:232-241, 1980.

82. Spodick DH and Bishop RL. Computer treason: intraobserver variability of an electrocardiographic computer system, *Am J Cardiol* 80:102-103, 1997.

PART TWO

General Appearance of the Patient

CHAPTER 4

Mental Status Examination

I. **INTRODUCTION.** Dementia is a clinical syndrome characterized by deteriorating cognition, behavior, and functional independence, which affects 3% to 11% of adults older than 65 years living in the community.[1] Before making the diagnosis of dementia, the clinician must exclude delirium (i.e., acute confusion; see Section IV below).

Of the many simple and rapid bedside tests developed to diagnose dementia, the most extensively investigated ones are the clock-drawing test and mini-mental status examination (MMSE).

II. **CLOCK-DRAWING TEST.** The clock-drawing test was originally developed in the early 1900s to evaluate soldiers who had suffered head wounds to the occipital or parietal lobes, which often caused subsequent difficulty composing images correctly with the appropriate number of parts of the correct size and orientation (i.e., constructional apraxia).[2] To correctly depict a clock, patients must be able to follow directions, comprehend language, visualize the proper orientation of an object, and execute normal movements, all tasks that may be disturbed in dementia.[3]

A. **Technique and scoring.** There are many methods for performing and scoring the clock-drawing test,[2,4] some of which involve intricate grading systems that defeat the test's simplicity.[3,5,6] The simplest and best-investigated method is that by Wolf-Klein.[7] In this method, the clinician gives the patient a piece of paper with a preprinted circle four inches in diameter and asks the patient to "draw a clock." If the patient has any questions, the clinician only repeats the same instructions and gives no other guidance. The patient may take as long as he wants to complete the task. Figure 4-1 describes how to score the patient's drawing.

B. Clinical significance. The data from Table 4-1 suggest that a positive clock-drawing test, without other known causes of constructional

Normal patterns:

Abnormal patterns:

FIGURE 4-1 The clock-drawing test. (Wolf-Klein method). The clock-drawing is normal if the patient has included most of the 12 numbers in the correct clockwise orientation. The patient does not need to draw the hands of the clock, and abnormal spacing of the numbers, however inappropriate, is still regarded normal as long as the numbers are in correct order and near the rim. Normal clock-drawing patterns, from left to right, are "normal," "missing one number," and "inappropriate spacing." Abnormal clock-drawing patterns, from left to right, are "irrelevant figures," "unusual arrangement" (i.e., vertical orientation of numbers), "counterclockwise rotation," and "absence of numbers." (Adapted with permission.[7])

TABLE 4-1 Dementia and delirium*

Finding (ref)	Sensitivity (%)	Specificity (%)	Positive LR	Negative LR
Dementia†				
Abnormal clock drawing test[7,8]	48-75	93-94	9.6	0.4
Mini-Mental Status Examination: Traditional Threshold				
23 or less[9-15]	69-100	78-99	9.0	0.2
Mini-Mental Status Examination: 3 Levels				
20 or less[11,13-15]	39-69	93-99	14.5	—
21-25[13-15]	26-51	—	2.2	—
26 or more[13-15]	4-10	14-27	0.1	—
Delirium				
Positive test using "Confusion Assessment Method"[16-18]†	46-94	92-98	8.8	0.2

*Diagnostic standards: For *dementia*, dementia by the NINCDS-ADRDA criteria,[7,8,19,20] the DMS-III criteria,[9,10,12,13,15] the CAMDEX instrument,[11] and a neurologist's opinion[14]; for *delirium*, the DMS criteria.[16-18]

†Definition of findings: For abnormal clock drawing test, see Figure 4-1; for Confusion Assessment Method, see text.

apraxia (e.g., parietal lobe lesion), strongly suggests the presence of dementia (likelihood ratio [LR] = 9.6). A normal clock-drawing test is not as useful, being elicited from up to half of patients having dementia as defined by other measures. The clock-drawing test differs from the MMSE in that the clock-drawing test is not affected by the patient's level of education.[8] Also, the clock-drawing test accurately predicts decline of the patient's MMSE score, as measured 4 years later, independent of the patient's age and the baseline MMSE score.[21]

III. THE MINI-MENTAL STATUS EXAMINATION (MMSE)

A. Introduction. The MMSE (Table 4-2) was introduced in 1975 by Folstein and others as an 11-part bedside test requiring only 5 to 10 minutes to administer, compared to the 1 to 2 hours of time demanded by more formal tests for dementia.[22] The MMSE combines questions that are highly specific but not sensitive (i.e., questions about orientation) with questions that are highly sensitive but not specific (i.e., poor recall or inability to perform serial 7's).[23]

B. Clinical significance. Table 4-1 illustrates that the traditional threshold for the MMSE (abnormal being scores of 23 or lower) performs very well, assuming there is no evidence of delirium (see Section IV below), scores from 0 to 23 argue strongly for the diagnosis of dementia (LR = 9.0), and scores from 24 to 30 argue against it (LR = 0.2). Nonetheless, because false-positive results become a concern when such a threshold is applied to large populations with a low incidence of dementia, such as persons living independently in the community, some experts prefer interpreting the MMSE score in three ranges (Table 4-1): a score of 20 or less rules-in dementia (LR = 14.5); one 26 or more rules-out dementia (LR = 0.1); and scores between 21 to 25

TABLE 4-2 Mini-mental status examination

Test	Maximum Score
Orientation	
1) What is the year? Season? Date? Day? Month?*	5
2) Where are we? State? County? City? Hospital? Floor?*	5
Registration	
3) Name 3 objects. Ask patient to name the items.*	3
Repeat the answers until the patient learns all three.	
Attention and Calculation	
4) Serial 7's (ask the patient to begin with 100 and count backward by 7's, stopping after 5 subtractions: 93, 86, 79, 72, 65)*	5
or	
Spell "world" backwards.*	
Recall	
5) Ask the patient to name the three objects learned under "registration" above.*	3
Language	
6) Point to a pencil and watch, asking the patient to name them.*	2
7) Have the patient repeat "no ifs, ands, or buts."	1
8) Have the patient follow a three-stage command (e.g., "Take a paper in your right hand. Fold the paper in half. Put the paper on the floor.").*	3
9) Have the patient read and obey the following sentence, written in large letters: "Close your eyes."	1
10) Have the patient write a sentence.†	1
11) Have the patient copy a picture of two intersecting pentagons.	1
Total	30

Adapted from references 15 and 22.

*Give one point for each correct answer.

†The sentence should make sense and contain a subject and object to earn the 1 point; spelling errors are ignored.

are regarded as less conclusive (LR = 2.2), indicating further investigation of the patient.

The MMSE score may be used to follow patients over time, but only changes of 4 points or more indicate a significant change of cognition (this is based on the standard deviation of results in stable patients).[10] The level of the patient's education also affects the MMSE score, whether or not dementia is present,[10,12,20,24,25] and some have suggested adjusting the threshold for a positive test downward slightly in more poorly educated persons.[10,20]

IV. DIAGNOSIS OF DELIRIUM ("CONFUSION ASSESSMENT METHOD"). Delirium is an acute and reversible confusional state, which affects up to 20% of elderly patients hospitalized with acute medical illnesses.[17,26] Of the several screening tools available to diagnose delirium,[17] one simple and well-investigated one is the "Confusion Assessment Method."[16]

A. Scoring. The clinician looks for the following 4 clinical features: (1) change in mental status (compared to the patient's baseline) that is *acute* and *fluctuating*, (2) difficulty focusing attention or trouble keeping track of what is being said, (3) disorganized thinking (e.g., rambling or irrelevant conversation, unpredictable switching between subjects, illogical flow of ideas), and (4) altered level of consciousness (e.g., lethargy, stupor, or hyperalert).

A positive test requires both features (1) and (2) *and* either (3) or (4).

B. Clinical significance. As illustrated in Table 4-1, a positive test argues strongly *for* delirium (Table 4-1, LR = 8.8), and a negative test argues *against* delirium (LR = 0.2). In any patient with delirium, positive bedside tests for *dementia* are meaningless because of the high false-positive rate.

REFERENCES

1. Knopman DS. The initial recognition and diagnosis of dementia, *Am J Med* 104:2S-12S, 1998.
2. Watson YI, Arfken CL, Birge SJ. Clock completion: an objective screening test for dementia, *J Am Geriatr Soc* 41:1235-1240, 1993.
3. Mendez MF, Ala T, and Underwood KL. Development of scoring criteria for the clock drawing task in Alzheimer's disease, *J Am Geriatr Soc* 40:1095-1099, 1992.
4. Sunderland T and others. Clock drawing in Alzheimer's disease: a novel measure of dementia severity, *J Am Geriatr Soc* 37:725-729, 1989.
5. Tuokko H and others. The clock test: a sensitive measure to differentiate normal elderly from those with Alzheimer disease, *J Am Geriatr Soc* 40:579-584, 1992.
6. Esteban-Santillan C and others. Clock drawing test in very mild Alzheimer's disease, *J Am Geriatr Soc* 46:1266-1269, 1998.
7. Wolf-Klein GP and others. Screening for Alzheimer's disease by clock drawing, *J Am Geriatr Soc* 37:730-734, 1989.
8. Ainslie NK and Murden RA. Effect of education on the clock-drawing dementia screen in non-demented elderly persons, *J Am Geriatr Soc* 41:249-252, 1993.
9. Grut M and others. Accuracy of the mini-mental status examination as a screening test for dementia in a Swedish elderly population, *Acta Neurol Scand* 87:312-317, 1993.
10. Tangalos EG and others. The mini-mental state examination in general medical practice: clinical utility and acceptance, *Mayo Clin Proc* 71:829-837, 1996.
11. O'Connor DW and others. The reliability and validity of the mini-mental state in a British community survey, *J Psychiatr Res* 23:87-96, 1989.
12. Gagnon M and others. Validity of the mini-mental state examination as a screening instrument for cognitive impairment and dementia in French elderly community residents, *Neuroepidemiology* 9:143-150, 1990.
13. Kay DWK and others. Dementia and depression among the elderly living in the Hobart community: the effect of the diagnostic criteria on the prevalence rates, *Psychol Med* 15:771-788, 1985.
14. Dick JPR and others. Mini-mental state examination in neurological patients, *J Neurol Neurosurg Psych* 47:496-499, 1984.

15. Anthony JC and others. Limits of the 'Mini-Mental State' as a screening test for dementia and delirium among hospital patients, *Psychol Med* 12:397-408, 1982.

16. Inouye SK and others. Clarifying confusion: the confusion assessment method. A new method for detection of delirium, *Ann Intern Med* 113:941-948, 1990.

17. Pompei P and others. Detecting delirium among hospitalized older patients, *Arch Intern Med* 155:301-307, 1995.

18. Zou Y and others. Detection and diagnosis of delirium in the elderly: psychiatrist diagnosis, confusion assessment method, or consensus diagnosis? *Int Psychoger* 10:303-308, 1998.

19. McKhann G and others. Clinical diagnosis of Alzheimer's disease: report of the NINCDS-ADRDA Work Group under the auspices of Department of Health and Human Services Task Force on Alzheimer's Disease, *Neurology* 34:939-944, 1984.

20. Uhlmann RF and Larson EB. Effect of education on the mini-mental state examination as a screening test for dementia, *J Am Geriatr Assoc* 39:876-880, 1991.

21. Ferrucci L and others. Does the clock drawing test predict cognitive decline in older persons independent of the mini-mental state examination? *J Am Geriatr Soc* 44:1326-1331, 1996.

22. Folstein MF, Folstein SE, and McHugh PR. "Mini-mental state": a practical method for grading the cognitive state of patients for the clinician, *J Psychiatr Res* 12:189-198, 1975.

23. Klein LE and others. Diagnosing dementia: univariate and multivariate analyses of the mental status examination, *J Am Geriatr Soc* 33:483-488, 1985.

24. O'Connor DW and others. The influence of education, social class and sex on Mini-Mental State scores, *Psychol Med* 19:771-776, 1989.

25. Brayne C and Calloway P. The association of education and socioeconomic status with the Mini Mental State examination and the clinical diagnosis of dementia in elderly people, *Age Ageing* 19:91-96, 1990.

26. Lewis LM and others. Unrecognized delirium in ED geriatric patients, *Am J Emerg Med* 13:142-145, 1995.

CHAPTER 5

Stance and Gait

I. INTRODUCTION. Observation of the patient's gait not only uncovers important neurologic problems (e.g., Parkinson's disease, hemiparesis) and musculoskeletal problems (e.g., spinal stenosis, hip disease), but it also provides information otherwise unavailable from the conventional examination, such as clues to the patient's emotions, overall function, and even prognosis. For example, the slowness of an elderly person's gait accurately predicts falls, future disability, and risk of institutionalization.[1-5] In a patient with congestive heart failure, the gait's speed and stride predict cardiac index, future hospitalization, and mortality as well as the ejection fraction and better than the performance on the treadmill.[6-8] Even depressed patients have a characteristic gait, marked by a shorter stride and weaker push-off with the heel, when compared with nondepressed persons.[9]

This chapter reviews both the musculoskeletal and neurologic causes of the abnormal gait. The phases of the normal gait are depicted in Figure 5-1.

II. ETIOLOGY OF GAIT DISORDERS. Which gait abnormalities a clinician is likely to see depends on the nature of his practice. Among patients presenting to neurologists, the most common causes of gait disorder are stroke and Parkinson's disease, followed by frontal gait disorder, myelopathy (e.g.,

FIGURE 5-1 Normal gait. This figure illustrates the phases of normal gait, focusing on the right leg (colored gray). Normal gait consists of the "stance phase" (the period during which the leg bears weight) and "swing phase" (the period during which the leg advances and does not bear weight). The stance and swing make up the "stride," which is the interval from the time one heel strikes the ground to when it again strikes the ground. During the normal stance phase, it is the *extensor* muscles that contract—the quadriceps in midstance, and the plantar flexors (soleus and gastrocnemius) in terminal stance—pushing off the heel. The healthy swing, in contrast, requires contraction of the *flexor* muscles, all of which are activated early in the swing phase: hip flexors (iliopsoas), knee flexors (hamstrings), and ankle flexors (tibialis anterior and toe extensors).[10,11] (Figure adapted with permission from reference 10.)

cervical spondylosis, B_{12} deficiency), peripheral neuropathy, and cerebellar disease.[12,13] Among patients presenting to general clinicians, most gait abnormalities are caused by arthritis, followed by orthostatic hypotension, stroke, Parkinson's disease, and intermittent claudication.[14]

III. TYPES OF GAIT DISORDERS AND THEIR SIGNIFICANCE.

Disorders of gait may occur because of one of 4 fundamental problems: pain, immobile joints, muscle weakness, or abnormal limb control. Abnormal limb control, in turn, may result from spasticity, rigidity, problems with proprioception, cerebellar diseases, or problems with cerebral control.

When analyzing disturbances of gait, the most important initial question is to ask whether the gait is symmetric or asymmetric. Pain, immobile joints, and muscle weakness are usually unilateral and therefore cause *asymmetric* gaits. Rigidity, proprioceptive and cerebellar diseases, and problems with central control all cause *symmetric* gaits. Spasticity may cause *asymmetric* (i.e., hemiplegia) or *symmetric* (i.e., paraplegia) gaits.

A. Painful gait ("antalgic gait"). If putting weight on one limb causes pain, patients adopt unusual gaits to minimize this pain (the word "antalgic" derives from the Greek *an* and *algesis,* meaning "against pain.") All antalgic gaits have one characteristic feature: the short contralateral step.

1. The short contralateral step. After bearing weight on the affected leg, patients with pain quickly step onto the sound leg. The short contralateral step produces an uneven cadence, which is identical to the gait persons adopt when there is a rock in one shoe.

2. Other characteristic features. Other features of the antalgic gait depend on whether the pain is located in the foot, knee, or hip. Each of these gaits has distinctive features, which allow diagnosis from a distance, although it is sometimes more efficient to simply ask the patient which joint is painful.

a. Foot pain. In patients with foot pain, the foot contacts the ground abnormally. For example, patients may bear weight during stance on their heel only, forefoot only, or along the lateral edge of the foot.

b. Knee pain. Patients with knee pain display a stiff knee that does not extend or flex fully during stride.[15,16]

c. Hip pain ("coxalgic gait"). Patients with hip pain limit the amount of hip extension toward the end of stance (normally, the hip extends 20 degrees). The most characteristic feature of the coxalgic gait, however, is an asymmetrical and excessive lateral shift of the patient's upper body toward the weight-bearing side when standing on the painful limb (i.e., the trunk leans and ipsilateral arm abducts).[17,18] This unusual movement is called "lateral lurch."[17,18]

Lateral lurch reduces the pain of patients with hip disease, because it minimizes the need to activate the ipsilateral hip abductor muscles. These muscles normally support the upper body during swing of the other leg, but when activated can easily put 400 pounds of pressure on the femoral head, a force patients with hip disease cannot tolerate. By leaning over the painful limb during stance, patients effectively balance their center of gravity over the painful limb and thus avoid activation of the hip abductors.

B. Immobile joints. Most clinicians do not consider immobile joints as a cause of abnormal gait, but the condition is well known to physiatrists. A common example is plantar flexion contracture, which may occur after prolonged periods of plaster immobilization or confinement to a chair or bed. Patients with a plantar flexion contracture may place their weight abnormally on the forefoot during initial stance, or, during midstance, lift their heel too early or lean their trunk forward. During swing phase, the abnormally flexed foot has difficulty clearing the floor, and the patient may drag the foot or develop an unusual movement to clear it, such as contralateral trunk lean or contralateral vaulting.[10,11]

The clinician can easily identify immobile joints as the cause of abnormal gait by testing the range of motion of hips, knees, and ankles of both legs.

C. **Weakness of specific muscles.** Weakness of the hip extensor and abductor muscles (i.e., gluteus maximus and medius/minimus), knee extensors (quadriceps) and foot and toe dorsiflexors (tibialis anterior and toe extensors) all cause specific abnormalities of gait. The gluteus maximus and quadriceps gait are much less prevalent today than they were in the days of poliomyelitis and diphtheria.

1. **Trendelenburg gait and sign (abnormal gluteus medius and minimus)**

a. **Definition of Trendelenburg gait** (or Trendelenburg's symptom; Friedrich Trendelburg [1844-1924]). The Trendelenburg gait occurs when the gluteus medius and minimus do not function properly. These two muscles abduct the hip, an action that supports the opposite pelvis and prevents it from dropping excessive amounts during the normal single-limb stance,[19] During walking, a slight dip of the opposite pelvis is normal during stance phase on one limb. The finding of *excessive drop* of the opposite pelvis, however, is the abnormal Trendelenburg gait. When the abnormality is bilateral, the pelvis waddles like that of a duck.

Like patients with the coxalgic gait (see previous Section III-A-2-c), patients with Trendelenburg gait may lean their trunk over the abnormal leg during stance, but the lean lacks the dramatic lurch seen in coxalgic gait, and the opposing sways of the ipsilateral shoulder and opposite pelvis make it appear as if patients with the Trendelenburg gait have a hinge between their sacrum and lumbar spine.[17,20]

   b. **Etiology of Trendelenburg gait.** Causes include the following: **(1) neuromuscular weakness of the hip abductors.** Although poliomyelitis and progressive muscular atrophy were important causes historically, this gait now occurs as a complication of hip arthroplasty using a lateral approach, which risks damage to the superior gluteal nerve or gluteus medius muscle[21-23]; **(2) hip disease**, especially congenital dislocation of the hip and coxa vara (i.e., "bent hip," a deformity in which the angle between femoral neck and body is significantly decreased). In both of these disorders, the abnormal upward displacement of the greater trochanter shortens the fibers of the gluteus medius and makes them more horizontal instead of vertical, thus abolishing their role as abductors.

   c. **Trendelenburg sign.** In 1895, before use of roentgenography, Friedrich Trendelenburg was the first to show that the waddling gait of patients with congenital dislocation of the hip was due to weak abductor function, not the upward movement of the femur during stance (which was what his contemporaries believed). He successfully argued this by inventing a simple test, now known as Trendelenburg's sign. In this test, the patient is asked to stand on one leg with the other hip flexed to 90 degrees (the clinician may help the patient balance by supporting the ipsilateral arm to align the ipsilateral shoulder over the hip being tested).[24] In patients with normal abductor strength, the contralateral buttock rises, but if the abductor muscles are weak, the contralateral buttock falls (the buttock falls until the ipsilateral femur and pelvis come into contact).

It is important to remember that the side being tested is the one bearing the weight. Some deformities of the leg, such as severe genu varum, may cause a false-positive result.[25]

2. **Gluteus maximus gait.** When the hip extensors are weak, the patient develops a characteristic abnormal backward trunk lean during early stance, which places the patient's center of gravity behind the hip joint line and removes the need for the gluteus maximus to contract.

3. **Weak quadriceps gait.** When the knee extensors are weak, some patients develop a characteristic hyperextension of the knee during stance. This at first seems paradoxical because the normal action of the quadriceps is knee extension, which should therefore be weak in these patients. However, the main role of the quadriceps during gait is to support the flexed knee during stance, and patients with weak quadriceps avoid bearing weight on a flexed knee by hyperextending the joint. They can fully extend the knee

because their hip flexes strongly during swing and then decelerates abruptly, which whips the tibia forward.[11]

Most patients with weak quadriceps muscles have great difficulty walking on uneven ground.

4. **Foot drop (weak tibialis anterior and toe extensors).** The characteristic features in these patients are (1) "foot slap," which is the uncontrolled slap of the forefoot immediately after the heel makes contact; (this causes two sounds instead of one when the abnormal foot contacts the ground, producing a the characteristic cadence (in a patient with *unilateral* foot drop) of "dada . . . da . . . dada . . . da") and (2) "steppage gait," in which the patient excessively flexes the hip and knee of the abnormal side during the swing phase to clear the foot from the ground.[10]

D. **Spasticity** is a feature of weakness of the upper motor neuron type (see Chapter 54). Characteristic gaits are the hemiplegic gait and diplegic (paraplegic) gait.

1. **Hemiplegic gait.**[26-28] The characteristic gait occurs because of poor control of the flexor muscles during swing phase and spasticity of the extensor muscles acting to lengthen the affected leg (compared to the healthy side). The ankle is abnormally flexed downward and inward (equinovarus deformity), and initial contact during stance is abnormal, along the lateral edge of the foot or forefoot. The knee is stiff, hyperextends during stance, and does not flex normally during swing. The contralateral step often advances just to meet the position of the weakened limb, instead of advancing normally beyond it.

Because the paralyzed leg is hyperextended, and therefore longer than the sound leg, the patient may drag the toe of the affected leg during swing or adopt abnormal movements to clear that limb during the swing phase. These movements include contralateral trunk lean, which raises the ipsilateral pelvis to clear the paralyzed leg, and circumduction, which describes the toe tracing a semicircle on the floor, first moving outward and then inward as it advances, instead of the normal straight forward movement.

According to classic teachings, the clinician may sometimes suspect mild hemiplegia because of asymmetric swinging of the arms, although one study has shown that asymmetric arm swinging occurs in 70% of normal persons.[29]

2. **Diplegic gait** affects patients with spinal cord disease (e.g., spinal cord trauma, cervical spondylosis, B_{12} deficiency), in whom both spasticity and abnormal proprioception cause a characteristic slow, laborious, and stiff-legged gait. In some spastic diplegias of childhood, adductor spasm causes the feet to cross in front of each other, a finding sometimes called "scissors gait."

E. **Rigidity.** Chapter 54 describes the characteristic features of rigidity and how it differs from spasticity. The most common gait abnormality due to rigidity is the Parkinsonian gait.

1. **The Parkinsonian gait.**[30,31] Characteristic features are (1) flexed posture of the arms, hips, trunk, and neck; (2) rigidity of movement (en bloc turning, difficulty initiating gait); (3) steps that are flat-footed, small, shuffling, and have a narrow base; (4) diminished arm swing (the normal excursion, measured at the wrist, averages 16 inches; the average value for patients with Parkinson's

disease is 5 inches); (5) involuntary hasten-
ing of gait (festination); and (6) poor postural
control (retropulsion).

2. **Differential diagnosis.** Patients with spinal stenosis superficially resemble those with
Parkinson's disease in that they have a flexed
stance ("simian stance"), which reduces the
tension on the lumbosacral nerves.[32] Patients
with spinal stenosis, however, complain of
pain and otherwise have a normal gait.

The distinguishing features of the frontal
gait disorder, which also may superficially
resemble the Parkinsonian gait, is discussed
in Section G-1 below.

F. **Ataxia.** The characteristic features of the ataxic
gait are a wide-based gait with irregular, uneven, and sometimes staggering steps (the normal base, measured when one limb swings past
the other at midstance is 2 to 4 inches). There are
two types of ataxia, sensory ataxia and cerebellar ataxia.

1. **Sensory ataxia.** Sensory ataxia affects patients with significant proprioceptive loss
(see Chapter 55). Characteristically, the patient looks down and walks as if throwing
his feet, which tend to slap on the ground.
Smooth, familiar routes cause less trouble
than uneven, rough ones.

2. **Cerebellar ataxia.** Patients place their feet
too far apart or too close together irregularly,
and sway, stagger, and reel in all directions
as if intoxicated by alcohol.[33,34] In contrast
to sensory ataxia, patients with cerebellar
ataxia have other cerebellar signs, including
dysmetria, hypotonia, intention tremor, dysarthria, and nystagmus (see Chapter 58).

3. **Romberg's sign**
   a. **Introduction.** In his famous textbook,
   written between 1840 and 1846, Moritz
   Romberg described the sign now bearing
   his name, as a finding in patients with

tabes dorsalis who have severe sensory ataxia from syphilitic damage to the dorsal columns of the spinal cord. Romberg wrote that, when a patient with tabes dorsalis stands and closes his eyes, "he immediately begins to move from side to side, and the oscillations soon attain such a pitch that unless supported, he falls to the ground."[35] Most authors claim that Romberg's sign is negative in patients with cerebellar ataxia, although it is important to know that Romberg did not make this claim, cerebellar disease having not yet been defined during his time (Duchenne and Babinski later added this diagnostic point).[36]

b. Definition of a positive Romberg's sign. A problem with Romberg's sign is that various authors differ on what constitutes a positive test: some state it is the increased swaying that occurs when the eyes close, while others require the patient to be on the verge of falling down.[35] Increased swaying alone seems to be a poor choice, because most normal persons sway more when they close their eyes, and increased swaying with eyes closed is well documented in patients with vestibular disease, cerebellar disease, and Parkinson's disease.[37-39]

The best definition of the positive Romberg's sign is inability to stand for 60 seconds with feet together and eyes closed. In one study, every healthy person and over half of the patients with cerebellar ataxia could maintain this position for 60 seconds, whereas half of the patients with sensory ataxia lasted only 10 seconds before beginning to topple over.[40]

A related sign, the sharpened Romberg's sign,[41] in which patients must stand with one foot in front of the other with eyes closed, has little proven diagnostic value. Many normal persons, especially elderly ones, are unable to stand like this for very long.[40,42]

G. Frontal gait disorder

1. **Definition.** "Frontal gait disorder" is an imprecise term describing a combination of findings seen in patients with cerebral tumors, subdural hematomas, dementing illness, normal pressure hydrocephalus, and multiple lacunar infarcts.[43,44] The characteristic findings are (1) slow, shuffling, wide-based gait ("marche a petis pas"), (2) hesitation in starting to walk ("ignition failure"), (3) difficulty in picking feet up off the floor ("magnetic foot" response), and (4) poor postural control. Motor function of the legs is sometimes much better when these patients are seated or lying, suggesting an element of gait apraxia.

Some of these findings resemble Parkinsonism, but the distinguishing features of the frontal gait disorder are its wide base, normal arm swing, lack of other features of Parkinsonism, more upright posture, and higher incidence of dementia and urinary incontinence.

2. **Clinical significance.** In studies of elderly patients undergoing computed tomography (CT) of the head because of neurologic problems, the finding of a frontal gait disorder[a] correlates strongly with the CT finding of ventricular enlargement.[13,45,46] Only a minority of these patients, however, met the criteria for normal pressure hydrocephalus,

---

[a] The specific definition of abnormal gait in these studies was a gait disturbance not attributable to muscle weakness, Parkinson's disease, or musculoskeletal problems.

suggesting that the findings of ventricular enlargement and gait disturbance are general ones occurring in many different forebrain disorders.[13,45]

IV. **EVALUATION OF GAIT DISORDERS.** The methods of evaluating gait range from very simple tests that require minutes to complete, which are most appropriate when screening elderly patients for their risk of falls, to the much more comprehensive observational gait analysis, which physiatrists use to break down complicated gait abnormalities into smaller components and to direct treatment.[11] Most clinicians adopt an intermediate approach and ask the patient first to walk back and forth several strides at a time, and then again on the toes, heels, and using tandem steps, all maneuvers that may bring out weak muscles or difficulties with balance.

Testing gait is essential, whatever the method, because it is common to find patients who have normal findings during conventional tests of motor, sensory, musculoskeletal, and visual function, yet who, when asked to stand and walk, demonstrate an abnormal gait.[47]

A. **Observational gait analysis.**[10,11] Using this method, the clinician watches the patient walk and focuses on one limb at a time, first observing the ankle, then the knee, hip, pelvis, and trunk. At each joint, the clinician considers each of the possible causes that contribute to abnormal gait: pain, immobile joints, muscle weakness, and abnormal limb control.

Each abnormal movement has a differential diagnosis. For "abnormal ipsilateral trunk lean during stance," possible causes include ipsilateral hip pain, ipsilateral short limb (more than 1 inch shorter), or intentional attempts to clear the contralateral limb during swing (e.g., drop foot or extended limb). Or, for "dragging of the foot or toe during swing," causes are weak ipsilateral ankle dorsiflexor muscles, ipsilateral plantar flexion contractures, inadequate ipsilateral hip or knee flexion, or impaired proprioception.

An excellent manual of observational gait analysis has been published.[10]

B. Simple tests of gait. These tests are especially useful in elderly patients to evaluate the risk of falls and to determine functional independence. Validated tests include the "timed 8-foot walk" test, the "timed up and go" test, and the "stops talking when walking" test.

   1. Timed 8-foot walk test.[1] The clinician measures the time it takes the patient to walk 8 feet using their normal pace. The measured time predicts future disability, as determined 4 years later.

   2. Timed "up and go" test.[3] The clinician measures the time it takes the patient to rise from a standard chair, walk to a line on the floor 3 meters away, turn, return, and sit down again. The measured time correlates with other accurate but more complex measures of functional independence.

   3. Stops talking when walking. In one study, the finding that a patient stopped walking when initiating conversation predicted subsequent falls during 6-month follow-up with a sensitivity of 48%, specificity of 95%, and positive LR of 8.8, and negative LR of 0.6.[2]

V. CANES. Physical examination of gait is not complete without considering the length of the patient's cane and which arm the patient uses to hold the cane.

   A. Length of cane. Twenty-three percent to 42% of the time, the cane is too long or too short by 5 cm or more.[48,49] An appropriately fitted cane should extend the distance from the distal wrist crease to the ground, when the patient is wearing everyday shoes and placing his or her arms at the sides.[50]

B. Contralateral vs. ipsilateral use of cane. In patients with hip and knee arthritis, the conventional teaching is for the patient to hold the cane in the contralateral hand, although compelling evidence for contralateral cane use exists only for patients with hip arthritis.[51-53] By placing just 20, 33, or 38 pounds of pressure on a cane contralateral to a diseased hip when standing on that hip, the patient can *reduce* the pressure on the diseased femoral head by 165, 272, or 319 pounds, respectively.[51]

REFERENCES

1. Guralnik JM and others. Lower-extremity function in persons over the age of 70 years as a predictor of subsequent disability, *N Engl J Med* 332:556-561, 1995.
2. Lundin-Olsson L, Nyberg L, and Gustafson Y. "Stops walking when talking" as a predictor of falls in elderly people, *Lancet* 349:617, 1997.
3. Podsiadlo D and Richardson S. The timed "up and go": a test of basic functional mobility for frail elderly persons, *J Am Geriatr Soc* 39:142-148, 1991.
4. Tinetti ME, Speechley M, and Ginter SF. Risk factors for falls among elderly persons living in the community, *N Engl J Med* 319:1701-1707, 1988.
5. Friedman PJ, Richmond DE, and Baskett JJ. A prospective trial of serial gait speed as a measure of rehabilitation in the elderly, *Age Ageing* 17:227-235, 1988.
6. Bittner V and others. Prediction of mortality and morbidity with a 6-minute walk test in patients with left ventricular dysfunction, *JAMA* 270:1702-1707, 1993.
7. Cowley AJ and others. Exercise capability in heart failure: is cardiac output important after all? *Lancet* 337:771-773, 1991.
8. Davies SW and others. Short-stepping gait in severe heart failure, *Br Heart J* 55:469-472, 1992.
9. Sloman L and others. Gait patterns of depressed patients and normal subjects, *Am J Psych* 139:94-97, 1982.

10. The Pathokinesiology Service and the Physical Therapy Department of Ranchos Los Amigos Medical Center. *Observational gait analysis*. Downey, Calif, 1993, Los Amigos Research and Education Institute, Inc.

11. Perry J. *Gait analysis: normal and pathological function*, Thorofare, NJ, 1992, SLACK, Inc.

12. Fuh JL and others. Neurologic diseases presenting with gait impairment in the elderly, *J Geriatr Psych Neurol* 7:89-92, 1994.

13. Sudarsky L and Ronthal M. Gait disorders among elderly patients, *Arch Neurol* 40:740-743, 1983.

14. Hough JC, McHenry MP, and Kammer LM. Gait disorders in the elderly, *Am Fam Phys* 35:191-196, 1987.

15. Murray MP and others. Antalgic maneuvers during walking in men with unilateral knee disability, *Clin Ortho Rel Res* 199:192-200, 1985.

16. Messier SP and others. Osteoarthritis of the knee: effects on gait, strength, and flexibility. *Arch Phys Med Rehabil* 73:29-36, 1992.

17. Calve J, Galland M, and de Cagny R. Pathogenesis of the limp due to coxalgia: the antalgic gait, *J Bone Joint Surg* 21:12-25, 1939.

18. Murray MP, Gore DR, and Clarkson BH. Walking patterns of patients with unilateral hip pain due to osteoarthritis and avascular necrosis, *J Bone Joint Surg* 53A:259-274, 1971.

19. Gottschalk F, Kourosh S, and Leveau B. The functional anatomy of tensor fasciae latae and gluteus medius and minimus, *J Anat* 166:179-189, 1989.

20. Peltier LF. Trendelenburg's test: 1895, *Clin Ortho Rel Res* 355:3-7, 1998.

21. Pai VS. Significance of the Trendelenburg test in total hip arthroplasty, *J Arthroplasty* 11:174-179, 1996.

22. Ramesh M and others. Damage to the superior gluteal nerve after the Hardinge approach to the hip, *J Bone Joint Surg* 78B:903-906, 1996.

23. Baker AS and Bitounis VC. Abductor function after total hip replacement, *J Bone Joint Surg* 71B:47-50, 1989.

24. Hardcastle P and Nade S. The significance of the Trendelenburg test, *J Bone Joint Surg* 67B:741-746, 1985.

25. Vasudevan PN, Vaidyalingam KV, and Nair PB. Can Trendelenburg's sign be positive if the hip is normal? *J Bone Joint Surg* 79B:462-466, 1997.

26. Brandstater ME and others. Hemiplegic gait: analysis of temporal variables, *Arch Phys Med Rehabil* 64:583-587, 1983.

27. Knutsson E and Richards C. Different types of disturbed motor control in gait of hemiparetic patients, *Brain* 102: 405-430, 1979.

28. Perry J. The mechanics of walking in hemiplegia, *Clin Orthoped* 63:23-31, 1969.

29. Riley TL, Ray WF, and Massey EW. Gait mechanisms: asymmetry of arm motion in normal subjects, *Military Med* 142:467-468, 1977.

30. Knutsson E. An analysis of parkinsonian gait, *Brain* 95:475-486, 1972.

31. Rogers MW. Disorders of posture, balance, and gait in Parkinson's disease, *Clin Geriatr Med* 12:825-845, 1996.

32. Simpkin PA. Simian stance: a sign of spinal stenosis, *Lancet* 2:652-653, 1982.

33. Gilman S, Bloedel JR, and Lechtenberg R. Disorders of the cerebellum. In Plum F, McDowell FH, and Baringer JR, editors. *Contemporary neurology series*, Philadelphia, 1981, FA Davis.

34. Holmes G. Clinical symptoms of cerebellar disease and their interpretation. Lecture 3, *Lancet* 2:59-65, 1922.

35. Rogers JH. Romberg and his test, *J Laryngol Otol* 94:1401-1404, 1980.

36. Schiller F. Staggering gait in medical history, *Neurology* 37:127-135, 1995.

37. Ojala M, Matikainen E, and Juntunen J. Posturography and the dizzy patient: a neurological study of 133 patients, *Acta Neurol Scand* 80:118-122, 1989.

38. Baloh RW and others. Static and dynamic posturography in patients with vestibular and cerebellar lesions, *Arch Neurol* 55:649-654, 1998.

39. Bronstein AM and others. Visual control of balance in cerebellar and Parkinsonian syndromes, *Brain* 113:767-779, 1990.

40. Notermans NC and others. Measuring ataxia: quantification based on the standard neurological examination, *J Neurol Neurosurg Psych* 57:22-26, 1994.

41. Graybiel A and Fregly AR. A new quantitative ataxia test battery, *Acta Otolaryngol (Stockh)* 61:292-312, 1966.

42. Heitmann DK and others. Balance performance and step width in noninstitutionalized, elderly, female fallers and nonfallers, *Phys Ther* 69:923-931, 1989.

43. Nutt JG, Marsden CD, and Thompson PD. Human walking and higher-level gait disorders, particularly in the elderly, *Neurology* 43:268-279, 1993.

44. Alexander NB. Gait disorders in older adults, *J Am Geriatr Soc* 44:434-451, 1996.

45. Koller WC and others. Senile gait: correlation with computed tomographic scans, *Ann Neurology* 13:343-344, 1983.

46. Fisher CM. Hydrocephalus as a cause of disturbances of gait in the elderly, *Neurology* 32:1358-1363, 1982.

47. Tinetti ME and Ginter SF. Identifying mobility dysfunctions in elderly patients: standard neuromuscular examination or direct assessment? *JAMA* 259:1190-1193, 1988.

48. George J and others. Aids and adaptations for the elderly at home: underprovided, underused, and undermaintained, *Br Med J* 296:1365-1366, 1988.

49. Sainsbury R and Mulley GP. Walking sticks used by the elderly, *Br Med J* 284:1751, 1982.

50. Mulley GP. Walking sticks, *Br Med J* 296:475-476, 1988.

51. Blount WP. Don't throw away the cane, *J Bone Joint Surg* 38A:695-708, 1956.

52. Edwards BG. Contralateral and ipsilateral cane usage by patients with total knee or hip replacement, *Arch Phys Med Rehabil* 67:734-740, 1986.

53. Vargo MM, Robinson LR, and Nicholas JJ. Contralateral vs. ipsilateral cane use: effects on muscles crossing the knee joint, *Am J Phys Med Rehabil* 71:170-176, 1992.

CHAPTER 6

Jaundice

I. INTRODUCTION. Jaundice is an abnormal yellowish discoloration of the skin and mucous membranes caused by accumulation of bile pigment. There are three forms of jaundice—(1) hemolytic (due to increased bilirubin production from excessive breakdown of red cells), (2) hepatocellular (due to disease of the liver parenchyma, sometimes referred to as "nonobstructive jaundice" or "medical jaundice"), and (3) obstructive (due to mechanical obstruction of the biliary ducts outside the liver, sometimes referred to as "surgical jaundice"). The most common causes of hepatocellular jaundice are viral hepatitis and alcoholic cirrhosis; the most common causes of obstructive jaundice are gallstone disease (i.e., choledocholithiasis) and pancreatic carcinoma.[1,2]

Because hemolytic disorders cause less than 2% of all jaundice[1,3] and because hemolysis usually causes obvious hematologic abnormalities and no other signs of liver disease, the clinician's usual task at the bedside of a jaundiced patient is to differentiate nonobstructive hepatocellular jaundice from obstructive jaundice.

II. THE FINDINGS

A. Jaundice. Jaundice is usually first noted in the conjunctiva of the eyes. Although the traditional term for this is "scleral icterus," this may be a misnomer because pathologic studies reveal most of the pigment to be deposited in the conjunctiva, not the avascular sclera.[4] As jaundice progresses and the serum bilirubin increases, the face, mucous membranes, and eventually the entire skin acquires a yellow or orange hue.

Prominent yellowish subconjunctival fat may be mistaken for conjunctival jaundice, but fat usually is limited to the conjunctival folds and, unlike jaundice, spares the area near the cornea. Patients with carotenemia (from excess carrot ingestion) also develop a yellowish discoloration of the skin, especially the palms, soles, and nasolabial fold; however, in contrast to jaundice, the conjunctiva are spared.[5]

B. Associated findings. Several findings traditionally distinguish hepatocellular from obstructive disease.

1. **Hepatocellular jaundice.** Findings characteristic of hepatocellular jaundice are spider telangiectasia, palmar erythema, dilated abdominal wall veins, splenomegaly, asterixis, and fetor hepaticus.

   a. **Spider telangiectasia ("spider angiomata").** Spider telangiectasia are dilated cutaneous blood vessels that have three components: (1) a central arteriole (the "body" of the spider), which, when compressed slightly with a glass slide, can be seen to pulsate; (2) multiple radiating "legs"; and (3) surrounding erythema, which may encompass the entire lesion or only its central portion.[6] After blanching, the returning blood fills the central arteriole first before traveling to the peripheral tips of each leg. Spiders are most numerous on the face and neck, followed by the shoulders, thorax, arms, and hands. They are rare on the palms, scalp, and below the umbilicus.[6] This peculiar distribution may reflect the neurohormonal properties of the microcirculation, because this distribution is also where blushing is most intense.[6]

Acquired vascular spiders are associated with three clinical conditions: liver disease, pregnancy, and malnutrition.[7] In patients with liver disease, the spiders advance and regress with disease severity, and their appearance correlates somewhat with an abnormally increased serum ratio of estradiol to testosterone levels.[8] In pregnant women, vascular spiders typically appear between the second and fifth months and usually disappear within days after delivery.[7] Vascular spiders also have been described in normal persons, but these lesions, in contrast to those of liver disease, are always small in number (average 3) and size.[6]

Vascular spiders were first described by the English physician Erasmus Wilson in 1867.[6]

d. Palmar erythema. Palmar erythema is a symmetric reddening of the surfaces of the palms, most pronounced over the hypothenar and thenar eminences.[7] Palmar erythema occurs in the same clinical conditions as vascular spiders, and the two lesions tend to come and go together.[7,9]

e. Dilated abdominal veins. In some patients with cirrhosis, high portal vein pressures lead to the development of collateral vessels connecting the portal venous and systemic venous systems. One group of collateral vessels develops around the umbilicus, connecting the left portal vein via paraumbilical vessels to abdominal wall veins.[10] These abdominal wall veins may become so prominent and numerous that they resemble a cluster of serpents, thus earning the name "caput medusae."[11] Dilated abdominal veins of portal hypertension may generate a continuous humming murmur heard during auscultation between the xiphoid and umbilicus.[12]

Dilated abdominal veins also occur in the superior vena cava syndrome (if the obstruction also includes the azygous system)[13] and inferior vena cava syndrome.[14] In these disorders, however, the collateral veins tend to appear on the lateral aspects of the abdominal wall. A traditional test to distinguish vena caval obstruction from portal hypertension is to strip abdominal wall veins located *below* the umbilicus and see which way blood is flowing (in portal-systemic collateral veins, flow should hypothetically flow away from the umbilicus; whereas vena caval collateral vein flow is reversed and toward the head.)[15] This test is unreliable, however, because most dilated abdominal vessels lack competent valves and the clinician can "demonstrate" blood to flow in both directions in both disorders.

d. Palpable spleen. Because a principal cause of splenomegaly is portal hypertension from severe hepatocellular disease,[16,17] a traditional teaching is that the finding of splenomegaly in a jaundiced patient argues for hepatocellular disease.

e. Asterixis. Asterixis, originally described by Adams and Foley in 1949,[18,19] is one of the earliest findings of hepatic encephalopathy and thus typical of hepatocellular jaundice. To elicit the sign, the patient holds his arms outstretched with fingers spread apart. After a short latent period, both fingers and hands commence to "flap" with abrupt movements occurring at irregular intervals of a fraction of a second to seconds (thus earning the name "liver flap"). The fundamental problem in asterixis is the inability to maintain a fixed posture ("asterixis" comes from the Greek *sterigma* meaning "to support"), and consequently, asterixis also can be demonstrated at other sites by having the patient elevate the leg and dorsiflex the foot, close the eyelids forcibly, or protrude the tongue.[18,20] Because some voluntary contraction of the muscles is necessary to elicit asterixis, the sign disappears once coma ensues (although in some comatose patients, the finding appears during the grasp reflex; see Chapter 56).[18]

Electromyograms reveal that the actual flap of asterixis is caused by an abrupt disappearance of electrical activity in the muscle.[20] Asterixis is therefore a form of negative myoclonus.

Asterixis is not a specific sign of liver disease and also appears in encephalopathy from hypercapnia, uremia, and other disorders.[21,22] Unilateral asterixis indicates structural disease in the contralateral brain.[23]

f. **Fetor hepaticus.** Fetor hepaticus is the characteristic breath of patients with severe parenchymal disease, which has been likened to "a mixture of rotten eggs and garlic."[24,25] Gas chromatography reveals that the compound causing the odor is dimethylsulphide. Fetor hepaticus is a sign of severe portal-systemic shunting, not encephalopathy per se, because levels of dimethylsulphide correlate best with the degree of portal-systemic shunting[26] and because alert patients with severe portal-systemic shunting also have the characteristic breath.[26]

2. **Obstructive jaundice: palpable gallbladder (Courvoisier's sign).** The presence of a smooth, nontender, distended gallbladder in a patient with jaundice is a traditional sign of obstructive jaundice. Courvoisier's sign refers to the association of the palpable gallbladder and malignant obstruction, a sign whose accuracy is discussed fully in Chapter 45.

III. CLINICAL SIGNIFICANCE

A. **Detection of jaundice.** Although the traditional teaching is that jaundice becomes evident once the serum bilirubin exceeds 2.5 to 3 mg/dl, clinical studies reveal that only 70% to 80% of observers detect jaundice at this threshold.[27,28] The sensitivity of examination increases to 83% if the serum bilirubin exceeds 10 mg/dl and 96% if the bilirubin exceeds 15 mg/dl.

B. **Hepatocellular vs. obstructive jaundice.** Several studies have shown that, just using the bedside and basic laboratory findings (i.e., before clinical imaging), clinicians accurately distinguish hepatocellular from obstructive jaundice more than 80% of the time.[29-31] Easy-to-use and accurate scoring charts that combine symptoms, signs, and laboratory values have been developed.[1]

Table 6-1 presents how well physical signs distinguish hepatocellular from obstructive jaundice. Because "disease" in this table was defined as hepatocellular jaundice, LRs with a large positive number argue for hepatocellular jaundice and those with an LR close to zero argue against hepatocellular jaundice and thus for obstructive jaundice.

These studies show that, in patients presenting with jaundice, the physical signs of portal

TABLE 6-1 Findings predicting hepatocellular jaundice, in patients with jaundice*

Finding (ref)	Sensitivity (%)	Specificity (%)	Positive LR	Negative LR
General Appearance				
Weight loss[30,32]	10-49	21-97	NS	NS
Skin				
Spider angiomata[30,32]	35-47	88-97	4.7	0.6
Palmar erythema[30]	49	95	9.8	0.5
Distended abdominal veins[30]	42	98	17.5	0.6
Abdominal Examination				
Ascites[30]	44	90	4.4	0.6
Palpable spleen[30,32]	29-47	83-90	2.9	0.7
Palpable gallbladder[30]	0†	69	0.04	1.4
Palpable liver[30,32]	71-83	15-17	NS	NS
Liver tenderness[30,32]	37-38	70-78	NS	NS

NS, Not significant.

*Diagnostic standard: For nonobstructive (vs. obstructive) jaundice, needle biopsy of liver, surgical exploration, or autopsy.

†None of the 41 patients with medical jaundice in this study had a palpable gallbladder; for calculation of the LRs, 0.5 was added to all cells of the 2 × 2 table.

TABLE 6-2 Findings predicting cirrhosis, in patients with chronic hepatitis*

Finding (ref)†	Sensitivity (%)	Specificity (%)	Positive LR	Negative LR
Spider angiomata[33]	67	48	NS	NS
Palpable spleen[33,34]	56-85	35-68	1.4	0.5
Ascites[33,34]	27-36	90-95	3.9	0.8
Jaundice[34]	14	99	14.2	0.9
Encephalopathy[33]	28	98	17.5	0.7

NS, Not significant.

*Diagnostic standard: For cirrhosis, needle biopsy of liver.

†Definition of findings: For encephalopathy, disordered consciousness and asterixis.[18]

hypertension (distended abdominal veins, LR = 17.5; ascites, LR = 4.4; and a palpable spleen, LR = 2.9), spider angiomata (LR = 4.7), and palmar erythema (LR = 9.8) all argue *for* hepatocellular jaundice. The only finding arguing strongly *against* hepatocellular jaundice is the palpable gallbladder (LR = 0.04; in other words, the finding of a palpable gallbladder argues *for* obstructed bile ducts with an LR of 26.0, the inverse of 0.04).

In these studies, weight loss occurred in all etiologies and did not discriminate well between hepatocellular and obstructive etiologies. Also unhelpful were the findings of liver tenderness and a palpable liver. The palpable liver remains unhelpful even when it is defined as a liver edge extending more than 4 to 5 fingerbreadths below the right costal margin.[30]

C. Chronic hepatitis vs. cirrhosis. The diagnosis of cirrhosis in a patient with chronic hepatitis has important prognostic and therapeutic implications. Table 6-2 shows which physical signs argue for cirrhosis, as applied in studies of 314 patients with chronic hepatitis. The findings of encephalopathy (irrational behavior, disordered consciousness, and asterixis; LR = 17.5; see Table 6-2) and jaundice (LR = 14.2) are compelling arguments that cirrhosis is present. The finding of ascites also argues for cirrhosis (LR = 3.9). The presence of a palpable spleen or spider angiomata has little or no diagnostic value, and no finding argues significantly *against* the presence of cirrhosis (i.e., no LRs <0.5).

REFERENCES

1. Lindberg G and others. Differential diagnosis of jaundice: applicability of the Copenhagen Pocket Chart proved in Stockholm patients, *Liver* 7:43-49, 1987.

2. Theodossi A and others. The value of clinical, biochemical, ultrasound and liver biopsy data in assessing patients with liver disease, *Liver* 3:315-326, 1983.

3. Matzen P. Diagnosis in jaundice: a contemporary approach, *Dig Dis* 4:220-230, 1986.

4. Tripathi RC and Sidrys LA. 'Conjunctival icterus,' not 'scleral icterus,' *JAMA* 242:2558, 1979.

5. Monk B. Carotenemia, *Int J Dermatol* 22:376-377, 1983.

6. Bean WB. *Vascular spiders and related lesions of the skin,* Springfield, Ill, 1958, Charles C Thomas.

7. Bean WB. Acquired palmar erythema and cutaneous vascular "spiders," *Am Heart J* 25:463-477, 1943.

8. Pirovino M and others. Cutaneous spider nevi in liver cirrhosis: capillary microscopical and hormonal investigations, *Klin Wochenschr* 66:298-302, 1988.

9. Morrison GR. Causative factors in palmar erythema, *Geriatrics* 30:59-61, 1975.

10. Lafortune M and others. The recanalized umbilical vein in portal hypertension: a myth. *AJR Am J Roengenol* 114:549-553, 1985.

11. Cohen SM. Caput medusae, *N Engl J Med* 341:419, 1999.

12. Armstrong EL and others. The Cruveilhier-Baumgarten syndrome: review of the literature and report of two additional cases, *Ann Intern Med* 16:113-151, 1942.

13. Nieto AF and Doty DB. Superior vena cava obstruction: clinical syndrome, etiology, and treatment, *Curr Probl Cancer* 10:442-484, 1986.

14. Missal ME, Robinson JA, and Tatum RW. Inferior vena cava obstruction: clinical manifestations, diagnostic methods, and related problems, *Ann Intern Med* 62:133-161, 1965.

15. Coetzee T. Clinical anatomy of the umbilicus, *S Afr Med J* 57:463-466, 1980.

16. Lipp WF, Eckstein EH, and Aaron AH. The clinical significance of the palpable spleen, *Gastroenterology* 3:287-291, 1944.

17. O'Reilly RA. Splenomegaly at a United States County hospital: diagnostic evaluation of 170 patients, *Am J Med Sci* 312:160-165, 1996.

18. Adams RD and Foley JM. The neurological disorder associated with liver disease, *Res Publ Assoc Nerv Ment Dis* 32:198-237, 1953.

19. Adams RD and Foley JM. The neurological changes in the more common types of severe liver disease, *Trans Am Neurol Assoc* 74:217-219, 1949.

20. Leavitt S and Tyler HR. Studies in asterixis, *Arch Neurol* 10:360-368, 1964.

21. Conn HO. Asterixis in non-hepatic disorders, *Am J Med* 29:647-661, 1960.

22. Conn HO. Asterixis: its occurrence in chronic obstructive pulmonary disease, with a commentary on its general mechanism, *N Engl J Med* 259:564-569, 1958.

23. Reinfeld H and Louis S. Unilateral asterixis: clinical significance of the sign, *N Y State J Med* 83:206-208, 1983.

24. Davidson LSP. Mercaptan in the breath of patients with severe liver disease, *Lancet* 2:197-198, 1949.

25. Challenger F and Walshe JM. Foetor hepaticus, *Lancet* 1:1239-1241, 1955.

26. Tangerman A, Meuwese-Arends MT, and Jansen JBM. Cause and composition of foetor hepaticus, *Lancet* 343:483, 1994.

27. Hung OL and others. Evaluation of the physician's ability to recognize the presence or absence of anemia, fever, and jaundice, *Acad Emerg Med* 7:146-156, 2000.

28. Ruiz MA, Saab S, and Rickman LS. The clinical detection of scleral icterus: observations of multiple examiners, *Mil Med* 162:560-563, 1997.

29. Martin WB, Apostolakos PC, and Roazen H. Clinical versus actuarial prediction in the differential diagnosis of jaundice, *Am J Med Sci* 240:571-578, 1960.

30. Shenker S, Balint J, and Schiff L. Differential diagnosis of jaundice: report of a prospective study of 61 proved cases, *Am J Dig Dis* 7:449-463, 1962.

31. O'Connor KW and others. A blinded prospective study comparing four current noninvasive approaches in the differential diagnosis of medical versus surgical jaundice, *Gastroenterology* 84:1498-1504, 1983.

32. Burbank F. A computer diagnostic system for the diagnosis of prolonged undifferentiating liver disease, *Am J Med* 46:401-415, 1969.

33. Czaja AJ, Wolf AM, and Baggenstoss AH. Clinical assessment of cirrhosis in severe chronic active liver disease: specificity and sensitivity of physical and laboratory findings, *Mayo Clin Proc* 55:360-364, 1980.

34. Cozzolino G and others. Differential diagnosis between hepatic cirrhosis and chronic active hepatitis: specificity and sensitivity of physical and laboratory findings in a series from the Mediterranean area, *Am J Gastroenterol* 78:442-445, 1983.

CHAPTER 7

Cyanosis

I. **DEFINITIONS.** Cyanosis is an abnormal bluish discoloration of the skin and mucous membranes, caused by blue-colored blood circulating in the superficial capillaries and venules. The blue color usually represents excessive amounts of deoxygenated hemoglobin, although in some patients it results from increased amounts of methemoglobin or sulfhemoglobin. Cyanosis may be "central" or "peripheral." In **central cyanosis** the blood leaving the heart is colored blue; in **peripheral cyanosis**, the blood leaving the heart is red although it becomes blue by the time it reaches the fingers and toes. **Pseudocyanosis,** in contrast, refers to a permanent bluish discoloration caused by deposition of blue pigments in the skin.

Cyanosis was described by Morgagni in 1761, who attributed it to pulmonic stenosis.[1] In 1869, Claude Bernard first described the qualitative difference in blood gases between blue venous blood and red arterial blood. The first person to quantify how much deoxygenated hemoglobin was necessary to produce the blue color was Lundsgaard in 1919.[1]

II. **PATHOGENESIS**
   A. **The blue color.** Blood becomes blue when an absolute amount of blue pigment (usually deoxyhemoglobin) accumulates, probably be-

cause only then is the blue color deep enough to be seen through the opaque epidermis.[1-4] Once this minimal amount of deoxyhemoglobin accumulates and cyanosis appears, the amount of additional red blood (or oxyhemoglobin) matters little to the overall skin color.

The color of the skin depends on the color of blood flowing through the dermal capillaries and subpapillary venous plexus, not the arteries and veins, which lie too deep to contribute to skin color.[1,5] There has been much confusion over the absolute concentration of deoxyhemoglobin required for cyanosis, primarily because some investigators have mistakenly equated arterial levels of deoxyhemoglobin, which are easy to measure, with capillary levels, which impart the blue color but must be higher than the measured arterial levels. In patients with central cyanosis, the *average* amount of *arterial* deoxyhemoglobin is 3.48 ±0.55 g/dl (or 5.3 g/dl in the capillaries and small venules). The *minimal* amount of *arterial* deoxyhemoglobin causing cyanosis is 2.38 g/dl (or 4.24 g/dl in the capillaries and small venules).[a4]

Because cyanosis depends on the absolute quantity of deoxyhemoglobin, not the relative amount, the level of oxygen saturation at which the finding appears depends on the patient's total hemoglobin concentration (i.e., 5 g/dl of deoxyhemoglobin in the capillaries represents a higher percent of oxygen desaturation for an anemic patient, who has less total hemoglobin, than it does for a polycythemic patient). This relationship is displayed in Table 7-1, showing that polycythemic patients may become cya-

---

[a] Levels of capillary deoxyhemoglobin were calculated assuming that the difference in oxygen content between the arteries and veins is 5 ml/dl and that the amount of deoxyhemoglobin in the capillaries is midway between that of the arteries and veins.

TABLE 7-1 Cyanosis and hemoglobin concentration

HEMOGLOBIN CONCENTRATION (G/DL)	CYANOSIS APPEARS AT:*	
	OXYGEN SATURATION (%) BELOW:	ARTERIAL P_{O_2} (MM HG) BELOW:
6	60	31
8	70	36
10	76	40
12	80	45
14	83	47
16	85	50
18	87	54
20	88	56

* These figures assume that central cyanosis begins to appear when 2.38 g/dl of deoxygenated hemoglobin accumulates in arterial blood (see text for calculations). The corresponding P_{O_2} was obtained from standard hemoglobin dissociation curves for oxygen.

notic with only mild hypoxemia (i.e., oxygen saturation of 88% if the total hemoglobin is 20 g/dl, which is an oxygen tension of 56 mm Hg), yet anemic patients do not develop the finding until hypoxemia is severe (i.e., oxygen saturation of 70% if the total hemoglobin is 8 g/dl, which is an oxygen tension of 36 mm Hg).[b]

B. Peripheral cyanosis. In peripheral cyanosis, blood leaving the heart is red, but because of increased extraction of oxygen by peripheral tissues, enough deoxyhemoglobin accumulates to turn it blue in the subepidermal blood vessels of the feet and hands. The clinician can easily demonstrate the phenomenon of peripheral cyanosis by wrapping a rubber band around a

[b] These figures are calculated as follows: for the polycythemic patient (total hemoglobin of 20 g/dl), 2.38 g/dl of arterial deoxyhemoglobin indicates that there is 20 − 2.38, or 17.62 g/dl of oxyhemoglobin. Oxygen saturation, therefore, is (17.62)/(20) = 0.88, or 88%. For the anemic patient, the calculation is (8 − 2.38)/8 = 0.7, or 70% saturation.

finger: Oxygen continues to be extracted from the stagnant blood, and within a minute or two, the distal digit turns blue.

III. **THE FINDING.** Cyanosis is best appreciated in areas of the body where the overlying epidermis is thin and subepidermal vessels are abundant, such as the lips, nose, cheeks, ears, hands, feet, and the mucous membranes of the oral cavity.[1,6] Cyanosis is more easily appreciated with fluorescent lighting than with incandescent lighting or daylight.[4]

A. **Central cyanosis.** Patients with central cyanosis have blue discoloration of the lips, tongue, and sublingual tissues in addition to the hands and feet. In patients with central cyanosis, the correlation between different levels of oxygen desaturation and severity of cyanosis is best when the color is determined from examination of the lips and buccal mucosa.[7,8] Some patients with longstanding central cyanosis also have clubbing of the digits.

When central cyanosis is suspected, yet administration of oxygen fails to diminish the blue color, the clinician should consider methemoglobinemia or sulfhemoglobinemia. Many patients with methemoglobinemia are described as having a characteristic brownish or "chocolate" hue ("chocolate cyanosis").[9]

Because cyanosis depends on blue blood being present in the underlying blood vessels, maneuvers that express blood out of the vessels, such as pressure on the skin, make the blue color temporarily disappear.

B. **Peripheral cyanosis.** Peripheral cyanosis causes blue hands and feet, although the mucous membranes of the mouth are pink. Warming the patient's limb skin often lessens the blue color of peripheral cyanosis because it improves flow of blood to that area, whereas in central cyanosis, warming of the skin causes either no change or makes the blue color deeper.

C. **Pseudocyanosis.** In patients with pseudocyanosis, the mucous membranes of the mouth are pink, and blanching of the skin by pressure does not make the color disappear.[6]

D. **Cyanosis and oximetry.** Cyanosis affects co-oximetry (i.e., blood gas analysis in the laboratory) differently than it affects pulse oximetry (i.e., equipment used at the bedside; see Chapter 18). Co-oximetry is able to distinguish deoxyhemoglobin from other abnormal hemoglobins and therefore indicates hypoxemia only in patients with central cyanosis (i.e., because it samples *arterial* blood, oxygen levels are normal in peripheral cyanosis). Pulse oximetry, in contrast, detects the *color* of the pulsatile waveform in the digit. Although it also indicates hypoxemia in patients with central cyanosis and high deoxyhemoglobin levels, pulse oximetry sometimes falsely indicates arterial hypoxemia in patients with peripheral cyanosis or with abnormal hemoglobins (see Chapter 18). Both co-oximetry and pulse oximetry indicate normal oxygen levels in pseudocyanosis.

IV. CLINICAL SIGNIFICANCE

A. **Central cyanosis.** Any disorder causing hypoxemia may cause enough deoxyhemoglobin to accumulate in the blood leaving the heart, thus producing central cyanosis. Typical etiologies are pulmonary edema, pneumonia, and intracardiac right-to-left shunts.

The finding of central cyanosis detects an arterial deoxyhemoglobin level of 2.38 g/dl or more with a sensitivity of 79% to 95%, specificity of 72% to 95%, positive LR of 7.4, and negative LR 0.2.[2,4] With knowledge of the patient's hemoglobin concentration, therefore, the clinician can be reasonably confident that the finding of central cyanosis indicates an arterial oxygen level below that indicated in Table 7-1.

B. Peripheral cyanosis. In clinical practice, common causes of peripheral cyanosis are low cardiac output, arterial disease or obstruction (e.g., Raynaud's disease), and venous disease.

C. Pseudocyanosis. Pseudocyanosis may occur after exposure to metals ("chrysiasis" of gold therapy; "argyria" from topical silver compounds) or drugs (amiodarone, minocycline, chloroquine, or phenothiazines).[6,10,11]

REFERENCES

1. Lundsgaard C and Van Slyke DD. Cyanosis, *Medicine* 2:1-76, 1923.
2. Goss GA, Hayes JA, and Burdon JGW. Deoxyhaemoglobin concentrations in the detection of central cyanosis, *Thorax* 43:212-213, 1988.
3. Martin L and Khalil H. How much reduced hemoglobin is necessary to generate central cyanosis? *Chest* 97:182-185, 1990.
4. Barnett HB, Holland JG, and Josenhans WT. When does central cyanosis become detectable? *Clin Invest Med* 5:39-43, 1982.
5. Lewis T. *The blood vessels of the human skin and their responses,* London, 1927, Shaw & Sons.
6. Carpenter KD. A comprehensive review of cyanosis, *Crit Care Nurs* 13:66-72, 1993.
7. Kelman GR and Nunn JF. Clinical recognition of hypoxaemia under fluorescent lamps, *Lancet* 1:1400-1403, 1966.
8. Medd WE, French EB, and Wyllie VM. Cyanosis as a guide to arterial oxygen desaturation, *Thorax* 14:247-250, 1959.
9. Whelan JF. Methemoglobin as a cause of cyanosis. *Can Med Assoc J* 130:1260, 1984.
10. Familton MJG and Armstrong RF. Pseudo-cyanosis: time to reclassify cyanosis? *Anaesthesiology* 44:257, 1989.
11. Timmins AC and Morgan GAR. Argyria or cyanosis, *Anaesthesiology* 43:755-756, 1988.

CHAPTER 8

Anemia

I. INTRODUCTION. Anemia refers to an abnormally low number of circulating red cells, caused by blood loss, hemolysis, or underproduction of cells by the bone marrow. In patients with acute blood loss, physical signs reflect the changing vital signs of hypovolemia (see Chapter 15). In chronic anemia, the subject of this chapter, physical examination focuses instead on the color of skin and conjunctiva. Chronic anemia is a feature of almost all chronic diseases.

II. THE FINDINGS. In chronic anemia, the skin and conjunctiva may appear abnormally pale because the amount of red-colored oxyhemoglobin circulating in the dermal and subconjunctival capillaries and venules is reduced.[1] This finding, however, is not always reliable, because the color of the skin also depends on the diameter of these minute vessels, the amount of circulating deoxyhemoglobin, and the patient's natural skin pigments.[1] Vasoconstriction from cold exposure or sympathetic stimulation also may cause pallor, and the pallor of anemia may be obscured by other colors, such as the red color of vasodilation (inflammatory response or permanent vascular injury from ischemia, cold, or radiation), the blue color of cyanosis (see Chapter 7), or the brown color of natural pigments of dark-skinned persons. Theoretically, examination of the conjunctiva, nail beds, and palms minimizes the effects of the patient's natural skin pigments.

Most clinicians assess for pallor subjectively, by comparing the patient's skin color with their own color or with some recollection of normal skin color. One definition of pallor, however, is more objective: **conjunctival rim pallor** is present if examination of the inferior conjunctiva reveals the color of the anterior rim to be the same pale fleshy color of the deeper posterior aspect of the palpebral conjunctiva.[2] Normally, in persons without anemia, the anterior rim has a bright red color that contrasts with the fleshy color of the posterior portion.

III. CLINICAL SIGNIFICANCE. Table 8-1 presents the diagnostic accuracy of physical signs for chronic anemia, as applied to hundreds of medical and surgical inpatients. These studies all excluded patients with acute bleeding and those who had received recent transfusions. As much as possible, the color of skin and conjunctiva was determined under natural lighting.

According to these studies, the most compelling findings arguing *for* anemia are conjunctival rim pallor (LR = 16.7), palmar crease pallor (LR = 7.9), pallor at multiple sites (LR = 4.5), and facial pallor (light-skinned persons only, LR = 3.8). Nail bed pallor has less diagnostic value (LR = 1.7), and another study[a] showed that nail bed pallor as determined by simple inspection and by "absence of nail bed blanching" were equivalent.[5] Importantly, no physical sign convincingly argues *against* the diagnosis of anemia (i.e., no LR is less than 0.5).

---

[a] This study was excluded from the table because the clinicians were aware of the patient's red cell count.

TABLE 8-1 Anemia*

Finding (ref)†	Sensitivity (%)	Specificity (%)	Positive LR	Negative LR
Pallor at multiple sites[3,4]	35-38	90-94	4.5	0.7
Facial pallor[3]	46	88	3.8	0.6
Nail bed pallor[3]	59	66	1.7	0.6
Palmar pallor[3]	64	74	2.5	0.5
Palmar crease pallor[3]	8	99	7.9	NS
Conjunctival rim pallor[2]				
Pallor present	10	99	16.7	—
Pallor borderline	36	—	2.3	—
Pallor absent	53	16	0.6	—

NS, Not significant.

*Diagnostic standard: For anemia, hematocrit <35%[3], hemoglobin <11 g/dl[2], or hemoglobin <11 g/dl in women and <13 g/dl in men.[4]

†Definition of findings: For pallor at multiple sites, examination of skin, nail beds, and conjunctiva[3]; or pallor of face, palms and conjunctiva[3]; for facial pallor, the study excluded black patients; for palmar crease pallor, examination after gentle extension of the patient's fingers; for conjunctival rim pallor, see text.

REFERENCES

1. Lewis T. *The blood vessels of the human skin and their responses,* London, 1927, Shaw & Sons.
2. Sheth TN and others. The relation of conjunctival pallor to the presence of anemia, *J Gen Intern Med* 12:102-106, 1997.
3. Nardone DA and others. Usefulness of physical examination in detecting the presence or absence of anemia, *Arch Intern Med* 150:201-204, 1990.
4. Gjorup T and others. A critical evaluation of the clinical diagnosis of anemia, *Am J Epidemiol* 124:657-665, 1986.
5. Strobach RS and others. The value of the physical examination in the diagnosis of anemia: correlation of the physical findings and the hemoglobin concentration, *Arch Intern Med* 148:831-832, 1988.

CHAPTER 9

Hypovolemia

I. INTRODUCTION. The term "hypovolemia" refers collectively to two distinct disorders: (1) "volume depletion," which is the loss of sodium from the extracellular space (intravascular and interstitial fluid) that occurs after gastrointestinal hemorrhage, vomiting, diarrhea, and diuresis; and (2) "dehydration," which refers to losses of intracellular water that ultimately cause cellular desiccation and elevates the plasma sodium concentration and osmolality.[1] Chapter 15 discusses the accuracy of abnormal vital signs in patients with volume depletion; this chapter discusses assorted additional findings.

II. THE FINDINGS AND THEIR PATHOGENESIS. Many of the traditional signs of hypovolemia—dry mucous membranes, sunken eyes, shriveled skin and tongue, confusion—originate in classic descriptions of cholera as findings of patients near vascular collapse.[2] Presumably, cellular dehydration, interstitial space dehydration, and poor perfusion contribute to these signs; however, studies of their pathogenesis are unavailable.

Poor skin turgor refers to the slow return of skin to its normal position after being pinched between the examiner's thumb and forefinger.[3,4] The protein elastin is responsible for the recoil of skin, and *in vitro* experiments show that its recoil time increases

TABLE 9-1 Hypovolemia*

Finding (ref)†	Sensitivity (%)	Specificity (%)	Positive LR	Negative LR
Skin, Eyes, and Mucous Membranes				
Dry axilla[5]	50	82	2.8	NS
Dry mucous membranes of mouth and nose[6]	85	58	NS	0.3
Longitudinal furrows on tongue[6]	85	58	NS	0.3
Sunken eyes[6]	62	82	NS	0.5
Neurologic Findings				
Confusion[6]	57	73	NS	NS
Weakness[6]	43	82	NS	NS
Speech not clear or expressive[6]	56	82	NS	0.5

NS, Not significant.

*Diagnostic standard: For hypovolemia, elevated serum urea nitrogen-creatinine ratio, osmolarity, or sodium level.

fortyfold after as little as 3.4% loss in wet weight.[3] Elastin also deteriorates with age, however, suggesting that poor skin turgor may be a less specific finding of hypovolemia in elderly patients.

III. CLINICAL SIGNIFICANCE. Table 9-1 presents clinical studies comparing traditional signs to laboratory tests of hypovolemia (i.e., serum urea-to-creatinine level, osmolarity, or sodium level). These studies enrolled elderly patients presenting to emergency departments with vomiting, decreased oral intake, or diarrhea. Few, if any, were as desperately hypovolemic as patients with classic cholera.

These studies show that only one finding, a dry axilla, argues somewhat *for* hypovolemia (LR = 2.8; see Table 9-1), and only two findings, the absence of tongue furrows and the presence of moist mucous membranes, argue *against* hypovolemia (LR = 0.3 for both findings). In these studies, the presence or absence of sunken eyes, confusion, weakness, or abnormal speech had little diagnostic value.

Another study confirms the association between dry axilla and hypovolemia.[7] Two studies have found poor skin turgor to have no diagnostic value in adults.[6,7] Although poor capillary refill time has been advanced as a reliable sign of hypovolemia, the only available studies either compare it to a questionable diagnostic standard (i.e., vital signs)[8] or find the sign has no diagnostic value.[6]

REFERENCES

1. Mange K and others. Language guiding therapy: the case of dehydration versus volume depletion, *Ann Intern Med* 127: 848-853, 1997.
2. Osler W. *The principles and practice of medicine* (facsimile by Classics of Medicine library), New York, 1892, D. Appleton and Co.

3. Dorrington KL. Skin turgor: do we understand the clinical sign? *Lancet* 1:264-265, 1981.

4. Aquilar OM and Albertal M. Images in clinical medicine. Poor skin turgor, *N Engl J Med* 338:25, 1998.

5. Eaton D and others. Axillary sweating in clinical assessment of dehydration in ill elderly patients, *Br Med J* 308:1271, 1994.

6. Gross CR and others. Clinical indicators of dehydration severity in elderly patients, *J Emerg Med* 10:267-274, 1992.

7. Levitt MA and others. Evaluation of the tilt test in an adult emergency medicine population, *Ann Emerg Med* 21:713-718, 1992.

8. Schriger DL and Baraff LJ. Capillary refill: is it a useful predictor of hypovolemic states? *Ann Emerg Med* 20:601-605, 1991.

CHAPTER 10

Protein-Energy Malnutrition and Weight Loss

PROTEIN-ENERGY MALNUTRITION

I. INTRODUCTION. Protein energy malnutrition occurs when the supply of protein, calories, or both is inadequate. Decreased oral intake is the most common cause worldwide, although in industrialized countries, increased nutrient loss (e.g., malabsorption, diarrhea, nephrotic syndrome) and increased nutrient requirements (e.g., fever, cancer, infection, or surgery) play a more important role. Among patients admitted to surgical services in industrialized nations, 9% to 27% have signs of severe malnutrition.[1,2]

II. THE FINDINGS. Two distinct syndromes of protein-energy malnutrition have been described in children of developing nations: *marasmus* (predominant caloric deficiency), characterized by weight loss, muscle and fat wasting, and *kwashiorkor* (predominant protein deficiency), characterized by ascites and edema. In industrialized countries, however, most malnourished patients present less dramatically with features of both syndromes, including low body weight, atrophy of muscle and subcutaneous fat, weakness, and various laboratory abnormalities (e.g., low albumin or other serum proteins).

A. **Arm muscle circumference.** Arm muscle circumference is a decades-old anthropometric measure designed to reflect the amount of muscle in the arm, which therefore provides an indirect measure of the total amount of muscle or protein in the body. After measuring the upper arm circumference with a flexible tape measure (C_a) and the triceps skinfold thickness with calipers (h), the clinician estimates arm muscle circumference (AMC) by using the following formula[a][3]:

$$AMC = C_a - \pi h$$

Age- and sex-standardized values of the normal AMC have been published.[5] Similar measurements are made to calculate the forearm muscle circumference.

B. **Grip strength.** Based on the hypothesis that skeletal muscle strength reflects total body protein stores, and that protein-malnutrition becomes particularly important during periods of stress, such as surgery, Klidjian in 1980 investigated the grip strength of 102 patients and showed that weakness accurately predicted postoperative complications.[6] In his method, the patient squeezed a simple hand-held spring dynamometer 3 times, resting 10 seconds between each attempt, and the clinician recorded

---

[a] This formula assumes that the arm is a cylinder and ignores the contribution of the humerus.[4] To derive this formula, $AMC = \pi d_1$, where d_1 is the diameter of the muscle component of the arm; $d_1 = d_2 - h$, where d_2 is the diameter of the arm and h is the skinfold thickness (which includes a double layer of skin and subcutaneous tissue). Therefore $AMC = \pi d_1 = \pi(d_2 - h) = \pi d_2 - \pi h = C_a - \pi h$. If the clinician desires to directly enter the skinfold thickness in mm (as it is measured), 0.314 is substituted for π in the formula (i.e., AMC and C_a are measured in cm).

the highest value obtained. The presence of arthritis, stroke, or other obvious reasons for reduced grip strength makes the test uninterpretable.

Age- and sex-standardized values of normal grip strength have been published.[7] Clinical studies of grip strength always test the nondominant arm, but this may be unnecessary because other studies show very little difference in strength between the two arms.[7]

III. CLINICAL SIGNIFICANCE. Table 10-1 applies the signs of weight loss, arm anthropometry, and grip strength to patients just before major surgery and addresses how accurately these signs predict significant postoperative complications, which are assumed in part to reflect the effects of malnutrition. "Significant complications" are those that prolong the hospital stay, threaten the patient's life, or cause death (e.g., sepsis, wound infections, myocardial infarction, stroke).

The findings of reduced arm or forearm muscle circumference (LR = 2.5 to 3.2), reduced grip strength (LR = 2.1), and low body weight (LR = 2.0) are all modest predictors of postoperative complications. Only one finding, a normal grip strength, argues *against* the development of complications (LR = 0.3). The presence of recent weight loss has little diagnostic value, presumably because this finding includes not only patients with significant ongoing weight loss but also obese patients who have lost weight (and thus reduced their complication rate)[11] and those who have lost weight but gained some of it back in the immediate preoperative period.

Another bedside tool, not reviewed in Table 10-1, is the "subjective global assessment," which combines elements from the patient's history (weight change, dietary history, gastrointestinal symptoms, and functional capacity) and physical examination (absence of subcutaneous fat, muscle

TABLE 10-1 Protein-energy malnutrition and major surgical complications*

Finding (ref)†	Sensitivity (%)	Specificity (%)	Positive LR	Negative LR
Body Weight				
Weight loss >10%[6,8-10]	16-75	47-88	1.4	NS
Low body weight[6,9-11]	11-35	83-97	2.0	NS
Anthropometry				
Upper arm muscle circumference <85% predicted[6,9,10]	26-38	83-91	2.5	0.8
Forearm muscle circumference <85% predicted[6,9,10]	14-42	85-97	3.2	0.8
Muscle Strength				
Reduced grip strength[6,7,9,10,12]	64-90	46-72	2.1	0.3

NS, Not significant.

Diagnostic standard: In each of these studies, *disease* is defined as a major postoperative complication, including those prolonging hospital stay, threatening the patient's life, or causing death.

†*Definition of findings* (all findings were assessed during the preoperative physical examination): For *weight loss* >10%, (recalled usual weight–measured weight)/(recalled usual weight) × 100; for *low body weight*, weight-for-height less than normal lower limit,[11] less than 90% of predicted,[6] or less than 85% of predicted[9,10]; for *predicted arm muscle circumference*, published standardized values[5]; for *forearm muscle circumference* <85%, <20 cm in men and <16.3 cm in women,[6,10] and; for *reduced grip strength*, specific thresholds differ but all correspond closely to published age- and sex-standardized abnormal values from reference 7.

wasting, edema, and ascites) to accurately predict postsurgical complications.[1,13] The components of this scoring tool, however, are imprecisely defined,[2] making it difficult for clinicians to duplicate the accuracy of the original investigators.

WEIGHT LOSS

I. INTRODUCTION. Involuntary weight loss reflects either diuresis, decreased caloric intake, or the increased caloric requirements of malabsorption, glucosuria, or a hypermetabolic state. In series of patients presenting with involuntary weight loss (exceeding 5% of their usual weight), organic disease is diagnosed in 65% of patients (most commonly cancer and gastrointestinal disorders, although virtually any chronic disease may cause weight loss) and psychiatric disorders in 10% (depression, anorexia nervosa, schizophrenia). In 25% of patients, the cause remained unknown despite at least 1 year follow-up.[14,15]

II. CLINICAL SIGNIFICANCE. Weight loss is rarely due to occult disease and most diagnoses are made during the initial evaluation, including the patient interview, physical examination, and basic laboratory testing.[14,15]

In patients who complain of weight loss, the patient's perceptions of the weight loss—whether they significantly underestimate or overestimate it—helps predict the final diagnosis. The patient is asked to estimate his weight before the illness (W) and the amount of weight he has lost (E). The observed weight loss (O) is the former weight (W) minus the current measured weight. Significant *underestimation* of weight loss, defined as (O–E) greater than 0.5 kg, predicts an *organic* cause of weight loss with a sensitivity of 40%, specificity of 92%, positive LR of 5.4 and negative LR of 0.6.[16] Significant *overestimation* of weight loss, defined as (E–O) greater than 0.5 kg, predicts a *nonorganic* cause of weight loss with a sensitivity of 70%, specificity of 81%, positive LR of 3.6, and negative LR of 0.4.[16]

REFERENCES

1. Baker JP and others. Nutritional assessment: a comparison of clinical judgment and objective measurements, *N Engl J Med* 306:969-972, 1982.
2. Detsky AS and others. What is subjective global assessment of nutritional status? *JPEN* 11:8-13, 1987.
3. Jelliffe DB. The assessment of the nutritional status of the community, *WHO Monograph Series* 53:1-271, 1966.
4. Hall JC and others. Upper limb anthropometry: the value of measurement variance studies. *Am J Clin Nutr* 33:1846-1851, 1980.
5. Frisancho AR. New norms of upper limb fat and muscle areas for assessment of nutritional status, *Am J Clin Nutr* 34:2540-2545, 1981.
6. Klidjian AM and others. Relation of anthropometric and dynamometric variables to serious postoperative complications, *Br Med J* 281:899-901, 1980.
7. Webb AR and others. Hand grip dynamometry as a predictor of postoperative complications reappraisal using age standardized grip strengths, *JPEN* 13:30-33, 1989.
8. Windsor JA and Hill GL. Weight loss with physiologic impairment: a basic indicator of surgical risk, *Ann Surg* 207:290-296, 1988.
9. Klidjian AM and others. Detection of dangerous malnutrition, *JPEN* 6:119-122, 1982.
10. Hunt DR, Rowlands BJ, and Johnston D. Hand grip strength—a simple prognostic indicator in surgical patients, *JPEN* 9:701-704, 1985.
11. Hickman DM and others. Serum albumin and body weight as predictors of postoperative course in colorectal cancer, *JPEN* 4:314-316, 1980.
12. Davies CWT, Jones DM, and Shearer JR. Hand grip—a simple test for morbidity after fracture of the neck of the femur, *J Roy Soc Med* 77:833-836, 1984.
13. Detsky AS, Smalley PS, and Chang J. Is this patient malnourished? *JAMA* 271:54-58, 1994.
14. Rabinovitz M and others. Unintentional weight loss: a retrospective analysis of 154 cases, *Arch Intern Med* 146:186-187, 1986.

15. Marton KI, Sox HC, and Krupp JR. Involuntary weight loss: diagnostic and prognostic significance, *Ann Intern Med* 95:568-574, 1981.
16. Ramboer C, Verhamme M, and Vermeire L. Patients' perception of involuntary weight loss: Implications of underestimation and overestimation, *Br Med J* 291:1091, 1985.

CHAPTER 11

Obesity

I. **INTRODUCTION.** Obesity increases the risk of coronary artery disease, diabetes, hypertension, osteoarthritis, cholelithiasis, certain cancers, and overall death.[1] Clinicians have recognized the hazards of obesity for thousands of years (according to one Hippocratic aphorism, "sudden death is more common in those who are naturally fat than in the lean").[2] At least one-third of U.S. adults are overweight.[3]

II. **THE FINDINGS AND THEIR SIGNIFICANCE.** Several different anthropometric parameters have been used to identify those patients at greatest risk for the medical complications of obesity. The most important ones are body-mass index, skinfold thickness, waist-to-hip ratio, waist circumference, and sagittal diameter.

A. **Body mass index (BMI)**

1. **The finding.** The BMI (or Quetelet index) is the patient's weight in kilograms divided by the square of his height in meters (kg/m^2). If pounds and inches are used, the quotient should be multiplied by 703.5 to convert the units to kg/m^2. An individual is overweight if the BMI exceeds 25 kg/m^2, and obese if the BMI exceeds 30 kg/m^2.[4,5]

   The BMI was derived by a seventeenth century Belgian mathematician and astronomer, Lambert-Adolphe-Jacques Quetelet, who discovered that this ratio best expressed the natural relationship between weight and height.[6]

2. **Clinical significance.** The BMI correlates well with precise measures of total body fat (r = 0.70 to 0.96),[7,8] much better than other formulas of weight (W) and height (H) (e.g., W/H, W/H^3, $W/H^{0.3}$, $W^{0.3}/H$).[8] The BMI also correlates significantly with the patient's cholesterol level,[9] blood pressure,[9] incidence of coronary events,[10-13] and overall mortality.[12-15]

The arbitrary cutoff of 25 kg/m² was chosen in part because it reflects the level at which there is a significant increase in mortality, although increased rates of some complications such as diabetes appear at lower cutoffs.[1] Early studies of BMI and mortality revealed a J-shaped relationship (i.e., both lean and overweight patients had increased mortality),[15] but the increased risk for lean individuals disappears after controlling for the patient's age, cigarette use, and illness-related weight loss.[12,14,16]

B. **Skinfold thickness.** Another measure of obesity is "total skinfold thickness," which is estimated by adding together the skinfold thickness (measured with calipers) of multiple sites (midbiceps, midtriceps, subscapular, and suprailiac area).[8] This sum is then converted using a formula into an estimate of total body fat, which correlates well with more precise measures (r = 0.7 to 0.8).[8,17] Skinfold measurements rarely are used today to assess obesity, partly because they are too complex, but mostly because relatively few studies[10] show the number is clinically significant.

C. **Waist-to-hip ratio**
1. **The finding.** The waist-to-hip ratio (WHR) is the circumference of the waist divided by

that of the hips. It is based on the premise that the most important characteristic of obesity is its distribution, not its quantity. "Abdominal" obesity (also called "android," "upper body," or "apple-shaped" obesity) has a much worse prognosis than "gluteal-femoral" obesity (also called "gynoid," "lower body," or "pear-shaped" obesity).

Although at least nine different methods of measuring WHR have been recommended,[9] most authorities measure the waist circumference at the midpoint between the lower costal margin and the iliac crest and the hip circumference at the widest part of the gluteal region.[18,19] Adverse health outcomes increase significantly when the WHR exceeds 1.0 in men and 0.85 in women,[18,20] values that are very close to the top quintiles in epidemiologic studies.[7,11,15,21]

The French diabetologist Jean Vague is usually credited with making the observation in the 1940s that abdominal obesity, common in men, is associated with worse health outcomes than obesity over the hips and thighs, more common in women (American life insurance companies, however, made the same observation in the late 1800s).[22,23] Vague's original "index of masculine differentiation," a complicated index based on skinfolds and limb circumferences,[24] is no longer used, having been replaced by the much simpler WHR in the 1980s.[25]

2. **Clinical significance.** The WHR predicts health outcomes better than any other anthropometric measure. Even after controlling for the effects of BMI, the WHR correlates significantly with blood pressure,[18,26] cholesterol level,[9,18,26] incidence of diabetes mellitus,[18,26] stroke,[10,21,26] coronary events,[10,11,18,26] and overall mortality.[10,15]

3. **Pathogenesis.** The main contributor to abdominal obesity is visceral fat (i.e., omental, mesenteric, and retroperitoneal fat), not subcutaneous fat. Visceral fat is metabolically very active, constantly releasing free fatty acids into the portal circulation,[22] which probably contributes to hyperlipidemia, atherogenesis, and hyperinsulinemia.[22] Gluteal-femoral fat, on the other hand, is metabolically inactive except during pregnancy and the postpartum period, which has led some to suggest that the role of lower body fat is to help guarantee the survival of the species, by providing a constant source of energy to the lactating female even when external nutrients are unavailable.

D. **Waist circumference.** Waist circumference is simply the numerator of the WHR calculation. It has the advantages of being simpler to measure and of avoiding attention to the hips, which, because they encompass bone and skeletal muscle as well as fat, should have no biologically plausible relationship to diabetes, hypertension, and atherosclerosis.[20] Nonetheless, very few studies have validated this measure,[9,27] and some studies show the waist circumference to be inferior to the WHR.[10,21] Recommended cutoffs for increased health risk are a waist circumference greater than 102 cm (40 in) for men and 88 cm (35 in) for women.[4]

E. **Sagittal diameter.** Because waist circumference encompasses both subcutaneous and visceral fat, investigators have looked for anthropometric measures that reflect more precisely just visceral fat. One proposed measure is the sagittal diameter, which is the total anterior-posterior distance between the anterior abdominal wall of the *supine* patient and the surface of the examining table. Theoretically, visceral fat maintains the abdominal depth in the supine patient, whereas subcutaneous fat allows the abdominal depth to partially collapse from the force of gravity.[19] Even so, there are few studies of this measure, and most that exist measure it by computed tomography (not during physical examination) and correlate it with variables of uncertain clinical significance (e.g., the amount of visceral fat visualized on computed tomography).[7,28]

REFERENCES

1. Willett WC, Dietz WH, and Colditz GA. Guidelines for healthy weight, *N Engl J Med* 341:427-434, 1999.
2. Hippocratic writings. Lloyd GER, editor. Harmondsworth, Middlesex, England, 1978 Penguin.
3. Kuczmarski RJ and others. Increasing prevalence of overweight among US adults: The National Health and Nutrition Examination Surveys 1960 to 1991, *JAMA* 272:205-211, 1994.
4. Executive summary of the clinical guidelines on the identification, evaluation, and treatment of overweight and obesity in adults, *Arch Intern Med* 158:1855-1867, 1998.
5. Bray GA and others. Evaluation of the obese patient. 2. Clinical findings, *JAMA* 235:2008-2010, 1976.
6. Jelliffe DB and Jeliffe EF. Underappreciated pioneers. Quetelet: man and index, *Am J Clin Nutr* 32:2519-2521, 1979.
7. Pouliot M and others. Waist circumference and abdominal sagittal diameter: best simple anthropometric indexes of abdominal visceral adipose tissue accumulation and related cardiovascular risk in men and women, *Am J Card* 73:460-468, 1994.
8. Womersley J and Durnin JVGA. A comparison of the skinfold method with extent of "overweight" and various weight-height relationships in the assessment of obesity, *Br J Nutr* 38:271-284, 1977.
9. Seidell JC and others. Fat distribution in European women: a comparison of anthropometric measurements in relation to cardiovascular risk factors, *Int J Epidemiol* 19:303-308, 1990.

10. Lapidus L and others. Distribution of adipose tissue and risk of cardiovascular disease and death: a 12 year follow up of participants in the population study of women in Gothenburg, Sweden, *Br Med J* 289:1257-1261, 1984.

11. Rimm EB and others. Body size and fat distribution as predictors of coronary heart disease among middle-aged and older US men, *Am J Epidemiol* 141:1117-1127, 1995.

12. Manson JE and others. Body weight and mortality among women, *N Engl J Med* 333:677-685, 1995.

13. Stevens J and others. The effect of age on the association between body-mass index and mortality, *N Engl J Med* 338:1-7, 1998.

14. Lee IM and others. Body weight and mortality: a 27-year follow-up of middle-aged men, *JAMA* 270:2823-2828, 1993.

15. Folsom AR and others. Body fat distribution and 5-year risk of death in older women. *JAMA* 269:483-487, 1993.

16. Calle EE and others. Body-mass index and mortality in a prospective cohort of U.S. adults. *N Engl J Med* 341:1097-1105, 1999.

17. Jebb SA and Elia M. Techniques for the measurement of body composition: a practical guide, *Int J Obes Relat Metab Disord* 17:611-621, 1993.

18. Bjorntorp P. Obesity, *Lancet* 350:423-426, 1997.

19. Van der Kooy K and Seidell JC. Techniques for the measurement of visceral fat: a practical guide, *Int J Obes Relat Metab Disord* 17:187-196, 1993.

20. Molarius A and Seidell JC. Selection of anthropometric indicators for classification of abdominal fatness—a critical review, *Int J Obes Relat Metab Disord*, 22:719-727, 1998.

21. Walker SP and others. Body size and fat distribution as predictors of stroke among US men, *Am J Epidemiol* 144:1143-1150, 1996.

22. Kaplan NM. Obesity: location matters, *Heart Dis Stroke* 1:148-150, 1992.

23. Kahn HS and Williamson DF. Abdominal obesity and mortality risk among men in nineteenth-century North America, *Int J Obes Relat Metab Disord* 18:686-691, 1994.

24. Vague J. The degree of masculine differentiation of obesities: a factor determining predisposition to diabetes, atherosclerosis, gout, and uric calculous disease, *Am J Clin Nutr* 4:20-34, 1956.

25. Krotkeiwski M and others. Impact of obesity on metabolism in men and women, *J Clin Invest* 72:1150-1162, 1983.

26. Egger G. The case for using waist to hip ratio measurements in routine medical checks, *Med J Aust* 156:280-285, 1992.
27. Lemieux S and others. A single threshold value of waist girth identifies normal-weight and overweight subjects with excess visceral adipose tissue, *Am J Clin Nutr* 64:685-693, 1996.
28. Seidell JC and Bouchard C. Visceral fat in relation to health: is it a major culprit or simply an innocent bystander? *Int J Obesity* 21:626-631, 1997.

CHAPTER 12

Cushing's Syndrome

I. INTRODUCTION. Cushing's syndrome refers to various clinical findings—hypertension, central obesity, weakness, hirsutism (in women), depression, skin striae, and bruises—that are caused by excess circulating glucocorticoids. The most common cause is exogenous administration of corticosteroid hormones.[1,2] Endogenous Cushing's syndrome results from pituitary tumors producing adrenocorticotropic hormone (ACTH) (i.e., "Cushing's disease," 70% of all endogenous cases), ectopic production of ACTH (usually by small cell carcinoma of the lung or carcinoid tumors of the lung or mediastinum, 10% of cases), adrenal adenomas (15% of cases), or adrenal carcinoma (5% of cases).[2-5] Cushing's disease and the ectopic ACTH syndrome are referred to as "ACTH-dependent," because the elevated cortisol levels are accompanied by inappropriately high ACTH levels. Adrenal tumors are "ACTH independent."

The bedside findings associated with Cushing's syndrome were originally described by Harvey Cushing in 1932.[6] Corticosteroid hormones were first used as therapeutic agents to treat patients with rheumatoid arthritis in 1949; within 2 years, clear descriptions of exogenous Cushing's syndrome appeared.[7]

TABLE 12-1 Cushing's syndrome—frequency of individual findings*

Physical Finding†	Frequency (%)‡
Vital Signs	
Hypertension	76
Body Habitus	
Moon facies	92
Central obesity	44-90
Buffalo hump	34-75
Skin Findings	
Thin skin	84
Plethora	28-94
Hirsutism, women	70
Ecchymoses	43-77
Red or purple striae	56
Acne	21-52
Extremity Findings	
Proximal muscle weakness	57
Edema	51
Other	
Significant depression	12-48

Information is based on 322 patients with endogenous Cushing's syndrome from references 2, 5, and 8 to 13.

*Diagnostic standard: For Cushing's syndrome, elevated daily cortisol or corticosteroid metabolites, or both, with loss of circadian rhythm of serum cortisol levels and with abnormal dexamethasone suppression tests.

†Definition of finding: For hypertension, systolic blood pressure >140 mm Hg[13] or 150 mm Hg,[9] diastolic blood pressure >90 mm Hg,[5,9,13] or not defined.

‡Results are overall mean frequency or, if statistically heterogenous, the range of values.

II. THE FINDINGS AND THEIR PATHOGENESIS.
Table 12-1 presents the physical signs found in 322 patients with Cushing's syndrome.

A. Body habitus. Patients with Cushing's syndrome develop central obesity (or "truncal obesity"), which means that fat accumulates centrally on the neck, chest, and abdomen, providing a striking visual contrast to the muscle atrophy that affects the extremities. The definitions of central obesity vary, depending on which clinical study is consulted: some define it subjectively as the appearance of obesity sparing the extremities.[8,13] Others define it more precisely using the "central obesity index," which is the sum of three truncal circumferences—neck, chest, and abdomen—divided by the sum of six limb circumferences—bilateral arms, thighs, and lower legs. A central obesity index exceeding 1 is abnormal.[14] A third definition of central obesity—an abnormal waist-to-hip circumference ratio (>1.0 in men and >0.8 in women; see Chapter 11)[1]—is not recommended because of the high false-positive rate.[15]

Other characteristic features of the Cushing's body habitus are accumulation of fat in the bitemporal region ("moon facies"),[16] between the scapulae and behind the neck ("dorsocervical fatpad" or "buffalo hump"), in the supraclavicular region (producing a "collar" around the base of the neck),[1] and in front of the sternum ("dewlap," named after the similarity to the hanging fold of skin at the base of the bovine neck).[17] Although many experts believe that the buffalo hump is not specific for Cushing's syndrome and may occur after weight gain from any cause,[4,18] this has not been formally tested. Morbid obesity (i.e., weight more than twice the ideal weight) is rare in Cushing's syndrome.[19]

The truncal obesity of Cushing's syndrome reflects an increase in intraabdominal visceral fat, not subcutaneous fat,[20] probably from glucocorticoid-induced reduction in lipolytic activity and activation of lipoprotein lipase, which allows tissues to accumulate triglyceride.[1,15]

B. Hypertension. Hypertension occurs in 3 of 4 patients with Cushing's syndrome. Proposed mechanisms are suppressed vasodepressor systems (prostaglandins, kallikrein-kinin), exaggerated pressor responses to vasoactive substances, and possible activation of the renin-angiotensin system.[21] Most patients do *not* have a positive salt and water balance.[1]

C. **Skin findings.** The characteristic skin findings are thin skin, striae, plethora, hirsutism (in women), acne, and ecchymoses.

Significant thinning of the skin, which affects most patients,[22-25] probably arises from corticosteroid-induced inhibition of epidermal cell division and dermal collagen synthesis.[1] To assess skin thickness, many experts recommend using calipers (either skinfold calipers or electrocardiograph calipers) to measure skinfold thickness on the back of the patient's hand, an area lacking significant subcutaneous fat and thus representing just epidermis and dermis.[22,25] In women of reproductive age, this skinfold should be thicker than 1.8 mm.[22] Precise cutoffs have not been established for men, whose skin is normally thicker than women's, or for elderly patients, whose skin is normally thinner than younger patients.[25]

The striae of Cushing's syndrome are wide (>1 cm) and are colored deep red or purple, in contrast to the thinner and paler pink or white striae that commonly occur in any individual after rapid weight gain.[8,26] Striae are usually found on the lower abdomen, but may occur on the buttocks, hips, lower back, upper thighs, and arms. In one of Cushing's original patients, wide striae extended from the lower abdomen to the axillae.[6] Pathologically, striae are dermal scars, with collagen fibers all aligned in the direction of stress, covered by an abnormally thin epidermis.[27] The pathogenesis of striae is not understood, but they may represent actual rupture of the weakened connective tissue of the skin, under tension from central obesity, which leaves a thin translucent window to the red and purple colored dermal blood vessels. Striae are more common in younger patients with Cushing's syndrome than older patients.[9,26]

Plethora is an abnormal diffuse purple or reddish color of the face.[8] Hirsutism and acne occur because of increased adrenal androgens.[1,26,28] Ecchymoses probably appear because the blood vessels, lacking connective tissue support and protection, are more easily traumatized.

The severity of striae, acne, and hirsutism correlate poorly with cortisol levels, indicating that other factors—temporal, biochemical, or genetic—play a role in these physical signs.[26]

D. Proximal weakness. Painless proximal weakness of the legs is common and prominent in Cushing's syndrome, especially elderly patients.[9,29-31] Because the weakness is a true myopathy, patients lack fasciculations, sensory, or reflex abnormalities.[29-31] Chapter 54 discusses how to assess proximal muscle strength.

E. Depression. Patients with Cushing's syndrome may have crying episodes, insomnia, impaired concentration, difficulty with memory, and suicide attempts.[12,32] The severity of depression correlates with the cortisol level,[32] and unless the depression antedates the endocrine symptoms by years, it usually improves dramatically after treatment.[12]

F. Pseudocushing's syndrome. Several disorders, including chronic alcoholism, depression, and HIV infection, may mimic the physical findings and biochemical findings of Cushing's syndrome and are referred to as "pseudocushing's syndrome." Patients with chronic alcoholism may develop the physical findings or the biochemical abnormalities, or both, probably because of overproduction of ACTH by the hypothalamic-pituitary axis, an abnormality that resolves after several weeks of abstinence.[33-36] Depressed patients may have the biochemical abnormalities of Cushing's syndrome, but they usually lack the physical findings.[37,38] Patients with HIV infection who are treated with protease inhibitors may develop some of the physical findings (especially the buffalo hump and truncal obesity) but rarely the biochemical abnormalities.[39-44]

III. CLINICAL SIGNIFICANCE

A. Diagnostic accuracy of finding.
Table 12-2 presents the diagnostic accuracy of individual physical signs for Cushing's syndrome, as applied to 247 patients with suspected Cushing's syndrome.[8,13,14,22] According to these studies, the findings arguing the most *for* Cushing's syndrome are thin skinfold (LR = 115.6), ecchymoses (LR = 4.5), central obesity (LR = 3.0), and plethora (LR = 2.7). (The astronomical LR for thin skinfold thickness (LR = 115.6) applies only to young women with suspected disease because of hirsutism and menstrual irregularity.) The findings arguing the most *against* the diagnosis of Cushing's syndrome are the presence of generalized obesity (LR = 0.1), absence of moon facies (LR = 0.1), the absence of central obesity (LR = 0.2), and the presence of normal skinfold thickness (LR = 0.2).

In these same studies, one of the most powerful predictors of Cushing's syndrome is clinically apparent osteoporosis (sensitivity of 61% to 63%, specificity of 94% to 97%, positive LR = 17.6, and negative LR = 0.4).[8,13] Although osteoporosis was identified radiographically in these studies, it is often apparent at the bedside because of vertebral fractures, kyphosis, and loss of height. Presumably, these bedside findings also would accurately identify patients with Cushing's syndrome.

TABLE 12-2 Cushing's syndrome*

Finding (ref)†	Sensitivity (%)	Specificity (%)	Positive LR	Negative LR
Vital Signs				
Hypertension[8,13]	25-38	83-94	2.3	0.8
Body Habitus				
Moon facies[13]	98	41	1.6	0.1
Central obesity[8,13,14]	72-90	62-97	3.0	0.2
Generalized obesity[8]	4	38	0.1	2.5
Skin Findings				
Thin skinfold[22]	78	99	115.6	0.2
Plethora[8]	83	69	2.7	0.3

Hirsutism, in women[8,13]	50-76	56-71	1.7	0.7
Ecchymoses[8,13]	54-71	69-94	4.5	0.5
Red or blue striae[8,13]	46-52	63-78	1.9	0.7
Acne[8]	52	76	2.2	0.6
Extremity Findings				
Proximal muscle weakness[8,13]	62-63	69-93	NS	0.4
Edema[8,13]	38-57	56-83	1.8	0.7

NS, Not significant.

*Diagnostic standard: For Cushing's syndrome, elevated daily cortisol or corticosteroid metabolites, or both, with loss of circadian rhythm of serum cortisol levels and with abnormal dexamethasone suppression tests.

†Definition of findings: For hypertension, diastolic blood pressure above 105 mm Hg; for central obesity, central obesity index exceeds 1[14] or subjective appearance of central obesity sparing the extremities[8,13]; for thin skinfold, skinfold thickness on back of hand <1.8 mm (women of reproductive age only).[22]

B. Etiology of Cushing's syndrome and bedside findings. Patients who take exogenous corticosteroids have the same frequency of central obesity, moon facies, and bruising as patients with endogenous Cushing's, but a significantly lower incidence of hypertension, hirsutism, acne, striae, and buffalo humps.[2]

Patients with the ectopic ACTH syndrome from small cell carcinoma are more often male, have Cushing's syndrome of rapid onset (over months instead of years), and present with prominent weight loss, myopathy, hyperpigmentation, and edema.[4,37,38,45,46] The irregular hepatomegaly of metastatic disease also may suggest this diagnosis.[46] In one study of patients with ACTH-dependent Cushing's syndrome, two findings strongly argued for the ectopic ACTH syndrome and against Cushing's disease: male gender (positive LR = 13.0) and symptom duration less than 18 months (positive LR = 15.0).[46]

Hirsutism and acne may occur in any woman with endogenous Cushing's syndrome, but the presence of virilization (i.e., male pattern baldness, deep voice, male musculature, clitoromegaly) argues strongly for adrenocortical carcinoma.[47-49]

REFERENCES

1. Yanovski JA and Cutler GB, Jr. Glucocorticoid action and the clinical features of Cushing's syndrome, *Endocrinol Metab Clin North Am* 23:487-509, 1994.
2. Liou TC, Lam HC, and Ho LT. Cushing's syndrome: analysis of 188 cases, *J Formosan Med Assoc* 88:886-893, 1989.
3. Invitti C and others. Diagnosis and management of Cushing's syndrome: results of an Italian multicentre study. Study Group of the Italian Society of Endocrinology on the Pathophysiology of the Hypothalamic-Pituitary-Adrenal Axis, *J Clin Endocrinol Metab* 84:440-448, 1999.

4. Newell-Price J and others. The diagnosis and differential diagnosis of Cushing's syndrome and pseudo-Cushing's states, *Endocr Rev* 19:647-672, 1998.

5. Ross EJ and Linch DC. Cushing's syndrome—killing disease: discriminatory value of signs and symptoms aiding early diagnosis, *Lancet* 2:646-649, 1982.

6. Cushing H. The basophil adenomas of the pituitary body and their clinical manifestations (pituitary basophilism), *Bull Johns Hopkins Hosp* 50:137-195, 1932.

7. Freyberg RH and others. Problems of prolonged cortisone treatment for rheumatoid arthritis: further investigation, *JAMA* 147:1538-1543, 1951.

8. Nugent CA and others. Probability theory in the diagnosis of Cushing's syndrome, *J Clin Endocrinol Metab* 24:621-630, 1964.

9. Urbanic RC and George JM. Cushing's disease—18 years' experience, *Medicine (Baltimore)*, 60:14-24, 1981.

10. Plotz CM, Knowlton AI, and Ragan C. The natural history of Cushing's syndrome, *Am J Med* 13:597-614, 1952.

11. Soffer LJ, Iannoccone A, and Gabrilove JL. Cushing's syndrome: a study of fifty patients, *Am J Med* 30:129-146, 1961.

12. Jeffcoate WJ and others. Psychiatric manifestations of Cushing's syndrome: response to lowering of plasma cortisol, *Q J Med* 48:465-472, 1979.

13. Streeten DHP and others. The diagnosis of hypercortisolism. Biochemical criteria differentiating patients from lean and obese normal subjects and from females on oral contraceptives, *J Clin Endocrinol* 29:1191-1211, 1969.

14. Hiramatsu R, Yoshida K, and Sato T. A body measurement to evaluate the pattern of fat distribution in central obesity. A screening and monitoring technique for Cushing's syndrome, *JAMA* 250:3174-3178, 1983.

15. Rebuffe-Scrive M and others. Muscle and adipose tissue morphology and metabolism in Cushing's syndrome, *J Clin Endocrinol Metab* 67:1122-1128, 1988.

16. Gottlieb NL. Temporal fat pad sign during corticosteroid treatment, *Arch Intern Med* 140:1507-1508, 1980.

17. Lucena GE, Bennett WM, and Pierre RV. "Dewlap": a corticosteroid-induced episternal fatty tumor, *N Engl J Med* 275:834-835, 1966.

18. Orth DN. Cushing's syndrome, *N Engl J Med* 332:791-803, 1995.

19. Printen KJ and Blommers TJ. Morbid obesity in Cushing's syndrome: a nonentity? *Am J Surg* 134:579-580, 1977.

20. Mayo-Smith W and others. Body fat distribution measured with CT: correlations in healthy subjects, patients with anorexia nervosa, and patients with Cushing syndrome, *Radiology* 170:515-518, 1989.
21. Saruto T and others. Multiple factors contribute to the pathogenesis of hypertension in Cushing's syndrome, *J Clin Endocrinol Metab* 62:275-279, 1986.
22. Corenblum B and others. Bedside assessment of skin-fold thickness: a useful measurement for distinguishing Cushing's disease from other causes of hirsutism and oligomenorrhea, *Arch Intern Med* 154:777-781, 1994.
23. Ferguson JK and others. Skin thickness in patients with acromegaly and Cushing's syndrome and response to treatment, *Clin Endocrinol (Oxf)* 18:347-353, 1983.
24. Greenwood BM. Capillary resistance and skin-fold thickness in patients with rheumatoid arthritis. Effect of corticosteroid therapy, *Ann Rheum Dis* 25:272-277, 1966.
25. Wright AD and Joplin GF. Skin-fold thickness in normal subjects and in patients with acromegaly and Cushing's syndrome, *Acta Endocrinol (Copenh)* 60:705-711, 1969.
26. Stratakis CA and others. Skin manifestations of Cushing disease in children and adolescents before and after the resolution of hypercortisolemia, *Pediatr Dermatol* 15:253-258, 1998.
27. Arem AJ and Kischer CW. Analysis of striae, *Plastic Reconstruct Surg* 65:22-29, 1980.
28. Smals AGH, Koppenborg PWC, and Benraad TJ. Plasma testosterone profiles in Cushing's syndrome, *J Clin Endocrinol Metab* 45:240-245, 1977.
29. Mueller R and Kugelberg E. Myopathy in Cushing's syndrome, *J Neurol Neurosurg Psychiatry* 22:314-319, 1959.
30. Olafsson E and others. Myopathy of endogenous Cushing's syndrome: a review of the clinical and electromyographic features in 8 patients, *Muscle Nerve* 17:692-693, 1994.
31. Pleasure DE, Walsh GO, and Engel WK. Atrophy of skeletal muscle in patients with Cushing's syndrome, *Arch Neurol* 22:118-125, 1970.
32. Starkman MN and Schteingart DE. Neuropsychiatric manifestations of patients with Cushing's syndrome. Relationship to cortisol and adrenocorticotropic hormone levels, *Arch Intern Med* 141:215-219, 1981.
33. Elias AN and others. Pseudo-Cushing's syndrome: the role of alcohol, *J Clin Gastroenterol* 4:137-139, 1982.

34. Kirkman S and Nelson DH. Alcohol-induced pseudo-Cushing's disease: a study of prevalence with review of the literature, *Metabolism* 37:390-394, 1988.

35. Rees LH and others. Alcohol-induced pseudo-Cushing's syndrome, *Lancet* 1:726-728, 1977.

36. Veldman RG and Meinders AE. On the mechanism of alcohol-induced pseudo-Cushing's syndrome, *Endocrine Rev* 17:262-268, 1996.

37. Trainer PJ and Grossman A. The diagnosis and differential diagnosis of Cushing's syndrome, *Clin Endocrinol (Oxf)* 34:317-330, 1991.

38. Howlett TA, Rees LH, and Besser G. Cushing's syndrome, *Clin Endocrinol Metab* 14:911-945, 1985.

39. Lo JC and others "Buffalo hump" in men with HIV-1 infection, *Lancet* 351:867-870, 1998.

40. Miller KD and others. Visceral abdominal-fat accumulation associated with use of indinavir, *Lancet* 351:871-875, 1998.

41. Aboulafia DM and Bundow D. Images in clinical medicine. Buffalo hump in a patient with the acquired immunodeficiency syndrome, *N Engl J Med* 339:1297, 1998.

42. Carr A and Cooper DA. Lipodystrophy associated with an HIV-protease inhibitor, *N Engl J Med* 339:1296, 1998.

43. De Luca A and others. "Buffalo hump" in HIV-1 infection, *Lancet* 352:320, 1998.

44. Miller KK and others. Pseudo-Cushing's syndrome in human immunodeficiency virus-infected patients, *Clin Infect Dis* 27:68-72, 1998.

45. Sowers JR and Lippman HR. Cushing's syndrome due to ectopic ACTH production: cutaneous manifestations, *Cutis* 36:351-353, 1985.

46. Blunt SB and others. An evaluation of the distinction of ectopic and pituitary ACTH dependent Cushing's syndrome by clinical features, biochemical tests and radiological findings, *Q J Med* 77:1113-1133, 1990.

47. Bertagna C and Orth DN. Clinical and laboratory findings and results of therapy in 58 patients with adrenocortical tumors admitted to a single medical center (1951 to 1978), *Am J Med* 71:855-875, 1981.

48. Hutter AM and Kayhoe DE. Adrenal cortical carcinoma: clinical features of 138 patients, *Am J Med* 41:572-580, 1966.

49. Luton JP and others. Clinical features of adrenocortical carcinoma, prognostic factors, and the effect of mitotane therapy, *N Engl J Med* 322:1195-1201, 1990.

PART THREE

Vital Signs

CHAPTER 13

Pulse Rate and Contour

PULSE RATE

I. INTRODUCTION. Taking the patient's pulse is one of the oldest physical examination techniques, practiced as long ago as 3500 B.C. by ancient Egyptian physicians, who believed a weakening pulse indicated advancing disease.[1] The pulse was one of Galen's (ca. 129-200 A.D.) favorite subjects, occupying several treatises, in which he instructed clinicians to observe the pulse's speed, force, and duration.[2,3] The first accurate observations of heart rate in disease were by John Foyer (1649-1734), who published his clinical observations in 1707 based on his invention, the "pulse-watch."[3] The first clinicians to establish the significance of bradycardia were Adams and Stokes, who, between 1827 and 1846, pointed out that not all seizures and fainting represented disease of the brain but instead could occur because of the slow pulse of heart block.[1]

II. TECHNIQUE. Most clinicians determine the pulse rate by palpating the radial pulse or, less often, by listening to the heart tones with the stethoscope (i.e., "apical rate"). Counting the pulse for 30 seconds and doubling the result is more accurate than 15 seconds of observation.[4] In patients with fast heart rates, especially if the patient has atrial fibrillation, counting the apical rate is more accurate than counting the radial pulse, and 60 seconds of observation is more accurate than shorter periods.[5]

A difference between the radial pulse rate and apical rate (the apical rate always being greater) is called the "pulse deficit." A pulse deficit has traditionally been associated with atrial fibrillation, although it is a common finding with extrasystoles and all fast heart rates and by itself has little diagnostic significance.

III. THE FINDING. Many textbooks state that the normal sinus rate ranges from 60 to 100 beats/min, but more recent information indicates that the heart rate of 95% of healthy persons instead ranges from 50 beats/min to 95 beats/min.[6] **Bradycardia** is a pulse rate less than 50 beats/min; **tachycardia** is a rate greater than 100 beats/min.

IV. CLINICAL SIGNIFICANCE. An important role of any vital sign is to provide the clinician an early indication that trouble is afoot for the patient. Table 13-1 shows that the finding of tachycardia serves this role well. In a wide variety of clinical disorders, including myocardial infarction, pneumonia, septic shock, gallstone pancreatitis, and pontine hemorrhage, the finding of tachycardia (variably defined as a rate >90 beats/min to >110 beats/min) predicts both increased complications (LR = 6.8) and worse survival (LR = 1.6 to 25.4). In patients with myocardial infarction, the increased risk of adverse outcome is a continuum, being greater for patients with higher heart rates and persisting whether or not the patient has a low ejection fraction, takes β-blocker medications, or receives thrombolytic therapy.[7,12-14] In patients with septic shock, the relationship between tachycardia and mortality is independent of whether the patient receives vasopressor medications,[8] and in patients with pontine hemorrhage, tachycardia is a better predictor of mortality than some other neurologic findings, such as extensor posturing or the absence of withdrawal to pain.[11]

TABLE 13-1 Tachycardia

Finding (ref)	Sensitivity (%)	Specificity (%)	Positive LR	Negative LR
Heart Rate ≥90 beats/min				
Predicting hospital mortality in patients with myocardial infarction[7]	41	75	1.6	0.8
Heart Rate >95 beats/min				
Predicting hospital mortality in patients with septic shock[8]	97	53	2.0	0.1
Heart Rate >100 beats/min				
Predicting complications in patients with gallstone pancreatitis[9]	86	87	6.8	NS
Predicting mortality in patients with pneumonia[10]	45	78	2.1	NS
Heart Rate >110 beats/min				
Predicting hospital mortality in patients with pontine hemorrhage[11]	70	97	25.4	0.3

NS, Not significant.

Heart rates less than 50 beats/min or greater than 120 beats/min also may indicate heart rhythms other than sinus rhythm (e.g., complete heart block, atrial flutter), a subject discussed in Chapter 14.

ABNORMALITIES OF PULSE CONTOUR

I. PULSUS ALTERNANS

A. The finding. Pulsus alternans describes a regular pulse that has alternating strong and weak beats. The pulse must be absolutely regular to diagnose pulsus alternans and to distinguish it from the bigeminal pulse, which also has beats of alternating strength although the rhythm is irregular (see below).[15] Rarely, in patients with pulsus alternans, the weak pulse is too small to feel and only half the beats reach the radial artery ("total alternans").[16] Pulsus alternans is often accompanied by alternation of the intensity of heart sounds and murmurs ("auscultatory alternans").[15,17]

Traube first described pulsus alternans in 1872.[18]

B. Technique. Palpating the radial pulse or using the blood pressure cuff is the best way to detect pulsus alternans. When using the blood pressure cuff, the clinician should stop deflating the cuff at the first appearance of Korotkoff sounds and hold the cuff pressure just below systolic level for several beats. In patients with pulsus alternans, only the Korotkoff sounds belonging to the strong beats are heard. After further deflation of the cuff, cuff pressure eventually falls below the systolic pressure of the weaker beats, causing the cadence of Korotkoff sounds to suddenly double. The usual difference in systolic pressure between the strong and weak beats is only 15 to 20 mm Hg.[16]

Pulsus alternans often is most prominent in the several beats immediately after a pause in the heart rhythm. Typically, the pause is caused by a premature beat or the abrupt termination of a paroxysmal tachycardia.[19]

C. Clinical significance. In patients with normal heart rates, the finding of pulsus alternans indicates severe left ventricular dysfunction, caused by ischemic or valvular heart disease, long-standing hypertension, or idiopathic cardiomyopathy.[20-22] In one series of patients presenting for cardiac catheterization, investigators specifically looked for pulsus alternans after premature beats or 10 seconds of pacemaker-induced atrial tachycardia: compared with patients without the finding, those with pulsus alternans had worse ejection fractions and higher left ventricular filling pressures.[19]

In patients with rapid heart rates, pulsus alternans has less significance because even patients with normal hearts sometimes develop the finding during paroxysmal tachycardia.[23]

D. Pathogenesis. There has been considerable debate over decades regarding whether the primary cause of pulsus alternans is alternation of intrinsic contractility of the heart ("contractility argument") or alternation of filling of the ventricles ("hemodynamic argument").

One version of the hemodynamic argument is particularly compelling.[18,24] In patients with a *regular* pulse, the sum of the length of systole and the length of the subsequent diastole must be constant. If systole lengthens for any reason, the subsequent diastole must be shorter; if systole shortens for any reason, the subsequent diastole must be longer. In patients with left ventricular dysfunction, a sudden increase in ventricular filling (such as that induced by a postextrasystolic pause) causes the subsequent systole to produce a strong beat, although it takes longer than normal for the weakened heart to eject this blood (i.e., thus lengthening systole). By prolonging systole, the strong beat thus shortens the next diastole, which reduces filling of the heart and causes the next beat to be weaker. The weaker beat is ejected more quickly, shortening systole and causing the next diastole to be longer, thus perpetuating the alternating pulse.

Nonetheless, the hemodynamic argument does not explain how pulsus alternans ever gets started when there is no pause in the rhythm from an extrasystole or termination of a tachycardia. Most experts now believe that alternation of intrinsic contractility is the fundamental problem in pulsus alternans, because alternation can even be demonstrated in vitro in isolated muscles at constant length and resting tension.[21,22] Once alternans begins, however, the hemodynamic effects probably contribute to the alternating amplitude of the pulse.

II. PULSUS BISFERIENS

A. The finding. Pulsus bisferiens (Latin *bis,* meaning "twice" and Latin *ferire*, meaning "to beat") has two beats per cardiac cycle, both of which occur in systole (the first beat is called the "percussion wave"; the second, the "tidal wave").[15] Descriptions of pulsus bisferiens appear in the writings of Galen.[25]

B. Technique. Pulsus bisferiens is detected by palpating the brachial or carotid pulse with moderate compression of the vessel, or by using the blood pressure cuff.[26] When using the blood pressure cuff, the clinician hears a quick double tapping sound instead of the typical single sound (the clinician can mimic the double sound by saying "pa-da . . . pa-da" as fast as possible).[27]

C. Clinical significance. Pulsus bisferiens is a finding in patients with moderate-to-severe aortic regurgitation.[25,27,28] Pulsus bisferiens also occurs in patients with combined aortic stenosis and regurgitation, although the principal lesion is usually the regurgitation and the stenosis is mild.[25,28,29] There are exceptional cases of the finding in severe aortic stenosis.[26]

Pulsus bisferiens is sometimes described in patients with hypertrophic cardiomyopathy,[30] although almost always as a finding seen on direct intraarterial pressure tracings, not as a finding palpated at the bedside.[31]

D. Pathogenesis. The bisferiens pulse probably results from rapid ejection of blood into a flexible aorta. Because of the Venturi effect, the rapidly moving blood stream temporarily draws the walls of the aorta together, reducing flow momentarily and producing a notch with two systolic peaks in the waveform (in hypertrophic cardiomyopathy, the Venturi effect draws the anterior leaflet of the mitral valve and the interventricular septum together).[26,32] Although this hypothesis was proposed over 30 years ago, direct evidence supporting it is difficult to find.

III. PULSUS PARADOXUS

A. The finding. Pulsus paradoxus is an exaggerated decrease of systolic blood pressure during inspiration.[15,33] Although the usual definition is an inspiratory fall in systolic blood pressure exceeding 10 mm Hg, a better threshold may be 12 mm Hg, which is the upper 95% confidence interval for inspiratory decline in normal persons (i.e., the average inspiratory decrease in systolic pressure of normal persons is 6 ±3 mm Hg).[34] In patients with pulsus paradoxus, the systolic blood pressure and pulse pressure fall dramatically during inspiration, although the diastolic blood pressure changes little.[33,34]

In 1873, Kussmaul first described pulsus paradoxus in three patients with pericardial disease.[35,36] Kussmaul called the finding "paradoxical" because the pulse of his patients disappeared during inspiration even though the apical beat persisted throughout the respiratory cycle. The term is unfortunate, because the finding is nothing more than an exaggeration of normal physiologic change.

B. Technique. When checking for pulsus paradoxus, the clinician should have the patient breathe quietly and regularly, because even normal persons can induce a pulsus paradoxus with vigorous respirations. Pulsus paradoxus is detected by palpating the pulse or using the blood pressure cuff, although only paradoxical pulses exceeding 15 to 20 mm Hg are palpable.[37,38] For this reason, most clinicians use the blood pressure cuff, which has the added advantage of quantifying the finding.

The clinician begins to check the blood pressure in the usual way, but tightens the stopcock and prevents further deflation of the cuff at the first appearance of Korotkoff sounds. In patients with pulsus paradoxus, these initial phase 1 Korotkoff sounds repeatedly come and go, disappearing every inhalation and reappearing every exhalation. The clinician notes this pressure and then again slowly deflates the cuff, noting the cuff pressure when Korotkoff sounds persist throughout the respiratory cycle and the cuff pressure when they disappear (i.e., diastolic pressure). For example, in a patient who has only expiratory Korotkoff sounds between cuff pressures of 140 mm Hg and 120 mm Hg but has sounds throughout the respiratory cycle between pressures of 120 mm Hg and 80 mm Hg, the blood pressure is "140/80 mm Hg with a paradox of 20 mm Hg" (i.e., 20 = 140 − 120).

Pulsus paradoxus also has been noted in pulse oximetry tracings, appearing as respiratory movement of the tracing's baseline.[39] The height of this oscillation correlates with severity of pulsus paradoxus.[39]

C. Clinical significance. Pulsus paradoxus is a common finding in two conditions, cardiac tamponade and acute asthma.

1. **Cardiac tamponade.** Pulsus paradoxus >10 mm Hg occurs in 98% of patients with cardiac tamponade (i.e., a pericardial effusion under high pressure compressing the heart and compromising cardiac output; see Chapter 42). Because it is one of three key findings of tamponade—the others being elevated neck veins (sensitivity = 100%) and tachycardia (sensitivity = 81% to 100%)—the clinician should consider tamponade and check for pulsus paradoxus in any patient suspected of having pericardial disease, such as those with elevated neck veins, unexplained dyspnea, pericardial rub, or known pericardial effusion.[38]

   In patients with pericardial effusions, the finding of pulsus paradoxus >12 mm Hg discriminates patients with tamponade from those without tamponade with a sensitivity of 98%, specificity of 83%, positive LR of 5.9, and negative LR of 0.03.[a][34]

2. **Cardiac tamponade without pulsus paradoxus.** In only 2% of patients with tamponade, pulsus paradoxus is absent. These patients usually have 1 of 5 associated disorders: (1) atrial septal defect, (2) severe left ventricular dysfunction (especially those with uremic pericarditis),[40] (3) regional tamponade (tamponade affecting only one or two heart chambers, a complication of cardiac surgery),[41] (4) severe hypotension,[42-44] and (5) aortic regurgitation. Knowing that aortic regurgitation may eliminate pulsus paradoxus is especially significant, because

---

[a] Tamponade was defined in this study as improvement in cardiac output of 20% or more following pericardiocentesis (see Chapter 42).

patients with proximal (type A) aortic dissection and hemopericardium usually lack the paradoxical pulse despite significant tamponade, and the unaware clinician may exclude the possibility of tamponade to the harm of the patient.

Section D below explains why pulsus paradoxus is missing in each of these clinical disorders.

3. **Asthma.** Table 13-2 shows that, in patients with acute asthma, pulsus paradoxus exceeding 20 mm Hg almost certainly indicates severe bronchospasm. Nonetheless, pulsus paradoxus has limited clinical utility in patients with acute asthma for two reasons: (1) Up to half of patients with severe bronchospasm lack a pulsus paradoxus greater than 10 mm Hg (see Table 13-2). The sensitivity is low because the pulsus paradoxus of asthma is notably dependent on respiratory rate and effort, even when the degree of airway obstruction remains constant,[46,48] (2) The best measure of bronchospasm (and the criterion standard in studies listed in Table 13-2) is the peak expiratory flow rate. In a busy emergency department with an anxious and dyspneic patient, it is much more convenient to measure peak flow rates using handheld flow-meters than trying to interpret the coming and going of Korotkoff sounds.

In patients being mechanically ventilated, the amount of pulsus paradoxus, as reflected in the changing baseline of the pulse oximeter tracing, correlates with the degree of the patient's auto-PEEP (a measure of expiratory difficulty in ventilated patients).[39]

4. **Pulsus paradoxus in other conditions.** Pulsus paradoxus has been described as an uncommon finding in constrictive pericardi-

TABLE 13-2 Pulsus paradoxus predicting severe asthma*

Finding (ref)	Sensitivity (%)	Specificity (%)	Positive LR	Negative LR
Pulsus paradoxus >10 mm Hg[37,45-47]	52-68	69-92	2.7	0.5
Pulsus paradoxus >20 mm Hg[37,45,46]	19-39	92-100	8.2	0.8
Pulsus paradoxus >25 mm Hg[47]	16	99	22.6	0.8

*Diagnostic standard: For severe asthma, a FEV₁/FVC <50%,[37] FEV₁ <1.0 L,[45] peak flow <200 L/min,[47] and peak flow <30% predicted.[46] All patients in these studies had acute asthma.

FEV₁, Forced expiratory volume in 1 second; FVC, forced vital capacity.

tis, right ventricular infarction, and pulmonary embolus (see Chapter 42).[33]

5. Reversed pulsus paradoxus.[49] Reversed pulsus paradoxus, which is a systolic blood pressure that falls more than 10 mm Hg *during expiration*, occurs in three clinical disorders: (1) hypertrophic cardiomyopathy, (2) isorhythmic dissociation (i.e., inspiration accelerates the sinus rate, which temporarily positions the P waves before the QRS complex, thus coordinating the atrial and ventricular contractions and raising blood pressure; expiration slows the sinus rate, removes atrioventricular coordination, and lowers blood pressure), and (3) intermittent inspiratory positive-pressure breathing in the presence of left ventricular failure (this is a variation of the Valsalva square wave response in heart failure; see Chapter 43).

D. Pathogenesis

1. Cardiac tamponade. Tamponade develops when the pressure of fluid inside the pericardial space exceeds the diastolic filling pressure of the heart chambers. Once this occurs, the diastolic pressure in the heart chambers, reflected in the neck veins, becomes a measurement of the force acting to compress the heart. The four chambers, now smaller in size, begin to compete for space, and an increase in the size of one comes at the expense of the size of another. Inspiration increases filling to the right side of the heart and shifts the interventricular septum to the left and posteriorly, thus obliterating the left ventricular chamber and causing the cardiac output to fall. During expiration, filling of the right side of the heart is less, which increases left ventricular size, and both cardiac output and blood pressure increase.[33,41,50-53]

This explains why pulsus paradoxus is

absent in regional tamponade and tamponade associated with atrial septal defect, severe left ventricular dysfunction, and aortic insufficiency (see Section III-C-2 above). Inspiratory movement of the interventricular septum is prevented when the right ventricle does not fill more during inspiration (atrial septal defect; see Chapter 35), when the left ventricular pressures are very high (severe left ventricular dysfunction), or when the left ventricle fills from some source other than the left atrium (aortic insufficiency). Regional tamponade, by definition, compresses only 1 or 2 chambers, enough to impair cardiac output but too confined to cause the heart chambers to compete for space.

2. **Asthma.** The mechanism of pulsus paradoxus in asthma is complex and not fully understood. Difficulty breathing causes wide swings of intrapleural pressure, which then are transmitted directly to the aorta, contributing to the paradoxical pulse. This is not a complete explanation, however, because the amount of pulsus paradoxus in asthma often exceeds the pressure shifts of these respiratory excursions.[48] Furthermore, the pulse pressure also declines during inspiration of some asthma patients, which would not happen if transmission of pressures were the only cause. Other proposed mechanisms are an inspiratory reduction in pulmonary venous return to the left heart[33,48,54,55] and the compressive action of the hyperinflated chest, which, like tamponade, may reduce the size of the heart chambers and cause them to compete for space.[46,56]

IV. PULSUS PARVUS ET TARDUS

A. **The finding and technique.** Pulsus parvus et tardus describes a carotid pulse with a small volume ("pulsus parvus") that rises slowly and has a delayed systolic peak ("pulsus tardus").[15] It is routinely detected by palpation.

B. Clinical significance. Pulsus parvus et tardus is a finding of aortic stenosis. Of its two components, pulsus tardus is the better discriminator, detecting severe aortic stenosis with a sensitivity of 31% to 90%, specificity of 68% to 93%, positive LR of 3.7, and negative LR of 0.4 (see Chapter 39).[57-60]

C. Pathogenesis. Pulsus tardus depends on both obstruction to flow and the compliance of the vessel distal to the obstruction. The pulse waveform rises rapidly in stiff vessels, but slowly in more compliant vessels, which act like low-pass filters and remove the high frequency components of the waveform.[61] That the delay in the pulse reflects the severity of obstruction is a principle also used by Doppler sonography to gauge the severity of renal artery stenosis.[61]

V. DICROTIC PULSE

A. The finding and technique. The dicrotic pulse has two beats per cardiac cycle, but, unlike pulsus bisferiens, one peak is systolic and the other is diastolic.[15] It is usually detected by palpation of the carotid artery.[62]

The second wave of the dicrotic pulse is identical in timing to the small dicrotic wave of normal persons, obvious on arterial pressure tracings but never palpable. The dicrotic wave is felt to represent rebound of blood against the closed aortic valve.

B. Clinical significance. The dicrotic pulse occurs in younger patients with severe myocardial dysfunction, low stroke volumes, and high systemic resistance.[62,63] In patients who have had valvular replacement surgery, the finding of a persistent dicrotic pulse is associated with a poor prognosis.[63]

C. Pathogenesis. The dicrotic pulse has two components: (1) low stroke volume, which significantly lowers the height of the pulse's initial systolic wave, thus increasing the chances that the dicrotic wave will be palpable[64]; and (2) a resilient arterial system, which amplifies the rebound of the pulse waveform during diastole. The importance of a resilient arterial system may explain why the dicrotic pulse usually occurs in young patients with cardiomyopathy, who have more compliant vessels than older patients.[62,63]

The importance of a low stroke volume to the dicrotic pulse is illustrated by the observation that the dicrotic pulse sometimes disappears with beats that have larger stroke volumes, such as the beat after a premature beat, the stronger beats of pulsus alternans, and the expiratory beats of pulsus paradoxus.[62,64] Vasodilators often cause the dicrotic pulse to disappear, perhaps because of better forward flow and a greater stroke volume.[62]

VI. HYPERKINETIC PULSE

A. **The finding.** The hyperkinetic pulse strikes the examiner's fingers with unusually abrupt and strong force. Hyperkinetic pulses may have either a normal pulse pressure (e.g., severe mitral regurgitation, hypertrophic obstructive cardiomyopathy) or increased pulse pressure (e.g., aortic insufficiency and other disorders with abnormal aortic runoff).[15] In both severe mitral regurgitation and hypertrophic obstructive cardiomyopathy, the blood is ejected rapidly from the left ventricle but the integrity of the aortic valve preserves a normal arterial diastolic and pulse pressure.[65] In aortic regurgitation, the rapid ejection of blood is accompanied by an incompetent aortic valve, which causes a very low diastolic pressure in the aortic root, thus increasing the pulse pressure and causing the "Corrigan" or "water-hammer" pulse characteristic of this disorder (see Chapter 40).

B. Clinical significance. Chapter 40 discusses the significance of the water hammer pulse and large pulse pressure of aortic regurgitation.

In patients with mitral stenosis, the pulse is characteristically normal or diminished. If the clinician instead finds a hyperkinetic pulse in these patients, the probability is high that additional valvular disease is present, such as significant mitral regurgitation (sensitivity 71%, specificity 95%, positive LR = 14.2, negative LR = 0.3).[66]

REFERENCES

1. Schechter DC, Lillehei CW, and Soffer A. History of sphygmology and of heart block. *Dis Chest* 55:535-579, 1969.
2. Galen. On the pulse. In: Clendening L, editor. *Source book of medical history,* New York, 1960, Dover.
3. Geddes LA. Perspectives in physiological monitoring, *Med Instrument* 10:91-97, 1976.
4. Hollerbach AD and Sneed NV. Accuracy of radial pulse assessment by length of counting interval, *Heart Lung* 19:258-264, 1990.
5. Sneed NV and Hollerbach AD. Accuracy of heart rate assessment in atrial fibrillation, *Heart Lung* 21:427-433, 1992.
6. Spodick DH. Normal sinus heart rate: appropriate rate thresholds for sinus tachycardia and bradycardia, *South Med J* 89:666-667, 1996.
7. Disegni E and others. The predictive value of admission heart rate on mortality in patients with acute myocardial infarction, *J Clin Epidemiol* 48:1197-1205, 1995.
8. Parker MM and others. Serial cardiovascular variables in survivors and nonsurvivors of human septic shock: heart rate as an early predictor of prognosis, *Crit Care Med* 15:923-929, 1987.
9. Arnell TD and others. Admission factors can predict the need for ICU monitoring in gallstone pancreatitis, *Am Surg* 62:815-819, 1996.
10. Starczewski AR and others. Clinical prognostic indices of fatality in elderly patients admitted to hospital with acute pneumonia, *Age Ageing* 17:181-186, 1988.

11. Wijdicks EFM and St. Louis E. Clinical profiles predictive of outcome in pontine hemorrhage, *Neurology* 49:1342-1346, 1997.

12. Hjalmarson A and others. Influence of heart rate on mortality after acute myocardial infarction, *Am J Cardiol* 65: 547-553, 1990.

13. Hathaway WR and others. Prognostic significance of the initial electrocardiogram in patients with acute myocardial infarction, *JAMA* 279:387-391, 1998.

14. Zuanetti G and others. Relevance of heart rate as a prognostic factor in patients with acute myocardial infarction: Insights from the GISSI-2 study, *Eur Heart J* 19(suppl F):F19-F26, 1998.

15. Feinstein AR and others. Glossary of cardiologic terms related to physical diagnosis: part IV. Arterial pulses, *Am J Card* 1971;27:708-709, 1971.

16. Liu CK, Luisada AA. Halving of the pulse due to severe alternans (pulsus bisectus), *Am Heart J* 50:927-932, 1955.

17. Tavel ME and Nasser WK. Murmur alternans in aortic stenosis, *Chest* 57:176-179, 1970.

18. Mitchell JH, Sarnoff SJ, and Sonnenblick EH. The dynamics of pulsus alternans: alternating end-diastolic fiber length as a causative factor, *J Clin Invest* 42:55-63, 1963.

19. Schaefer S and others. Clinical and hemodynamic characteristics of patients with inducible pulsus alternans, *Am Heart J* 115:1251-1257, 1988.

20. Swanton RH and others. An analysis of pulsus alternans in aortic stenosis, *Eur J Cardiol* 4:39-47, 1976.

21. Lab MJ and Seed WA. Pulsus alternans, *Cardiovasc Res* 27:1407-1412, 1993.

22. Surawicz B and Fisch C. Cardiac alternans: diverse mechanisms and clinical manifestations, *J Am Coll Cardiol* 20:483-499, 1992.

23. Saunders DE and Ord JW. The hemodynamic effects of paroxysmal supraventricular tachycardia in patients with the Wolff-Parkinson-White syndrome, *Am J Cardiol* 9:223-236, 1962.

24. Gleason WL and Braunwald E. Studies on Starling's law of the heart: relationships between left ventricular end-diastolic volume and stroke volume in man with observations on the mechanism of pulsus alternans, *Circulation* 25:841-848, 1962.

25. Fleming PR. The mechanism of the pulsus bisferiens, *Br Heart J* 19:519-524, 1957.

26. MacAlpin RN, and Kattus AA. Brachial-artery bruits in aortic-valve disease and hypertrophic subaortic stenosis, *N Engl J Med* 273:1012-1018, 1965.

27. Ciesielski J and Rodbard S. Doubling of the arterial sounds in patients with pulsus bisferiens, *JAMA* 175:475-477, 1961.

28. Ikram H, Nixon PGF, and Fox JA. The hemodynamic implications of the bisferiens pulse, *Br Heart J* 26:452-459, 1964.

29. Wood P. Aortic stenosis, *Am J Cardiol* 1:553-571, 1958.

30. Frank S and Braunwald E. Idiopathic hypertrophic subaortic stenosis: clinical analysis of 126 patients with emphasis on the natural history, *Circulation* 37:759-788, 1968.

31. Perloff JK. Clinical recognition of aortic stenosis: the physical signs and differential diagnosis of the various forms of obstruction to left ventricular outflow, *Prog Cardiovasc Dis* 10:323-352, 1968.

32. Constant J. *Bedside cardiology*, Boston, 1985, Little, Brown & Co.

33. Shabetai R. *The pericardium*, New York, 1981, Grune & Stratton.

34. Curtiss EI and others. Pulsus paradoxus: definition and relation to the severity of cardiac tamponade, *Am Heart J* 115:391-398, 1988.

35. Kussmaul A. Ueber schwielige Mediastino-Pericarditis und den paradoxen Puls, *Berl Klin Wochenschrift* 38:445-449, 1873.

36. Shapiro E and Salick AI. A clarification of the paradoxical pulse: Adolf Kussmaul's original description, *Am J Cardiol* 16:426-431, 1965.

37. Knowles GK and Clark TJH. Pulsus paradoxus as a valuable sign indicating severity of asthma, *Lancet* 2:1356-1359, 1973.

38. Fowler NO. Pulsus paradoxus, *Heart Dis Stroke* 3:68-69, 1994.

39. Hartert TV, Wheeler AP, and Sheller JR. Use of pulse oximetry to recognize severity of airflow obstruction in obstructive airway disease: correlation with pulsus paradoxus, *Chest* 115:475-481, 1999.

40. Reddy PS and others. Cardiac tamponade: hemodynamic observations in man, *Circulation* 58:265-272, 1978.

41. Shabetai R. Changing concepts of cardiac tamponade, *J Am Coll Cardiol* 12:194-195, 1988.

42. Antman EM and Cargill V. Low-pressure tamponade, *Ann Intern Med* 91:403-406, 1979.

43. Himelman RB and others. Inferior vena cava plethora with blunted respiratory response: A sensitive echocardiographic sign of cardiac tamponade, *J Am Coll Cardiol* 12:1470-1477, 1988.

44. Hayes SN, Freeman WK, and Gersh BJ. Low pressure cardiac tamponade: diagnosis facilitated by Doppler echocardiography, *Br Heart J* 63:136-140, 1990.

45. Carden DL and others. Vital signs including pulsus paradoxus in the assessment of acute bronchial asthma, *Ann Emerg Med* 12:80-83, 1983.

46. Shim C and Williams MH. Pulsus paradoxus in asthma, *Lancet* 1:530-531, 1978.

47. Pearson MG and others. Value of pulsus paradoxus in assessing acute severe asthma, *Br Med J* 307:659, 1993.

48. Martin J and others. Factors influencing pulsus paradoxus in asthma, *Chest* 80:543-549, 1981.

49. Massumi RA and others. Reversed pulsus paradoxus, *N Engl J Med* 289:1272-1275, 1973.

50. Savitt MA and others. Physiology of cardiac tamponade and paradoxical pulse in conscious dogs, *Am J Physiol* 265:H1996-H2008, 1993.

51. Settle HP and others. Echocardiographic study of cardiac tamponade, *Circulation* 56:951-959, 1977.

52. Yeh E. Varying ejection fractions of both ventricles in paradoxical pulses: demonstration by radionuclide study, *Chest* 74:687-689, 1978.

53. Santoro IH and others. Pulsus paradox: a definition revisited, *J Am Soc Echocardiogr* 4:409-412, 1991.

54. Squara P and others. Decreased paradoxic pulse from increased venous return in severe asthma, *Chest* 97:377-383, 1990.

55. Settle HP and others. Echocardiographic study of the paradoxical arterial pulse in chronic obstructive lung disease, *Circulation* 62:1297-1307, 1980.

56. Rebuck AS and Pengelly LD. Development of pulsus paradoxus in the presence of airways obstruction, *N Engl J Med* 288:66-69, 1973.

57. Aronow WS and Kronzon I. Prevalence and severity of valvular aortic stenosis determined by doppler echocardiography and its association with echocardiographic and electrocardiographic left ventricular hypertrophy and physical signs of aortic stenosis in elderly patients, *Am J Cardiol* 67:776-777, 1991.

58. Forssell G, Jonasson R, and Orinius E. Identifying severe aortic valvular stenosis by bedside examination, *Acta Med Scand* 218:397-400, 1985.

59. Hoagland PM and others. Value of noninvasive testing in adults with suspected aortic stenosis, *Am J Med* 80:1041-1050, 1986.

60. Aronow WS and Kronzon I. Correlation of prevalence and severity of valvular aortic stenosis determined by continuous-wave doppler echocardiography with physical signs of aortic stenosis in patients aged 62 to 100 years with aortic systolic ejection murmurs, *Am J Cardiol* 60:399-401, 1987.

61. Bude RO and others. Pulsus tardus: its cause and potential limitations in detection of arterial stenosis, *Radiology* 190:779-784, 1994.

62. Ewy GA, Rios JC, and Marcus FI. The dicrotic arterial pulse, *Circulation* 39:655-661, 1969.

63. Orchard RC and Craige E. Dicrotic pulse after open heart surgery, *Circulation* 62:1107-1114, 1980.

64. Smith D and Craige E. Mechanisms of the dicrotic pulse, *Br Heart J* 56:531-534, 1986.

65. Perloff JK. The physiologic mechanisms of cardiac and vascular physical signs, *J Am Coll Cardiol* 1:184-198, 1983.

66. Wood P. An appreciation of mitral stenosis: Part 1. Clinical features. Part 2. Investigations and results, *Br Med J* 1:1051-63, 1113-1124, 1954.

Abnormalities of Pulse Rhythm

I. **INTRODUCTION.** In the late nineteenth and early twentieth century, before the introduction of electrocardiography, clinicians could examine the patient's arterial pulse, heart tones, and jugular venous waveforms, and, from these observations alone, diagnose atrial and ventricular premature contractions, atrial flutter, atrial fibrillation, complete heart block, Mobitz 1 and 2 atrioventricular block, and sinoatrial block.[1-3] In fact, clinicians were familiar enough with the bedside findings of these arrhythmias that early textbooks of electrocardiography included tracings of the arterial and venous pulse to help explain the electrocardiogram (ECG).[4]

The bedside diagnosis of arrhythmias today is probably little more than an intellectual game, because all significant arrhythmias require electrocardiography for confirmation and monitoring. Nonetheless, bedside diagnosis of arrhythmias is still possible, using the principles discovered 100 years ago by Mackenzie, Wenckebach, and Lewis. These principles, based on extensive investigation and many polygraph recordings of the arterial and venous pulse,[1-4] allow diagnosis of simple arrhythmias when the electrocardiograph is not nearby.

II. TECHNIQUE. The first step in diagnosing arrhythmias is to determine the basic rhythm of the patient's radial pulse. Most arrhythmias can be classified into 1 of 5 basic abnormalities: (1) the pause, (2) regular bradycardia, (3) regular tachycardia, (4) irregular rhythm that varies with respiration, and (5) irregularly irregular (or "chaotic") rhythm.

The radial pulse may not correspond to the ventricular pulse (or "apical pulse"), as determined by auscultation of the heart tones or palpation of the cardiac impulse, because some ventricular contractions are too weak to propel blood to the radial artery. Although the clinician must compare the radial pulse with the ventricular pulse to diagnose arrhythmias, the difference in *rate* between the two by itself indicates no particular diagnosis.

After the basic rhythm of the radial pulse is identified, analysis of the jugular venous waveforms, heart tones, and response of the heart rhythm to vagal maneuvers may further distinguish the various causes.

III. THE FINDINGS AND THEIR CLINICAL SIGNIFICANCE

　A. The pause. The pause has two important causes, premature contractions (common) and heart block (uncommon).

　　1. Terminology. When the radial pulse consists of the regular repetition of two beats followed by a pause, the term "bigeminal pulse" or "bigeminal rhythm" is used. When there are three radial pulse beats between each pause, the appropriate term is "trigeminal" pulse or rhythm. The finding of several beats between each pause is usually called "group beating," and much longer periods of regular rhythm interrupted by the rare pause is sometimes referred to as "pulse intermissions." The basic mechanism for all of these rhythm disturbances is the same, only the frequency of premature beats or heart block differs among them.

Because the cadence of these rhythms becomes predictable after short periods of observation, the term "regularly irregular" is sometimes used. This term, however, inaccurately conveys to others what actually is going on, and it is best discarded.

2. **Basic mechanism of the pause.** The pause has three basic mechanisms, illustrated in Figure 14-1. The two most important questions that distinguish these mecha-

Premature beat opens aortic valve:

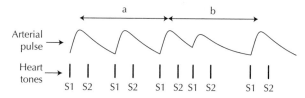

Premature beat fails to open aortic valve:

Heart block:

FIGURE 14-1 Mechanism of the pause. The radial pulse tracing and heart tones are presented, illustrating the three mechanisms for the pause: (1) premature contraction that opens the aortic valve, (2) premature contraction that fails to open the aortic valve, and (3) heart block. See text.

nisms are (1) Is there a premature radial pulse immediately preceding the pause? and (2) Do additional ventricular beats (identified by listening to the heart tones or palpating the apical pulse) occur during the pause?

a. Premature beat. Patients with premature contractions (the first two examples in Figure 14-1) have evidence of a premature ventricular beat during or immediately preceding the pause in the radial pulse. This early beat is always evident in the form of a palpable apical impulse or additional heart tones, although it may not be felt in the radial artery.

Some premature contractions are strong enough to open the aortic valve (first example in Figure 14-1). If so, the clinician will feel a quick beat in the radial pulse just preceding the pause, although the quick beat is usually not as strong as a normal sinus beat. When listening to the heart tones, the clinician will hear both the first and second heart sounds of the early beat, which produces the following characteristic cadence:

lub dup   lub dup   lub dup lub dup   lub dup

(In this and the following two examples, "*lub*" is the first heart sound and "*dup*" is the second sound; each rhythm begins with three normal beats, i.e., three "*lub dups*").

If the premature contraction is too weak to open the aortic valve (second example in Figure 14-1), the clinician palpating the pulse will not detect the quick beat but will only feel the pause. Listening to the heart, he or she will hear only the first sound of the premature beat (S2 is absent because the aortic valve never opens):

lub dup   lub dup   lub dup lub   lub dup

b. Heart block. Patients with heart block (third example in Figure 14-1), whether sinoatrial or atrioventricular, have no palpable apical impulse or extra heart tones during the pause. The cadence of heart tones contrasts with those of the premature beat:

lub dup   lub dup   lub dup   lub dup

3. **Bigeminal and trigeminal rhythms, and grouped beating.** Based on the mechanisms previously discussed, there are three causes of the bigeminal rhythm: (1) alternating normal and premature contractions (in this case, the second beat of the couplet is weaker); (2) premature contractions occurring every third beat, although the premature contraction is too weak to open the aortic valve; and (3) 3:2 heart block (atrioventricular or sinoatrial). In cases (2) and (3), both beats of the couplet are strong, but (2) has evidence of a ventricular contraction during the pause, whereas (3) does not.

The same analysis is used for trigeminal rhythms (i.e., possible causes are premature contractions after every 2 or 3 normal beats or 4:3 heart block) and grouped beating.

4. **Atrial vs. ventricular premature contractions.** Two helpful bedside findings distinguish atrial premature contractions from ventricular ones:

a. Compensatory pause. Beats that originate in the ventricle usually do not upset the underlying sinus rhythm, causing the beat immediately following the pause to fall exactly where the clinician anticipates it would. Tapping the foot during the normal regular rhythm helps determine this. In Figure 14-1, the distance "b" equals "a," meaning there is a "complete compensatory pause."

Beats that originate in the atria, in contrast, often reset the sinus node, causing the next beat to appear early. In Figure 14-1, "b" would be less than "a," and the clinician tapping the foot would find that the basic meter of rhythm changes.

This rule is much more helpful when the pause is not compensatory (i.e., "b" < "a," indicating the beat is atrial), because many atrial premature contractions also seem to have a complete compensatory pause at the bedside.

b. **Cannon A waves.** The appearance of a sudden prominent venous wave in the neck (cannon A wave) *during the pause* indicates that the premature beat was ventricular (see also Chapter 31). This occurs because the right atrium, still beating under the direction of the uninterrupted sinus impulses, contracts after the ventricular premature contraction has closed the tricuspid valve. Rarely, very early atrial premature beats also have a cannon A wave, but this wave precedes the first heart sound of the premature contraction, whereas cannon A waves from ventricular premature contractions always follow the first heart sound of the premature beat.

B. **Regular bradycardia** (rate <50 beats/min). There are three causes of regular bradycardia recognizable at the bedside: sinus bradycardia, complete heart block, and "halved pulse."

1. **Sinus bradycardia.** This arrhythmia resembles the normal rhythm in every way except for the abnormally slow rate: the venous waveforms in the neck are normal, the intensity of the first heart sound is the same with each beat, and there is no evidence of ventricular contractions between

radial pulsations (as determined by palpation of apical impulse or auscultation of the heart tones).

2. **Complete heart block.** In complete heart block, the atria and ventricles beat independently of each other (i.e., atrioventricular dissociation). Sometimes the atrial and ventricular contractions are contiguous and sometimes they are far apart. Atrioventricular dissociation causes two important bedside findings: changing intensity of the first heart sound and intermittent cannon A waves in the venous pulse.

   a. **Changing intensity of the first heart sound.** In complete heart block, the first heart sound of most beats is faint. Intermittently, however, the atrium contracts just before the ventricle contracts, which results in a first heart sound of booming intensity (named "bruit de canon" for its explosive quality; see Chapter 35 for pathophysiology of S1 intensity).[5]

   The finding of a changing first heart sound is only significant when the pulse is regular, because in irregular rhythms its intensity varies with the length of the previous diastole (i.e., long diastoles cause next first heart sound to be loud; short ones cause it to be soft). If the ventricular pulse is regular, however, a changing first heart sound (or intermittent "booming" of the first heart sound) indicates only one diagnosis, atrioventricular dissociation.

   b. **Intermittent appearance of cannon A waves in the venous pulse.** When the atrial contraction falls intermittently just after a ventricular contraction in complete heart block, the right atrium is contracting against a closed tricuspid valve, causing an abrupt systolic outward wave in the jugular venous pulse (i.e., cannon A wave; see also Chapter 31).

Cannon A waves appearing with every arterial pulse occur in many different arrhythmias. If the cannon A wave appears *intermittently*, however, in a patient whose ventricular pulse is regular, the only diagnosis is atrioventricular dissociation.

   c. Other evidence of atrioventricular dissociation. Other uncommon signs of atrioventricular dissociation are regular small A waves in the venous pulse; regular muffled fourth heart sounds at the apex; or, in patients with mitral stenosis, regular short murmurs from the atrium pushing blood across the stenotic valve. All of these findings represent regular atrial contractions that continue during the long ventricular diastoles.

  3. Halved pulse. "Halved pulse" refers to the finding of twice as many ventricular beats as radial pulse beats. This is almost always due to premature contractions, which appear every other beat but are too weak to open the aortic valve and reach the radial pulse. Rarely, pulsus alternans may be the cause ("total alternans"),[6] although in these patients the heart tones at the apex are regular, whereas in premature contractions they are bigeminal.

C. Regular tachycardia. The regular tachycardias that *sometimes* are recognizable at the bedside include sinus tachycardia, atrial flutter, paroxysmal supraventricular tachycardia, and ventricular tachycardia. The bedside observations that distinguish these arrhythmias are response to vagal maneuvers, signs of atrioventricular dissociation, and abnormalities of the neck veins. Even so, bedside examination is diagnostic in only the minority of patients with rapid rates, and the careful clinician always relies on electrocardiography for diagnosis.

1. **Vagal maneuvers.** The usual maneuvers are the Valsalva maneuver and carotid artery massage.

   a. **Technique.** Both maneuvers are performed when the patient is supine. To perform the Valsalva maneuver, the clinician asks the patient to bear down and strain against a closed glottis as if "having a bowel movement." Patients who have difficulty following this instruction sometimes respond better when asked to put the tip of their own thumb in their mouth and to pretend it is a balloon to blow up. In patients with supraventricular tachycardia, 15 seconds of straining is as effective as 30 seconds.[7] The maneuver increases vagal tone and has its maximal effect on tachycardias *after* the release of the Valsalva, not while the patient is straining.[7]

   In carotid artery massage, the clinician finds the bifurcation of one carotid artery, located just below the angle of the jaw, and massages or presses on it for 5 seconds.[7,8]

   The Valsalva maneuver is preferred for two reasons: (1) it tends to be more efficacious, terminating supraventricular tachycardia 20% to 50% of the time, compared with only a 10% efficacy with carotid massage,[7,9] and (2) in elderly patients with carotid artery disease, carotid artery massage risks causing strokes.[8]

   b. **Response of regular tachycardias to vagal maneuvers.**[8] Transient slowing of the pulse during a vagal maneuver indicates sinus tachycardia. **Abrupt termination** of the tachycardia indicates paroxysmal supraventricular tachycardia (this occurs with both nodal reentry tachycardias and reciprocating tachycardias using an accessory pathway). **Abrupt halving** of the rate may occur in atrial flutter. **No response** is unhelpful, being characteristic of ventricular tachycardia[10] but also occurring with every other regular tachycardia.[7,9]

2. **Atrioventricular dissociation.** Any finding of atrioventricular dissociation in patients with regular tachycardia indicates the rhythm is ventricular tachycardia. These findings include the *intermittent* appearance of cannon A waves in the neck veins, changing intensity of the first heart sound, and changing systolic blood pressure (usually detected with the blood pressure cuff).[11] In one study of patients with ventricular tachycardia, in which atrioventricular association or dissociation was determined by pacing (Table 14-1), the finding of a changing S1 argued strongly *for* atrioventricular dissociation (LR = 24.4) and the *absence* of intermittent cannon A waves argued convincingly *against* atrioventricular dissociation (LR = 0.1).

Even so, these LRs are somewhat misleading because some patients with ventricular tachycardia lack atrioventricular dissociation and instead have 1:1 retrograde conduction or atrial fibrillation.[10] Given the serious consequences of misdiagnosing this arrhythmia, an ECG should always be obtained.

3. **Flutter waves in the venous pulse.** In elderly patients with a ventricular pulse of 130 to 160 beats/min, the clinician should suspect atrial flutter with 2:1 conduction. In addition to performing vagal maneuvers, the clinician may see rapid, small undulations (with a rate about 300/min) in the venous

TABLE 14-1 Atrioventricular dissociation and ventricular tachycardia*

Finding (ref)†	Sensitivity (%)	Specificity (%)	Positive LR	Negative LR
Varying arterial pulse[12]	63	70	NS	NS
Intermittent cannon A waves, neck veins[12]	96	75	3.8	0.1
Changing intensity S1[12]	58	98	24.4	0.4

NS, Not significant.

*Diagnostic standards: For atrioventricular dissociation, ventricular-paced rhythm at a rate independent of the atrial rate.

† Definition of findings: For varying arterial pulse, varying amplitude of radial or carotid pulse by palpation.

pulse, which are called flutter waves (or f waves) and which correspond to the wave of the same name on the ECG.[13]

4. **Sensation of pounding in the neck.** In one study of 244 consecutive patients referred for electrophysiologic testing, all of whom had intermittent rapid palpitations, the history of feeling rapid and regular pounding in the neck during the palpitations discriminated atrioventricular nodal reentrant tachycardia from other causes of tachycardia, with a sensitivity of 92%, specificity of 100%, positive LR of 350.7, and negative LR of 0.1.[14] The pounding occurs because both the carotid pulsation and cannon A waves arrive in the neck simultaneously (atrial and ventricular pulsations practically coincide in these patients). Patients with reciprocating tachycardias using an accessory pathway, another common supraventricular tachycardia, lack these pounding sensations, because the atrial contraction is delayed until well after the ventricular contraction.

D. **Irregular rhythm that varies with respiration.** This rhythm is sinus arrhythmia, an especially common and prominent arrhythmia of younger patients. The pulse characteristically quickens during inspiration and slows during exhalation.[15] The slowing during expiration is sometimes so conspicuous it mimics the finding of a pause.

E. **Irregularly irregular rhythm ("chaotic" rhythm).** This term describes a cadence of ventricular and radial beats that is completely irregular and unpredictable. The diagnosis is usually atrial fibrillation. Frequent premature contractions may sometimes seem chaotic at the bedside, but two findings distinguish this rhythm from atrial fibrillation: **(1) Venous pulse.** In atrial fibrillation, the venous pulse is very simple and consists of only one wave per cardiac cycle (i.e., there is no A wave and the X' descent is diminished; see Chapter 31). In frequent premature contractions, in contrast, the venous pulse is complex and consists of intermittent cannon A waves superimposed on two venous movements per cardiac cycle. **(2) Rhythm of ventricular pulse.** In atrial fibrillation, the interval between ventricular beats is random, and it is quite common to have one pause followed by an even longer pause. In frequent premature contractions, this is impossible because the pause must be followed by another quick beat or the normal sinus interval. This difference in rhythm, which again focuses on the ventricular rhythm at the apex, not the radial pulse, is quite conspicuous once the clinician is aware of it.

REFERENCES

1. Mackenzie J. *The study of the pulse: arterial, venous, and hepatic and of the movements of the heart* (facsimile by the Classics of Cardiology Library), Edinburgh, 1902, Young J. Pentland.

2. Wenckebach KF. *Arrhythmia of the heart: a physiological and clinical study* (facsimile by the Classics of Cardiology Library), Edinburgh, 1904 William Green & Sons.

3. Lewis T. *Clinical disorders of the heart beat,* ed 4, London, 1918, Shaw & Sons.

4. Lewis T. The mechanism and graphic registration of the heart beat, ed 3, London, 1925, Shaw & Sons Ltd.

5. Burggraf GW and Craige E. The first heart sound in complete heart block: phono-echocardiographic correlations, *Circulation* 50:17-24, 1974.

6. Liu CK and Luisada AA. Halving of the pulse due to severe alternans (pulsus bisectus), *Am Heart J,* 50:927-932, 1955.

7. Mehta D and others. Relative efficacy of various physical manoeuvres in the termination of junctional tachycardia, *Lancet* 1:1181-1185, 1988.

8. Schweitzer P and Teichholz LE. Carotid sinus massage: its diagnostic and therapeutic value in arrhythmias, *Am J Med* 78:645-654, 1985.

9. Lim SH and others. Comparison of treatment of supraventricular tachycardia by Valsalva maneuver and carotid sinus massage, *Ann Emerg Med* 31:30-35, 1998.

10. Armbrust CA and Levine SA. Paroxysmal ventricular tachycardia: a study of one hundred and seven cases, *Circulation* 1:28-40, 1950.

11. Wilson WS, Judge RD, and Siegel JH. A simple diagnostic sign in ventricular tachycardia, *N Engl J Med* 270:446-448, 1964.

12. Garratt CJ and others. Value of physical signs in the diagnosis of ventricular tachycardia, *Circulation* 90:3103-3107, 1994.

13. Hartman H. The jugular venous tracing, *Am Heart J* 59:698-717, 1960.

14. Gursoy S and others. The hemodynamic mechanism of pounding in the neck in atrioventricular nodal reentrant tachycardia, *N Engl J Med* 327:772-774, 1992.

15. van Ravenswaaij-Arts CMA and others. Heart rate variability, *Ann Intern Med* 118:436-447, 1993.

CHAPTER 15

Blood Pressure

I. **INTRODUCTION.** Systolic blood pressure is the maximal pressure within the artery during ventricular systole, **diastolic blood pressure** is the lowest pressure in the vessel just before the next systole, and **pulse pressure** is the difference between them. Pulse pressure may be normal, abnormally small ("narrow"), or abnormally large ("wide"; see Section III-F below). The mean arterial pressure can be estimated by (S + 2D)/3, where S is systolic blood pressure and D is diastolic blood pressure.[1]

The first person to measure blood pressure was Stephen Hales, an English clergyman of creative genius, who in 1708 directly connected the left crural artery of a horse to a nine-foot tall glass manometer using brass tubes and a trachea of goose.[2,3] Vierordt of Germany introduced the indirect method of measuring blood pressure in 1855, based on the principle that blood pressure is equal to the amount of external pressure necessary to obliterate the distal pulse. Indirect measurements required cumbersome mechanical devices and were not widely accepted until 1896, when the Italian Riva-Rocci invented the blood pressure cuff.[2,3]

Blood pressure was the last of the four traditional vital signs to be routinely monitored in hospitalized patients. In 1901, after Harvey Cushing first brought the blood pressure cuff to America and encouraged its use in neurosurgical patients, most clinicians resisted using it because they believed palpation of pulse revealed much more information, characterized by the pulse's "fullness," "tension," "rate," "rhythm," "size," "force," and "duration."[4,5] Two events were responsible for clinicians eventually accepting the blood pressure cuff: (1) Korotkoff described his sounds in 1905, which allowed clinicians to easily measure systolic and diastolic blood pressure; and (2) Janeway published his book *Clinical Study of Blood Pressure* in 1907, which proved that monitoring blood pressure was clinically useful (Janeway showed, for example, that the first sign of intestinal perforation or hemorrhage in typhoid fever was a falling blood pressure).[6] By the first World War, blood pressure was routinely recorded by most clinicians along with the patient's pulse, respirations, and temperature.[5,7,8]

II. TECHNIQUE

A. **Recommended method of measuring blood pressure.**[9,10] Published recommendations for measuring blood pressure are based on the consensus opinion of expert committees who have reviewed all available scientific evidence. These recommendations, however, are designed to avoid misdiagnosis of hypertension and may not be as relevant to clinicians using the blood pressure cuff to diagnose other abnormalities, such as hypotension or abnormalities of pulse contour (see below).

   The important elements of the correct technique are as follows: (1) The patient should sit in a chair with his or her back supported and should rest for at least 5 minutes before the blood pressure is measured. (2) The patient's arm should be at heart level. (3) The length of the blood pressure cuff's bladder should encircle at least 80% of the arm's circumference. (4) The clinician should inflate the cuff to a pressure 20 to 30 mm Hg above systolic pressure, as first identified by palpation of the distal pulse (i.e., the pulse disappears when cuff pressure exceeds systolic pressure). (5) The pressure in the cuff should be released at a rate of 2 mm Hg per second. (6) The clinician should obtain at least 2 readings separated by at least 30 seconds and average them; if these differ by more than 5 mm Hg, additional readings are necessary. (7) The readings should be rounded off to the nearest 2 mm Hg.

These recommendations also state that the bell of the stethoscope should be used, because Korotkoff sounds contain primarily low-frequency sound, although this technique is often inconvenient and one study showed that measurements made by the bell and diaphragm were the same.[11]

In some clinical scenarios, described in Section III below, additional measurements are necessary, including those of the opposite arm or the legs, or measurements taken with the patient in different positions.

B. Korotkoff sounds

1. Definition of systolic and diastolic blood pressure.
As the cuff is slowly deflated from a point above systolic pressure, the first appearance of sound (Korotkoff phase 1) indicates systolic blood pressure.[a] Clinicians have debated for decades whether the muffling of sound (Korotkoff phase 4) or disappearance of sound (Korotkoff phase 5) better indicates diastolic blood pressure, although

---

[a] There are five Korotkoff phases, numbered in order as they appear during deflation of the cuff. The initial tapping sound at systolic blood pressure is phase 1, a swishing murmur is phase 2, the reappearance of a softer tapping sound is phase 3, the disappearance of the tapping and appearance of a much softer murmur ("muffling") is phase 4, and the disappearance of all sound is phase 5.[2] Korotkoff described only four of these sounds (phases 1, 2, 3, and 5). Ettinger added the muffling point (phase 4) in 1907.[7,10,12]

now all experts favor using phase 5 for the following reasons: (1) in most studies phase 5 sounds correlate better with intra-arterial measurements of diastolic blood pressure[13,14]; (2) many persons lack phase 4 sounds[13,15]; (3) interobserver agreement is better for phase 5 sounds than phase 4 sounds[13,15]; and, most importantly, (4) long-term studies showing that hypertension increases the risk of cardiovascular events and that treatment reduces this risk have used phase 5 sounds as the definition of diastolic blood pressure.[16-18]

2. **Pathogenesis.** Korotkoff sounds are produced underneath the *distal* half of the blood pressure cuff.[19] The sounds occur with cuff pressures between the systolic and diastolic blood pressure, because the underlying artery is collapsing completely and then re-opening with each heart beat. The artery collapses because cuff pressure exceeds diastolic pressure; it opens again with each beat because cuff pressure is less than systolic pressure. The sound represents the sudden deceleration of the rapidly opening arterial walls, which causes a snapping or tapping sound just like the sail of a boat snaps when it suddenly tenses after tacking in the wind or a handkerchief snaps when its ends are suddenly drawn taut.[19-23] Once cuff pressure falls below the diastolic blood pressure, the sound disappears because the vessel wall no longer collapses but instead gently ebbs and expands with each beat, being held open by diastolic pressure.

The genesis of the Korotkoff sounds, therefore, is similar to the genesis of other snapping or tapping sounds produced by the sudden deceleration of other biologic membranes, such as the normal first and second heart sounds or the femoral pistol shot sounds of aortic regurgitation (see Chapters 35 and 40).

C. **Measurement using palpation.** Even before the discovery of Korotkoff sounds, clinicians used the blood pressure cuff to measure both systolic and diastolic blood pressure.[6] Systolic blood pressure was simply the amount of cuff pressure necessary to obliterate the pulse. Clinicians still use this technique to measure the pressure of patients with hypotension, when Korotkoff sounds are faint, or to determine whether the patient has an auscultatory gap (see below).

To identify diastolic pressure, clinicians can use 1 of 2 methods. In the first method the clinician applies light pressure to palpate the brachial artery just below the blood pressure cuff. As the cuff is deflated, the first appearance of a pulse indicates systolic blood pressure. As the cuff pressure falls more and approaches diastolic pressure, the pulsatile forces distending the artery distal to the cuff progressively grow, eventually causing a sudden shock to strike the clinician's fingers as the artery abruptly opens and then completely collapses with each beat (this abrupt tapping sensation is similar to the "water-hammer pulse" of aortic regurgitation).[20] At the moment the cuff pressure falls below diastolic blood pressure, the shocking sensations disappear, being replaced by a much gentler pulse because the underlying artery no longer collapses completely between beats. The cuff pressure at this "lower limit of maximal pulsation" indicates the diastolic blood pressure.[6]

A second method requires a rigid and tightly applied cuff, so that the arterial pulsations under the cuff are actually transmitted to the manometer. As the cuff pressure decreases, the mercury column of a mercury manometer or the indicator needle of an aneroid manometer starts to bob with increasing amplitude, until the bobbing suddenly disappears at the moment cuff pressure falls below diastolic pressure.[6] Many patients with tightly applied cuffs also experience a similar pounding sensation in their arm near the diastolic pressure, which abruptly disappears the moment cuff pressure falls below diastolic blood pressure.

Measurements of systolic and diastolic blood pressure by palpation differ from readings by auscultation by only 6 to 8 mm Hg or less.[24,25]

D. Postural vital signs.[26] When obtaining postural vital signs (i.e., comparison of measurements when the patient is supine with those when the patient is upright), clinicians should wait 2 minutes before measuring the supine vital signs and 1 minute after standing before measuring the upright vital signs. These recommendations are based on the following observations: (1) Shorter periods of supine rest significantly reduce the sensitivity of postural vital signs for detecting blood loss, and (2) After normal persons stand, the pulse change stabilizes after 45 to 60 seconds and the blood pressure stabilizes after 1 to 2 minutes. Counting the heart rate first, beginning at 1 minute, allows more time for the blood pressure to stabilize.

Supine vital signs should always be compared with standing vital signs, because sitting instead of standing significantly reduces the clinician's ability to detect postural changes after blood loss.[27,28]

E. Common errors. Biologic variation of blood pressure is common, and many studies show that blood pressure measurements vary with physical activity, smoking, caffeine ingestion, emotional state, temperature of the room, and season.[18,29,30] In addition, the blood pressure measurement may be inaccurate because of inappropriate technique, improper equipment, or other biases related to the observer.[10,30]

1. **Wrong cuff size.** In 1901, von Reckling-hausen discovered that Riva-Rocci's original blood pressure cuff, whose bladder was about the size of a bicycle tire, was too narrow and often overestimated the true blood pressure, especially in larger arms.[7,31,32] Subsequent investigations have shown that both the bladder width and length affect the measurement, although if the bladder encircles at least 80% of the arm's circumference, the effect of width is minimized.[14,31,33] The bladder of the standard cuff measures 12 × 23 cm and thus is appropriate only for arm circumferences up to 28 cm, which includes only 60% to 70% of the European adult population.[31]

   Cuffs that are too short overestimate blood pressure because they transmit cuff pressure inefficiently to the underlying soft tissues. Much higher cuff pressures are then necessary to cause collapse of the artery, leading the clinician to misdiagnose hypertension when it is not present.[33] This error is greater the farther the *center* of the bladder is positioned from the brachial artery.[14]

   The significance of the opposite error—underestimation of true blood pressure by using too large a cuff—is controversial, although most studies show that such an error is small. Table 15-1 presents the mean errors resulting from using cuffs too small or large. These data are based on measurements of blood pressure in the same individual with three cuffs of different sizes, assuming that the most accurate measurement is the one made with the smallest cuff encircling 80% of the arm. The greatest errors, according to these data, occur from using too small of a cuff; the risk of underestimating true pressure with too large a cuff is relatively small.

2. **Auscultatory gap.** Up to 20% of elderly patients with hypertension have an auscul-

TABLE 15-1　Blood pressure cuff size and error in measurement*

| Cuff Bladder Size | Arm Circumference | | |
	28 cm or Less	29 to 42 cm	43 cm or More
Regular (12 × 23 cm)	Accurate	Overestimates SBP by 4-8 mm Hg DBP by 3-6 mm Hg	Overestimates SBP by 16-17 mm Hg DBP by 10-11 mm Hg
Large (15 × 33 cm)	Underestimates SBP by 2-3 mm Hg DBP by 1-2 mm Hg	Accurate	Overestimates SBP by 5-7 mm Hg DBP by 2-4 mm Hg
Thigh (18 × 36 cm)	Underestimates SBP by 5-7 mm Hg DBP by 1-3 mm Hg	Underestimates SBP by 5-7 mm Hg DBP by 2-4 mm Hg	Accurate

DBP, Diastolic blood pressure reading; *SBP,* systolic blood pressure reading.

*"Overestimation" means that hypertension may be diagnosed in someone with normal blood pressure; "underestimation" means that hypertension may be overlooked in someone who actually has high blood pressure. See text for further discussion. Data from reference 34.

tatory gap, which means that the phase 1 Korotkoff sounds normally appear at systolic pressure but then disappear for varying lengths of time before they reappear above the diastolic pressure.[35] This "auscultatory gap" is important because inflation of the cuff only to the initial disappearance of sounds (i.e., auscultatory gap) significantly underestimates the true systolic blood pressure. Because the distal pulse persists during the auscultatory gap, however, clinicians can avoid this mistake by palpating the systolic pressure before using the stethoscope.

The cause of the auscultatory gap remains a mystery. Patients with auscultatory gaps have twice as much arterial atherosclerotic plaque as those without a gap, suggesting perhaps that the gap is somehow related to arterial stiffness.[35] Venous congestion also seems to promote auscultatory gaps, because slow cuff inflation (which increases venous congestion) sometimes makes auscultatory gaps appear and elevation of the arm before inflating the cuff makes them disappear.[32]

Krylov discovered the auscultatory gap in 1906, 1 year after Korotkoff's discovery.[12] In part, the discovery of the auscultatory gap was responsible for the initial reluctance of clinicians to adopt Korotkoff's method of indirect blood pressure measurement.[7]

3. **Stethoscope pressure too firm.** Excessive pressure with the stethoscope artificially lowers the diastolic reading, sometimes by 10 mm Hg or more, although the systolic reading is usually unaffected.[36] This error occurs because the stethoscope pressure then contributes to the collapse of the underlying artery (i.e., the total tissue pressure around the artery represents the sum of both cuff and stethoscope pressure). If the clinician applies 10 mm Hg of stethoscope pressure to

the arm of a patient whose intraarterial diastolic pressure is 80 mm Hg, the diastolic reading will be 70 mm Hg (i.e., Korotkoff sounds disappear at a tissue pressure of 80 mm Hg = 70 mm Hg cuff pressure, the basis for the reading, and 10 mm Hg of stethoscope pressure).

4. **Inappropriate level of the arm.** The recommended position of the patient's elbow is the "level of the heart," which is usually regarded to be the fourth intercostal space at the sternum. If the patient's arm is instead 6 to 7 cm higher (e.g., level of the sternomanubrial junction), both the systolic and diastolic readings will be about 5 mm Hg lower. If the arm is 7 to 8 cm lower (e.g., level of the xiphosternal junction), the pressures will be about 6 mm Hg higher.[37]

   These errors are completely explained by the hydrostatic effect. When the arm is at the lower position, for example, the measured pressure is the sum of the blood pressure in the artery plus the weight of a column of blood 8 cm high (i.e., 8 cm blood = (8 ÷ 13.6) × 1.06 = 0.6 cm or 6 mm Hg; 13.6 = density of mercury; 1.06 = density of blood).

5. **Terminal digit preference.**[29,30] Clinicians often tend to round off blood pressure readings to the nearest "0," "5," or other preferred number, a bias called terminal digit preference. Clinical studies minimize this and other observer biases by using a random zero sphygmomanometer, which blinds the clinician to the true reading.[18,38]

III. THE FINDINGS AND THEIR CLINICAL SIGNIFICANCE
A. Hypertension
1. **Essential hypertension.** Essential hypertension is defined as three or more blood pressure readings taken over three visits

separated by weeks whose average exceeds 140/90 (i.e., systolic blood pressure of 140 mm Hg and diastolic blood pressure of 90 mm Hg).[9] Detecting essential hypertension is the reason blood pressure should be measured in every person, even when asymptomatic, because the disorder is common and treatable and because treatment reduces cardiovascular morbidity and overall mortality.

2. **Pseudohypertension and Osler's sign.** "Pseudohypertension" describes the finding of elevated indirect measurements in persons who have normal intraarterial pressure. The traditional explanation for pseudohypertension is that the artery under the cuff is so stiff and calcified it remains open long after the cuff pressure exceeds systolic blood pressure, continuing to produce Korotkoff sounds.

The diagnosis of pseudohypertension requires direct cannulation of the patient's artery, which is of course inappropriate and impractical during daily routine. A single study from 1985 proposed that a simple physical finding, Osler's sign, accurately identifies patients with pseudohypertension.[39] This sign is positive if the patient's radial or brachial artery distal to the cuff remains palpable after inflation of the cuff above systolic blood pressure.

Osler's sign, however, has limited clinical value. It occurs commonly in elderly individuals, whether or not they have hypertension (11% over the age of 75 years and 44% over 85 years have a positive Osler's sign).[40] Other investigators have shown that almost all patients with Osler's sign do not have pseudohypertension, but instead actually have direct measurements that exceed the indirect ones.[41,42]

Although pseudohypertension remains an important problem in blood pressure measurements of the legs, especially in diabetic patients with intermittent claudication (see Chapter 48), undue emphasis on pseudohypertension in the brachial artery misses the point that all clinical studies showing that treatment of essential hypertension is beneficial used the blood pressure cuff and indirect measurements, not intraarterial measurements.

B. Hypotension. In patients with acute illness, hypotension is ominous. It predicts death in patients hospitalized in the intensive care unit (LR = 4.0, Table 15-2), in patients with pneumonia (LR = 10.0) or myocardial infarction (LR = 15.5), and presumably in many other acute disorders as well. The APACHE scoring system, which predicts the risk of hospital mortality among patients in the intensive care unit, assigns more points (and thus a higher risk) to severe hypotension than to any other physiologic variable.[48] In patients with myocardial infarction, a systolic blood pressure less than 80 mm Hg also predicts a much higher incidence of congestive heart failure, ventricular tachycardia and fibrillation, and complete heart block.[47]

C. Differences in pressure between the arms. The average difference in systolic blood pressure between the two arms is about 10 mm Hg.[49] Differences of 20 mm Hg or more are uncommon and usually indicate obstructed flow in the subclavian artery leading to the arm with the lower pressure. This is a significant finding in the following two clinical settings:

1. Subclavian steal syndrome. The finding of one weak radial pulse in a patient with symptoms of vertebral-basilar ischemia (episodic vertigo, visual complaints, hemiparesis, ataxia, or diplopia) suggests the subclavian steal syndrome. In this syndrome,

TABLE 15-2 Hypotension

Finding (ref)	Sensitivity (%)	Specificity (%)	Positive LR	Negative LR
Systolic Blood Pressure <90 mm Hg				
Predicting mortality in intensive care unit[43]	21	95	4.0	0.8
Predicting mortality in patients with pneumonia[44-46]	11-35	97-99	10.0	NS
Systolic Blood Pressure ≤80 mm Hg				
Predicting mortality in patients with acute myocardial infarction[47]	32	98	15.5	0.7

NS, Not significant.

stenosis or occlusion of one subclavian artery proximal to the vertebral artery causes a reduction of pressure distally, with the result that blood, instead of travelling normally up the vertebral artery to perfuse the brain, courses down the vertebral artery to perfuse the arm.[50] Ninety-four percent of affected patients have a systolic blood pressure that is 20 mm Hg or more lower on the affected side than on the opposite arm (the mean difference between the arms is 45 mm Hg).[51] Most patients have an ipsilateral radial pulse that is diminished or absent and a systolic bruit over the ipsilateral subclavian artery.[51] The left side is affected in 70% and the right side in 30%.[51]

2. **Aortic dissection.** The finding of a difference in blood pressure between the two arms in a patient with acute chest pain suggests aortic dissection. The frequency of blood pressure discrepancy in aortic dissection is unknown, although the complete absence of a pulse on one side (e.g., one carotid, radial, or femoral artery) occurs in 6% to 31% of patients.[52-54] In aortic dissection, other signs are the murmur of aortic regurgitation (10% to 32% of patients), hemiparesis (1% to 6%), spinal stroke (3%), pulsatile sternoclavicular joint (1%), and unilateral femoral pistol shot sounds (rare). All of these findings are relatively uncommon compared with an abnormal chest radiograph revealing an increased aortic diameter and widened mediastinum, which is found in 86% of patients.[52-55]

   In patients with known aortic dissection, a murmur of aortic insufficiency argues strongly for proximal involvement of the aorta (i.e., type A dissection vs. type B, positive LR = 11.9); the absence of a peripheral pulse also favors type A dissection, although less so (positive LR = 3.3).[52,53] The absence of either of these findings is diagnostically unhelpful.

D. Differences in pressure between arms and legs. This finding is valuable in the following two clinical settings:

    1. Chronic ischemia of the lower extremities. Chapter 48 describes calculation of the ankle-arm index, which is the principal bedside tool used in patients with intermittent claudication.

    2. Coarctation of the aorta. In young patients with hypertension, the finding of an unobtainable blood pressure in the legs or a blood pressure that is much lower than in the arms suggests the diagnosis of coarctation of the aorta.[56,57] These patients also have hypertension of the arms (96% have a blood pressure >140/90), femoral pulses that are absent or diminished and delayed (100%), augmented carotid pulsations, various murmurs (usually a systolic murmur at the sternal border and a continuous murmur posteriorly over the upper spine), and visible collateral arteries (usually around the scapula, intercostal spaces, or axilla).[56,57]

    During simultaneous palpation of the femoral and radial arteries of healthy persons, it is impossible to tell which comes first. In patients with coarctation, however, the femoral pulse is delayed, due both to delay in arrival at the legs and to more rapid than normal conduction of the wave to the arms.[58]

E. Abnormal pulse contour. The three abnormalities of pulse contour—pulsus paradoxus, pulsus alternans, and pulsus bisferiens—are easily detectable using the blood pressure cuff (see Chapter 13)

F. Abnormal pulse pressure

    1. Abnormally small pulse pressure. Since the pulse pressure depends on stroke volume, clinicians have tried for decades to use it as a way to quantify cardiac output. This relationship has been validated in only one setting, in patients with known left ventricular dysfunction: In these patients, the finding of a proportional pulse pressure (i.e., the pulse pressure divided by the systolic pressure) less than 0.25 detects a cardiac index less than 2.2 L/min/m^2 with a sensitivity of 91%, specificity of 83%, positive LR of 5.4, and negative LR of 0.1.[59]

In contrast to conventional teachings, many patients with significant aortic stenosis have a normal pulse pressure (see Chapter 39).[60]

2. **Abnormally large pulse pressure.** In patients with the murmur of aortic insufficiency, a pulse pressure of 80 mm Hg or more argues that the regurgitation is moderate or severe, with a sensitivity of 57%, specificity of 95%, and positive LR of 10.9 (see Chapter 40).[61]

G. **Orthostatic hypotension.** When a person stands, about 350 to 600 ml of blood shifts to the lower body. Normally, the blood pressure remains relatively stable during this shift because of compensatory increases in cardiac output, heart rate, and systemic vascular resistance and transfer of blood from the pulmonary circulation to the systemic side.[26] Orthostatic hypotension, usually defined as a fall in systolic blood pressure of 20 mm Hg or more when the patient stands from the supine position, may occur if (1) compensatory mechanisms fail (i.e., "autonomic insufficiency"), or (2) the patient has lost excessive amounts of fluid from the vascular space (e.g., acute blood loss).

1. **Postural vital signs in healthy persons.** As normovolemic persons stand up from the supine position, the pulse increases on average by 10.9 beats/min, systolic blood pres-

sure decreases by 3.5 mm Hg, and diastolic blood pressure increases by 5.2 mm Hg.[26] Postural hypotension, defined as a decrement in systolic blood pressure of 20 mm Hg or more, occurs in 10% of normovolemic individuals younger than 65 years and in 11% to 30% older than 65 years.[26] As persons age, the postural pulse increment diminishes ($r = -0.50$, $p < .02$); this phenomenon and the observation that older persons have more postural hypotension suggests that autonomic reflexes decline as persons age.

2. **Vital signs and hypovolemia.** Table 15-3 presents the vital signs from normal persons before and after phlebotomy of 450 to 630 ml (moderate blood loss) or 630 to 1150 ml (large blood loss).[b] Chapter 9 reviews the other physical findings of hypovolemia.

   a. **Postural change in pulse.** Table 15-3 shows that the most valuable observation is *either* a postural pulse increment of 30/min or more *or* the inability of the patient to stand long enough for vital signs because of severe dizziness. Most persons have one or both of these findings after large amounts of blood loss (sensitivity = 98%), but only 1 of 5 persons develops either of them after moderate blood loss.[26] These findings are durable after hemorrhage, lasting at least 12 to 72 hours if intravenous fluids are withheld.[28,69,70]

---

[b] Calculating LRs for these data is not appropriate, because "acute blood loss" has endless gradations of severity, many of which are important to the clinician. For example, the LRs of physical signs for moderate blood loss are of little use to the clinician who, when taking care of the patient with melena, regards blood loss of 400 mL ("disease-negative" according to the LR) as significant as a loss of 500 ml ("disease-positive"). Table 15-3 instead just illustrates the general trends of vital signs with increasing amounts of blood loss.

TABLE 15-3 Vital signs and acute blood loss

Physical Finding (ref)*	Moderate Blood Loss, Sensitivity (%)	Large Blood Loss, Sensitivity (%)	Specificity (%)
Postural pulse increment ≥30/min or severe postural dizziness[27,62,63]	7-57	98	99
Postural hypotension (>20 mm Hg decrease in SBP)[62,63]	9	—	90-98
Supine tachycardia (pulse >100/min)[28,64-66]	0	10	98
Supine hypotension (SBP <95 mm Hg)[28,64,65,67,68]	13	31	98

SBP, Systolic blood pressure.

Data obtained from 568 normal persons, mostly young and healthy, after "moderate" blood loss (phlebotomy of 450-630 ml) or "large" blood loss (phlebotomy of 630-1150 ml). Specificity is from same patients when euvolemic, before blood loss. Results are overall mean frequency or, if statistically heterogenous, the range of values. Adapted from reference 26.

Definition of finding: For *postural*, supine measurement minus standing measurement; for *postural hypotension (>20 mm Hg decrease in SBP)*, the finding applies only to patients able to stand without severe dizziness.

b. **Postural change in blood pressure.**
After excluding those patients unable to
stand for vital signs (which includes almost all patients after large amounts of
blood loss), the finding of postural hypotension (>20 mm Hg postural decrement
in systolic blood pressure) has no proven
value, being found just as often in patients before blood loss as after it. For
example, in persons younger than 65
years, postural hypotension is found in
8% before moderate blood loss and 9%
after blood loss. In persons 65 years or
older, postural hypotension is detected in
11% to 30% before blood loss and about
25% after blood loss.[26,63]

Obviously, because severe dizziness
with standing is a valuable finding, but
postural hypotension of 20 mm Hg is not,
there must be an intermediate level of
postural fall (e.g., 30 mm Hg, 40 mm Hg,
or another value), not yet identified, that
better discriminates between patients
with and without blood loss.

c. **Supine pulse and supine blood pressure.** In patients with suspected blood
loss, both supine tachycardia and supine
hypotension are specific indicators of
significant blood loss, although both
are infrequent. After moderate blood loss,
0% have tachycardia in the supine position and only 13% have supine hypotension; after large blood loss, only
10% have tachycardia and 31% have
hypotension.

Sinus bradycardia, in contrast, is a
common arrhythmia after blood loss and
frequently precedes the drop in blood
pressure that causes patients to faint.[26]

H. **Capillary fragility test (Rumpel-Leede test).**
Traditionally, the blood pressure cuff also was

used to test capillary fragility, although measurements of blood pressure were not part of the test. Capillary fragility tests were designed to detect abnormally weakened capillary walls in the skin that would burst when distended, resulting in appearance of high numbers of petechiae. The diseases associated with capillary fragility were legion, ranging from coagulopathies, vitamin deficiencies (e.g., scurvy), infectious diseases (e.g., scarlet fever), and endocrine disorders (e.g., hyperthyroidism), to dermatologic disorders (e.g., Osler-Weber-Rendu syndrome).[71] Both negative and positive pressure methods were used. The negative pressure technique applied suction to a defined area of the skin, a technique whose undoing was the eventual demonstration that the number of resulting petechiae depended on not only the age of patient, but also on the time of day, season, and psychic influences.[72] Positive pressure methods, introduced at the turn of the century by Drs. Rumpel and Leede, consisted of raising the venous pressure by a tourniquet or blood pressure cuff around the arm and counting petechiae that subsequently developed in a defined area distally. This test was eventually standardized,[72] but interest fell after the introduction of better diagnostic tests for coagulation and the other associated disorders. Recently, increased capillary fragility was believed to represent a sign of diabetic retinopathy,[73] but this was soon disproved.[74]

REFERENCES

1. Thulin T, Andersson G, and Schersten B. Measurement of blood pressure: a routine test in need of standardization, *Postgrad Med J* 51:390-395, 1975.
2. Burch GE and DePasquale NP. *Primer of clinical measurement of blood pressure*, St Louis, 1962, CV Mosby Co.

3. Major RH. The history of taking the blood pressure, *Ann Med Hist* 2:47-55, 1930.

4. Gibson GA and Russell W. *Physical diagnosis: a guide to methods of clinical investigation,* ed 2, New York, 1893, D. Appleton & Co.

5. Crenner CW. Introduction of the blood pressure cuff into U.S. medical practice: technology and skilled practice, *Ann Intern Med* 128:488-493, 1998.

6. Janeway TC. *The clinical study of blood-pressure: a guide to the use of the sphygmomanometer,* New York, 1907, D Appleton & Co.

7. Geddes LA, Hoff HE, and Badger AS. Introduction of the auscultatory method of measuring blood pressure— including a translation of Korotkoff's original paper, *Cardiovasc Res Center Bull* 5:57-74, 1966.

8. Geddes LA. Perspectives in physiological monitoring, *Med Instrument* 10:91-97, 1976.

9. Joint National Committee on Prevention and the National High Blood Pressure Education Program Coordinating Committee. The sixth report of the Joint National Committee on prevention, detection, evaluation, and treatment of high blood pressure, *Arch Intern Med* 157:2413-2446, 1997.

10. Perloff D and others. Human blood pressure determination by sphygmomanometry, *Circulation* 88:2460-2470, 1993.

11. Cushman WC and others. Effect of back support and stethoscope head on seated blood pressure determination, *Am J Hypertension* 3:240-241, 1990.

12. Askey JM. The auscultatory gap in sphygmomanometry, *Ann Intern Med* 80:94-97, 1974.

13. London SB and London RE. Critique of indirect diastolic end point, *Arch Intern Med* 119:39-49, 1967.

14. Karvonen MJ, Telivuo LJ, and Jarvinen EJK. Sphygmomanometer cuff size and the accuracy of indirect measurement of blood pressure, *Am J Cardiol* 13:688-693, 1964.

15. Penny J, Shennan A, and De Swiet M. The reproducibility of Korotkoff 4 and 5, *Am J Hypertension* 9:839, 1996.

16. Medical Research Council Working Party. MRC trial of treatment of mild hypertension: principal results, *Br Med J* 291:97-104, 1985.

17. Hypertension Detection and Follow-up Program Cooperative Group. Five-year findings of the hypertension detection and follow-up program. I. Reduction in mortality of persons with high blood pressure, including mild hypertension, *JAMA* 242:2562-2571, 1979.

18. Bailey RH and Bauer JH. A review of common errors in the indirect measurement of blood pressure (sphygmomanometry), *Arch Intern Med* 153:2741-2748, 1993.

19. Tavel ME and others. Korotkoff sounds: observations on pressure-pulse changes underlying their formation, *Circulation* 39:465-474, 1969.

20. Enselberg CD. Measurement of diastolic blood pressure by palpation, *N Engl J Med* 265:272-274, 1961.

21. Dock W. Korotkoff's sounds, *N Engl J Med* 302:1264-1267, 1980.

22. Ur A and Gordon M. Origin of Korotkoff sounds, *Am J Physiol* 218:524-529, 1970.

23. McCutcheon EP and Rushmer RF. Korotkoff sounds: an experimental critique, *Circ Res* 20:149-161, 1967.

24. Segall HN. A note on the measurement of diastolic and systolic blood pressure by the palpation of arterial vibrations (sounds) over the brachial artery, *Can Med Assoc J* 42:311-313, 1940.

25. Putt AM. A comparison of blood pressure readings by auscultation and palpation, *Nurs Res* 15:311-316, 1966.

26. McGee S, Abernethy WB, and Simel DL. Is this patient hypovolemic? *JAMA* 281:1022-1029, 1999.

27. Knopp R, Claypool R, and Leonardi D. Use of the tilt test in measuring acute blood loss, *Ann Emerg Med* 9:72-75, 1980.

28. Wallace J and Sharpey-Schafer EP. Blood changes following controlled haemorrhage in man, *Lancet* 241:393-395, 1941.

29. Rose GA, Holland WW, and Crowley EA. A sphygmomanometer for epidemiologists, *Lancet* 1:296-300, 1964.

30. Reeves RA. Does this patient have hypertension? How to measure blood pressure, *JAMA* 273:1211-1218, 1995.

31. O'Brien E. Review: a century of confusion; which bladder for accurate blood pressure measurement? *J Human Hypertension* 10:565-572, 1996.

32. Ragan C and Bordley J. The accuracy of clinical measurements of arterial blood pressure. *Bull Johns Hopkins Hosp* 69:504-528, 1941.

33. King GE. Errors in clinical measurement of blood pressure in obesity, *Clin Sci* 32:223-237, 1967.

34. Maxwell MH and others. Error in blood-pressure measurement due to incorrect cuff size in obese patients, *Lancet* 2:33-35, 1982.

35. Cavallini MC and others. Association of the auscultatory gap with vascular disease in hypertensive patients, *Ann Intern Med* 124:877-883, 1996.

36. Londe S and Klitzner TS. Auscultatory blood pressure measurement: Effect of pressure on the head of the stethoscope, *West J Med* 141:193-195, 1984.

37. Mitchell PL, Parlin RW, and Blackburn H. Effect of vertical displacement of the arm on indirect blood-pressure measurement, *N Engl J Med* 271:72-74, 1964.

38. Wright BM and Dore CF. A random-zero sphygmomanometer, *Lancet* 1:337-338, 1970.

39. Messerli FH, Ventura HO, and Amodeo C. Osler's maneuver and pseudohypertension, *N Engl J Med* 312:1548-1551, 1985.

40. Tsapatasaris NP, Napolitana BT, and Rothchild J. Osler's maneuver in an outpatient clinic setting, *Arch Intern Med* 151:2209-2211, 1991.

41. Kuwajima I and others. Pseudohypertension in the elderly, *J Hypertension* 8:429-432, 1990.

42. Belmin J and others. Osler's maneuver: absence of usefulness for the detection of pseudohypertension in an elderly population, *Am J Med* 98:42-49, 1995.

43. Lemeshow S and others. Mortality probability models (MPM II) based on an international cohort of intensive care unit patients, *JAMA* 270:2478-2486, 1993.

44. Allen SC. Lobar pneumonia in Northern Zambia: clinical study of 502 adult patients, *Thorax* 39:612-616, 1984.

45. Conte HA and others. A prognostic rule for elderly patients admitted with community-acquired pneumonia, *Am J Med* 106:20-28, 1999.

46. Fedullo AJ and Swinburne AJ. Relationship of patient age to clinical features and outcome for in-hospital treatment of pneumonia, *J Gerontol* 40:29-33, 1985.

47. Goldberg RJ and others. Cardiogenic shock after acute myocardial infarction: incidence and mortality from a community-wide perspective, 1975 to 1988, *N Engl J Med* 325:1117-1122, 1991.

48. Knaus WA and others. The APACHE III prognostic system: risk prediction of hospital mortality for critically ill hospitalized adults, *Chest* 100:1619-1636, 1991.

49. Singer AJ and Hollander JE. Blood pressure: assessment of interarm differences, *Arch Intern Med* 156:2005-2008, 1996.

50. Fisher CM. A new vascular syndrome—"the subclavian steal," *N Engl J Med* 265:912-913, 1961.

51. Fields WS and Lemak NA. Joint study of extracranial arterial occlusion. VII. Subclavian steal—a review of 168 cases, *JAMA* 222:1139-1143, 1972.

52. Slater EE and DeSanctis RW. The clinical recognition of dissecting aortic aneurysm, *Am J Med* 60:625-633, 1976.

53. Spittell PC and others. Clinical features and differential diagnosis of aortic dissection: experience with 236 cases (1980 through 1990), *Mayo Clin Proc* 68:642-651, 1993.

54. Hirst AE, Johns VJ, and Kime SW. Dissecting aneurysm of the aorta: a review of 505 cases, *Medicine* 37:217-279, 1958.

55. McGee SR and Adcox M. Unilateral femoral pistol-shot sounds: a clue to aortic dissection, *West J Med* 162:547-548, 1995.

56. Ostermiller WE and others. Coarctation of the aorta in adult patients, *J Thor Cardiovasc Surg* 61:125-130, 1971.

57. Cleland WP and others Coarctation of the aorta, *Br Med J* 2:379-390, 1956.

58. Lewis T. Material relating to coarctation of the aorta of the adult type, *Heart* 16:205-261, 1933.

59. Stevenson LW and Perloff JK. The limited reliability of physical signs for estimating hemodynamics in chronic heart failure, *JAMA* 261:884-888, 1989.

60. Hancock EW and Abelmann WH. A clinical study of the brachial arterial pulse form: with special reference to the diagnosis of aortic valvular disease, *Circulation* 16:572-581, 1957.

61. Frank MJ and others. The clinical evaluation of aortic regurgitation, *Arch Intern Med* 116:357-365, 1965.

62. Baraff LJ and Schriger DL. Orthostatic vital signs: variation with age, specificity, and sensitivity in detecting a 450-mL blood loss, *Am J Emerg Med* 10:99-103, 1992.

63. Witting MD, Wears RL, and Li S. Defining the positive tilt test, *Ann Emerg Med* 23:1320-1323, 1994.

64. Skillman JJ and others. The hemodynamic effect of acute blood loss in normal man, with observations on the effect of the Valsalva maneuver and breath holding, *Ann Surg* 166:713-738, 1967.

65. Shenkin HA and others. On the diagnosis of hemorrhage in man, *Am J Med Sci* 208:421-436, 1944.

66. Ralston LA, Cobb LA, and Bruce RA. Acute circulatory effects of arterial bleeding as determined by indicator-dilution curves in normal human subjects, *Am Heart J* 61:770-776, 1961.

67. Bergenwald L, Freyschuss U, and Sjostrand T. The mechanism of orthostatic and haemorrhage fainting, *Scand J Clin Lab Invest* 37:209-216, 1977.

68. Warren JV and others. The effect of venesection and the pooling of blood in the extremities on the atrial pressure and cardiac output in normal subjects with observations on acute circulatory collapse in three instances, *J Clin Invest* 24:337-344, 1945.

69. Green DM and Metheny D. The estimation of acute blood loss by the tilt test, *Surg Gynecol Obstet* 84:1045-1050, 1947.

70. Ebert RV, Stead EA, and Gibson JG. Response of normal subjects to acute blood loss, *Arch Intern Med* 68:578-590, 1941.

71. Peck SM and Copley AL. Diagnosis and treatment of skin manifestations of capillary fragility, *N Engl J Med* 235:900-906, 1946.

72. Beaser SB, Rudy A, and Seligman AM. Capillary fragility in relation to diabetes mellitus, hypertension, and age, *Arch Intern Med* 73:18-22, 1944.

73. Reynolds WA. Identification of diabetic retinopathy, *JAMA* 249:1267, 1983 (letter).

74. Williams R and Jones L. The tourniquet test and screening for diabetic retinopathy *JAMA* 254:235, 1985 (letter).

CHAPTER 16

Temperature

I. INTRODUCTION. Fever is a fundamental sign of almost all infectious diseases and many noninfectious disorders. Clinicians began to monitor the temperature of febrile patients in the 1850s and 1860s, after Traube introduced the thermometer to hospital wards and Wunderlich published an analysis based on observation of an estimated 20,000 subjects that convinced clinicians of the value of graphing temperature over time.[1-3] These temperature charts, the first vital sign to be routinely recorded in hospitalized patients, were originally named "Wunderlich curves."[4]

II. TECHNIQUE

A. Site of measurement. Thermometers are used to measure the temperature of the patient's oral cavity, rectum, axilla, or, using infrared technology, tympanic membrane. Rectal temperatures are on average 0.4 to 0.5° C (0.7 to 1.0° F) higher than oral temperatures,[5-8] which in turn are 0.4 to 0.7° C (0.7 to 1.3° F) higher than axillary measurements[9,10] and 0.4° C (0.7° F) higher than tympanic membrane measurements.[7] These differences, however, are only average values; the difference between rectal and oral measurements in one person on successive days may vary from –0.4 to 1.3° C (–0.8 to 2.4° F).[8]

Tympanic measurements are potentially

ideal because they are rapid, convenient, and theoretically best reflect core temperature (i.e., the core temperature is the temperature of the hypothalamus, which is supplied by the same artery as the tympanic membrane).[11] Nonetheless, tympanic measurements of a single person vary over time much more than do oral or rectal measurements,[7,9,11,12] and some studies question their precision, demonstrating that the correlation between the right and left tympanic temperatures in the same person, measured only minutes apart, is poor ($r = 0.57$).[12]

B. Variables affecting the temperature measurement

1. Eating and smoking.[7,13] The *oral* temperature measurement increases about 0.3° C after sustained chewing and stays elevated for up to 20 minutes, probably because of increased blood flow to the muscles of mastication. Drinking hot liquids also increases oral readings about 0.9° C, for up to 15 minutes, and smoking a cigarette increases oral readings about 0.2° C for 30 minutes. Drinking ice water causes the oral reading to fall 0.3 to 1.2° C, a reduction lasting about 10 to 15 minutes.

2. Tachypnea. Tachypnea reduces the *oral* temperature reading about 0.5° C for every 10 breaths/min increase in the respiratory rate.[5,6] This phenomenon probably explains why marathon runners, at the end of their race, often have a large discrepancy between normal oral temperatures and high rectal temperatures.[14]

In contrast, administration of oxygen by nasal cannula does not affect oral temperature.[15]

3. Cerumen. Cerumen lowers *tympanic* temperature readings, simply because it obstructs radiation of heat from the tympanic membrane.[7]

4. Hemiparesis. In patients with hemiparesis, *axillary* temperature readings are about
0.5° C lower on the weak side compared with
the healthy side. The discrepancy between
the two sides correlates poorly with the
severity of the patient's weakness, suggesting that it is not due to difficulty holding the
thermometer under the arm, but instead to
other factors, such as differences in cutaneous blood flow between the two sides.[16]

III. THE FINDING

A. Normal temperature and fever. In healthy
persons, the mean oral temperature is 36.8° C
(98.2° F),[17] a value slightly lower than Wunderlich's original estimate of 37° C (98.6° F), which
in turn had been established using foot-long
axillary thermometers that may have been calibrated higher than the thermometers used today.[1] The temperature is usually lowest at 6 AM
and highest at 4 to 6 PM (a variation called
"diurnal variation").[17] Fever is defined as the
99th percentile of maximum temperatures in
healthy persons, which is an oral temperature
greater than 37.7° C (99.9° F).[17]

B. Fever patterns. In the early days of clinical
thermometry, clinicians observed that prolonged fevers could be categorized into 1 of
4 fever patterns—sustained, intermittent, remittent, and relapsing.[3,18-20] **(1) Sustained fever.** In
this pattern the fever varies little from day to
day (the modern definition is variation <0.3° C
[0.5° F] each day). **(2) Intermittent fever.** In this
pattern the temperature returns to normal between exacerbations. If the exacerbations occur
daily, the fever is "quotidian"; if they occur
every 48 hours, it is "tertian" (i.e., they appear
again on the third day); and if they occur every
72 hours, it is "quartan" (i.e., they appear again
on the fourth day). **(3) Remittent.** Remittent
fevers vary at least 0.3° C (0.5 ° F) each day but

do not return to normal. **Hectic fevers** are intermittent or remittent fevers with wide swings in temperature, usually greater than 1.4° C (2.5° F) each day. **(4) Relapsing fevers.** These fevers are characterized by periods of fever lasting days interspersed by equally long afebrile periods.

Each of these patterns was associated with prototypic diseases: for sustained fever—lobar pneumonia (lasting 7 days until it disappeared abruptly by "crisis" or gradually by "lysis"), for intermittent fever—malarial infection; for remittent fever—typhoid fever (causing several days of ascending remittent fever, whose curve resembles climbing steps, before becoming sustained), for hectic fever—chronic tuberculosis or pyogenic abscesses, and for relapsing fever—relapse of a previous infection (e.g., typhoid fever). Other causes of relapsing fever are the Pel-Ebstein fever of Hodgkin's disease,[21] rat-bite fever (*Spirillum minus* or *Streptobacillus moniliformis*),[22] and *Borrelia* infections.[23]

Despite these etiologic associations, early clinicians recognized that the diagnostic significance of fever patterns was limited.[24] Instead, they used these labels more often to communicate a specific observation at the bedside rather than imply a specific diagnoses, much like we use the words "systolic murmur" or "lung crackle" today.

C. Associated findings

1. **Focal findings.** Over 80% of patients with bacterial infections have specific focal signs or symptoms that point the clinician to the correct diagnosis.[25] There are countless focal signs associated with febrile illness (e.g., the tender swelling of an abscess or the diastolic murmur of endocarditis), which are reviewed in detail in infectious diseases textbooks. One potentially misleading focal sign, however, is jaundice. Although fever and

jaundice are often due to hepatitis or cholangitis, jaundice is also a nonspecific complication of bacterial infection distant to the liver, occurring in 1% of all bacteremias.[26,27] This "reactive hepatopathy of bacteremia" was recognized over a century ago by Osler, who wrote that jaundice appeared in pneumococcal pneumonia with curious irregularity in different outbreaks.[24]

2. **Relative bradycardia.** Relative bradycardia, a traditional sign of intracellular bacterial infections (e.g., typhoid fever), refers to a pulse rate that is inappropriately slow for the patient's temperature. The best definition is a pulse rate that is lower than the 95% confidence limit for the patient's temperature, which can be estimated by multiplying the patient temperature in degrees Celsius times 10 and then subtracting 323.[28] For example, if the patient's temperature is 39° C, relative bradycardia would refer to pulse rates below 67/min (i.e., 390 − 323).[a]

3. **Anhidrosis.** Classically, patients with heat stroke have "bone-dry skin," but most modern studies show that anhidrosis appears very late in the course and has a sensitivity of only 3% to 60%.[29-31] In contrast, 91% of patients with heat stroke have extreme pyrexia (exceeding 40° C), and 100% have abnormal mental status.

4. **Muscle rigidity.** Muscle rigidity suggests the diagnosis of neuroleptic malignant syndrome, a febrile complication that develops in patients taking antidopaminergic medications or in those withdrawing from dopaminergic medications. In studies of neuroleptic

---

[a] This formula combines separate formulas for women (<11 × T° C − 359) and men (<10.2 × T° C − 333) provided in reference 28, which in turn were based on observations of 700 febrile patients.

syndrome, 92% have muscle rigidity, 73% have depressed mental status, and 54% have labile blood pressure.[32]

IV. CLINICAL SIGNIFICANCE

A. Detection of fever. Studies show that the patient's subjective report of fever is a slightly more accurate indicator of a measured temperature >38° C than the clinician's impression from palpating the patient's forehead at the bedside (LR = 4.9 for patient's report and 2.5 for palpation; Table 16-1).

B. Predictors of bacteremia. In febrile patients, the best predictors of bacterial infection are the patient's focal findings and the results of microscopic examination of relevant clinical specimens. In febrile patients *who lack focal findings,* however, the best bedside predictors of bacterial infection are (1) older age, (2) the presence of underlying conditions such as diabetes mellitus, and (3) the degree of elevation of white blood cell count.[25,35-37]

Other findings have relatively little value in predicting bacteremia. Although the temperature value is significantly higher in bacterial infection than in other causes of their fever, the differences are small and of little help in the individual patient (e.g., mean temperatures of 38.7° C for bacterial infection vs. 38.1° C for nonbacterial infection).[35,36,38] The presence of "shaking chills" discriminates only weakly between bacteremia and other causes of fever (sensitivity 27% to 58%; specificity 65% to 87%; positive LR 1.8, negative LR not significant),[36,39] and the "toxic appearance" fails to discriminate serious infection from trivial illness.[25,40]

C. Extreme pyrexia and hypothermia. Extreme pyrexia (i.e., temperature exceeding 41.1° C or 106° F) has diagnostic significance because the cause is usually gram-negative bacteremia or problems with temperature regulation

TABLE 16-1 Detection of fever*

FINDING (REF)†	SENSITIVITY (%)	SPECIFICITY (%)	POSITIVE LR	NEGATIVE LR
Patient's report of fever[33]	83	83	4.9	0.2
Patient's forehead abnormally warm[34]	71	72	2.5	0.4

*Diagnostic standard: For fever, measured temperature >38° C.

(heat stroke, intracranial hemorrhage, severe burns).[31]

In a wide variety of disorders, the finding of a very high or very low temperature indicates a worse prognosis.[41,42] For example, in pontine hemorrhage, a fever greater than 39° C predicts hospital mortality with a sensitivity of 66%, specificity of 97%, positive LR of 23.7, and negative LR of 0.4.[43] In elderly patients hospitalized with pneumonia, an admission temperature <36.1° C predicts hospital mortality with a sensitivity of 14%, specificity of 93%, and positive LR of 2.0.[44]

D. Fever patterns. Most fevers today, whether infectious or noninfectious in origin, are intermittent or remittent and lack any other characteristic feature.[45,46] Antibiotic medications have changed many traditional fever patterns. For example, the fever of lobar pneumonia, which in the preantibiotic era was sustained and lasted 7 days, now lasts only 2 to 3 days.[47,48] The double quotidian fever pattern (i.e., 2 daily fever spikes), a feature of gonococcal endocarditis present in 50% of cases during the preantibiotic era, is consistently absent in reported cases from the modern era.[49] The characteristic tertian or quartan intermittent fever of malaria infection also is uncommon today, because most patients are treated before the characteristic synchronization of the malaria cycle.[50]

Nonetheless, although traditional fever patterns may be less common, they still have some significance. For example, in a modern study of typhoid fever, 96% of patients had a remittent or sustained pattern; the intermittent pattern was rare.[51] Among travelers with malarial infection who reported a tertian pattern, most were infected with *Plasmodium vivax* (traditionally the most common cause of this pattern).[52]

Moreover, the antibiotic era has given fever patterns a new significance, because once antibiotics have been started, the finding of an unusually prolonged fever is an important sign indicating either that the diagnosis of infection was incorrect (e.g., the patient instead has a connective tissue disorder or neoplasm) or that the patient has one of several complications, such as resistant organisms, superinfection, drug fever, or an abscess requiring surgical drainage.

E. Relative bradycardia. Clinical studies demonstrate that some intracellular bacterial infections, such as typhoid fever and Legionnaire's disease, produce less tachycardia than other infections, but, because very few patients with these infections actually have a relative bradycardia (as previously defined), the clinical utility of this observation is limited.[28]

REFERENCES

1. Mackowiak PA and Wordern G. Carl Reinhold August Wunderlich and the evolution of clinical thermometry, *Clin Inf Dis* 18:458-467, 1994.

2. Wright-St. Clair RE. Go to the bedside, *J Roy Coll Gen Pract* 21:442-452, 1971.

3. Guttman P. *A handbook of physical diagnosis: comprising the throat, thorax, and abdomen,* New York, 1880, William Wood & Co.

4. Geddes LA. Perspectives in physiological monitoring, *Med Instrument* 10:91-97, 1976.

5. Tandberg D and Sklar D. Effect of tachypnea on the estimation of body temperature by an oral thermometer, *N Engl J Med* 308:945-946, 1983.

6. Durham ML, Swanson B, and Paulford N. Effect of tachypnea on oral temperature estimation: a replication, *Nurs Res* 35:211-214, 1986.

7. Rabinowitz RP and others. Effects of anatomic site, oral stimulation, and body position on estimates of body temperature, *Arch Intern Med* 156:777-780, 1996.

8. Horvath SM, Menduke H, and Piersol GM. Oral and rectal temperatures of man, *JAMA* 144:1562-1565, 1950.

9. Nichols GA and others. Oral, axillary, and rectal temperature determinations and relationships, *Nurs Res* 15:307-310, 1966.

10. Erickson RS and Kirklin SK. Comparison of ear-based, bladder, oral, and axillary methods for core temperature measurement, *Crit Care Med* 21:1528-1534, 1993.

11. Klein DG and others. A comparison of pulmonary artery, rectal, and tympanic membrane temperature measurement in the ICU, *Heart Lung* 22:435-441, 1993.

12. Chu A and Burnham RS. Reliability and validity of tympanic temperature measurement in persons with high spinal cord injuries, *Paraplegia* 33:476-479, 1995.

13. Terndrup TE, Allegra JR, and Kealy JA. A comparison of oral, rectal, and tympanic membrane-derived temperature changes after ingestion of liquids and smoking, *Am J Emerg Med* 7:150-154, 1989.

14. Maron MB. Effect of tachypnea on estimation of body temperature, *N Engl J Med* 309:612-613, 1983 (letter).

15. Lim-Levy F. The effect of oxygen inhalation on oral temperature, *Nurs Res* 31:150-152, 1982.

16. Mulley G. Axillary temperature differences in hemiplegia, *Postgrad Med J* 56:248-249, 1980.

17. Mackowiak PA, Wasserman SS, and Levine MM. A critical appraisal of 98.6 degrees F, the upper limit of the normal body temperature, and other legacies of Carl Reinhold August Wunderlich, *JAMA* 268:1578-1580, 1992.

18. Sahli H. *A treatise on diagnostic methods of examination,* Philadelphia, 1911, WB Saunders.

19. Gibson GA and Russell W. *Physical diagnosis: a guide to methods of clinical investigation,* ed 2, New York, 1893, D. Appleton & Co.

20. Brown JG. *Medical diagnosis: a manual of clinical methods,* New York, 1884, Bermingham and Co.

21. Reimann HA. Periodic (Pel-Ebstein) fever of lymphomas, *Ann Clin Lab Sci* 7:1-5, 1977.

22. Beeson PB. The problem of the etiology of rat bite fever: report of 2 cases due to spirillum minus, *JAMA* 123:332-334, 1943.

23. Bennett IL. The significance of fever in infections, *Yale J Biol Med* 26:491-505, 1954.

24. Osler W. *The principles and practice of medicine* (facsimile by Classics of Medicine library), Birmingham, 1892, Gryphon Editions.

25. Mellors JW and others. A simple index to identify occult bacterial infection in adults with acute unexplained fever, *Arch Intern Med* 147:666-671, 1987.

26. Franson TR, Hierholzer WJ, and LaBrecque DR. Frequency and characteristics of hyperbilirubinemia associated with bacteremia, *Rev Infect Dis* 7:1-9, 1985.

27. Vermillion SE and others. Jaundice associated with bacteremia, *Arch Intern Med* 124:611-618, 1969.

28. Ostergaard L, Huniche B, and Andersen PL. Relative bradycardia in infectious diseases, *J Infect* 33:185-191, 1996.

29. Costrini AM and others. Cardiovascular and metabolic manifestations of heat stroke and severe heat exhaustion, *Am J Med* 66:296-302, 1979.

30. Shibolet S and others. Heatstroke: its clinical picture and mechanism in 36 cases, *Quart J Med* 36:525-548, 1967.

31. Simon HB. Extreme pyrexia, *JAMA* 236:2419-2421, 1976.

32. Kurlan R, Hamill R, and Shoulson I. Neuroleptic malignant syndrome, *Clin Neuropharmacol* 7:109-120, 1984.

33. Buckley RG and Conine M. Reliability of subjective fever in triage of adult patients, *Ann Emerg Med* 27:693-695, 1996.

34. Hung OL and others. Evaluation of the physician's ability to recognize the presence or absence of anemia, fever, and jaundice, *Acad Emerg Med* 7:146-156, 2000.

35. Arbo MJ and others. Fever of nosocomial origin: etiology, risk factors, and outcomes, *Am J Med* 95:505-512, 1993.

36. Bates DW and others. Predicting bacteremia in hospitalized patients: a prospectively validated model, *Ann Intern Med* 113:495-500, 1990.

37. Leibovici L, Cohen O, and Wysenbeek AJ. Occult bacterial infection in adults with unexplained fever: validation of a diagnostic index, *Arch Intern Med* 150:1270-1272, 1990.

38. Bor DH and others. Fever in hospitalized medical patients: characteristics and significance, *J Gen Intern Med* 3:119-125, 1988.

39. Van Dissel JT and others. Implications of chills, *Lancet* 352:374, 1998.

40. Marantz PR and others. Inability to predict diagnosis in febrile intravenous drug abusers, *Ann Intern Med* 106:823-828, 1987.

41. Fine MJ and others. Prognosis of patients hospitalized with community-acquired pneumonia, *Am J Med* 88:5-1N-8N, 1990.

42. Knaus WA and others. The APACHE III prognostic system: risk prediction of hospital mortality for critically ill hospitalized adults, *Chest* 100:1619-1636, 1991.

43. Wijdicks EFM and St. Louis E. Clinical profiles predictive of outcome in pontine hemorrhage, *Neurology* 49:1342-1346, 1997.

44. Conte HA and others. A prognostic rule for elderly patients admitted with community-acquired pneumonia, *Am J Med* 106:20-28, 1999.

45. Mackowiak PA and LeMaistre CF. Drug fever: a critical appraisal of conventional concepts, *Ann Intern Med* 106: 728-733, 1987.

46. Musher DM and others. Fever patterns: their lack of clinical significance, *Arch Intern Med* 139:1225-1228, 1979.

47. Halm EA and others. Time to clinical stability in patients hospitalized with community-acquired pneumonia: Implications for practice guidelines, *JAMA* 279:1452-1457, 1998.

48. van Metre TE. Pneumococcal pneumonia treated with antibiotics: The prognostic significance of certain clinical findings, *N Engl J Med* 251:1048-1052, 1954.

49. Fernandez GC and others. Gonococcal endocarditis: a case series demonstrating modern presentation of an old disease, *Am Heart J* 108:1326-1334, 1984.

50. Stanley J. Malaria, *Emerg Med Clin North Am* 15:113-155, 1997.

51. Gupta SP and others. Current clinical patterns of typhoid fever: a prospective study, *J Trop Med Hygiene* 88:377-381, 1985.

52. Svenson JE and others. Imported malaria: clinical presentation and examination of symptomatic travelers, *Arch Intern Med* 155:861-868, 1995.

CHAPTER 17

Respiratory Rate and Abnormal Breathing Patterns

RESPIRATORY RATE

I. **INTRODUCTION.** The respiratory rate (i.e., number of breaths per minute) is one of the four traditional vital signs, the others being heart rate, blood pressure, and temperature.

One of the first clinicians to recommend routine measurement of the respiratory rate was Stokes in 1825,[1] although routine charting of this vital sign was infrequent until the late nineteenth century.[2,3]

II. **TECHNIQUE.** The respiratory rate is usually measured while the clinician is holding the patient's wrist and ostensibly measuring the pulse, primarily because the respiratory rate may change if attention is drawn to it. This practice seems reasonable, because the respiratory rate is the only vital sign that is under voluntary control.

As routinely recorded in the patient's hospital record, the respiratory rate is often inaccurate.[4,5] In one study of patients whose actual respiratory rates ranged from 11 to 33 breaths/min, the recorded rate 98% of the time was from 18 to 22 breaths/min.[5] Some of these errors represent too short a period of observation (i.e., the clinician counting the number of breaths in 10 seconds multiplying the result times 6). Consequently, it is probably good practice to observe respirations for at least 30 to 60 seconds, which not only may make the measured rate more accurate but also allows detection of unusual breathing patterns, such as Cheyne-Stokes respirations (see below).

III. FINDING

A. The normal respiratory rate. The normal respiratory rate averages 20 breaths per minute (range 16 to 25 breaths/min), based on careful measurement in persons without fever, heart disease, or lung disease.[6,7] This estimate is identical to that made over 150 years ago by Lambert Quetelet, who was the first to compile and analyze vital and social statistics.[a8] For unclear reasons, many textbooks, citing no data, mistakenly record the normal rate as 12 to 18 breaths/min.[6]

B. Tachypnea. Definitions of tachypnea vary, but the most reasonable one, based on the normal range and clinical studies, is a respiratory rate of 25 breaths/min or more.

C. Bradypnea. Bradypnea is defined as a respiratory rate less than 8 breaths/min, a threshold derived from studies of patients taking opioid medications, because this rate best predicts respiratory depression and correlates well with level of sedation.[9]

IV. CLINICAL SIGNIFICANCE

A. Tachypnea. The finding of tachypnea has both diagnostic and prognostic value. As a diagnostic sign, it argues modestly for the diagnosis of pneumonia in outpatients with cough

---

[a] Quetelet's 1835 monumental treatise also provided our current formula for body mass index, known as the Quetelet index (see Chapter 11).

and fever (LR = 2.0). Tachypnea also argues for pneumonia in hospitalized patients, the abnormal sign sometimes appearing as early as 1 to 2 days before the diagnosis is apparent by other means.[7,10]

One characteristic of a vital sign is that it accurately predicts the patient's prognosis, and Table 17-1 shows that tachypnea predicts subsequent cardiopulmonary arrest in hospitalized patients (LR = 3.0), much better than does tachycardia or abnormal blood pressure.[12] During trials of weaning from a ventilator, tachypnea also is a significant although modest predictor of weaning failure (LR = 2.9).[11,18] In patients hospitalized with pneumonia, severe tachypnea (i.e., rate >30 breaths/min) predicts subsequent hospital death (LR = 2.0).[14-17]

B. Tachypnea and oxygen saturation. The respiratory rate correlates poorly with the patient's level of oxygen desaturation ($r = 0.16$).[19] Although this at first seems surprising (i.e., the lower the oxygen level, the harder a patient should breathe), this actually is expected because some hypoxemic patients, by breathing rapidly, are able to bring their oxygen level back up to normal (i.e., hyperventilation raises arterial oxygen levels) and because other patients are hypoxemic simply because they have a primary hypoventilatory disorder. Consequently, the respiratory rate and oxygen saturation are both valuable to the clinician, each providing information independent from the other.

ABNORMAL BREATHING PATTERNS

I. CHEYNE-STOKES BREATHING ("PERIODIC BREATHING")

A. Introduction. Cheyne-Stokes breathing consists of alternating periods of apnea and hyperpnea (Figure 17-1). Some authors equate the

TABLE 17-1 Tachypnea

Finding (ref)	Sensitivity (%)	Specificity (%)	Positive LR	Negative LR
Rate > 24/min				
Predicting failure of weaning from the ventilator, in intubated patients[11]	94	68	2.9	NS
Rate > 27/min				
Predicting cardiopulmonary arrest, in medical inpatients[12]	54	82	3.0	0.6
Rate > 28/min				
Detecting pneumonia, in outpatients with cough and fever[13]	36	82	2.0	0.8
Rate > 30/min				
Predicting hospital mortality, in patients with pneumonia,[14-17]	41-85	63-81	2.0	0.6

NS, Not significant.

*Diagnostic standard: For failure of weaning, progressive hypoxemia or respiratory acidosis; for pneumonia, infiltrate on chest radiograph

FIGURE 17-1 Cheyne-Stokes respiration. There are alternating cycles of hyperpnea and apnea. During the hyperpnea phase only the tidal volume oscillates; the respiratory frequency is constant.

term "periodic breathing" with Cheyne-Stokes breathing,[20,21] while others reserve "periodic breathing" for oscillations of tidal volume that lack intervening periods of apnea.[22]

Cheyne-Stokes breathing was described by John Cheyne in 1818 and William Stokes in 1854.[23]

B. The finding

1. The breathing pattern. At the end of each apneic period, breathing commences with excursions of the chest that initially are small but gradually increase for several breaths and then diminish until apnea returns. The respiratory rate is constant during the hypernea phase and does not gradually increase and then decrease as often surmised.[24] Cheyne-Stokes breathing often first appears when the patient lies down, probably because this position reduces the patient's functional residual capacity, thus diminishing the lung's ability to buffer changes in carbon dioxide (see "Pathogenesis" below).[21,25]

The time between two consecutive peaks of hyperpnea is called the "cycle length" or "period." Each cycle length is divided into a hyperpnea phase (lasting about 30 seconds on average in patients with congestive heart failure) and an apnea phase (lasting about 25 seconds on average).[26]

2. Associated bedside observations. Several additional findings appear in patients with Cheyne-Stokes breathing. During the hyperpnea phase, the patient is alert and sometimes agitated, with dilated pupils, hyperactive muscle stretch reflexes, and increased muscle tone. During the apnea phase, the patient appears motionless and asleep with constricted pupils, hypoactive reflexes, and reduced muscle tone.[27,28] The agitation of the hyperpnea phase can easily startle a patient out of sleep, a nocturnal symptom that clinicians can mistake for the paroxysmal nocturnal dyspnea of heart failure caused by transient pulmonary edema.[29,30]

C. Clinical significance

  1. Associated conditions. Cheyne-Stokes breathing affects 30% of patients with stable congestive heart failure.[22] The breathing pattern also appears in many neurologic disorders, including hemorrhage, infarction, tumors, meningitis, and head trauma involving the brainstem or higher levels of the central nervous system.[27,28,31,32] Normal persons often develop Cheyne-Stokes breathing during sleep[20] or at high altitudes.[27]

  2. Prognostic importance. Modern studies confirm Dr. Stokes' original impression that, in patients with heart disease, this breathing pattern carries a poor prognosis. Compared with heart failure patients with normal breathing, patients with Cheyne-Stokes breathing have lower cardiac outputs, higher pulmonary capillary wedge pressures, and shorter survival.[22,33-35]

D. Pathogenesis. The fundamental problem causing Cheyne-Stokes breathing is enhanced sensitivity to carbon dioxide. The circulatory delay between the lungs and systemic arteries, caused by poor cardiac output, also contributes to the waxing and waning of breaths. Cerebral blood flow increases during hyperpnea and decreases during apnea, perhaps explaining the fluctuations of mental status.[26,36]

1. **Enhanced sensitivity to carbon dioxide.** Whether because of congestive heart failure or neurologic disease, patients with Cheyne-Stokes breathing have two to three times the normal sensitivity to carbon dioxide.[27,36-38] This causes patients to hyperventilate excessively, eventually driving the carbon dioxide level so low that central apnea results. After they stop breathing, carbon dioxide levels again rise, eliciting another hyperventilatory response and thus perpetuating the alternating cycles of apnea and hyperpnea.

   Mountain climbers develop Cheyne-Stokes breathing because hypoxia induces hypersensitivity to carbon dioxide. In contrast, their native Sherpa guides, who are acclimated to hypoxia, lack an exaggerated ventilatory response and do not develop Cheyne-Stokes breathing.[27]

2. **Circulatory delay between lungs and arteries.** Ventilation is normally controlled by the medullary respiratory center, which monitors arterial carbon dioxide levels and directs the lungs to ventilate more if carbon dioxide levels are too high and less if levels are too low. The medulla signals the lungs almost immediately, the message travelling via the nervous system. The feedback to the medulla, however, is much slower because it requires circulation of blood from lungs back to systemic arteries.

   In Cheyne-Stokes breathing, the carbon dioxide levels in the alveoli and those of the systemic arteries are precisely out of sync. During peak hyperpnea, carbon dioxide levels in the alveoli are very low, yet the medulla is just beginning to sample blood containing high carbon dioxide levels from the previous apnea phase and thus still directs the lungs to continue breathing deeply.[27] The delay in feedback to the medulla contributes to the gradual waxing and waning of tidal volume.

The length of circulatory delay also governs the cycle length of Cheyne-Stokes breathing, the two correlating closely ($r = 0.80$ between cycle length and circulation time from lung to arteries, $p < .05$).[26,36] The cycle length is about two times the circulation time, just as would be expected from the observation that carbon dioxide levels in the lungs and arteries are precisely out of sync. This suggests that the clinician should be able to take a stopwatch to the bedside and time the patient's cycle length, using this number as a rough guide to the patient's cardiac output. This idea, however, has never been formally tested.

II. KUSSMAUL'S RESPIRATION.
Kussmaul's respirations are rapid and deep and appear in patients with metabolic acidosis. The unusually deep respirations are distinctive, because other causes of tachypnea, such as heart and lung disease reduce vital capacity and thus cause rapid, *shallow* respirations.

III. GRUNTING RESPIRATIONS
A. Definition. Grunting respirations are short, explosive sounds of low-to-medium pitch produced by vocal cord closure during expiration. The actual sound is the rush of air that occurs when the glottis opens and suddenly allows air to escape. Grunting respirations are more common in children,[39] although the finding also has been described in adults as a sign of respiratory muscle fatigue[40] and, in the pre-antibiotic era, as a cardinal sign of lobar pneumonia, usually appearing after 4 to 6 days of illness.[3,41]

B. Pathogenesis. Grunting respirations slow down expiration and allow more time for maximal gas exchange.[40] In animal experiments, artificial mimicking of grunting respirations causes the Po_2 to increase by 10% and the Pco_2 to fall by 11%, whether or not the animal has pneumonia.[42] Grunting respirations also produce positive pressure exhalation that may reduce exudation of fluid into the alveoli, based on an old observation that administration of morphine to patients with pneumonia often reduced the grunting respirations but was sometimes followed immediately by fatal pulmonary edema.[41]

IV. ABNORMAL ABDOMINAL MOVEMENTS

A. Normal abdominal movements. In the absence of massive gaseous distention, the abdominal viscera are noncompressible and act like hydraulic coupling fluid that directly transmits movements of the diaphragm to the anterior abdominal wall.[43] Abdominal respiratory movements, therefore, indicate indirectly how the diaphragm is moving. During normal respiration, the chest and abdomen move synchronously: both out during inspiration and both in during expiration (Figure 17-2). The chest wall moves more when the person is upright, and the abdomen moves more when the person is supine.[44,45]

B. Abnormal abdominal movements. Three abnormal abdominal movements are all signs of chronic airflow obstruction or respiratory muscle weakness: asynchronous breathing, respiratory alternans, and paradoxical abdominal movements.

1. Asynchronous breathing

a. Findings. Asynchronous breathing is an abnormal *expiratory* movement that sometimes develops in patients with chronic airflow obstruction. In these patients, the

Chest wall movements:

Abdominal wall movements:

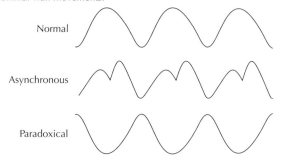

FIGURE 17-2 Respiratory abdominal movements. Chest movements are depicted in the first row. "I" denotes inspiration and "E," expiration. Upward sloping lines on the drawing indicate outward body wall movements; downward sloping lines, inward movements. In normal persons, the abdominal and chest wall movements are completely in sync. In asynchronous breathing, only expiratory abdominal movements are abnormal. In paradoxical abdominal movements, both inspiratory and expiratory abdominal movements are abnormal. See text.

normal smooth inward abdominal movement during expiration is replaced by an abrupt inward and then outward movement (Figure 17-2).[46,47]

b. Clinical significance. In patients with chronic airflow obstruction, asynchronous breathing correlates with lower forced expiratory volumes and a much poorer prognosis.[47] Among patients with chronic airflow obstruction who develop acute respiratory symptoms, the presence of an asynchronous breathing pattern predicted subsequent hospital death or the need for artificial ventilation with a sensitivity of 64%, specificity of 80%, and positive LR of 3.2 (negative LR not significant).[46]

  c. **Pathogenesis.** The outward abdominal movement during expiration probably reflects the strong action of chest wall accessory muscles during expiration, which push the flattened diaphragm temporarily downward, and thus the abdomen abruptly outward.[44,46]

2. **Respiratory alternans.** Respiratory alternans describes a breathing pattern that alternates between inspiratory movements that are mostly abdominal and inspiratory movements that are mostly thoracic.[18]

3. **Paradoxical abdominal movements**

  a. **Finding.** Paradoxical abdominal movements are completely out of sync with the those of the chest wall. During inspiration the abdomen moves in as the chest wall moves out; during expiration, the abdomen moves out as chest moves in.[43,48-50]

  b. **Clinical significance.** The finding of paradoxical abdominal movements is a sign of bilateral diaphragm weakness. Most of these patients also complain of severe orthopnea. In one study of patients with dyspnea and neuromuscular disease, the finding of paradoxical abdominal movements detected diaphragm weakness with a sensitivity of 95%, specificity of 71%, and positive LR of 3.3 (in this study, the definition of paradoxical movements was any inspiratory inward abdominal movement, and the definition of diaphragm weakness was a maximal transdiaphragmatic pressure of 30 cm H_2O or less; the normal sniff transdiaphragmatic pressure is >98 cm H_2O).[48]

   c. Pathogenesis. If the diaphragm is totally paralyzed, the inspiratory outward movement of the chest wall will draw the diaphragm upward, and thus the abdomen inward. The weight of the abdominal viscera probably also plays a role, because paradoxical movements are most obvious in affected patients who are positioned supine and are often absent when the patient is upright.[48]

V. ORTHOPNEA, TREPOPNEA, AND PLATYPNEA.

These terms describe tachypnea (and dyspnea) that appears abruptly in particular positions: when the patient is supine (orthopnea), lying on a side (trepopnea), or upright (platypnea). These findings are often first diagnosed during observation of the patient's respirations at the bedside.

A. Orthopnea

   1. Finding. Orthopnea describes dyspnea that appears when the patient lies down but is relieved when the patient sits up (from the Greek words *ortho,* meaning "straight" or "vertical," and *pnea,* meaning "to breathe").

   2. Clinical significance. Orthopnea occurs in a variety of disorders, including massive ascites, bilateral diaphragm paralysis, pleural effusion, and severe pneumonia, although its most important clinical association is congestive heart failure.[48,49,51] In one study of patients with known chronic obstructive pulmonary disease, the finding of orthopnea distinguished between those patients with abnormally low ejection fraction (<0.50) and those with normal ejection fraction with a sensitivity of 97%, specificity of 64%, positive LR of 2.7 and negative LR of 0.04.[52] This suggests that, in patients with lung disease, the *presence* of orthopnea has limited value (i.e., occurs in both lung and heart disease), but the *absence* of orthopnea is more compelling, arguing *against* the presence of associated left ventricular dysfunction (LR = 0.04).

3. **Pathogenesis.** In patients with orthopnea, lung compliance and vital capacity fall significantly after moving from the upright to supine position. This explains in part why dyspnea worsens in the supine position and why orthopnea is a finding common to so many different clinical conditions.[51,53] Nonetheless, orthopnea cannot be entirely caused by postural changes in lung mechanics, for several reasons. First, orthopnea is uncommon in other disorders with similar reductions of vital capacity and compliance (e.g., interstitial fibrosis). Second, in patients with congestive heart failure, orthopnea correlates poorly with the pulmonary artery wedge pressure, which should have some relation to interstitial edema and pulmonary mechanics.[54] Finally, elevation of the head alone brings prompt relief to some orthopneic patients. It was once believed that elevation of the head relieved dyspnea because it reduced intracranial venous pressure and thus improved cerebral perfusion, although this hypothesis has been experimentally disproved.[51]

B. Trepopnea

1. **Finding.** Trepopnea[b] (from Greek *trepo*, meaning "twist" or "turn") describes dyspnea that is worse in one lateral decubitus position and relieved in the other.

---

[b] In 1937, Drs. Wood and Wolferth first described trepopnea in patients with congestive heart failure.[55] In searching for a name for the finding, a patent lawyer suggested to them "rolling relief," which they translated into "rotopnea," until a Dr. Kern pointed out that "roto" was a Latin root and the pure Greek term "trepopnea" would be better.[56]

2. **Clinical significance.** There are three causes of trepopnea.
   a. **Unilateral lung disease.**[57,58] Affected patients usually prefer to position their healthy lung down, which improves oxygenation because blood preferentially flows to the lower lung.
   b. **Congestive heart failure from dilated cardiomyopathy.**[55,56] Patients usually prefer to have their right side down. Whether this is due to a position-dependent deterioration of oxygenation (e.g., the large heart compresses the left lung, leading to more unfavorable gas exchange when the left side is dependent) or mechanical compression of airways is not clear.
   c. **Mediastinal or endobronchial tumor.** Tumors may compress the airway in one position but not the other.[59,60] A clue to this diagnosis is a localized wheeze that appears in the position causing symptoms.[59]

C. **Platypnea**
   1. **Finding.** Platypnea (from the Greek *platus*, meaning "flat") is the opposite of orthopnea: patients experience worse dyspnea when they sit up and relief when they lie down (a related term, "orthodeoxia," described a similar deterioration of oxygen saturation in the upright position). This rare syndrome was first described in 1949, and the term "platypnea" was first coined in 1969.[61,62]
   2. **Clinical significance.** Platypnea occurs in patients with right-to-left shunting of blood through intracardiac or intrapulmonary shunts.
      a. **Right-to-left shunting** of blood through a **patent foramen ovale** or atrial septal defect. These patients often first develop the finding after undergoing pneumo-

nectomy or developing a pulmonary embolus or pericardial effusion, which for unclear reasons promotes right-to-left shunting in the upright position.[63-67]

b. Right-to-left shunting of blood through **intrapulmonary shunts** located in the bases of the lungs, which occurs in the hepatopulmonary syndrome, a complication of chronic liver disease.[68] In these patients, the upright position causes more blood to flow to the bases, thus aggravating the right-to-left shunting of blood and the patient's hypoxemia.

REFERENCES

1. Stokes W. *An introduction to the use of the stethoscope* (facsimile edition by the Classics of Cardiology Library), Edinburgh, 1825, Maclachlin & Stewart.

2. Geddes LA. Perspectives in physiological monitoring, *Med Instrument* 10:91-97, 1976.

3. Osler W. *The principles and practice of medicine* (facsimile by Classics of Medicine library), Birmingham, 1892, Gryphon Editions.

4. Krieger B and others. Continuous noninvasive monitoring of respiratory rate in critically ill patients, *Chest* 90:632-634, 1986.

5. Kory RC. Routine measurement of respiratory rate: An expensive tribute to tradition. *JAMA* 165:448-450, 1957.

6. Hooker EA and others. Respiratory rates in emergency department patients, *J Emerg Med* 7:129-132, 1989.

7. McFadden JP and others. Raised respiratory rate in elderly patients: a valuable physical sign, *Br Med J* 284:626-627, 1982.

8. Quetelet LAJ. *A treatise on man and the development of his faculties* (1969 facsimile by Scholars facsimiles and reprints), Edinburgh, 1842, William and Robert Chambers.

9. Mulroy MF. Monitoring opioids, *Reg Anesthesia* 21:89-93, 1996.

10. Gravelyn TR and Weg JG. Respiratory rate as an indicator of acute respiratory dysfunction, *JAMA* 244:1123-1125, 1980.

11. Tobin MJ and others. The pattern of breathing during successful and unsuccessful trials of weaning from mechanical ventilation, *Am Rev Respir Dis* 134:1111-1118, 1986.

12. Fieselmann JF and others. Respiratory rate predicts cardiopulmonary arrest for internal medicine inpatients, *J Gen Intern Med* 8:354-360, 1993.

13. Heckerling PS. The need for chest roentgenograms in adults with acute respiratory illness: clinical predictors, *Arch Intern Med* 146:1321-1324, 1986.

14. Research Committee of the British Thoracic Society. Community-acquired pneumonia in adults in British hospitals in 1982-1983: a survey of aetiology, mortality, prognostic factors and outcome, *Quart J Med* 62:195-220, 1987.

15. Conte HA and others. A prognostic rule for elderly patients admitted with community-acquired pneumonia, *Am J Med* 106:20-28, 1999.

16. Farr BM, Sloman AJ, and Fisch MJ. Predicting death in patients hospitalized for community-acquired pneumonia, *Ann Intern Med* 115:428-436, 1991.

17. Brancati FL and others. Is pneumonia really the old man's friend? Two-year prognosis after community-acquired pneumonia, *Lancet* 342:30-33, 1993.

18. Cohen CA and others. Clinical manifestations of inspiratory muscle fatigue, *Am J Med* 73:308-316, 1982.

19. Mower WR and others. A comparison of pulse oximetry and respiratory rate in patient screening, *Resp Med* 90:593-599, 1996.

20. Webb P. Periodic breathing during sleep, *J Appl Physiol* 37:899-903, 1974.

21. Altschule MD and Iglauer A. The effect of position on periodic breathing in chronic cardiac decompensation, *N Engl J Med* 259:1064-1066, 1958.

22. Mortara A and others. Association between hemodynamic impairment and Cheyne-Stokes respiration and periodic breathing in chronic stable congestive heart failure secondary to ischemic or idiopathic dilated cardiomyopathy, *Am J Cardiol* 84:900-904, 1999.

23. Sternbach GL. John Cheyne and William Stokes: periodic respiration, *J Emerg Med* 3:233-236, 1985.

24. Morse SR, Chandrasekhar AJ, and Cugell DW. Cheyne-Stokes respiration redefined, *Chest* 66:345-346, 1974.

25. Lange RL and Hecht HH. The mechanism of Cheyne-Stokes respiration, *J Clin Invest* 41:42-52, 1962.

26. Franklin KA and others. Hemodynamics, cerebral circulation, and oxygen saturation in Cheyne-Stokes respiration, *J Appl Physiol* 83:1184-1191, 1997.

27. Tobin MJ and Snyder JV. Cheyne-Stokes respiration revisited: controversies and implications, *Crit Care Med* 12:882-887, 1984.

28. Dowell AR and others. Cheyne-Stokes respiration: a review of clinical manifestations and critique of physiological mechanisms, *Arch Intern Med* 127:712-726, 1971.

29. Harrison TR and others. Congestive heart failure: XX. Cheyne-Stokes respiration as the cause of paroxysmal dyspnea at the onset of sleep, *Arch Intern Med* 53:891-910, 1934.

30. Rees PJ and Clark TJH. Paroxysmal nocturnal dyspnea and periodic respiration, *Lancet* 2:1315-1317, 1979.

31. Lee MC and others. Respiratory rate and pattern disturbances in acute brainstem infarction, *Stroke* 7:382-385, 1976.

32. Brown HW and Plum F. The neurologic basis of Cheyne-Stokes respiration, *Am J Med* 30:849-860, 1961.

33. Andreas S and others. Cheyne-Stokes respiration and prognosis in congestive heart failure, *Am J Cardiol* 78:1260-1264, 1996.

34. Hanly PJ and Zuberi-Khokhar NS. Increased mortality associated with Cheyne-Stokes respiration in patients with congestive heart failure, *Am J Respir Crit Care Med* 153:272-276, 1996.

35. Findley LJ and others. Cheyne-Stokes breathing during sleep in patients with left ventricular heart failure, *South Med J* 78:11-15, 1985.

36. Karp HR, Sieker HO, and Heyman A. Cerebral circulation and function in Cheyne-Stokes respiration, *Am J Med* 30:861-870, 1961.

37. Javaheri S. A mechanism of central sleep apnea in patients with heart failure, *N Engl J Med* 341:949-954, 1999.

38. Naughton MT. Pathophysiology and treatment of Cheyne-Stokes respiration, *Thorax* 53:514-518, 1998.

39. Poole SR, Chetham M, and Anderson M. Grunting respirations in infants and children, *Pediatr Emerg Care* 11:158-161, 1995.

40. Grinman S and Whitelaw WA. Pattern of breathing in a case of generalized respiratory muscle weakness, *Chest* 84:770-772, 1983.

41. Barach AL. Physiologic advantages of grunting, groaning, and pursed-lip breathing: adaptive symptoms related to the development of continuous positive pressure breathing, *Bull NY Acad Med* 49:666-673, 1973.

42. Knelson JH, Howatt WF, and DeMutyh GR. The physiologic significance of grunting respiration, *Pediatrics* 44:393-400, 1969.

43. Loh L, Goldman M, and Newsome Davis J. The assessment of diaphragm function, *Medicine* 56:165-169, 1977.

44. Goldman MD and others. Asynchronous thoracoabdominal movements in chronic airflow obstruction (CAO), *Adv Exp Med Biol* 393:95-100, 1995.

45. Sharp JT and others. Relative contributions of rib cage and abdomen to breathing in normal subjects, *J Appl Physiol* 39:608-618, 1975.

46. Gilbert R and others. Prospective study of controlled oxygen therapy: poor prognosis of patients with asynchronous breathing, *Chest* 71:456-462, 1977.

47. Ashutosh K and others. Asynchronous breathing movements in patients with chronic obstructive pulmonary disease, *Chest* 67:553-557, 1975.

48. Mier-Jedrzejowicz A and others. Assessment of diaphragm weakness, *Am Rev Respir Dis* 137:877-883, 1988.

49. Chan CK and others. Bilateral diaphragmatic paralysis: clinical spectrum, prognosis, and diagnostic approach, *Arch Phys Med Rehabil* 69:976-979, 1988.

50. Newsom Davis J and others. Diaphragm function and alveolar hypoventilation, *Quart J Med* 45:87-100, 1976.

51. Calhoun JA and others. Studies in congestive heart failure. XIV. Orthopnea: its relation to ventilation, vital capacity, oxygen saturation and acid-base condition of arterial and jugular blood, *J Clin Invest* 10:833-855, 1931.

52. Zema MJ, Masters AP, and Margouleff D. Dyspnea: the heart or the lungs? Differentiation at bedside by use of the simple Valsalva maneuver, *Chest* 85:59-64, 1984.

53. Sharp JT, Rakowski D, and Keefer D. The effect of body position change on lung compliance in normal subjects and in patients with congestive heart failure, *J Clin Invest* 38:659-667, 1959.

54. Chakko S and others. Clinical, radiographic, and hemodynamic correlations in chronic congestive heart failure: conflicting results may lead to inappropriate care, *Am J Med* 90:353-359, 1991.

55. Wood FC and Wolferth CC. The tolerance of certain cardiac patients for various recumbent positions (trepopnea), *Am J Med Sci* 193:354-378, 1937.

56. Wood FC. Trepopnea, *Arch Intern Med* 104:966-973, 1959.

57. Zack MB, Pontoppidan H, and Kazemi H. The effect of lateral positions on gas exchange in pulmonary disease: a prospective evaluation, *Am Rev Respir Dis* 110:49-55, 1974.

58. Remolina C and others. Positional hypoxemia in unilateral lung disease, *N Engl J Med* 304:523-525, 1981.

59. Acosta J, Khan F, and Chitkara R. Trepopnea resulting from large aneurysm of sinus of Valsalva and descending aorta, *Heart Lung* 11:342-344, 1982.

60. Mahler DA and others. Positional dyspnea and oxygen desaturation related to carcinoma of the lung: up with the good lung, *Chest* 83:826-827, 1983.

61. Altman M and Robin ED. Platypnea (diffuse zone 1 phenomenon?), *N Engl J Med* 281:1347-1348, 1969.

62. Robin ED and McCauley RF. An analysis of platypnea-orthodeoxia syndrome, including a "new" therapeutic approach, *Chest* 112:1449-1451, 1997.

63. LaBresh KA and others. Platypnea syndrome after left pneumonectomy, *Chest* 79:605-607, 1981.

64. Seward JB and others. Platypnea-orthodeoxia: clinical profile, diagnostic workup, management, and report of seven cases, *Mayo Clin Proc* 59:221-231, 1984.

65. Wright RS and others. Eosinophilic endomyocardial disease presenting as cyanosis, platypnea, and orthodeoxia, *Ann Intern Med* 117:482-483, 1992.

66. Adolph EA and others. Reversible orthodeoxia and platypnea due to right-to-left intracardiac shunting related to pericardial effusion, *Ann Intern Med* 116:138-139, 1992.

67. Begin R. Platypnea after pneumonectomy, *N Engl J Med* 293:342-343, 1975.

68. Robin ED and others. Platypnea related to orthodeoxia caused by true vascular lung shunts, *N Engl J Med* 294:941-943, 1976.

CHAPTER 18

Pulse Oximetry

I. INTRODUCTION. Pulse oximetry measures the arterial oxygen saturation rapidly and conveniently. It is now regarded the fifth vital sign,[1,2] although some clinicians argue that pulse oximetry is a diagnostic test, not a physical sign, because it requires special equipment. Measurement of oxygen saturation, however, is no different from the other vital signs whose measurement requires a thermometer, sphygmomanometer, or stopwatch.

Takuo Aoyagi of Japan discovered the basic principle of pulse oximetry—pulsatile transmission of light through tissue depends on the patient's arterial saturation—in the mid-1970s. The first pulse oximeters were successfully marketed in the 1980s.[3]

II. THE FINDING. Measurements are obtained by using a self-adhesive or clip-type probe attached to the patient's finger or ear. The oximeter makes several hundred measurements each second and then displays an average value based on the previous 3 to 6 seconds, which is updated about every second.[4] Although the digital display of pulse oximeters creates a sense of precision, studies show that, between oxygen saturation levels of 70% to 100%, pulse oximeters are only accurate within 5% (i.e., ±2 standard deviations) of measurements made by in vitro arterial blood gas analysis using co-oximetry.[3,5,6]

The most common causes of inadequate oximeter signals are poor perfusion due to cold or hypotension, excessive ambient light, and motion artifact. The clinician can sometimes correct these problems and thus improve the signal by warming or rubbing the patient's hand, repositioning the probe, or resting the patient's hand on a soft surface.[4] If inadequate signals persist, the clinician should try obtaining measurements with the clip probe attached to the lobule or pinna of the patient's ear.

III. CLINICAL SIGNIFICANCE

A. Advantages of pulse oximetry. As a sign of low oxygen levels, pulse oximetry is superior to the physical sign of cyanosis, because oximetry is more sensitive and because readings do not depend on the patient's hemoglobin level (see Chapter 7). Consequently, pulse oximetry has become indispensable in the monitoring of patients in emergency departments, recovery and operating rooms, pulmonary clinics, and intensive care units, where measurements often reveal unsuspected oxygen desaturation, leading to changes in diagnosis and treatment.[7] Oxygen therapy prolongs survival of some hypoxemic patients, such as patients chronically hypoxemic from lung disease.[8,9] Presumably, oxygen therapy benefits patients with acute hypoxemia as well.

B. Limitations of pulse oximetry.[3,5,10] Because pulse oximetry readings indicate only the degree of oxygen saturation of hemoglobin, they fail to detect problems of poor oxygen delivery (e.g., anemia, poor cardiac output), hyperoxia, and hypercapnia. Other limitations of pulse oximetry measurements are discussed below.

1. Dyshemoglobinemias. The pulse oximeter interprets carboxyhemoglobin to be oxyhemoglobin and therefore seriously underestimates the degree of oxygen desaturation in patients with carbon monoxide poisoning. In patients with methemoglobinemia, the pulse oximetry readings decrease initially but eventually plateau at around 85%, despite true oxyhemoglobin levels that continue to decrease to much lower levels.

2. **Dyes.** Methylene blue causes a spurious decrease in oxygen saturation readings. Hyperbilirubinemia and jaundice, however, do not affect the pulse oximeter's accuracy.

3. **Low perfusion pressure.** In patients with hypotension or peripheral vascular disease, the arterial pulse may be so weak that the pulse oximeter is unable to pick up the arterial signal, thus making measurements difficult or impossible.

4. **Exaggerated venous pulsations.** In patients with right-sided heart failure or tricuspid regurgitation, the oximeter may mistake the venous waveform for the arterial one, leading to spuriously low oxygen saturation readings.

5. **Excessive ambient light.** Excessive ambient light (or malposition of the probe allowing ambient light to reach the sensor) also may interfere with the oximeter's accuracy, falsely lowering the value in patients with normal oxygen saturation and, more importantly, overestimating it in patients with significant hypoxemia.

REFERENCES

1. Tierney LM, Whooley MA, and Saint S. Oxygen saturation: a fifth vital sign? *West J Med* 166:285-286, 1997.
2. Neff TA. Routine oximetry: a fifth vital sign? *Chest* 94:227, 1988.
3. Tremper KK and Barker SJ. Pulse oximetry, *Anesthesiology* 70:98-108, 1989.

4. Hanning CD and Alexander-Williams JM. Pulse oximetry: a practical review, *Br Med J* 311:367-370, 1995.

5. Sinex JE. Pulse oximetry: principles and limitations, *Am J Emerg Med* 17:59-66, 1999.

6. Jensen LA, Onyskiw JE, and Prasad NGN. Meta-analysis of arterial oxygen saturation monitoring by pulse oximetry in adults, *Heart Lung* 27:387-408, 1998.

7. Mower WR and others. Pulse oximetry as a fifth vital sign in emergency geriatric assessment, *Acad Emerg Med* 5:858-865, 1998.

8. Medical Research Council Working Party. Long-term domiciliary oxygen therapy in chronic hypoxic cor pulmonale complicating chronic bronchitis and emphysema, *Lancet* 1:681-686, 1981.

9. Nocturnal Oxygen Therapy Trial Group. Continuous or nocturnal oxygen therapy in hypoxemic chronic obstructive lung disease: a clinical trial, *Ann Intern Med* 93:391-398, 1980.

10. Schnapp LM and Cohen NH. Pulse oximetry: uses and abuses, *Chest* 98:1244-1250, 1990.

PART FOUR

Head and Neck

CHAPTER 19

The Pupils

NORMAL PUPIL

I. INTRODUCTION. The integrity of the pupil depends on the iris, cranial nerves 2 and 3, and the sympathetic nerves innervating the eye.

II. SIZE. The size of the normal pupil decreases as persons grow older ($r = -0.75$, $p < .001$): At 10 years of age the mean diameter is 7 mm, at 30 years it is 6 mm, and at 80 years it is 4 mm.[1,2] Throughout human history, large pupils have been associated with youth, beauty, and vigor, explaining why the plant yielding the pupillary dilator atropine was named *belladonna*, which literally means "beautiful lady."

III. HIPPUS. Under steady illumination, the normal pupil is in continual motion, repeatedly dilating and contracting small amounts. This restless undulation, called "hippus" or "pupillary unrest," is more prominent in younger patients and during exposure to bright light. Clinicians of the nineteenth century associated hippus with all sorts of diseases, from myasthenia gravis to brain tumors, but hippus is now known to be a normal phenomenon.[3] The oscillations of the right and left pupil are synchronous, which suggests hippus is under central control.

IV. SIMPLE ANISOCORIA. Simple anisocoria, a normal finding, is defined as a 0.4 mm or more difference in size of the right and left pupil that cannot be attributed to any of the abnormal pupils discussed below, intraocular drugs, ocular injury, or ocular inflammation.[2] Simple anisocoria occurs in up to 38% of healthy persons (only half of these patients have anisocoria at any given moment) and affects 3% of persons all of the time. When simple anisocoria waxes and wanes, the same eye usually displays the larger pupil.[2]

The difference in pupil size in simple anisocoria rarely exceeds 1 mm.[2] Other features distinguishing it from pathologic anisocoria are described later under "abnormal pupils."

V. NORMAL LIGHT REFLEX

A. Anatomy. Figure 19-1 illustrates the nerves responsible for the normal light reflex. Because both pupillary constrictor muscles normally receive identical signals from the midbrain, they constrict the same amount, which may be small or large depending on the *summation* of light intensity coming into *both* eyes. For example, both pupils dilate the same amount in darkness, constrict an identical small amount when a dim light is held in front of one eye, and constrict an identical larger amount when a bright light is held in front of one eye.

With a light held in front of one eye, ipsilateral pupillary constriction is called "direct reaction" to light and contralateral constriction is called "consensual reaction."

B. Clinical significance. The anatomy of the normal light reflex has two important clinical implications:

1. Anisocoria is absent in disorders of the optic nerve or retina (i.e., the afferent connections). Because the signal in both

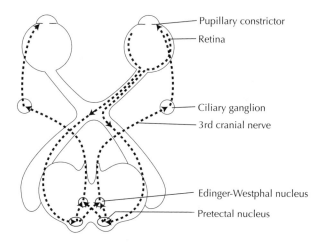

FIGURE 19-1 Anatomy of the pupillary light reflex. The dotted lines show how nerve impulses from the retina and optic nerve on one side (right eye in this example), contribute to the nerve impulses of both third nerves, via the crossing of the nerve impulses from the nasal retina in the optic chiasm and the abundant interconnections between both pretectal nuclei and both Edinger-Westphal nuclei. Unless there is asymmetric disease of the efferent pathway (i.e., third nerve, ciliary ganglion and postganglionic fibers, iris), the pupils are thus symmetric.

outgoing third nerves is identical in these disorders, representing the summation of light intensity from both eyes, the pupils are the same size. Unilateral afferent disease is similar to the experiment previously described of holding a bright light in front of one eye (i.e., the eye not being illuminated is similar to an eye with an afferent defect: despite receiving less light on one side, the pupils are the same).

2. **Anisocoria indicates asymmetric disease of the iris, third nerve, or sympathetic nerves (i.e., efferent connections and iris).** Asymmetric disease of the efferent connections guarantees that the signals arriving at the pupil are different and that the pupil size, therefore, will be different.

VI. NEAR SYNKINESIS REACTION. The near synkinesis reaction occurs when a person focuses on a near object. The reaction has three parts: (1) constriction of the pupils (pupilloconstrictor muscle), (2) convergence of eyes (medial rectus muscles), and (3) accommodation of the lenses (ciliary body).

ABNORMAL PUPILS

I. RELATIVE AFFERENT PUPILLARY DEFECT (MARCUS GUNN PUPIL)

A. Introduction. The relative afferent pupillary defect is the most common abnormal pupillary finding, more common than all other pupillary defects combined.[4]

Although the relative afferent pupillary defect was described by R. Marcus Gunn in 1904, it is clear from his report that the sign was generally known to clinicians of his time. Kestenbaum named the finding in 1946 after Marcus Gunn,[4] and in 1959, Levatin introduced the "swinging flashlight test," which is how most clinicians now elicit the finding.[5]

B. The finding. Because the pupils are equal in patients with disorders of the retina and optic nerves (see Normal Pupils above and Figure 19-1), the swinging flashlight test is necessary to uncover disorders of the afferent half of the light reflex. This test compares the amount of pupilloconstriction produced by illuminating one eye with that produced by illuminating the other.

To perform the test, the clinician swings the flashlight back and forth from eye to eye, holding it over each pupil 1 to 2 seconds at a time before immediately shifting it to the other. Both pupils constrict strongly when the light is shining into the normal eye, but, as the light moves to illuminate the abnormal eye, both pupils dilate (dilation occurs because the pupils respond as if the light were much dimmer, producing a smaller bilateral constriction—or net dilation—compared to when the light is shining in the normal eye).[4,6] As long as the clinician swings the light back and forth, the reaction persists—pupils constrict with light into the normal eye and dilate with light into the abnormal eye. Because the clinician usually just focuses on the illuminated pupil, the one that dilates is labeled as having a "relative afferent pupillary defect" or the "Marcus Gunn pupil."

There has been some debate whether eyes with afferent defects also display abnormal pupillary release (pupillary release occurs during steady illumination and is the small amount of pupillary dilation that immediately follows initial constriction).[7] Two careful studies, however, have shown that only the swinging flashlight test reliably uncovers the afferent defect.[8,9]

Light reflecting off the cornea may sometimes obscure the movements of the pupils. To overcome this, the clinician should angle the light to come from a point slightly below the horizontal axis.

Interpreting the swinging flashlight test has three caveats[6,10]:

1. **Correct interpretation of the test ignores hippus**, which otherwise can make interpretation difficult.

2. **The clinician should avoid the tendency to linger with the flashlight on the eye suspected to have disease.** Uneven swinging of the light may temporarily bleach the retina being illuminated more, thus eventually producing a relative pupillary defect and erroneously confirming the initial suspicion. To avoid this and ensure equal illumination of both retinas, the clinician should count to himself: "one, two, switch, one two, switch," and so on.

3. **Only one working iris is required to interpret this pupillary sign.** If the patient has only one pupil that reacts to light (see

Anisocoria below), the test is performed the same way, although the clinician focuses only on the normal iris to interpret the results.

C. Clinical significance. A relative afferent defect implies optic nerve or severe retinal disease of the ipsilateral eye.

1. **Optic nerve disease (e.g., optic neuritis, ischemic optic neuropathy).** Patients with optic nerve disease have the most prominent relative afferent pupillary defects. If the disease is asymmetric, the sensitivity of the finding is 92% to 98%, much higher than that for any other test of afferent function, including visual acuity, pupil cycle times, appearance of optic disc during fundoscopy, and visual evoked potentials.[11,12] The finding depends, however, on *asymmetric* optic nerve function (hence the word "relative" in its label); consequently, in patients with suspected unilateral disease but without the afferent pupillary finding, bilateral optic nerve disease is eventually found two thirds of the time.[12]

2. **Retinal disease.** Severe retinal disease may cause a relative afferent pupillary defect, although the retinal disease must be markedly asymmetric to produce the finding and, once the finding appears, it is subtle compared with that seen in optic nerve disease.[13]

3. **Cataracts do not cause the relative afferent pupillary defect.**[14] Although this seems surprising, it is because the retina, if healthy, compensates over minutes for any diminished brightness, just as it does when a person walks into a dark movie theater. In fact, in Galen's time it was known that an intact pupillary light reaction was a good prognostic sign for vision if cataract couching was being considered (i.e., the retina and optic nerve behind the cataract are intact).[4]

II. ARGYLL ROBERTSON PUPILS

A. The finding.[15,16] Argyll Robertson pupils have four characteristic findings: (1) bilateral involvement, (2) small pupils that fail to dilate fully in dim light, (3) no light reaction, and (4) brisk constriction to near vision and brisk redilation to far vision.

Originally described by Douglas Moray Cooper Lamb Argyll Robertson in 1868, this finding had great significance a century ago because it settled a long-standing debate whether general paresis and tabes dorsalis were the same disease. The pupillary abnormality was found in a high proportion of patients with both diseases and was limited to these diseases, arguing for a common syphilitic origin of both. The introduction of Wasserman's serologic test for syphilis in 1906 confirmed that the two diseases had the same cause.

B. Clinical significance

1. Associated disorders. In addition to neurosyphilis, there are rare, scattered reports of Argyll Robertson pupils in patients with various other disorders, including diabetes mellitus, neurosarcoidosis, and Lyme disease (see Diabetic Pupil below).[15] The responsible lesion is probably located in the dorsal midbrain, where damage would interrupt the light reflex fibers but spare the more ventrally located fibers innervating the Edinger-Westphal nuclei that control the near reaction.[17]

2. Differential diagnosis of light-near dissociation. Argyll Robertson pupils display light-near dissociation, that is, they fail to react to light but constrict during near vision. Several other causes of light-near dissociation include the following:

a. Adie's tonic pupil (see below)

b. Optic nerve or severe retinal disease. Either of these disorders may eliminate the light reaction when light is directed into the abnormal eye, although the pupils still constrict with the near synkinesis. In contrast to other causes of light-near dissociation, however, optic nerve and retinal disease severely impair vision.

c. **Dorsal midbrain syndrome** (also known as "Parinaud's syndrome," "Sylvian aqueduct syndrome," or "pretectal syndrome"). Characteristic findings of dorsal midbrain syndrome are light-near dissociation, vertical gaze palsy, lid retraction, and convergence-retraction nystagmus (a rhythmic inward movement of both eyes from cocontraction of the extraocular muscles, usually elicited during convergence or upward gaze; most neuroophthlamologists use a optokinetic drum rotating downward to elicit the finding). Common causes of the dorsal midbrain syndrome are pinealoma in younger patients and multiple sclerosis and basilar artery strokes in older patients.[18]

d. **Aberrant regeneration of the third nerve.** After damage to the third nerve (from trauma, aneurysms, or tumors but *not* ischemia), regenerating fibers originally destined for the medial rectus muscle may instead reinnervate the pupillary constrictor, thus causing pupillary constriction during convergence but no reaction to light. Unlike Argyll Robertson pupils, however, this finding is unilateral, and most patients also have anisocoria, ptosis, and diplopia.[19,20]

3. **"Near-light dissociation."** The phenomenon opposite to light-near dissociation, "near-light dissociation" describes pupils that react to light but not during the near synkinesis.

Near-light dissociation was historically described as a finding of von Economo's encephalitis lethargica, although now it usually
means the patient is not trying hard enough
to focus on a near object.[15] For this reason,
many neuroophthalmologists save time during their examination and skip testing the
near response unless the patient demonstrates no pupillary light reaction.

III. **OVAL PUPIL.** There are three causes of the oval
pupil.
   A. **Evolving third nerve palsy from brain
      herniation.** These patients are invariably co-
      matose from cerebral catastrophes causing ele-
      vated intracranial pressure.[21,22] As the pupil
      marches on to become fully round, dilated, and
      fixed, it may appear oval for a short time.
   B. **Adies tonic pupil** (see below) may sometimes
      appear oval from segmental iris palsy.[23] These
      patients are alert and, if complaining of any-
      thing, describe only blurring of vision in the in-
      volved eye (from paralysis of accommodation).
   C. **Previous surgery or trauma to the iris**

IV. **ANISOCORIA**
   A. **Definition.** Anisocoria is defined as a differ-
      ence of 0.4 mm or more in the diameter of the
      pupils. It represents either a problem with the
      pupillary constrictor muscle (parasympathetic
      denervation, iris disorder, pharmacologic pupil)
      or the pupillary dilator muscle (sympathetic
      denervation, simple anisocoria).
   B. **Technique.** Figure 19-2 summarizes the ap-
      proach to anisocoria. The most important initial
      questions follow:
      1. **Is the anisocoria old or new?** Examina-
         tion of driver's license photograph or other
         facial photograph, magnified with the direct
         ophthalmoscope (using the +10 lens), may
         reveal a preexisting pupillary inequality.[26]

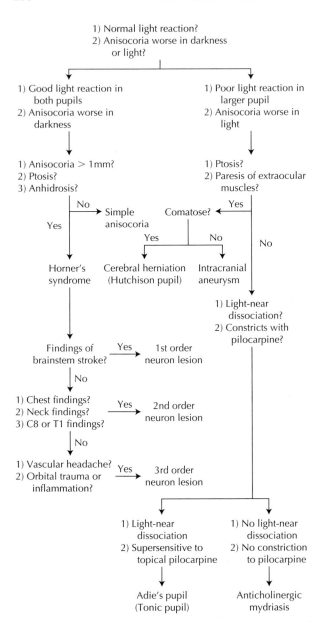

FIGURE 19-2 For legend see opposite page.

FIGURE 19-2 Summary of approach to anisocoria. The first two questions (Is there a normal light reaction? and Is anisocoria worse in darkness or light?) distinguish problems with the pupillary dilator muscle (i.e., Horner's syndrome, simple anisocoria; *left side* of Figure 19-2) from problems with the pupillary constrictor muscle (i.e., third cranial nerve, iris; *right side* of Figure 19-2). Two other tests distinguish Horner's syndrome from simple anisocoria: the cocaine test (see text) and pupillary dilator lag (i.e., the pupil dilates slowly in darkness, as documented by photographs). (Figure 19-2 is based on references 24 and 25.)

---

2. **Do both pupils constrict normally during the light reflex?** If there is a poor light reaction in the eye with the larger pupil, the pupillary constrictor of that eye is abnormal. If there is a good light reaction in both eyes, the pupillary dilator of the eye with the smaller pupil is abnormal.

3. **Is the anisocoria worse in bright light or dim light/darkness?** If anisocoria is worse in light than darkness, the pupillary constrictor of the eye with the larger pupil is abnormal. If anisocoria is worse in darkness than light, the pupillary dilator of the eye with the smaller pupil is abnormal.[a][27]

C. **Abnormal pupillary constrictor (the "fixed, dilated pupil," due to parasympathetic defect, iris disorder, or pharmacologic blockade).** The most important questions in these patients are (1) Is there a full third nerve palsy or are the findings confined to the pupillary constrictor? and (2) Is there altered mental status or other neurologic findings?

---

[a] To determine the amount of anisocoria in darkness, neuroophthalmologists often take a flash picture of the patient in darkness. Because there is a delay of about 1.5 seconds between the flash of light and subsequent pupillary constriction, such a picture actually reflects pupil size in darkness (this delay explains why cameras designed to reduce "red eye" actually flash repeatedly *before* the picture is taken).[4]

1. **Full third nerve palsy: Associated ptosis and paralysis of ocular movements.** Because the third cranial nerve controls the levator palpebrae (which lifts the eyelid) and four of the six eye muscles (medial, inferior, and superior recti, and inferior oblique), a full third nerve palsy causes a dilated pupil, ptosis, ophthalmoplegia, and an eye that is deviated outward and downward. In patients with anisocoria, this has two important causes:

   a. **Ipsilateral brain herniation (Hutchinson pupil).**[28,29] These patients are in the midst of a neurologic catastrophe from an expanding unilateral cerebral mass that causes coma, damage to the ipsilateral third nerve (dilated pupil, ptosis, and ophthalmoplegia), and eventually, damage to the contralateral cerebral peduncle (hemiplegia on the *same* side of the lesion). Although the involvement of the ocular muscles may be difficult to recognize, most patients have a narrowed palpebral fissure and an eye that, if not dysconjugate, moves poorly during the vestibuloocular reflex. The expanding mass is on the same side as the dilated pupil 77% to 96% of the time.[30-32]

   b. **Posterior communicating artery aneurysm.** Posterior communicating artery aneurysms are the most common of all intracranial aneurysms. Twenty to 61% of patients present with a ipsilateral third nerve palsy, which dilates the pupil. It is essential to recognize this disorder promptly because of the risk of subsequent devastating subarachnoid hemorrhage. Importantly, the abnormal pupil is almost always accompanied by ptosis and ophthalmoplegia (i.e., full third nerve palsy): In reports of 332 aneurysms that

give details of the third nerve paresis,
71% had dilated pupil and complete ophthalmoplegia, 25% had dilated pupil and
partial ophthalmoplegia, 4% had sparing
of the pupil with partial ophthalmoplegia, and only 1 patient had isolated
involvement of the pupil.[33-41]

2. The tonic pupil

a. The finding. The tonic pupil has five
important features: (1) unilateral dilation
of a pupil; (2) poor or absent response to
light; (3) extensive, slow (over seconds),
and long-lasting constriction during near
vision (this is why the pupil is "tonic,"
that is, it is analogous to "myotonia");
(4) disturbances of accommodation,
which causes the main concern for many
patients, (i.e., an inability to focus vision in the involved eye) and (5) super-
sensitivity of pupillary constriction to
pilocarpine.[23,42,43]

Although both the Argyll Robertson
pupil and the tonic pupil display light-
near dissociation, they are easily distinguished by the characteristics in Table 19-1.

b. Pathogenesis. The tonic pupil occurs
because of injury to the ciliary ganglion

**TABLE 19-1 Comparison between tonic and Argyll
Robertson pupil**

FINDING	TONIC PUPIL	ARGYLL ROBERTSON PUPILS
Pupil size	Large	Small
Laterality	Mostly unilateral	Mostly bilateral
Reaction to near vision	Extremely slow and prolonged with slow redilation	Normal with brisk redilation

Based on reference 42.

and postganglionic fibers (see Figure 19-1) and subsequent misdirection of nerve fibers as they regenerate from the ciliary ganglion to the eye. In the normal eye, the ciliary ganglion sends 30 times the number of nerve fibers to the ciliary body (the muscle that focuses the lens during the near synkinesis) as to the iris (i.e., the pupillary constrictor).[44] Once these fibers are disrupted, odds are 30 to 1 that the iris will receive regenerating fibers that were originally intended for the ciliary body instead of the normal ones that participate in the light reaction. The pupil of these patients thus fails to respond to light, although during near vision, which normally activates the ciliary body, the misdirected fibers to the iris cause the pupil to constrict (i.e., light-near dissociation).

c. Clinical significance. Because the ciliary ganglion and postganglionic fibers are contiguous to the eyeball, any of various injuries may cause the tonic pupil, including orbital trauma, orbital tumors, or *Varicella zoster* infections of the ophthalmic division of the trigeminal nerve. Most cases, however, are idiopathic, which has been dubbed "Adie's pupil" (named after William John Adie, although the syndrome was more thoroughly and accurately described by others before his 1931 paper).[42]

3. Disorders of the iris

a. Pharmacologic blockade of the pupil with topical anticholinergic drugs. Pharmacologic blockade causes an isolated fixed, dilated pupil without paralysis of eye movements. Not all patients with this problem are surreptitiously instilling mydriatic drops. Causes include

unintended exposure of the eye to anticholinergic nebulizer treatments,[45] scopol-
amine patches,[46] and plants containing
anticholinergic substances (blue nightshade, angel's trumpet, jimsonweed).[47-49]
Nebulizer treatments are an important
cause to recognize in the intensive care
unit, where metabolic encephalopathy is
also common, leading clinicians to misdiagnose the Hutchison pupil in patients with pharmacologic anisocoria and
unresponsiveness.

The pharmacologic pupil characteristically fails to constrict to topical pilocarpine (see below).

4. **The poorly reactive pupil—response to
pilocarpine.** In difficult diagnostic problems, especially when pharmacologic blockade is a consideration, the pupil's response
to topical pilocarpine solution is very helpful. Pilocarpine constricts Adie's pupil and
the dilated pupil from parasympathetic denervation (Hutchinson pupil, aneurysm), but
not the dilated pupil from pharmacologic
blockade.[50]

D. **Abnormal pupillary dilator**
1. **Definition.** The most important cause of an
abnormal pupillary dilator muscle is sympathetic denervation of the pupil, or **Horner's
syndrome**, which has three characteristics:
(1) ipsilateral miosis (paralyzed pupillodila-
tor muscle), (2) ipsilateral ptosis (paralyzed
superior tarsal muscle), and (3) ipsilateral
anhidrosis of the face (from damage to sudomotor fibers). Figure 19-3 describes the neuroanatomy of the sympathetic pathways innervating the eye.

Horner's syndrome is named after the
Swiss ophthalmologist Johann Horner, who
published a description of the syndrome in
1869. Like other eponymous pupillary find-

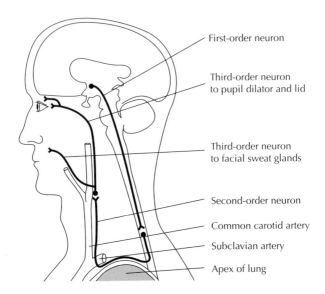

First-order neuron

Third-order neuron
to pupil dilator and lid

Third-order neuron
to facial sweat glands

Second-order neuron

Common carotid artery

Subclavian artery

Apex of lung

FIGURE 19-3 Anatomy of sympathetic pathways to the eye. The sympathetic innervation of the eye consists of three neurons connected in series: first-order neurons, second-order neurons, and third-order neurons. The first-order neurons ("central" neurons) extend from the posterior hypothalamus to the C8-T2 level of the spinal cord. The second-order neurons ("preganglionic" neurons) leave the spinal cord and travel over the lung apex, around the subclavian artery, and along the carotid artery to the superior cervical ganglion. The third-order neurons ("postganglionic neurons") diverge and take two paths: those to the pupil and lid muscles travel along the internal carotid artery through the cavernous sinus to reach the orbit; those to the facial sweat glands travel with the external carotid artery to the face. Lesions in any of these neurons cause Horner's syndrome and distinct physical signs (see Figure 19-2 and text).

ings (Adie and Marcus Gunn), other clinicians had published earlier descriptions of the same finding.[51]

2. **Horner's syndrome vs. simple anisocoria.** When evaluating a pupil that dilates abnormally (left half of Figure 19-2), the findings of anisocoria greater than 1 mm, associated ptosis, or asymmetric facial sweating all indicate Horner's syndrome.

In difficult cases, the definitive test of sympathetic denervation is the cocaine test (cocaine drops diminish the anisocoria of simple anisocoria but aggravate that of Horner's syndrome).[b] In one study of 169 persons, postcocaine anisocoria of 1 mm or more detected Horner's syndrome with a sensitivity of 95%, specificity of 99%, and positive LR of 96.8, and negative LR of 0.1.[52,53]

3. **Clinical significance of Horner's syndrome**

   a. **Etiology.** Which etiologies of Horner's syndrome a clinician is likely to see depends on the clinician's specialty. On a neurologic service, 70% of patients with Horner's syndrome have lesions in the first-order neuron, usually strokes in the brainstem (see Table 55-2 in Chapter 55).[54] On a medical service, 70% of patients have a lesion in the second-order neuron, usually from tumors (e.g., lung and thyroid) or trauma (e.g., to the neck, chest, spinal nerves, subclavian or carotid arteries).[51] Causes of lesions in the third-order neuron are vascular headache, skull fracture, and cavernous sinus syndrome.[55,56]

   b. **Localizing the lesion**

      (1) **Associated findings.** Helpful features are (1) findings from the ipsilateral brainstem (e.g., lateral medullary syndrome), pointing to a first-order neuron lesion (see Table 55-2 in Chapter 55); (2) abnormal chest or neck findings, a supraclavicular mass, or motor, reflex, or sensory findings of the ipsilateral C_8-T_1 spinal roots, all

---

[b] Cocaine eye drops block the reuptake of norepinephrine at the myoneural junction of the iris dilator, causing the pupil to dilate unless norepinephrine is absent because of sympathetic denervation.

pointing to the second order neuron lesion; and (3) orbital trauma, orbital inflammation, migraine or neck pain, pointing to a third order neuron lesion.

(2) *Facial sweating.* The sudomotor sympathetic fibers to the face diverge from the sympathetic pathway at the bifurcation of the carotid artery and therefore do not accompany the sympathetic nerves to the pupil and lid. Theoretically, therefore, Horner's syndrome from third-order neuron lesions would preserve facial sweating, whereas Horner's syndrome from first- and second-order neurons would cause asymmetric facial sweating. In one study, however, this finding lacked diagnostic value: the finding of asymmetric facial sweating argued *for* a first- or second-order lesion and *against* a third-order lesion with a sensitivity of only 53%, a specificity of 78%, and a positive LR that was not significant.[57]

(3) *Paredrine test.* In rare patients whose Horner's syndrome remains unexplained, the "Paredrine test" was historically used to identify the site of the lesion. In first- and second-order neuron lesions, but not third-order neuron lesions, topical Paredrine (hydroxyamphetamine) causes pupillary dilation.[55,56] Paredrine is no longer readily available; however, the homologous compound Pholedrine (hydroxymethylamphetamine) may serve as a substitute.[58,59]

E. Intraocular inflammation. As part of the eye's response to intraocular inflammation, the ipsilateral pupil often constricts. In one study of

317 patients with the unilaterally red eye, anisocoria of 1 mm or more with the small pupil in the red eye detected serious eye diseases (i.e., corneal foreign body or abrasion, keratitis, and uveitis) and distinguished it from more benign problems (i.e., subconjunctival hemorrhage, conjunctivitis) with a sensitivity of 19%, specificity of 97%, positive LR of 6.5, and negative LR of 0.8.[60]

V. DIABETES AND THE PUPIL. The pupils of patients with long-standing diabetes show signs of sympathetic denervation (small size and poor dilation in darkness)[1,61-66] and parasympathetic denervation (sluggish light reaction).[1,61,64,65,67] Diabetes also reduces the amplitude of hippus.[1,68] Denervation alone, however, does not explain all of the diabetic pupillary abnormalities, because the pupils of many patients also respond poorly to dilating and constricting eye drops, which suggests an additional disorder of the iris itself (i.e., denervated pupils are classically supersensitive to eye drops).[63] Some reviews state that diabetes causes the Argyll Robertson pupil, but the data for this are meager and what exists suggests that the finding is rare.[15,69,70]

REFERENCES

1. Smith SE and others. Pupillary signs in diabetic autonomic neuropathy, *Br Med J* 2:924-927, 1978.
2. Lam BL, Thompson HS, and Corbett JJ. The prevalence of simple anisocoria, *Am J Ophthalmol* 104:69-73, 1987.
3. Thompson HS, Franceschetti AT, and Thompson PM. Hippus: semantic and historic considerations of the word, *Am J Ophthalmol* 71:1116-1120, 1971.
4. Thompson HS. Afferent pupillary defects: pupillary findings associated with defects of the afferent arm of the pupillary light reflex arc, *Am J Ophthalmol* 62:861-871, 1966.
5. Levatin P. Pupillary escape in disease of the retina or optic nerve, *Arch Ophthalmol* 62:768-779, 1959.

6. Thompson HS, Corbett JJ, and Cox TA. How to measure the relative afferent pupillary defect, *Surv Ophthalmol* 26: 39-42, 1981.

7. Landau WM. The Marcus Gunn phenomenon: loose canon of neuro-ophthalmology, *Neurology* 38:1141-1142, 1988.

8. Cox TA. Pupillary escape, *Neurology* 42:1271-1273, 1992.

9. Enyedi LB, Dev S, and Cox TA. A comparison of the Marcus Gunn and alternating light tests for afferent pupillary defects, *Ophthalmology* 105:871-873, 1998.

10. Thompson HS and Corbett JJ. Swinging flashlight test, *Neurology* 38:154-156, 1989.

11. Cox TA and others. Visual evoked potential and pupillary signs: a comparison in optic nerve disease, *Arch Ophthalmol* 100:1603-1606, 1982.

12. Cox TA, Thompson HS, and Corbett JJ. Relative afferent pupillary defects in optic neuritis, *Am J Ophthalmol* 92:685-690, 1981.

13. Newsome DA and Milton RC. Afferent pupillary defect in macular degeneration, *Am J Ophthalmol* 92:396-402, 1981.

14. Sadun AA, Bassi CJ, and Lessell S. Why cataracts do not produce afferent pupillary defects, *Am J Ophthalmol* 110: 712-714, 1990.

15. Loewenfeld IE. The Argyll Robertson pupil, 1869-1969: a critical survey of the literature, *Surv Ophthalmol* 14:199-299, 1969.

16. Dacso CC. Significance of the Argyll Robertson pupil in clinical medicine, *Am J Med* 86:199-202, 1989.

17. Poole CJM. Argyll Robertson pupils due to neurosarcoidosis: evidence for site of lesion, *Br Med J* 289:356, 1984.

18. David NJ. Optokinetic nystagmus: a clinical review, *J Clin Neuro-ophthalmol* 9:258-266, 1989.

19. Ford FR, Walsh FB, and King A. Clinical observations on the pupillary phenomena resulting from regeneration of the third nerve with especial reference to the Argyll Robertson pupil, *Bull Johns Hopkins Hosp* 68:309-318, 1941.

20. Spector RH and Faria MA. Aberrant regeneration of the inferior division of the oculomotor nerve, *Arch Neurol* 38:460-461, 1981.

21. Marshall LF and others. The oval pupil: clinical significance and relationship to intracranial hypertension, *J Neurosurg* 58:566-568, 1983.

22. Fisher CM. Oval pupils, *Arch Neurol* 37:502-503, 1980.

23. Thompson HS. Segmental palsy of the iris sphincter in Adie's syndrome, *Arch Ophthalmol* 96:1615-1620, 1978.

24. Czarnecki JSC, Pilley SFJ, and Thompson HS. The analysis of anisocoria: the use of photography in the clinical evaluation of unequal pupils, *Can J Ophthalmol* 14:297-302, 1979.

25. Thompson HS and Pilley SFJ. Unequal pupils. A flow chart for sorting out the anisocorias, *Surv Ophthalmol* 21:45-48, 1976.

26. Zito G and Gennaro P. Clinical evaluation of anisocoria, *Arch Neurol* 39:604, 1982 (letter).

27. Lam BL, Thompson HS, and Walls RC. Effect of light on the prevalence of simple anisocoria, *Ophthalmology* 103:790-793, 1996.

28. Sunderland S and Bradley KC. Disturbances of oculomotor function accompanying extradural haemorrhage, *J Neurol Neurosurg Psych* 16:35-46, 1953.

29. Ropper AH. The opposite pupil in herniation, *Neurology* 40:1707-1709, 1990.

30. Mitsumoto H, Conomy JP, and Regula G. Ophthalmologic aspects of subdural hematoma, *Cleve Clin Q* 44:101-105, 1977.

31. Stone JL and others. Subdural hematomas I. Acute subdural hematoma: progress in definition, clinical pathology, and therapy, *Surg Neurol* 19:216-231, 1983.

32. Talalla A and Morin MA. Acute traumatic subdural hematoma: a review of one hundred consecutive cases, *J Trauma* 11:771-777, 1971.

33. Fujiwara S and others. Oculomotor nerve palsy in patients with cerebral aneurysms, *Neurosurg Rev* 12:123-132, 1989.

34. Kissel JT and others. Pupil-sparing oculomotor palsies with internal carotid-posterior communicating artery aneurysms, *Ann Neurol* 13:149-154, 1983.

35. Capo H, Warren F, and Kupersmith MJ. Evolution of oculomotor nerve palsies, *J Clin Neuro-ophthalmol* 12:12-15, 1992.

36. Cogan DG and Mount HTJ. Intracranial aneurysms causing ophthalmoplegia, *Arch Ophthalmol* 70:757-771, 1963.

37. Green WR, Hackett ER, and Schlezinger NS. Neuro-ophthalmologic evaluation of oculomotor nerve paralysis, *Arch Ophthalmol* 72:154-167, 1964.

38. Rucker CW. The causes of paralysis of the third, fourth and sixth cranial nerves, *Am J Ophthalmol* 61:1293-1298, 1966.

39. Keane JR. Aneurysms and third nerve palsies, *Ann Neurol* 14:696-697, 1983.

40. Raja IA. Aneurysm-induced third nerve palsy, *J Neurosurg* 36:548-551, 1972.

41. Botterell EH, Lloyd LA, and Hoffman HJ. Oculomotor palsy due to supraclinoid internal carotid artery berry aneurysm, *Am J Ophthalmol* 54:609-616, 1962.

42. Loewenstein O and Loewenfeld IR. Pupillotonic pseudo-tabes (syndrome of Markus-Weill and Reys-Holmes-Adie): a critical review of the literature, *Surv Ophthalmol* 10:129-185, 1967.

43. Loewenfeld IR and Thompson HS. The tonic pupil: a re-evaluation, *Am J Ophthalmol* 63:46-87, 1967.

44. Warwick R. The ocular parasympathetic nerve supply and its mesencephalic sources, *J Anat* 88:71-93, 1954.

45. Helprin GA and Clarke GM. Unilateral fixed dilated pupil associated with nebulised ipratropium bromide, *Lancet* 2:1469, 1986.

46. Riddick FA and Jordan JD. Cruise ship anisocoria, *Ann Intern Med* 117:95, 1992.

47. Rubinfeld RS and Currie JN. Accidental mydriasis from blue nightshade "lipstick," *J Clin Neuro-ophthalmol* 7:34-37, 1987.

48. Savitt DL, Roberts JR, and Siegel EG. Anisocoria from jimsonweed, *JAMA* 255:1439-1440, 1986.

49. Voltz R and others. Gardener's mydriasis, *Lancet* 339:752, 1992.

50. Thompson HS, Newsome DA, and Loewenfeld IE. The fixed dilated pupil: sudden iridoplegia or mydriatic drops? A simple diagnostic test, *Arch Ophthalmol* 86:21-27, 1971.

51. Giles CL and Henderson JW. Horner's syndrome: an analysis of 216 cases, *Am J Ophthalmol* 46:289-296, 1958.

52. Kardon RH and others. Critical evaluation of the cocaine test in the diagnosis of Horner's syndrome, *Arch Ophthalmol* 108:384-387, 1990.

53. Kardon RH and others. The cocaine test and Horner's syndrome, *Arch Ophthalmol* 108:1667-1668, 1990.

54. Keane JR. Oculosympathetic paresis: analysis of 100 hospitalized patients, *Arch Neurol* 36:13-16, 1979.

55. Cremer SA and others. Hydroxyamphetamine mydriasis in Horner's syndrome, *Am J Ophthalmol* 110:71-76, 1990.

56. Van der Wiel HL and Van Gijn J. Localization of Horner's syndrome: use and limitations of the hydroxyamphetamine test, *J Neurol Sci* 59:229-235, 1983.

57. Rosenberg ML. The friction sweat test as a new method for detecting facial anhidrosis in patients with Horner's syndrome, *Am J Ophthalmol* 108:443-447, 1989.

58. Bates AT and others. Pholedrine: a substitute for hydroxyamphetamine as a diagnostic eyedrop test in Horner's syndrome, *J Neurol Neurosurg Psych* 58:215-217, 1995.

59. Burde RM and Thompson HS. Hydroxyamphetamine. A good drug lost? *Am J Ophthalmol* 111:100-102, 1991.

60. Rose GE and Pearson RV. Unequal pupil size in patients with unilateral red eye, *Br Med J* 302:571-572, 1991.

61. Hreidarsson AB and Gundersen HJG. The pupillary response to light in type 1 (insulin-dependent) diabetes, *Diabetologia* 28:815-821, 1985.

62. Hreidarsson AB. Pupil size in insulin-dependent diabetes: relationship to duration, metabolic control, and long-term manifestations, *Diabetes* 31:442-448, 1982.

63. Alio J and others. Pupil responsiveness in diabetes mellitus, *Ann Ophthalmol* 21:132-137, 1989.

64. Smith SA and Smith SE. Reduced pupillary light reflexes in diabetic autonomic neuropathy, *Diabetologia* 24:330-332, 1983.

65. Lanting P and others. Assessment of pupillary light reflex latency and darkness adapted pupil size in control subjects and in diabetic patients with and without cardiovascular autonomic neuropathy, *J Neurol Neurosurg Psych* 53:912-914, 1990.

66. Smith SA and Smith SE. Evidence for a neuropathic aetiology in the small pupil of diabetes mellitus, *Br J Ophthalmol* 67:89-93, 1983.

67. Friedman SA and others. Pupillary abnormalities in diabetic neuropathy, *Ann Intern Med* 67:977-983, 1967.

68. Hreidarsson AB and Gundersen HJG. Reduced pupillary unrest: autonomic nervous system abnormality in diabetes mellitus, *Diabetes* 37:446-451, 1988.

69. Waite JH and Beetham WP. The visual mechanism in diabetes mellitus (A comparative study of 2002 diabetics and 457 non-diabetics for control), *N Engl J Med* 212:367-379, 1935.

70. Martin MM. Diabetic neuropathy: a clinical study of 150 cases, *Brain* 76:594-624, 1953.

CHAPTER 20

Diabetic Retinopathy

I. **INTRODUCTION.** Diabetic retinopathy is the leading cause of blindness in adults between the ages of 25 and 74.[1] Whether a patient develops proliferative retinopathy depends to a large extent on the type and duration of diabetes: patients with type 1 diabetes have a 0% risk of proliferative retinopathy at 5 years after diagnosis, 4% at 10 years and 50% at 20 years, whereas those with type 2 diabetes, the risk is 3% to 4% at the time of diagnosis, 10% at 10 years and 20% at 15 years.[2] Once retinopathy develops, however, one of the best predictors of progression to sight-threatening retinopathy is the extent of retinopathy during the baseline examination: The higher the grade of retinopathy during the initial examination, the greater the risk of progression (Table 20-1). In type 1 diabetics, pregnancy increases the risk of progression 2.3-fold.[2]

In large cross-sectional surveys of diabetic patients examined by general practitioners, sight-threatening retinopathy (i.e., proliferative retinopathy and more severe forms of nonproliferative retinopathy) is found in 5% to 15% of patients.[7-11]

II. **THE FINDINGS.** The findings of diabetic retinopathy are divided into nonproliferative changes, which occur *within* the retina, and proliferative changes, which are located on the inner surface of

TABLE 20-1 Progression to high-risk proliferative diabetic retinopathy*

GRADE OF BASELINE RETINOPATHY	PRINCIPLE CLINICAL FINDINGS	CUMULATIVE RISK (%) OF HIGH-RISK PROLIFERATIVE RETINOPATHY AT VISIT:	
		1 YEAR	5 YEARS
Nonproliferative Retinopathy			
Mild	Microaneurysms	1	16
	Dot and blot hemorrhages		
	Soft exudates		
Moderate	Extensive microaneurysms and hemorrhages	3-8	27-39
	IRMA		
	Venous beading		
Severe	Same as moderate†	15	56
Very severe	Same as moderate†	45	71
Proliferative Retinopathy‡			
	Neovascularization	22-46	64-75
	Preretinal/vitreous hemorrhages		
	Fibrovascular proliferation		

IRMA, Intraretinal microvascular abnormalities (see text).

*High-risk proliferative retinopathy is NVD >1/4 disc area in size, NVD <1/4 disc area *and* vitreous or preretinal hemorrhage, or NVE >1/2 disc area *and* vitreous or preretinal hemorrhage.[3] These figures, based on references 4 and 5, assume that the patient is untreated.

†Moderate, severe, and very severe nonproliferative retinopathy share the same fundoscopic findings, although they differ in severity (based on standardized photographs)[6] and the number of retinal quadrants involved.[5]

‡Percentages are for patients whose baseline evaluation reveals proliferative retinopathy with less than high-risk characteristics.

the retina or in the vitreous.[12] The terms "background retinopathy" and "preproliferative retinopathy" are outdated and no longer recommended, having been replaced by the grades of retinopathy shown in Table 20-1.[13] Diabetic retinopathy progresses in an orderly fashion through these grades.

A. Nonproliferative changes. The earliest changes to appear in diabetic retinopathy are **microaneurysms**, which are distinct red, round spots that are less than 1/12 the diameter of an average optic disc, or 125 μm in its longest dimension (a long-standing convention assumes the average optic disc is 1500 μm in diameter; 125 μm is approximately the width of an average major vein at the disc margin).[6] **Dot hemorrhages** are larger red dots with sharp borders; red spots with indistinct borders are **blot hemorrhages.** Both dot and blot hemorrhages are located in the inner retinal layers. **Hard exudates** (deposition of lipid in the inner retina) are small, white or yellowish-white deposits with sharp margins that often have a waxy or glistening appearance.[6] **Soft exudates** (or "cotton wool" exudates) are ischemic swellings of the superficial nerve fiber layer, which appear as white, round, or oval patches with ill-defined (feathery) edges.[6] As retinal ischemia progresses, two other abnormalities appear: venous beading (veins sometimes resemble a string of beads) and intraretinal microvascular abnormalities (IRMA—extra tortuous vessels *within* the retina, which may be either new vessels or dilated preexisting capillaries).[6,14]

B. Proliferative retinopathy. Proliferative retinopathy is new vessel formation on the inner surface of the retina or vitreous, which subsequently can threaten vision by causing retinal detachment or vitreous hemorrhage. These new vessels, or **neovascularization**, often resemble a small wagon wheel, the new vessels radiating like spokes to a circumferential vessel forming the rim.[12] New vessel formation is subdivided into neovascularization of the disc (within one disc diameter of the optic disc, abbreviated "NVD") and neovascularization elsewhere ("NVE"). Of the two, NVD has a much worse visual prognosis.[5]

C. Macular edema. Macular edema may accompany any stage of nonproliferative or proliferative retinopathy. It is very difficult to visualize using the direct ophthalmoscope, although important clues are rings of hard exudates, often surrounding the edematous area, and diminished visual acuity.[12]

III. CLINICAL SIGNIFICANCE. In patients with high-risk proliferative retinopathy or those with clinically significant macular edema, laser photocoagulation reduces the risk of subsequent visual loss by at least 50% (the footnote to Table 20-1 defines high-risk proliferative retinopathy).[3] Retinal examination is the only way to detect these lesions, thereby making diabetic retinopathy one of the best examples of a disorder in which careful, attentive physical examination has profound positive effects on a patient's health.

The findings that best predict subsequent proliferative retinopathy are venous beading, intraretinal microvascular abnormalities, and the extent of microaneurysms and hemorrhages. Soft exudates are less predictive, and the extent of hard exudates correlates poorly with subsequent proliferative retinopathy.[5]

A. Diagnostic accuracy of ophthalmoscopy. Table 20-2 presents the accuracy of ophthalmoscopy for sight-threatening retinopathy (i.e., proliferative changes and macular edema), using as the diagnostic standard retinal photographs through dilated pupils or slit-lamp biomicroscopy. Not surprisingly, specialists per-

TABLE 20-2 Ophthalmoscopy and diabetic retinopathy*

Finding (ref)†	Sensitivity (%)	Specificity (%)	Positive LR	Negative LR
Detecting Sight-Threatening Retinopathy, Using the Following Technique:				
Nondilated pupils[15]	50	91	5.8	0.5
Dilated pupils, general providers[8,10,11,16]	53-69	91-96	10.0	0.4
Dilated pupils, specialists[9-11,17]	48-81	90-99	18.1	0.3

*Diagnostic standard: For sight-threatening retinopathy, retinal photographs through dilated pupils or slit-lamp biomicroscopy.

†Definition of findings: For sight-threatening retinopathy, proliferative retinopathy and macular edema.

form better than general clinicians, and dilated examinations are superior to nondilated ones. If general providers examine with ophthalmoscopy and also review retinal photographs of the patient, sensitivity improves to over 80%, suggesting that this approach may become the most effective screening strategy when access to specialists is limited.[8,10,16]

Macular edema is rarely detected by general providers using direct ophthalmoscopy (sensitivity is close to 0%).[18] Because many patients with macular edema have normal visual acuity (i.e., for the finding "visual acuity less than 20/30," the sensitivity is only 38%),[18] clinicians who exclude macular edema because visual acuity is normal are missing many patients who would benefit from laser photocoagulation.

B. Screening recommendations. Diabetic retinopathy is a common and treatable problem that is detectable during a long asymptomatic period using simple tools. Consequently, it meets every criteria for a disease that benefits from screening. Screening programs are cost saving, being less expensive than the disability payments that otherwise would go to people who develop blindness.[1,2] Table 20-3 reviews the screening schedule recommended by the American Diabetes Association, American College of Physicians, and American Academy of Ophthalmology.[1,14] Given the stakes of missing serious retinopathy and the less than optimal performance of general clinicians using just direct ophthalmoscopy, only clinicians with training and experience—in most cases, optometrists and ophthalmologists—should screen patients. Any patient with macular edema, more than moderate nonproliferative retinopathy, or proliferative retinopathy should be seen by eye care providers with experience in the management of diabetic retinopathy.[1]

TABLE 20-3 Recommended schedule for eye examination in patients with diabetes mellitus

TIME OF ONSET OF DIABETES	RECOMMENDED TIME OF INITIAL EYE EXAMINATION	MINIMAL INTERVAL BETWEEN ROUTINE FOLLOW-UP VISITS
Less than 30 years of age*	5 years after onset or at puberty	12 months
30 years of age or older*	At time of diagnosis	12 months
Before pregnancy	Just before or soon after conception	At least every 3 months

*Less than 30 years and greater than 30 years are operational definitions of type 1 and type 2 diabetes used in the Wisconsin Epidemiologic Study of Diabetic Retinopathy.

REFERENCES

1. American Diabetes Association. Diabetic retinopathy, *Diabetes Care* 21:S47-S49, 1998.
2. Singer DE and others. Screening for diabetic retinopathy, *Ann Intern Med* 116:660-671, 1992.
3. Aiello LM and Cavallerano J. Diabetic retinopathy, *Curr Ther Endocrinol Metab* 6:475-485, 1997.
4. Early Treatment Diabetic Retinopathy Study Research Group. Early photocoagulation for diabetic retinopathy, *Ophthalmology* 98:766-785, 1991.
5. Early Treatment Diabetic Retinopathy Study Research Group. Fundus photographic risk factors for progression of diabetic retinopathy, *Ophthalmology* 98:823-833, 1991.
6. Early Treatment Diabetic Retinopathy Study Research Group. Grading diabetic retinopathy from stereoscopic color fundus photographs: an extension of the modified Airlie House Classification, ETDRS report number 10, *Ophthalmology* 98:786-806, 1991.
7. Lee VS and others. The diagnosis of diabetic retinopathy: ophthalmoscopy versus fundus photography, *Ophthalmology* 100:1504-1512, 1993.
8. O'Hare JP and others. Adding retinal photography to screening for diabetic retinopathy: a prospective study in primary care, *Br Med J* 312:679-682, 1996.
9. Harding SP and others. Sensitivity and specificity of photography and direct ophthalmoscopy in screening for sight threatening eye disease: the Liverpool Diabetic Eye Study, *Br Med J* 311:1131-1135, 1995.
10. Gibbons RL and others. Practical application of the European Field Guide in screening for diabetic retinopathy by using ophthalmoscopy and 35 mm slides, *Diabetologia* 41:59-64, 1998.
11. Buxton MJ and others. Screening for treatable diabetic retinopathy: a comparison of different methods, *Diab Med* 8:371-377, 1991.
12. Fonseca V and others. Diabetic retinopathy: a review for the primary care physician, *South Med J* 89:839-846, 1996.
13. Aiello LP and others. Diabetic retinopathy, *Diabetes Care* 21:143-156, 1998.
14. Ferris FL, Davis MD, and Aiello LM. Treatment of diabetic retinopathy, *N Engl J Med* 341:667-677, 1999.
15. Klein R and others. Diabetic retinopathy as detected using ophthalmoscopy, a nonmydriatic camera and a standard fundus camera, *Ophthalmology* 92:485-491, 1985.

16. Owens DR and others. Screening for diabetic retinopathy by general practitioners: ophthalmoscopy or retinal photography as 35 mm colour transparencies? *Diabet Med* 15:170-175, 1998.

17. Moss SE and others. Comparison between ophthalmoscopy and fundus photography in determining severity of diabetic retinopathy, *Ophthalmology* 92:62-67, 1985.

18. Nathan DM and others. Role of diabetologist in evaluating diabetic retinopathy, *Diab Care* 14:26-33, 1991.

CHAPTER 21

Hearing

I. INTRODUCTION. Hearing loss, which affects 25% to 40% of persons over the age of 65, is associated with depression, difficulty communicating, and reduced mobility.[1] Clinicians using casual assessment in the office overlook significant hearing loss about half the time.[2] The causes of hearing loss are either "neurosensory" (i.e., damage to the auditory nerve) or "conductive" (i.e., damage to the parts of the ear that conduct sound from air to the cochlea). Most neurosensory hearing loss is due to presbyacusis (the degenerative hearing loss of aging).[3] Less common causes are Meniere's disease and acoustic neuroma. The most common causes of conductive loss are impacted cerumen, otitis media, and otosclerosis.[4,5]

II. TECHNIQUE

    A. Whispered voice test. Many tests of hearing are available to general clinicians, some more formal (hand-held audiometer) than others (listening to whisper, watch, or tuning fork).[1,6] The only validated test not requiring special tools is the "whispered voice test." In this test, the clinician whispers a combination of three letters or numbers (e.g., "5, B, 6") while standing arm's length (i.e., about 2 feet) behind the patient, and then asks the patient to repeat the sequence. If the patient answers correctly, hearing is considered normal and testing is stopped. If the patient misidentifies any of the three items, the clinician repeats different triplets of numbers or letters one or two more times. If 50% or more of the items in the two or three triplets are incorrect, the test is abnormal.[2,7,8]

The clinician stands behind the patient to prevent lip-reading. Only one ear is tested at a time, the other being masked by the examiner's finger occluding the external auditory canal and making a continuous circular rubbing motion (occlusion without rubbing is insufficient masking). The clinician should quietly exhale before whispering to produce the quietest whisper possible.[7]

B. Tuning fork tests

1. **Introduction.** Once hearing loss is identified, tuning forks can distinguish neurosensory from conductive loss. All tuning fork tests are based on the fundamental principle, discovered almost 500 years ago,[a] that sound conducts through bone preferentially to an ear with conductive hearing loss. Tuning fork tests were introduced into clinical otology in the early 1800s, and at one time were the otologist's favorite tool consisting of over 15 distinct tests.[10] After introduction of audiometry, however, enthusiasm for these tests waned, and only two are commonly used today, the Weber and Rinne test.[11]

2. **The frequency of the tuning fork.** Most authorities recommend using the 512 Hz tuning fork for tuning fork tests[12] because frequencies above 512 Hz detect conductive hearing loss less well[5,13-15] and because frequencies of 128 Hz or lower generate so

---

[a] The Italian physician Capivacci made this fundamental observation after connecting his subject's teeth to a zither and then plucking the zither's strings.[9]

many vibrations that even patients without hearing can sense them.[5] The 512 Hz fork is preferred to the 256 Hz fork because the 256 Hz fork, in some studies of tuning fork tests, is less specific.[16,17]

3. **Method of striking the fork.** Most authorities recommend striking the fork against a soft surface, such as a rubber pad or the muscles of the forearm.[12] The principal tone produced is the same whether the tines are struck on a soft or harder surface, but the harder surface generates multiple overtones, which may confound interpretation of the test.[10] Weights, sometimes added to the tines to minimize overtones, also shorten the time of vibration and are not recommended.[10]

4. **Weber test.** In this test, the clinician strikes the fork, places it in the middle of the patient's vertex, forehead, or bridge of nose, and asks the patient "Where do you hear the sound?" In patients *with unilateral hearing loss*, the sound is heard preferentially in the *good* ear if the loss is neurosensory and in the *bad* ear if the loss is conductive.[12,18] Weber himself recommended placing the vibrating fork on the incisors[19] and subsequent studies do show this is the most sensitive technique,[20] although concerns of transmitting infectious diseases prohibit using this method now.

According to traditional teachings, persons with normal hearing perceive the sound in the midline or inside their head, but studies show that up to 40% of normal-hearing persons also lateralize the Weber test.[15] Therefore, the Weber test should be interpreted only in patients with hearing loss.

5. **Rinne test** (pronounced "RIN-neh"). In this test, the clinician tests each ear individually to determine whether that ear detects sound better through air or bone. Air conduction

(AC) is tested by holding the vibrating fork about 2.5 cm away from the ear, with the axis joining the tips of the tines in line with the axis through both external auditory canals.[b] Bone conduction (BC) is tested by holding the stem of the vibrating fork against the mastoid (excessive force should not be used because it causes sounds to be heard longer and diminishes the test's specificity).[21] The clinician compares air and bone conduction by either the (1) loudness comparison technique, in which the fork is held about 2 seconds in each position and the patient indicates which position is louder; or the (2) threshold technique, in which the clinician uses a stopwatch to time how long the patient hears the sound, from the moment the fork is struck to when the sound disappears, first for air conduction and then bone conduction.[12,18,20]

Patients with normal hearing or neurosensory hearing loss perceive the sound better through air conduction than through bone conduction. Patients with conductive hearing loss, in contrast, perceive the sound better (i.e., louder or longer) through bone conduction: According to a confusing tradition, this result is recorded "Rinne negative," although it is more explicit to record "BC > AC" for the abnormal result.

Table 21-1 presents some examples of

---

[b] During air conduction, the orientation of the tines of the fork is important because the sound waves emanate in two directions from the fork: one direction is parallel to the axis of the tines and the other is perpendicular to it. If the tines are held at an oblique angle, these sound waves may actually cancel each other out and diminish the sound.[10] Clinicians can easily convince themselves of this by rotating the stem of a vibrating fork near their own ear, noting that the sound intermittently disappears.

TABLE 21-1 Tuning fork tests—traditional interpretation

WEBER TEST	RINNE TEST	POSSIBLE INTERPRETATIONS
Midline	AC > BC, bilateral	1) Normal hearing, bilateral
		2) Neurosensory loss, bilateral
Louder in left	BC > AC, left	1) Conductive loss, left
	AC > BC, right	
Louder in left	AC > BC, bilateral	1) Normal hearing, bilateral
		2) Neurosensory loss, worse on right
Louder in right	BC > AC, bilateral	1) Conductive loss, bilateral but worse on right
		2) Conductive loss on right and severe neurosensory loss on left*

From reference 12.

AC, Air conduction; BC, bone conduction.

*Some patients with severe neurosensory loss have the finding BC > AC because the BC stimulus is cross-heard by the better cochlea on the nontest side.

different results from the Weber and Rinne test, and their possible interpretations.

III. CLINICAL SIGNIFICANCE

A. Whispered voice test. Table 21-2 reveals that the whispered voice test is an accurate test, arguing strongly for significant hearing loss (i.e., >30 dB) when it is positive (LR = 6.0) and practically excluding significant hearing loss when it is negative (LR = 0.03).

B. Tuning fork tests. Table 21-2 shows that the Rinne test (by the loudness comparison technique) is an accurate test of conductive hearing loss. The finding of "BC > AC" argues strongly for an air-bone gap greater than 20 dB on audiometry (LR = 16.8); the finding of "AC > BC" argues against an air-bone gap this large (LR = 0.2). The larger the patient's air-bone gap on audiometry, the more likely the Rinne test will reveal "BC > AC" (for comparison, the mean air-bone gap in otosclerosis and otitis media is 21 to 27 dB).[4,17,22]

The Weber test, on the other hand, is less accurate, arguing only somewhat for neurosensory hearing loss when it lateralizes to the good ear (LR = 2.7). The Weber test performs poorly because many patients with unilateral hearing loss, whether neurosensory or conductive, hear the tuning fork in the midline.[15]

Tuning fork tests cannot distinguish normal hearing from bilateral neurosensory losses (see Table 21-1), and therefore, they should always follow hearing tests. Moreover, tuning fork tests cannot distinguish a pure conductive loss from a mixed conductive and neurosensory defect (see Table 21-1).[23]

TABLE 21-2 Hearing tests*

Finding (ref)†	Sensitivity (%)	Specificity (%)	Positive LR	Negative LR
Hearing Tests				
Abnormal whispered voice test[2,7,8]	90-99	80-87	6.0	0.03
Tuning Fork Tests (Patients With Unilateral Hearing Loss)				
Rinne test, detecting conductive hearing loss[4,17]	60-90	95-98	16.8	0.2
Weber test lateralizes to good ear, detecting neurosensory loss[15]	58	79	2.7	NS
Weber test lateralizes to bad ear, detecting conductive loss[15]	54	92	NS	0.5

NS, Not significant.

*Diagnostic standard: For hearing loss (whispered voice test), mean pure tone threshold greater than 30 dB on audiometry; for conductive hearing loss (Rinne test), air-bone gap on audiometry 20 dB or more.

†Definition of findings: For abnormal whispered voice test, see text; for Rinne test, bone conduction (BC) greater than air conduction (AC), using the loudness comparison technique; all tuning fork tests used 512 Hz tuning fork.

REFERENCES

1. Lichtenstein MJ, Bess FH, and Logan SA. Validation of screening tools for identifying hearing-impaired elderly in primary care, *JAMA* 259:2875-2878, 1988.
2. Macphee GJA, Crowther JA, and McAlpine CH. A simple screening test for hearing impairment in elderly patients, *Age Ageing* 17:347-351, 1988.
3. Nadol JB. Hearing loss, *New Engl J Med* 329:1092-1102, 1993.
4. Burkey JM and others. Clinical utility of the 512-Hz Rinne tuning fork test, *Am J Otol* 19:59-62, 1998.
5. Gelfand SA. Clinical precision of the Rinne test, *Acta Otolaryngol* 83:480-487, 1977.
6. Arbit E. A sensitive bedside hearing test, *Ann Neurol* 2:250-251, 1977.
7. Swan IRC and Browning GB. The whispered voice as a screening test for hearing impairment, *J Roy Coll Gen Pract* 35:197, 1985.
8. Eekhof JAH and others. The whispered voice: the best test for screening for hearing impairment in general practice? *Br J Gen Pract* 46:473-474, 1996.
9. Ng M and Jackler RK. Early history of tuning-fork tests, *Am J Otolaryngol* 14:100-105, 1993.
10. Samuel J, Eitelberg E, and Habil I. Tuning forks: the problem of striking, *J Laryngol Otol* 103:1-6, 1989.
11. Johnson EW. Tuning forks to audiometers and back again, *Laryngoscope* 80:49-68, 1970.
12. British Society of Audiology. Recommended procedure for Rinne and Weber tuning-fork tests, *Br J Audiol* 21:229-230, 1987.
13. Crowley H and Kaufman RS. The Rinne tuning fork test, *Arch Otolaryngol* 84:70-72, 1966.
14. Jacob V and others. Can Rinne's test quantify hearing loss? *ENT J* 72:152-153, 1993.
15. Stankiewicz JA and Mowry HJ. Clinical accuracy of tuning fork tests, *Laryngoscope* 89:1956-1973, 1979.
16. Browning GG and Swan IRC. Sensitivity and specificity of Rinne tuning fork test, *Br Med J* 297:1381-1382, 1988.
17. Chole RA and Cook GB. The Rinne test for conductive deafness: a critical reappraisal. *Arch Otolaryngol Head Neck Surg* 114:399-403, 1988.
18. Sheehy JL, Gardner G, and Hambley WM. Tuning fork tests in modern otology, *Arch Otolaryngol* 94:132-138, 1971.

19. Huizing EH. The early description of the so-called tuning fork tests of Weber and Rinne I. the "Weber test" and its first description by Schmalz, *ORL J Otorhinolaryngol Relat Spec* 35:278-282, 1973.

20. Golabek W and Stephens SDG. Some tuning fork tests revisited, *Clin Otolaryngol* 4:421-430, 1979.

21. Johnston DF. A new modification of the Rinne test, *Clin Otolaryngol* 17:322-326, 1992.

22. Wilson WR and Woods LA. Accuracy of the Bing and Rinne tuning fork tests, *Arch Otolaryngol* 101:81-85, 1975.

23. Doyle PJ, Anderson DW, and Pijl S. The tuning fork: an essential instrument in otologic practice, *J Otolaryngol* 13:83-86, 1984.

CHAPTER 22

The Thyroid and Its Disorders

GOITER

I. INTRODUCTION. In industrialized areas of the world, goiter (i.e., enlarged thyroid) occurs in up to 10% of women and 2% of men, the usual causes being multinodular goiter, Hashimoto's thyroiditis, or Graves' disease (the most common cause worldwide is endemic goiter, largely from inadequate iodine intake).[1] About 80% of patients with goiter are clinically euthyroid, 10% are hypothyroid, and 10% are hyperthyroid.[1,2] Most patients are asymptomatic or present for evaluation of a neck mass. A few, especially those with substernal goiters, present with dyspnea, stridor, hoarseness, or dysphagia.[3,4]

Endemic goiter has been described for millennia, although it is unclear whether early clinicians distinguished goiter from other causes of neck swelling such as tuberculous lymphadenitis. The first person to clearly differentiate cystic goiter from cervical lymphadenopathy was Celsus, the Roman physician, writing in AD 30.[5]

II. TECHNIQUE

  A. Normal thyroid. The important landmarks for locating the thyroid gland are the "V" at the top of the thyroid cartilage (the *laryngeal prominence* of the thyroid cartilage) and the cricoid cartilage (Figure 22-1). These two structures, which are usually 3 cm apart, are the most conspicuous structures in the midline of the neck. The isthmus of the normal thyroid lies just below the cricoid cartilage and is usually 1.5 cm wide, covering the second, third, and fourth tracheal rings.[6,7] Each lateral lobe of the thyroid is 4 to 5 cm long and hugs the trachea tightly, extending from the middle of the thyroid cartilage down to the fifth or sixth tracheal rings.[7] A pyramidal lobe is found in up to 50% of anatomic dissections, usually on the left side, and is palpable in 10% of nontoxic goiters but seldom in normal-sized glands.[7,8]

The thyroid has a constant relationship with the laryngeal prominence (which is about 4 cm above the thyroid isthmus) and the cricoid cartilage (which is just above the isthmus), but the position of these structures in the neck (and thus of the thyroid in the neck) varies considerably among patients (Figure 22-1).[9] If the laryngeal prominence and suprasternal notch of the manubrium are far apart (e.g., 10 to 12 cm), the patient has a "high-lying" thyroid, which is sometimes so conspicuous it suggests goiter even though it is normal-sized (see Pseudo-

Laryngeal prominence of thyroid cartilage
Cricoid cartilage
Thyroid gland
Suprasternal notch

FIGURE 22-1 The normal thyroid. The thyroid gland has a constant relationship with the two most prominent landmarks of the middle of the neck—the laryngeal prominence of the thyroid cartilage and the cricoid cartilage. On the left is the usual position of the thyroid gland. On the right is a "low-lying" thyroid, most of which is hidden behind the clavicles and inaccessible to palpation.

goiter below). If the laryngeal prominence is close to the suprasternal notch (e.g., 5 cm or less apart), the patient has a "low-lying" thyroid, which may be concealed behind the sterno-cleidomastoid muscles and clavicles, making complete palpation of the gland impossible.[9-11] Low-lying thyroids are more common in elderly patients.[11]

In areas of the world with iodine-replete diets, the normal thyroid is less than 20 ml in volume.[12,13]

B. Examination for goiter

   1. Inspection. Two maneuvers make the thyroid more conspicuous: (1) extending the patient's neck, which lifts the trachea (and thyroid) about 3 cm away from the suprasternal notch and stretches the skin against the thyroid and (2) inspecting the patient's neck from the side. In patients with normal- or high-lying thyroids, the line between the cricoid prominence and suprasternal notch, when viewed from the side, should be straight. Anterior bowing of this line suggests a goiter.[14]

   2. Palpation. The clinician may stand in front or behind the patient when palpating the thyroid, whichever position is most comfortable and effective, because no study has shown the superiority of either method.[13] Most authorities recommend palpating the thyroid with the patient's neck slightly flexed, to relax the sternocleidomastoid and sternohyoid muscles. A firm technique should be used. Special features to note during palpation are thyroid size, consistency (whether it is soft, firm, or hard; a "soft" thyroid has the consistency of the surrounding tissue in the neck), and texture (diffuse or nodular), and whether there is thyroid tenderness, tracheal deviation (a clue to asymmetric goiter), or cervical lymphadenopathy.

3. **Observing the patient swallow.** Because the thyroid and trachea are firmly attached by ligaments and must move together, observation of the patient swallowing helps distinguish the thyroid from other neck structures. During a normal swallow, both the thyroid and trachea make an initial upward movement of 1.5 to 3.5 cm; the larger the oral bolus, the greater the movement.[15] The thyroid and trachea then hesitate 0.2 to 0.7 seconds before returning to their original position.

Therefore, a neck mass is probably *not* in the thyroid, if (1) the mass does not move during a swallow, or it moves less than the thyroid cartilage; (2) the mass does not hesitate before descending to its original position; or (3) the mass returns to its original position before complete descent of the thyroid cartilage.[15]

III. THE FINDINGS

A. **Cervical goiter.** Some of the more common definitions of goiter include the following: **(1) The "rule of thumb,"** which states that a lateral lobe is enlarged if it is larger than the distal phalanx of the patient's thumb. **(2) Estimates of thyroid volume from palpation.** For example, a thyroid whose lateral lobes each measure 3 cm wide, 2 cm deep, and 5 cm long would have an estimated volume of 60 ml (i.e., $2 \times 3 \times 2 \times 5 = 60$). Any estimate greater than 20 ml is classified as a goiter (i.e., each lateral lobe is normally less than 10 ml). **(3) Epidemiologic definitions of goiter.** These definitions are designed for clinicians who rapidly survey large numbers of persons in areas of endemic goiter (these clinicians sometimes perform as many as 150 to 200 examinations per hour).[16] Table 22-1 presents an epidemiologic definition developed by the World Health Organization.

B. Substernal and retroclavicular goiters.[22-27] Large goiters may extend from the neck to the superior mediastinum, passing through the inflexible thoracic inlet (i.e., the bony ring formed by the upper sternum, first ribs, and first thoracic vertebral body). At the thoracic inlet, a goiter may compress the trachea, esophagus, or neck veins and cause dyspnea, dysphagia, facial plethora, cough, and hoarseness. Sometimes, when these patients flex or elevate the arms, the thoracic inlet is pulled up into the cervical goiter, just as if the thyroid were a cork and the thoracic inlet were the neck of a bottle. This causes a characteristic sign, **Pemberton's sign**, which is congestion of the face, cyanosis, and eventual distress induced by arm elevation.[25,28,29] The exact frequency of Pemberton's sign is unknown. In two small series of patients with substernal goiter, it was positive in every

TABLE 22-1 World Health Organization definition of goiter*

Classification	Inspection: Thyroid Visible?	Palpation: Thyroid Lobe Larger Than Distal Phalanx of Patient's Thumb?
Grade 0	No	No
Grade 1a	No	Yes
Grade 1b	Yes, only when neck extended	Yes
Grade 2	Yes, head in normal position	Yes
Grade 3	Yes, at a considerable distance	Yes

*Grades 1a and above are classified as "goiter." Some authors[17,18] label the grades differently than the more widely used system presented here.[16,19-21]

patient[24,25]; two other larger series did not mention it at all.[26,27]

Other findings in patients with substernal goiters are cervical goiter (i.e., palpable goiter above the thoracic inlet, 86% of patients), tracheal deviation (33%), distention of neck veins (22%), and stridor (10%) (for comparison, 75% have tracheal deviation on the chest radiograph).

C. **Thyroglossal cyst.**[30-33] Thyroglossal cysts are cystic swellings of the thyroglossal duct, an epithelium-lined remnant marking the embryologic descent of thyroid tissue from the base of the tongue to its final location anterior to the larynx. Thyroglossal cysts present at any age, appearing as tense, nontender (unless infected or after acute hemorrhage into the capsule), mobile, nonlobulated round tumors, usually at the level of the hyoid bone or just below it (the hyoid bone is *above* the thyroid cartilage). They are in the midline in the neck, unless they are so low they lie to one side of the thyroid cartilage. Despite their cystic structure, they do not usually transilluminate. If the cyst remains attached to the base of the tongue or hyoid bone, a characteristic physical sign of thyroglossal cysts is upward movement when the patient protrudes the tongue, just as if the two structures were connected by a string. Thyroglossal cysts account for three quarters of congenital neck masses, the other one quarter being branchial cleft cysts, which are located more laterally, usually anterior to the sternocleidomastoid muscle at the level of the hyoid bone.[34,35]

D. **Pseudogoiter.** Pseudogoiter refers to thyroid glands that appear enlarged even though they are normal sized. There are three causes: (1) **High-lying thyroid gland**, which, although normal sized, lies so high in the neck it is unusually conspicuous after neck extension. This diagnosis is suggested when the patient's laryngeal prominence is more than 10 cm above the suprasternal notch and both thyroid lobes are smaller than the distal phalanx of the patient's thumb. In one study, high-lying but normal-sized thyroids accounted for 8% of suspected goiters referred to an endocrinology service.[9] **(2) Other cervical masses**, such as adipose tissue, cervical lymphadenopathy, branchial cleft cysts, and pharyngeal diverticula. Observation during swallowing helps identify these lesions. **(3) Modigliani syndrome**, which describes a normal-sized thyroid lying in front of an exaggerated cervical spine lordosis,[36] named after the painter Amedeo Modigliani, whose portraits had subjects with long, curved necks.

E. The Delphian node. The Delphian node, a lymph node that drains the thyroid gland and larynx, lies directly anterior to the cricothyroid ligament (just cephalad to the thyroid isthmus).[37,38] When enlarged, the node is readily palpable because of its superficial location and the fact that it lies against the unyielding trachea. The node is called "Delphian" because it is the first one exposed during surgery, and its appearance often foretells what the surgeon will find in the thyroid (e.g., carcinoma), just as the oracle at Delphi foretold the future.[a][39] The Delphian node enlarges in some patients with thyroid cancer, Hashimoto's thyroiditis, and laryngeal cancer.[37] Its involvement in laryngeal cancer carries an ominous prognosis,[38,40,41] but no studies of its significance in thyroid cancer could be found.

IV. CLINICAL SIGNIFICANCE

A. Detecting goiter. The findings listed in Table 22-2 are categorized into three levels: (1) no

---

[a] The word "delphian" was originally suggested by Raymond Randall, a fourth-year medical student attending the thyroid clinic at The Massachusetts General Hospital.[39]

TABLE 22-2 Goiter*

Finding (ref)†	Sensitivity (%)	Specificity (%)	Positive LR
No goiter by palpation or inspection[14,20,42-45]	5-57	0-26	0.4
Goiter by palpation, visible only after neck extension[42]	13	—	NS
Goiter by palpation and inspection with neck in normal position[42-45]	43-82	88-100	26.3

NS, Not significant.

*Diagnostic standard: For goiter, ultrasound volume greater than 20 ml[42-45] or greater than 18 ml (women) or 25 ml (men),[20] or surgical weight greater than 23 g.[14]

†Definition of finding: For thyroid gland enlarged by palpation and visible with neck in normal position, WHO grade 2 or 3,[42] two observers agreeing that thyroid is visible and palpably enlarged,[43,44] or two observers agreeing that goiter is present.[45]

goiter by palpation or inspection (including inspection of the extended neck); (2) goiter by palpation, although the gland is visible only after extending the neck, and; (3) goiter by palpation and inspection of neck in the normal position. The first finding, absence of goiter by inspection and palpation, argues somewhat *against* the presence of an enlarged thyroid (LR = 0.4, Table 22-2; enlarged thyroid defined as thyroid volume more than 20 to 25 ml). Up to half of patients with an enlarged gland by ultrasonography have this finding; however, presumably these goiters are small. The intermediate finding (i.e., goiter by palpation but visible only after neck extension) fails to distinguish goiter from normal-sized glands (LR not significant). Although this finding was tested in only one study, it suggests that subtle enlargement by palpation, not confirmed by inspection of the neck in the normal position, is not a reliable sign of goiter. The most compelling finding arguing for an enlarged thyroid is a gland that is both enlarged by palpation and visible with the neck in the normal position (LR = 26.3).

B. Etiology of goiter. Multinodular goiter and Hashimoto's thyroiditis are the most common causes in a clinically euthyroid patient; Hashimoto's thyroiditis, in a hypothyroid patient; and Graves' disease and multinodular goiter, in a hyperthyroid patient. The associated finding of ophthalmopathy (tearing, diplopia, proptosis) or dermopathy (pretibial myxedema) indicates Graves' disease (see below).

Although thyroid cancer can also cause a goiter, it usually presents instead as a thyroid nodule (see Thyroid Nodule below).[46,47] Three findings argue strongly that a goiter contains carcinoma: vocal cord paralysis (LR = 45.2, Table 22-3), cervical adenopathy (LR = 13.4), and fixation of the goiter to surrounding tissues (LR = 9.7).

TABLE 22-3 Goiter and thyroid nodules—findings predicting carcinoma*

Finding (ref)†	Sensitivity (%)	Specificity (%)	Positive LR	Negative LR
Goiter[8]				
Vocal cord paralysis	24	99	45.2	0.8
Cervical adenopathy	45	97	13.4	0.6
Fixation to surrounding tissues	60	94	9.7	0.4
Goiter nodular (vs. diffuse)	78	49	1.5	0.5
Pyramidal lobe present	3	90	NS	NS
Thyroid Nodule[48]				
Vocal cord paralysis	14	99	12.0	NS
Cervical adenopathy	31	96	7.4	0.7
Fixation to surrounding tissues	14	98	7.2	NS
Very firm nodule	4	99	NS	NS

NS, Not significant.

*Diagnostic standard: For carcinoma, pathologic examination of tissue.[8,48]

†Definition of findings: For vocal cord paralysis, direct visualization of vocal cords.

Silent and postpartum thyroiditis also cause goiter, but goiter is present in only 50% or less of patients and it is rarely prominent, the clinician's attention instead directed toward the findings of hyperthyroidism.[49] The finding of a painful or tender thyroid gland, sometimes mimicking pharyngitis, suggests subacute thyroiditis[50-52] or hemorrhage into a cyst or nodule (although most thyroid hemorrhage is painless).[53] In subacute thyroiditis, the thyroid is modestly enlarged, usually 1.5 to 3 times the normal size.

THYROID NODULES

I. INTRODUCTION. Palpable thyroid nodules occur in about 5% of women and 1% of men, most of whom are clinically euthyroid.[54-56] Although thyroid nodules raise concerns about thyroid cancer, over 95% are benign disorders, including colloid cysts, adenomas, or dominant nodules of a multinodular gland.[57]

II. OCCULT NODULES. Because thyroid nodules are palpable in only 1% to 5% of persons but they are found in up to 50% of patients during ultrasound and autopsy surveys,[58-60] it is clear that most thyroid nodules are "occult" (i.e., detectable by clinical imaging but not by palpation). Furthermore, when the clinician feels a single *palpable* nodule in the patient's thyroid gland, ultrasonography reveals multiple nodules half the time.[61] Occult nodules are not palpable either because the patient's neck is too short or thick,[62] the nodules are buried in the posterior parts of the gland,[63] or the nodules are too small (The mean diameter of a *palpable* nodule is 3 cm; palpation fails to detect 50% of nodules less than 2 cm in diameter and over 90% of nodules less than 1 cm in diameter).[58,61,62] Although the large number of occult nodules raises the concern that palpation of the thyroid misses many thyroid cancers, it is important to emphasize that occult nodules rarely contain clinically important carcinoma[54,60,62] and that the most common presentation for thyroid carcinoma remains the *palpable* thyroid nodule.[46,47,64,65]

III. CLINICAL SIGNIFICANCE. The most important diagnostic test for thyroid nodules is fine needle aspiration. Nonetheless, a few physical signs, if present, argue strongly that the thyroid nodule contains carcinoma (Table 22-3): vocal cord paralysis (LR = 12.0), cervical adenopathy (LR = 7.4), and fixation of the nodule to surrounding tissues (LR = 7.2). Fewer than 1 of 3 patients with thyroid carcinoma, however, has any of these findings.

HYPOTHYROIDISM (MYXEDEMA)

I. INTRODUCTION. Hypothyroidism is a clinical syndrome that results from diminished levels of thyroid hormone, which slows the patient's metabolic rate and neuromuscular reactions and causes accumulation of mucopolysaccharides in the skin and other tissues throughout the body. In areas of the industrialized world with iodine-replete diets, hypothyroidism affects 9% of women and 1% of men.[1] The usual cause is disease in the thyroid gland itself (primary hypothyroidism), usually from Hashimoto's thyroiditis (60% to 70% of cases) or previous radioiodine treatment for Grave's disease (20% to 30% of cases).[1]

The diagnosis of hypothyroidism relies on laboratory tests, which have been available for over 100 years.[b] Nonetheless, bedside diagnosis still has two

---

[b] The first thyroid test was measurement of the basal metabolic rate (BMR) (i.e., oxygen consumption), introduced in the 1890s. Radioactive iodine uptake appeared in the 1940s, serum protein-bound iodide (PBI) in the 1950s, serum total thyroxine (T4) in the 1960s, and sensitive assays for thyroid stimulating hormone in the 1980s.[66,67]

important roles: (1) it estimates the likelihood of thyroid disease, which then can be used to identify subgroups of patients with high or low probability of abnormal thyroid function, thus increasing the yield of laboratory testing[68]; and (2) it is essential to the diagnosis of subclinical hypothyroidism or sick euthyroid syndrome, conditions which, by definition, describe patients with abnormal laboratory tests but no bedside findings of thyroid disease.

All of the classic bedside findings of hypothyroidism—the puffy skin, slow reflexes, thick speech, and sluggish thinking—were first described by William Gull and William Ord in the 1870s.[69-71]

II. FINDINGS AND THEIR PATHOGENESIS

A. Skin and soft tissue. The nonpitting puffiness of hypothyroidism results from dermal accumulation of mucopolysaccharides (mostly hyaluronic acid and chondroitin sulfate), which freely bind water.[32] These changes cause a "jelly-like swelling (and) overgrowth of mucus-yielding cement," which led Ord to coin the term "myxedema" in 1877.[71] Even after effective thyroid replacement, these changes may persist for months or longer.[72]

Some myxedematous patients also have a yellow tint to their skin, which occurs because of diminished conversion of carotenoids to retinol and subsequent hypercarotenemia.[73,74] The apparent coolness of the skin is attributed to diminished dermal blood flow,[75] and dryness results in part from decreased sebum production.[76] The loss of hair from the lateral eyebrows occurs in about a third of hypothyroid patients and is one of the least specific signs, commonly found in euthyroid patients.[77]

B. The Achilles Reflex. The ankle jerk has been investigated more extensively than any other physical finding of thyroid disease. By the 1970s, at least nine different pieces of equipment had been designed to precisely measure the duration of reflex to the nearest millisecond (ms).[78,79]

Both the contraction and relaxation phase of the ankle jerk are prolonged in hypothyroidism,[79-82] although prolonged relaxation seems most prominent to the human eye (and on many of the tracings of the reflex). In one study, the mean half-relaxation time (i.e., the time from the hammer tap to the moment the Achilles tendon has returned halfway to its original position) for hypothyroid patients was 460 ms (standard deviation [SD] 40 ms), compared to 310 ms (SD 30 ms) for euthyroid patients.[82] Experiments in hypothyroid rats suggest that the prolongation results from diminished calcium transport by the sarcoplasmic reticulum and subsequent slowing of the interaction between actin and myosin.[83]

When testing for hypothyroidism, clinicians usually elicit the ankle jerk by tapping on the Achilles tendon with the patient kneeling on a chair.[80,82,84] The force of the tap does not affect the duration of the reflex, although slightly more force is necessary in hypothyroid patients to generate a reflex than in hyperthyroid patients.[80]

C. **Hypothyroid speech.** Hypothyroid speech, seen in 39% of patients in one study,[85] has a slow rate and rhythm and is characteristically deep, low-pitched, and hyponasal (i.e., as if the patient has a cold).[86-88] Some patients even slur their words slightly, leading one clinician to describe the hypothyroid voice as "a bad gramophone record of a drowsy, slightly intoxicated person with a bad cold and a plum in the mouth."[89] Biopsies of vocal cords have revealed deposition of mucinous material.[90]

D. **Obesity is no more common in hypothyroid patients than euthyroid patients.**[91]

III. **CLINICAL SIGNIFICANCE.** Table 22-4 summarizes the diagnostic accuracy of physical signs associated with hypothyroidism, as applied to over 1500 patients with suspected thyroid disease. The

TABLE 22-4 Hypothyroidism*

Finding (ref)	Sensitivity (%)	Specificity (%)	Positive LR	Negative LR
Skin				
Coarse skin[92]	29	95	5.6	0.7
Cool and dry skin[93]	16	97	4.7	0.9
Cold palms[92]	37	77	NS	NS
Dry palms[92]	42	73	NS	NS
Periorbital puffiness[92]	53	81	2.8	0.6
Puffiness of wrists[92]	39	86	2.9	0.7
Hair loss of eyebrows[92]	29	85	1.9	NS
Speech				
Hypothyroid speech[92]	37	93	5.4	0.7

Pulse				
Pulse <70 beats/min[93]	29	93	4.1	0.8
Thyroid				
Enlarged thyroid[93]	46	84	2.8	0.6
Billewicz Score[94,95]				
Less than –15 points	3-4	28-68	0.1	—
–15 to +29 points	35-39	—	NS	—
+30 points or more	57-61	90-99	18.8	—

NS, Not significant.

*Diagnostic standard: For *hypothyroidism*, low free T4 level and high thyroid stimulating hormone (TSH),[95] or low protein-bound iodide (PBI) level.[92-94] The PBI level and total T4 level correlate closely, except in patients with thyroiditis and those who ingest exogenous iodides (e.g., radio-contrast dye, cough suppressants), diagnoses in which the PBI level may be falsely high.[96] These diagnoses, however, were largely excluded from the studies reviewed here.

Billewicz scoring scheme, which appears on the bottom of Table 22-4, is fully described in Table 22-5.

In patients with suspected thyroid disease, the findings arguing the most *for* hypothyroidism are coarse skin (LR = 5.6), hypothyroid speech (LR = 5.4), cool *and* dry skin (LR = 4.7), bradycardia (LR = 4.1 for pulse <70/min), puffiness of the wrist (LR = 2.9), periorbital puffiness (LR = 2.8), and a goiter (LR = 2.8). Hair loss of the eyebrows was one of the least compelling diagnostic signs (LR =

TABLE 22-5 Billewicz diagnostic index for hypothyroidism

	Points scored if finding:	
Finding*	Present	Absent
Symptoms		
Diminished sweating	+6	−2
Dry skin	+3	−6
Cold intolerance	+4	−5
Weight increase	+1	−1
Constipation	+2	−1
Hoarseness	+5	−6
Paresthesiae	+5	−4
Deafness	+2	0
Physical Signs		
Slow movements	+11	−3
Coarse skin	+7	−7
Cold skin	+3	−2
Periorbital puffiness	+4	−6
Pulse rate <75/min	+4	−4
Slow ankle jerk	+15	−6

From reference 94.

*Definition of findings: For *weight increase,* recorded increase in weight or tightness in clothing; for *slow movements,* observations while patient removing and replacing a buttoned garment; for *coarse skin,* roughness and thickening of skin of hands, forearms, and elbows; for *slow ankle jerk,* reflex appears slow with patient kneeling on a chair, grasping its back.

1.9), and isolated coolness or isolated dryness of the palms is not significant. No single finding, when absent, argues convincingly *against* hypothyroidism (i.e., negative LRs range from 0.6 to 1.0).

Precise measurements of the ankle jerk discriminate well between patients with and without hypothyroidism (sensitivity 91% to 99%, specificity 94% to 97%, positive LR = 18.7, negative LR = 0.1),[82,84,93] although only 25% to 33% of hypothyroid patients have prolonged reflexes when they are assessed using the naked eye.[77,85]

A Billewicz score of +30 points or more argues convincingly *for* hypothyroidism (LR = 18.8), whereas a score less than –15 points argues convincingly *against* hypothyroidism (LR = 0.1). The mean ages of the patients in these studies is unknown[c]; the Billewicz score may perform less well in elderly patients, who, as a rule, have fewer findings than younger patients.[97]

HYPERTHYROIDISM

I. INTRODUCTION. Hyperthyroidism is a clinical syndrome due to increased production or release of thyroid hormone, which elevates the metabolic rate and causes characteristic findings of the skin, thyroid, eyes, and neuromuscular system. The most common causes of hyperthyroidism are Graves' disease (60% to 90% of cases), toxic nodular goiter, thyroiditis (subacute, silent, or postpartum), and iatrogenic overtreatment with thyroid replacement.[98] Hyperthyroidism affects women (4% prevalence) more than men (0.2% prevalence).

Three clinicians—Caleb Parry, Robert Graves, and Adolf von Basedow—all writing between 1825 and 1840, independently described the classic physical signs associated with thyrotoxicosis. All three

---

[c] One study[95] presented the range of ages (17 to 73 years) but the other study[94] presented no information about age.

were especially impressed with the triad of goiter, prominent eyes, and forceful tachycardia.[99]

II. FINDINGS AND THEIR PATHOGENESIS

A. The thyroid. A goiter is present in 70% to 93% of patients with hyperthyroidism.[100-102] The goiter is diffuse and symmetric in patients with Graves' disease and thyroiditis, but nodular in those with toxic nodular goiter.[49,102]

A thyroid bruit is a common feature of Grave's disease (73% of patients in one study).[10] Nonetheless, the finding also was noted in 30% of elderly patients with toxic nodular goiter,[104] suggesting that the finding is not as specific for Graves' disease as is classically taught. Bruits often radiate far from their source, and perhaps the "thyroid bruit" in the elderly with toxic nodular goiter is actually a carotid bruit made prominent by the increased cardiac output of hyperthyroidism.[d]

B. Eye findings. Three distinct eye findings are associated with hyperthyroidism: lid lag (von Graefe's sign, 1864), lid retraction (Dalrymple's sign, 1849),[e] and Graves' ophthalmopathy. Graves' ophthalmopathy afflicts exclusively patients with Graves' disease, whereas lid lag and lid retraction may occur in hyperthyroidism from any etiology.[52,108]

1. Lid lag. This sign describes the appearance of white sclera between the margin of the upper eyelid and corneal limbus as the patient looks downward. In von Graefe's

---

[d] The opposite phenomenon—a "carotid bruit" actually emanating from a superior thyroid artery—has also been described.[105]

[e] The British eye surgeon John Dalrymple (1803-1852) apparently thought so little of his sign that he never published a description of it. Writing in 1849, W. White Cooper attributed the sign to his friend Dalrymple.[106] Albrecht von Graefe (1828-1870) described his sign in 1864.[99] Ruedemann coined the term "lid lag" in 1932.[107]

words, ". . . as the cornea looks down, the upper eyelid does not follow."[99]

2. **Lid retraction.** This sign describes a peculiar staring appearance of the eyes, caused by a widened palpebral fissure. As the patient looks straight ahead, the upper eyelid is positioned abnormally high, revealing white sclera between the lid margin and superior limbus. Normally the margin of the upper eyelid rests just below the edge of the corneal limbus and covers about 1 mm of the iris.[109,110]

Both lid lag and lid retraction are attributed to the sympathetic hyperactivity of hyperthyroidism, which causes excess contraction of Mueller's muscle (the involuntary lid elevator whose paralysis causes the ptosis of Horner's syndrome). Although the findings improve after treatment with β-blocking medications,[111] mechanisms other than sympathetic hyperactivity must contribute to the lid findings of patients with Graves' disease (even those without exophthalmos or obvious ophthalmopathy, see below), because the lid findings of Graves' disease are often unilateral and persist after the patient becomes euthyroid, and because the pupils of patients with lid findings are usually normal sized (instead of the dilated pupils of sympathetic hyperactivity).[112-115]

Other common causes of lid retraction are unilateral ptosis, facial muscle weakness, previous eyelid surgery, or the irritation of wearing contact lenses.[116] Ptosis causes contralateral lid retraction because attempts to elevate the weakened lid generate excessive neural signals to the motor neuron of the healthy lid, thus elevating it.[117] A simple test confirming ptosis as the cause is to occlude the eye that has ptosis, which then causes the lid retraction in the opposite eye to resolve.

Facial weakness causes retraction of the ipsilateral eyelid because the lid elevators are no longer opposed by the orbicularis oculi muscle.[118]

3. **Graves' ophthalmopathy.** Graves' ophthalmopathy is a constellation of findings, apparent in 25% to 50% of patients with Graves' disease,[113,119] that results from edema and lymphocytic infiltration of orbital fat, connective tissue, and eye muscles.[120] Characteristic physical findings are lid edema, limitation of eye movements, conjunctival chemosis and injection, and exophthalmos (as measured with an exophthalmometer).[110] Clinicians should suspect Graves' ophthalmopathy when patients complain of gritty sensation in the eyes, tearing, eye discomfort, or diplopia. The orbital swelling of Graves' ophthalmopathy may threaten the optic nerve and vision. The bedside findings best predicting incipient optic neuropathy are lid edema and limitation of eye movements—not, surprisingly, the degree of proptosis (proptosis does not predict incipient optic neuropathy perhaps because intraocular pressure is relieved by the outward protrusion).[115,121]

C. **Cardiovascular findings.** Hyperthyroidism causes a fast heart rate, a loud snapping first heart sound, a midsystolic flow murmur, and an increase in supraventricular arrhythmias.[103,122-125]

D. **Skin findings.** The skin of hyperthyroid patients is warm, moist, and smooth,[32] probably because of increased sympathetic tone to sweat glands and increased dermal blood flow. These skin findings often resolve after treatment with β-blocker medications.[75,103,122]

Up to 4% of patients with Graves' disease develop a skin lesion with the confusing name "pretibial myxedema," characterized by bi-

lateral, asymmetric raised, firm plaques or
nodules, which are pink to purple-brown in
color and usually distributed over the anterior shins.[32,126]

E. Neuromuscular findings. The neuromuscular findings of hyperthyroidism are weakness
and diminished exercise tolerance, tremor, and
brisk ankle jerks. The diminished exercise tolerance (affecting 67% of patients) is due to an
inability to increase cardiac output appropriately with exercise and to proximal muscle
wasting and weakness from accelerated protein
catabolism.[102,125,127-129] The fine tremor of hyperthyroidism occurs because of increased sympathetic tone and resolves with β-blocking
medications.[103,122] Brisk reflexes are noted at
the bedside in only 25% of patients or less,[77]
and even precise measurements of the half-
relaxation time (see Hypothyroidism for definition) reveal considerable overlap between normal values (range 230 to 420 ms) and hyperthyroid values (range 200 to 300 ms).[82]

III. CLINICAL SIGNIFICANCE. Table 22-6 presents
the diagnostic accuracy of physical signs for hyperthyroidism, as applied to over 1700 patients with
suspected thyroid disease. At the bottom of Table
22-6 is the accuracy of the Wayne index, a diagnostic scoring scheme described in Table 22-7.

The findings that argue *for* the diagnosis of
hyperthyroidism, in descending order of their LRs,
are lid retraction (LR = 31.5), lid lag (LR = 17.6), fine
finger tremor (LR = 11.4), moist and warm skin (LR
= 6.7), and tachycardia (LR = 4.4, pulse ≥90 beats/
min). Those findings arguing convincingly *against*
hyperthyroidism are normal thyroid size (LR =
0.1), pulse less than 90 beats/min (LR = 0.2), and
absence of finger tremor (LR = 0.3).

A Wayne index score of 20 or more points argues
for hyperthyroidism (LR = 18.2) and one of 10 or
fewer points argues *against* hyperthyroidism (LR =

TABLE 22-6 Hyperthyroidism*

FINDING (REF)†	SENSITIVITY (%)	SPECIFICITY (%)	POSITIVE LR	NEGATIVE LR
Pulse				
Pulse ≥90 beats/min[102]	80	82	4.4	0.2
Skin				
Skin moist and warm[102]	34	95	6.7	0.7
Thyroid				
Enlarged thyroid[102]	93	59	2.3	0.1
Eyes				
Eyelid retraction[102]	34	99	31.5	0.7
Eyelid lag[102]	19	99	17.6	0.8
Neurologic				
Fine finger tremor[102]	69	94	11.4	0.3
Wayne Index[130,131]				
Less than 11 points	1-6	13-32	0.1	—
11-19 points	12-30	—	NS	—
20 points or more	66-88	92-99	18.2	—

NS, Not significant.

*Diagnostic standards: For hyperthyroidism, high levels of PBI for patients evaluated in the 1960s, total T4 for those in the 1970s, and total T4 and TSH for those in the 1980s and 1990s (see footnote to Table 22-4 for discussion of PBI).

TABLE 22-7 Wayne diagnostic index for hyperthyroidism*

Symptoms of Recent Onset or Increased Severity	Present	Signs	Present	Absent
Dyspnea on effort	+1	Palpable thyroid	+3	−3
Palpitations	+2	Bruit over thyroid	+2	−2
Tiredness	+2	Exophthalmos	+2	
Preference for heat (irrespective of duration)	−5	Lid retraction	+2	
Preference for cold	+5	Lid lag	+1	
Excessive sweating	+3	Hyperkinetic movements	+4	−2
Nervousness	+2	Hands:		
Appetite increased	+3	Hot	+2	−2
Appetite decreased	−3	Moist	+1	−1
Weight increased	−3	Casual pulse rate:		
Weight decreased	+3	Atrial fibrillation	+4	
		<80, regular	−3	
		80-90, regular	0	
		>90, regular	+3	

*From reference 130.

0.1). This index, however, may be less useful in elderly patients,[132] who, as a rule, have less goiter and tachycardia than younger patients.[133-135] In one study, 36% of elderly hyperthyroid patients had scores less than 11.[104] Elderly patients also have more weight loss and atrial fibrillation than younger patients,[102,104,136,137] but the frequency of lid retraction and lid lag is the same.[102,104]

REFERENCES

1. Vanderpump MPJ and others. The incidence of thyroid disorders in the community: a twenty-year follow-up of the Whickham Survey, *Clin Endocrinol* 43:55-68, 1995.
2. Hurley DL and Gharib H. Evaluation and management of multinodular goiter, *Otolaryngol Clin North Am* 29:527-540, 1996.
3. Zorrilla L, Tsai J, and Freedman M. Airway obstruction due to goiter in older patients, *J Am Geriatr Soc* 37:1153-1156, 1989.
4. Close LG, Costin BS, and Kim EE. Acute symptoms of the aerodigestive tract caused by rapidly enlarging thyroid neoplasms, *Otolaryngol* 91:441-445, 1983.
5. Celsus. *De Medicina.* De Medicina (English translation of Latin edition written between A.D. 25 and 35, printed in 1478). Cambridge, 1953, Harvard University Press, pp. 140-141, 374-375.
6. Calhoun KH and others. Management of the thyroid isthmus in tracheostomy: a prospective and retrospective study, *Otolaryngol Head Neck Surg* 111:450-452, 1994.
7. Hansen JT. Embryology and surgical anatomy of the lower neck and superior mediastinum. In Falk SA, editor. *Thyroid disease: endocrinology, surgery, nuclear medicine, and radiotherapy*, ed 2, Philadelphia, 1997, Lippincott-Raven, pp. 15-27.
8. Boyle JA and others. Construction of a model for computer-assisted diagnosis: application to the problem of non-toxic goiter, *Q J Med* 35:565-588, 1966.
9. Gwinup G and Morton ME. The high lying thyroid: a cause of pseudogoiter, *J Clin Endocrinol Metab* 40:37-42, 1975.
10. Dobyns BM. Goiter, *Curr Prob Surg* 2-60, 1969.

11. Slater S. Cricoid cartilage and suprasternal notch: the "low-lying thyroid," *South Med J* 72:1621-1622, 1979.

12. Hegedus L and others. The determination of thyroid volume by ultrasound and its relationship to body weight, age, and sex in normal subjects, *J Clin Endocrinol Metab* 56:260-263, 1983.

13. Siminoski K. The rational clinical examination: does this patient have a goiter? *JAMA* 273:813-817, 1995.

14. Silink K and Reisenauer R. Geographical spread of endemic goitre and problems of its mapping. In Silink K and Cerny K, editors. *Endemic goitre and allied diseases*, Bratislava, 1966, Publishing House of the Slovak Academy of Sciences, pp. 33-47.

15. Siminoski K. Differential movement during swallowing as an aid in the detection of thyroid pseudonodules, *Head Neck* 16:21-24, 1994.

16. Perez D, Scrimshaw NS, and Munoz JA. Classification of goitre and technique of endemic goitre surveys, *Bull World Health Org* 18:217-232, 1958.

17. Stanbury JB and others. Endemic goitre and cretism: public health significance and prevention, *WHO Chronicle* 28:220-228, 1974.

18. Berghout A and others. Determinants of thyroid volume as measured by ultrasonography in healthy adults in a non-iodine deficient area, *Clin Endocrinol* 26:273-280, 1987.

19. Fenzi G and others. Clinical approach to goiter, *Balliere Clin Endocrinol Metab* 2:671-682, 1988.

20. Hintze G and others. Thyroid volume and goitre prevalence in the elderly as determined by ultrasound and their relationships to laboratory indices, *Acta Endocrinol (Copenh)* 124:12-18, 1991.

21. Lisboa HRK and others. Clinical examination is not an accurate method of defining the presence of goitre in schoolchildren, *Clin Endocrinol* 45:471-475, 1996.

22. Sherman PH and Shahbahrami F. Mediastinal goiter: review of ten cases, *Am Surg* 32:137-142, 1966.

23. Singh B, Lucente FE, and Shaha AR. Substernal goiter: a clinical review, *Am J Otolaryngol* 15:409-416, 1994.

24. Klassen-Udding LM, van Lijf JH, and Napel HHT. Substernal goitre, deep venous thrombosis of the arm, and Pemberton's sign, *Neth J Med* 26:228-231, 1983.

25. Blum M, Biller BJ, and Bergman DA. The thyroid cork. Obstruction of the thoracic inlet due to retroclavicular goiter, *JAMA* 227:189-191, 1974.

26. Katlic MR, Grillo HC, and Wang C. Substernal goiter: analysis of 80 patients from Massachusetts General Hospital, *Am J Surg* 149:283-287, 1985.

27. Reeve TS and others. The investigation and management of intrathoracic goiter, *Surg Gynecol Obstet* 115:223-229, 1962.

28. Wallace C and Siminoski K. The Pemberton sign, *Ann Intern Med* 125:568-569, 1996.

29. Pemberton HS. Sign of submerged goiter, *Lancet* 251:509, 1946.

30. Pounds LA. Neck masses of congenital origin, *Pediatr Clin North Am* 28:841-844, 1981.

31. Girard M and Deluca SA. Thyroglossal duct cyst, *Am Fam Phys* 42:665-668, 1990.

32. Heymann WR. Cutaneous manifestations of thyroid disease, *J Am Acad Derm* 26:885-902, 1992.

33. Marshall SF and Becker WF. Thyroglossal cysts and sinuses, *Ann Surg* 129:642-651, 1949.

34. Liston SL and Siegel LG. Branchial cysts, sinuses, and fistulas, *ENT J* 58:504-509, 1979.

35. Himalstein MR. Branchial cysts and fistulas, *ENT J* 59:23-29, 1980.

36. Mercer RD. Pseudo-goiter: the Modigliani syndrome, *Cleve Clin J Med* 42:319-326, 1975.

37. Cope O and others. What thyroid nodules are to be feared? *J Clin Endocrinol Metab* 9:1012-1022, 1949.

38. Olsen KD, DeSanto LW, and Pearson BW. Positive Delphian lymph node: clinical significance in laryngeal cancer, *Laryngoscope* 97:1033-1037, 1987.

39. Cope O. The surgery of the thyroid. In: Means JH, editor. *The thyroid and its diseases*, ed 2, Philadelphia, 1948, JB Lippincott Co.

40. Foote RL and others. Patterns of failure after total laryngectomy for glottic carcinoma, *Cancer* 64:143-149, 1989.

41. Thaler ER and others. Delphian lymph node in laryngeal carcinoma: a whole organ study. *Laryngoscope* 107:332-334, 1997.

42. Berghout A and others. The value of thyroid volume measured by ultrasonography in the diagnosis of goiter, *Clin Endocrinol* 28:409-414, 1988.

43. Hegedus L and others. High frequency of goitre in cigarette smokers, *Clin Endocrinol* 22:287-292, 1985.

44. Hegedus L and others. Increased frequency of goitre in epileptic patients on long-term phenytoin or carbamazepine treatment, *Clin Endocrinol* 23:423-429, 1985.

45. Perrild H and others. Thyroid function and ultrasonically determined thyroid size in patients receiving long-term lithium treatment, *Am J Psychiatry* 147:1518-1521, 1990.

46. Christensen SB, Ljungberg O, and Tibblin S. Thyroid carcinoma in Malmo, 1960-1977: epidemiologic, clinical, and prognostic findings in a defined urban population, *Cancer* 53:1625-1633, 1984.

47. Mazzaferri EL and others. Papillary thyroid carcinoma: the impact of therapy in 576 patients, *Medicine* 56:171-196, 1977.

48. Hamming JF and others. The value of fine-needle aspiration biopsy in patients with nodular thyroid disease divided into groups of suspicion of malignant neoplasms on clinical grounds, *Arch Intern Med* 150:113-116, 1990.

49. Woolf PD. Transient painless thyroiditis with hyperthyroidism: a variant of lymphocytic thyroiditis? *Endocrinol Rev* 1:411-1420, 1980.

50. Greene JN. Subacute thyroiditis, *Am J Med* 51:97-108, 1971.

51. Murray IPC, Stewart RDH, and Indyk JS. The diagnosis of the painful thyroid, *Med J Austral* 2:1055-1061, 1970.

52. Volpe R and Johnston MW. Subacute thyroiditis: a disease commonly mistaken for pharyngitis, *Can Med Assoc J* 77:297-307, 1957.

53. Mizokami T and others. Acute spontaneous hemorrhagic degeneration of the thyroid nodule with subacute thyroiditis-like symptoms and laboratory findings, *Endocrine J* 42:683-689, 1995.

54. Vander JB, Gaston EA, and Dawber TR. The significance of nontoxic thyroid nodules: Final report of a 15-year study of the incidence of thyroid malignancy, *Ann Intern Med* 69:537-540, 1968.

55. Tunbridge WMG and others. The spectrum of thyroid disease in a community: the Whickham survey, *Clin Endocrinol* 7:481-493, 1977.

56. Wang C and Crapo LM. The epidemiology of thyroid disease and implications for screening, *Endocrinol Metab Clin North Am* 26:189-218, 1997.

57. Hermus AR and Huysmans DA. Treatment of benign nodular thyroid disease, *N Engl J Med* 338:1438-1446, 1998.

58. Tomimori E and others. Prevalence of incidental thyroid disease in a relatively low iodine intake area, *Thyroid* 5:273-276, 1995.

59. Ridgeway EC. Clinical review 30: clinician's evaluation of a solitary thyroid nodule, *J Endocrinol Clin Metab* 74:231-235, 1992.

60. Ezzat S and others. Thyroid incidentalomas: prevalence by palpation and ultrasonography, *Arch Intern Med* 154:1838-1840, 1994.

61. Brander A and others. Clinical versus ultrasound examination of the thyroid gland in common clinical practice, *J Clin Ultrasound* 20:37-42, 1992.

62. Witterick IJ and others. Incidence and types of non-palpable thyroid nodules in thyroids removed for palpable disease, *J Otolaryngol* 22:294-300, 1993.

63. Schneider AB and others. Thyroid nodules in the follow-up of irradiated individuals: Comparison of thyroid ultrasound with scanning and palpation, *J Clin Endocrinol Metab* 82:4020-4027, 1997.

64. Brennan MD and others. Follicular thyroid cancer treated at the Mayo Clinic, 1946 through 1970: initial manifestations, pathologic findings, therapy, and outcome, *Mayo Clin Proc* 66:11-22, 1991.

65. McConahey WM and others. Papillary thyroid cancer treated at the Mayo Clinic, 1946 through 1970: initial manifestations, pathologic findings, therapy, and outcome, *Mayo Clin Proc* 61:978-996, 1986.

66. Gruhn JG, Barsano CP, and Kumar Y. The development of tests of thyroid function, *Arch Pathol Lab Med* 111:84-100, 1987.

67. Dubois EF. *Basal metabolism in health and disease,* Philadelphia, 1927, Lea & Febiger.

68. White GH. Can the initial clinical assessment of thyroid function be improved? *Lancet* 2:933-935, 1978.

69. Beahrs OH. American Association of Endocrine Surgeons. Presidential address: lest we forget, *Surgery* 102:893-897, 1987.

70. Hoffenberg R. The thyroid and Osler, *J Roy Coll Physic Lond* 19:80-84, 1985.

71. Rolleston HD. The endocrine organs in health and disease with an historical review, London, 1936, Oxford University Press.

72. Gabrilove JL and Ludwig AW. The histogenesis of myxedema, *J Clin Endocrinol Metab* 17:925-932, 1957.

73. Al-Jubouri MA and others. Xanthoderma: an unusual presentation of hypothyroidism, *J Clin Pathol* 47:850-851, 1994.

74. Escamilla RF. Carotinemia in myxedema: explanation of the typical slightly icteric tint, *J Clin Metab Endocrinol* 2:33-35, 1942.

75. Thomson JA. Alterations in capillary fragility in thyroid disease, *Clin Sci* 26:55-60, 1964.

76. Goolamali SK, Evered D, and Shuster S. Thyroid disease and sebaceous function, *Br Med J* 1:432-433, 1976.

77. Danowski TS. *Clinical endocrinology,* Baltimore, 1962, William & Wilkins.

78. Chaney WC. Tendon reflexes in myxedema: a valuable aid in diagnosis, *JAMA* 82:2013-2016, 1924.

79. Rives KL, Furth ED, and Becker DV. Limitations of the ankle jerk test: intercomparison with other tests of thyroid function, *Ann Intern Med* 62:1139-1146, 1965.

80. Lawson JD. The free Achilles reflex in hypothyroidism and hyperthyroidism. *N Engl J Med* 259:761-764, 1958.

81. Sherman L. The Achilles reflex, *Lancet* 2:942-943, 1963 (letter).

82. Sherman M and Larson FC. The Achilles reflex: a diagnostic test of thyroid function, *Lancet* 1:243-245, 1963.

83. Fanburg BL. Calcium transport by skeletal muscle sarcoplasmic reticulum in the hypothyroid rat, *J Clin Invest* 47:2499-2506, 1968.

84. Reinfrank RF and others. Observations of the Achilles reflex test, *JAMA* 199:59-62, 1967.

85. Cassidy CE and Eddy RL. Hypothyroidism in patients with goiter, *Metabolism* 19:751-759, 1970.

86. Lloyd WH. Value of the voice in diagnosis of myxoedema in the elderly, *Br Med J* 1:1208-1211, 1959.

87. Maragos NE. Vocal abnormalities: what listening can tell you, *Postgrad Med* 76:25-34, 1984.

88. Wolf S. Hypothyroiditis, *J Fam Pract* 37:225, 1993 (letter).

89. Asher R. Myxoedematous madness, *Br Med J* 2:555-562, 1949.

90. Bicknell PG. Mild hypothyroidism and its effects on the larynx, *J Laryngol Otol* 87:123-127, 1973.

91. Plummer WA. Body weight and spontaneous myxedema, *West J Surg* 50:85-92, 1942.

92. Barker DJ and Bishop JM. Computer-based screening system for patients at risk of hypothyroidism, *Lancet* 2:835-838, 1969.

93. Nordyke RA, Kulikowski CA, and Kulikowski CW. A comparison of methods for the automated diagnosis of thyroid dysfunction, *Comput Biomed Res* 4:374-389, 1971.

94. Billewicz WZ and others. Statistical methods applied to the diagnosis of hypothyroidism, *Q J Med* 38:255-266, 1969.

95. Seshadri MS and others. Clinical scoring system for hypothyroidism: is it useful? *J Gen Intern Med* 4:490-492, 1989.

96. Sisson JC. Principles of, and pitfalls in, thyroid function tests, *J Nuc Med* 6:853-901, 1965.

97. Doucet J and others. Does age play a role in clinical presentation of hypothyroidism? *J Am Geriatr Soc* 42:984-986, 1994.

98. Franklyn JA. The management of hyperthyroidism, *N Engl J Med* 330:1731-1738, 1994.

99. Major RH. *Classic descriptions of disease: with biographical sketches of the authors,* Springfield, 1932, Charles C Thomas.

100. Hegedus L, Hansen JM, and Karstrup S. High incidence of normal thyroid gland volume in patients with Graves' disease, *Clin Endocrinol* 19:603-607, 1983.

101. Hegedus L and others. Thyroid size and goitre frequency in hyperthyroidism, *Dan Med Bull* 34:121-123, 1987.

102. Nordyke RA, Gilbert FI, and Harada ASM. Graves' disease: influence of age on clinical findings, *Arch Intern Med* 148:626-631, 1988.

103. Chapdelain A, Coulombe R, and LeLorier J. The effects of propranolol, practolol, and placebo on the clinical manifestations of thyrotoxicosis, *Int J Clin Pharm* 14:308-312, 1976.

104. Davis PJ and Davis FB. Hyperthyroidism in patients over the age of 60 years: clinical features in 85 patients, *Medicine* 53:161-181, 1974.

105. Healy JF and Brault T. Enlargement of the superior thyroid artery: an unusual cause for a cervical bruit, *Angiology* 35:579-580, 1984.

106. Cooper WW. On protrusion of the eyes, in connexion with anaemia, palpitation, and goiter, *Lancet* 1:551-554, 1849.

107. Ruedemann AD. Ocular changes associated with hyperthyroidism. In: Crile G, editor. *Diagnosis and treatment of diseases of the thyroid gland*, Philadelphia, 1932, WB Saunders, pp. 196-208.

108. Miller NR. *Walsh and Hoyt's clinical neuro-ophthalmology*, ed 4, Baltimore, 1985, Williams & Wilkins, pp. 945-957.

109. Duke-Elder S. Lid-retraction. In Duke-Elder S, editor. *System of ophthalmology, neuro-ophthalmology*, London, 1971, Henry Kimpton, pp. 905-915.

110. Gladstone GJ. Ophthalmologic aspects of thyroid-related orbitopathy, *Endocrinol Metab Clin North Am* 27:91-100, 1998.

111. Murchison L and others. Comparison of propanolol and practolol in the management of hyperthyroidism, *Br J Clin Pharm* 3:273-277, 1976.

112. Hall R, Storey E, and Farmer FT. Ophthalmic Graves' disease: clinical and laboratory features, *Proc Roy Soc Med* 61:1305-1306, 1968.

113. Bartley GB and others. Clinical features of Graves' ophthalmopathy in an incidence cohort, *Am J Ophthalmol* 121:284-290, 1996.

114. Feldon SE and Levin L. Graves' ophthalmopathy: V. Aetiology of upper eyelid retraction in Graves' ophthalmopathy, *Br J Ophthalmol* 74:484-485, 1990.

115. Hallin ES and Feldon SE. Graves' ophthalmopathy: II. Correlation of clinical signs with measures derived from computed tomography, *Br J Ophthalmol* 72:678-682, 1988.

116. Bartley GB. The differential diagnosis and classification of eyelid retraction, *Ophthalmology* 103:168-176, 1996.

117. Lepore FE. Unilateral ptosis and Hering's law, *Neurology* 38:319-322, 1988.

118. Schmidtke K and Buettner-Ennever JA. Nervous control of eyelid function: a review of clinical, experimental and pathological data, *Brain* 115:227-247, 1992.

119. Bahn RS and Heufelder AE. Pathogenesis of Graves' ophthalmopathy, *N Engl J Med* 329:1468-1475, 1993.

120. Grove AS. Evaluation of exophthalmos, *N Engl J Med* 292:1005-1013, 1974.

121. Feldon SE, Muramatsu S, and Weiner JM. Clinical classification of Graves' ophthalmopathy: identification of risk factors for optic neuropathy, *Arch Ophthalmol* 102:1469-1472, 1984.

122. Shanks RG and others. Controlled trial of propranolol in thyrotoxicosis, *Lancet* 1:993-994, 1969.

123. Woeber KA. Thyrotoxicosis and the heart, *N Engl J Med* 327:94-98, 1992.

124. van Olshausen K and others. Cardiac arrhythmias and heart rate in hyperthyroidism, *Am J Cardiol* 63:930-933, 1989.

125. Forfar JC and others. Abnormal left ventricular function in hyperthyroidism: evidence for a possible reversible cardiomyopathy, *N Engl J Med* 307:1165-1170, 1982.

126. Fatourechi V, Pajouhi M, and Fransway AF. Dermopathy of Graves' disease (pretibial myxedema), *Medicine* 73:1-7, 1994.

127. Engel AG. Neuromuscular manifestations of Graves' disease, *Mayo Clin Proc* 47:919-925, 1972.

128. Williams RH. Thiouracil treatment of thyrotoxicosis: I. The results of prolonged treatment, *J Clin Endocrinol* 6:1-22, 1946.

129. Martin WH and others. Mechanism of impaired exercise capacity in short duration experimental hyperthyroidism, *J Clin Invest* 88:2047-2053, 1991.

130. Crooks J, Murray IPC, and Wayne EJ. Statistical methods applied to the clinical diagnosis of thyrotoxicosis, *Q J Med* 28:211-234, 1959.

131. Gurney C and others. Newcastle thyrotoxicosis index, *Lancet* 2:1275-1278, 1970.

132. Harvey RF. Indices of thyroid function in thyrotoxicosis, *Lancet* 2:230-233, 1971.

133. Klein I and others. Symptom rating scale for assessing hyperthyroidism, *Arch Intern Med* 148:387-390, 1988.

134. Trzepacz PT and others. Graves' disease: an analysis of thyroid hormone levels and hyperthyroid signs and symptoms, *Am J Med* 87:558-561, 1989.

135. Trivalle C and Doucet J. Differences in the signs and symptoms of hyperthyroidism in older and younger patients, *J Am Geriatr Soc* 44:50-53, 1996.

136. Martin FIR and Deam DR. Hyperthyroidism in elderly hospitalised patients: clinical features and treatment outcomes, *Med J Austral* 164:200-203, 1996.

137. Tibaldi JM and others. Thyrotoxicosis in the very old, *Am J Med* 81:619-622, 1986.

CHAPTER 23

Meninges

I. **THE FINDINGS.** The terms "meningeal signs" and "meningismus" refer to the physical findings that develop after meningeal irritation from inflammation, tumor, or hemorrhage. Those most widely known are neck stiffness (or "nuchal rigidity"), Kernig's sign, and Brudzinski's sign.

A. **Neck stiffness.** Neck stiffness denotes involuntary resistance to neck flexion, which the clinician perceives when trying to bend the patient's neck, bringing the chin down to the chest. Occasionally, the aggravated extensor tone of the neck and spine is so severe that the patient's entire spine is hyperextended, leaving the torso of the supine patient supported only by occiput and heels. This extreme posture is called "opisthotonus."

B. **Kernig's sign** (described by Vladimir Kernig in 1882). With the patient's hips and knees flexed, Kernig's sign is positive when the patient resists extension of the knee. Kernig called this a "contracture" of the hamstrings that prevented extension of the knee beyond an angle of 135 degrees, even though he found the knee extended fully if the hip was first positioned in the fully extended position.[1] Most clinicians perform this test in the supine patient, although Kernig described the test being performed in the seated patient.

C. Brudzinski's sign. Jozef Brudzinski described several meningeal signs between 1909 and 1916. In his most popular sign, flexion of the supine patient's neck causes the patient to flex both hips and knees, thus retracting the legs toward the chest.[1]

II. PATHOGENESIS OF MENINGEAL SIGNS.

The basis for all meningeal signs is the patient's natural rejection of any movement that stretches spinal nerves, all of which pass through the irritated subarachnoid space. Experiments with cadavers show that flexion of the neck pulls the spinal cord toward the head, thus stretching spinal nerves, whereas flexion of the hips with knees extended pulls on the sciatic nerve, thus displacing the conus of the spinal cord downward toward the sacrum.[2] Flexion of the hips with knees flexed, in contrast, does not stretch the sciatic nerve.

These experiments explain why patients with meningeal irritation have neck stiffness and a positive Kernig's sign, and also show that Kernig's sign does not differ from the straight-leg raising test for sciatica (see Chapter 57). Brudzinski's sign, however, is more difficult to understand. At first, it seems logical that patients with meningeal irritation would want to extend their hips and flex their knees when their neck is flexed (i.e., the position opposite Kernig's sign). Although this position removes tension from the sciatic nerve, it stretches the femoral nerve,[2] explaining why Brudzinski's test causes the patient to flex both hips and knees, thus relieving tension on both nerves.

III. CLINICAL SIGNIFICANCE

A. Acute bacterial meningitis. Table 23-1 summarizes the frequency of individual findings of 1100 adults with acute bacterial meningitis (the major organisms in these studies were *Streptococcus pneumoniae*, *Neisseria meningitidis*, and *Lis-*

**TABLE 23-1 Acute bacterial meningitis
and subarachnoid hemorrhage***

Finding	Frequency (%)†
Acute Bacterial Meningitis	
Neck stiffness	57-92
Fever	66-100
Altered mental status	44-96
Kernig's or Brudzinski's sign	61
Focal neurologic signs	9-37
Seizures	9-23
Petechial rash	3-52
Subarachnoid Hemorrhage	
Neck stiffness	21-86
Seizures	32
Altered mental status	29
Focal neurologic findings	13-36
Fever	8
Preretinal hemorrhages	2

Data obtained from 1100 patients with meningitis from references 3-11 and 583 patients with subarachnoid hemorrhage from references 12-14.

Diagnostic standard: For *meningitis*, cerebrospinal fluid pleocytosis and appropriate microbiologic data or postmortem examination; for *subarachnoid hemorrhage*, computed tomography or lumbar puncture.

†Results are overall mean frequency or, if statistically heterogeneous, the range of values.

teria monocytogenes; cases of tuberculosis were excluded). This table reveals that the most frequent findings in bacterial meningitis are neck stiffness, fever, and altered mental status. Neck stiffness is a more common sign than Kernig's or Brudzinski's sign (sensitivity is 84% for neck stiffness vs. 61% for Kernig/Brudzinski's signs), although this difference is not significant and may reflect in part the clinician's diligence in looking for these findings. Eighty percent of patients with petechial rash have infection with *Neisseria meningitidis.*

Some of the heterogeneity in these studies (Table 23-1) is due to the ages of the patients. Compared to younger patients, elderly patients (defined as >65 years old for 3 of 4 studies, >50 years for one study) have a higher frequency of mental status change (90% vs. 72%), focal neurologic signs (30% vs. 17%), and fever (94% vs. 84%), but no difference in the frequency of neck stiffness.[4,9-11]

None of these studies address the specificity of these findings. A positive Kernig's sign is seen in patients with sciatica and those with subarachnoid or epidural hemorrhage or tumor of the cauda equina.[15] In a study of hospitalized elderly patients (mean age 79 years), none of whom had meningitis, nuchal rigidity was found in 35%.[16]

B. Subarachnoid hemorrhage. Table 23-1 summarizes the findings of over 500 patients with subarachnoid hemorrhage, 80% of whom presented with a severe precipitous headache. The most common physical finding in these patients was neck stiffness (sensitivity 21% to 86%). Only 29% had altered mental status.

In another study of 197 patients admitted to the hospital within 24 hours of a sudden global or focal neurologic impairment (Table 23-2), two findings argued strongly *for* subarachnoid hemorrhage and *against* cerebral infarction or intracranial hemorrhage: neck stiffness (LR = 10.3) and the absence of focal neurologic findings (LR = 5.9).[14]

TABLE 23-2 Subarachnoid Hemorrhage*

Finding	Sensitivity (%)	Specificity (%)	Positive LR	Negative LR
Neck stiffness	59	94	10.3	0.4
Neurologic findings not focal	64	89	5.9	0.4
Age ≤60 years	86	52	1.8	0.3
Seizures	32	86	2.2	NS

NS, Not significant.

*Diagnostic standard: For subarachnoid hemorrhage, computed tomography or lumbar puncture.[14]

REFERENCES

1. Verghese A and Gallemore G. Kernig's and Brudzinski's signs revisited, *Rev Inf Dis* 9:1187-1192, 1987.
2. O'Connell JEA. The clinical signs of meningeal irritation, *Brain* 69:9-21, 1946.
3. Sigurdardottir B and others. Acute bacterial meningitis in adults: a 20-year overview, *Arch Intern Med* 157:425-430, 1997.
4. Gorse GJ and others. Bacterial meningitis in the elderly, *Arch Intern Med* 144:1603-1607, 1984.
5. Aronin SI, Peduzzi P, and Quagliarello VJ. Community-acquired bacterial meningitis: risk stratification for adverse clinical outcome and effect of antibiotic timing, *Ann Intern Med* 129:862-869, 1998.
6. Hosoglu S and others. Acute bacterial meningitis in adults: analysis of 218 episodes, *Ir J Med Sci* 166:231-234, 1997.
7. Durand ML and others. Acute bacterial meningitis in adults: a review of 493 episodes, *N Engl J Med* 328:21-28, 1993.
8. Magnussen CR. Meningitis in adults: ten-year retrospective analysis at community hospital, *N Y State J Med* 80:901-906, 1980.
9. Behrman RE and others. Central nervous system infections in the elderly, *Arch Intern Med* 149:1596-1599, 1989.
10. Domingo P and others. Acute bacterial meningitis in the elderly, *Arch Intern Med* 150:1546-1548, 1990.
11. Massanari RM. Purulent meningitis in the elderly: when to suspect an unusual pathogen, *Geriatrics* 32:55-59, 1977.
12. Sengupta RP and McAllister VL. *Subarachnoid haemorrhage,* Berlin, 1986, Springer-Verlag.
13. Seet CM. Clinical presentation of patients with subarachnoid haemorrhage at a local emergency department, *Sing Med J* 40:383-385, 1999.
14. Talavera JO and others. Predictive value of signs and symptoms in the diagnosis of subarachnoid hemorrhage among stroke patients, *Arch Med Res* 27:353-357, 1996.
15. Wartenberg R. The signs of Brudzinski and of Kernig, *J Pediatr* 37:679-684, 1950.
16. Puxty JAH, Fox RA, and Horan MA. The frequency of physical signs usually attributed to meningeal irritation in elderly patients, *J Am Geriatr Soc* 31:590-592, 1983.

PART FIVE

The Lungs

CHAPTER **24**

Inspection of the Chest

This chapter discusses the findings of clubbing, barrel chest, pursed-lips breathing, accessory muscle use, and inspiratory "white noise." Other relevant findings that may be detected during inspection of the respiratory system include cyanosis (Chapter 7) and abnormal respiratory rate or breathing pattern (Chapter 17).

I. CLUBBING ("ACROPACHY," "HIPPOCRATIC FINGERS")

A. Introduction.
Clubbing is a painless focal enlargement of the connective tissue in the terminal phalanges of the digits.[1] Clubbing is usually symmetric, affecting the fingers more prominently than the toes. Although some persons have hereditary clubbing, the finding usually indicates serious underlying disease (see Clinical Significance below).

Hippocrates first described clubbing in the third century B.C. He noted it in patients with empyema, commenting that "the fingernails become curved and the fingers become warm, especially at their tips."[2]

B. The finding.
Precise definitions of clubbing were developed in the 1960s and 1970s, prompted by reports that clinicians of that time were using at least a dozen different definitions[3] and by the observation that clubbing regresses after effective treatment of the underlying dis-

order, thus making accurate measures of this physical finding an important end point to follow. There are two substantiated definitions of clubbing: (1) an interphalangeal depth ratio exceeding 1 and (2) a hyponychial angle exceeding 190 degrees (Figure 24-1). Both definitions are valid in patients of all ages, heights, and weights.

1. **Interphalangeal depth ratio.** Measurement of the interphalangeal depth ratio is described in Figure 24-1. If this ratio exceeds 1, clubbing is present, a conclusion supported by two observations: (1) the interphalangeal depth ratio of normal persons is 0.895 ± 0.041, making the threshold of 1.0 more than 2.5 standard deviations above the normal,[4] and (2) a ratio of 1.0 distinguishes digits of healthy persons from those of patients with disorders traditionally associated with clubbing (such as cyanotic heart disease and cystic fibrosis). In one study, for example, 91% of patients with cystic fibrosis

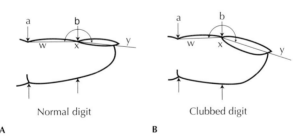

Normal digit   Clubbed digit

A   B

FIGURE 24-1 Clubbing. A, Normal digit. **B.** Clubbed digit. The middle of the distal interphalangeal joint is denoted by *a*; the junction of the nail and skin at the midline is denoted by *b*. The interphalangeal depth ratio is the ratio of the digit's depth measured at *b* divided by that at *a*. The hyponychial angle is the angle *wxy*. In the figure, the depth ratio is 0.9 for the normal digit and 1.2 for the clubbed digit (a ratio >1 indicates clubbing), and the hyponychial angle is 185 degrees for the normal digit and 200 degrees for the clubbed digit (a hyponychial angle exceeding 190 degrees indicates clubbing).

had an interphalangeal depth ratio exceeding 1 but only 1.5% of normal persons did.[4]

2. **Hyponychial angle.** Measurement of the hyponychial angle is described in Figure 24-1. If this angle exceeds 190 degrees, clubbing is present, a conclusion supported by three observations: (1) the normal hyponychial angle is 180 ± 4.2 degrees, and thus this definition is almost 2.5 standard deviations above normal[4,5]; (2) the hyponychial angle is the best parameter distinguishing plaster casts of digits labeled "definitely clubbed" by experienced clinicians from those labeled "definitely normal"[6]; and (3) one study showed that 69% of patients with cystic fibrosis had a hyponychial angle greater than 190 degrees, but no normal person did.[5]

A disadvantage to using the hyponychial angle is that precise measurement requires an apparatus called the shadowgraph, which projects the silhouette of the finger against a screen fitted with a movable protractor and which is no longer widely available.[7]

3. **Shamroth's sign.** After watching his own clubbing come and go during an episode of endocarditis, the renowned electrocardiographer Leo Shamroth suggested another definition of clubbing in 1976.[8] He noted that when clubbing was absent, placing the terminal phalanges of similar fingers back to back (especially the ring fingers) formed a small diamond-shaped window, its contour outlined by the bases of the nail beds. When clubbing developed, this window disappeared. Shamroth recommended that others subject his sign to more rigorous study, but thus far this has not occurred.

4. **Other definitions.** Parameters found to be not as accurate definitions of clubbing (compared with the hyponychial angle and interphalangeal depth ratio) are the distal

interphalangeal *width* ratio, the longitudinal curvature of nail, the transverse curvature of the nail, and the profile angle (i.e., the angle between line *wx* in Figure 24-1 and a second line extending from *x* to a point on the top of nail about a third of the distance from nail fold to nail tip).[6,9]

C. Clinical significance

1. **Etiology.** In one study of 350 patients with clubbed fingers, 80% had underlying respiratory disorders (e.g., lung tumor, bronchiectasis, lung abscess, empyema, interstitial fibrosis), 10% to 15% had miscellaneous disorders (congenital cyanotic heart disease, liver cirrhosis, chronic diarrhea, subacute endocarditis), and 5% to 10% were hereditary or idiopathic.[10]

2. **Relationship to hypertrophic osteoarthropathy.** Clubbing is sometimes associated with hypertrophic osteoarthropathy, which consists of painful edema and arthritis of the distal arms and legs, and periosteal elevation of the diaphysis of the distal long bones.[11] The usual cause is intrathoracic neoplasm (e.g., lung cancer or mesothelioma).

D. Pathogenesis.

The increased volume of the clubbed digit is primarily due to increased amounts of vascular connective tissue,[12] although the cause of this fibrovascular proliferation is still debated. According to one hypothesis, clubbing results from large megakaryocytes and clumps of platelets that become trapped in the distal digits and then release growth factors causing soft tissue growth.[13] Normally, megakaryocytes do not appear in arterial blood: they leave the bone marrow and travel in the systemic veins to the pulmonary capillaries, where they become trapped because of their large size (20 to 50 microns in diameter) and fragment into smaller platelets. In most patients with clubbing, the pulmonary capillaries are either damaged (e.g., as in many inflammatory and neoplastic pulmonary disorders) or a right-to-left shunt exists (e.g., as in congenital heart disease, or the hepatopulmonary syndrome of cirrhosis), which allows the large megakaryocytes to travel freely through the lung into arterial blood and the distal digits, where they become wedged in the digital capillaries and release growth factors, causing fibrovascular proliferation and clubbing.

This hypothesis explains why clubbing accompanies endocarditis and why it is sometimes found unilaterally in the digits distal to an infected dialysis shunt. In both examples, platelet clumps are presumably released from the infected surface to travel to the digits, where they become embedded within capillaries and release growth factors.[13]

II. BARREL CHEST

A. The finding. The normal chest is shaped like an oval cylinder, its anteroposterior diameter being less than its lateral diameter. The ratio of the anteroposterior to lateral diameter (called the "thoracic ratio," "thoracic index," or "chest index") is normally about 0.70 to 0.75 in adults and increases as persons grow older. The upper normal limit is about 0.9.[14-16]

The "barrel chest deformity" refers to a chest whose transverse section is more round than oval. It is traditionally a finding of chronic obstructive lung disease (i.e., chronic bronchitis, emphysema). Most patients also have dorsal kyphosis, a prominent sternum, widened intercostal spaces, elevated clavicles, and a shortened neck.[14] According to traditional teachings, the thoracic ratio of these patients exceeds 0.90, presumably because overactivity of the scalene and sternocleidomastoid muscles lifts the upper ribs and sternum (see Accessory Muscle Use below).

B. **Clinical significance.** Evidence linking the barrel chest deformity with chronic obstructive lung disease is conflicting. Two studies did find a significant correlation between the barrel chest deformity with more severe airflow obstruction,[17,18] although another two studies found no relationship between the finding and measures of obstruction.[14,19] Additional problems with this physical sign are that the barrel chest is not specific for obstruction and also occurs in elderly persons without lung disease,[14] and that, in some patients, the large anteroposterior dimension of the barrel chest is an illusion: the actual anteroposterior dimension is normal, but it appears abnormally large because it contrasts with an abnormally thin abdominal dimension, caused by weight loss.[20]

III. **PURSED-LIPS BREATHING.** Many patients with chronic obstructive lung disease instinctively learn that pursing the lips during expiration reduces dyspnea. The exact cause of the relief of dyspnea is still debated. Pursed-lips breathing significantly reduces the respiratory rate (from about 20 breaths/min to 12 to 15 breaths/min), increases tidal volume (by about 250 to 800 ml), decreases $Paco_2$ (by 5%), and increases oxygen saturation (by 3%).[21-23] Dyspnea may be diminished because there is less work of breathing (from slower rate), less expiratory airway collapse (the pressure drop across the lips, 2 to 4 cm of H_2O, provides continuous expiratory positive pressure), or recruitment of respiratory muscles in a way that is less fatiguing to the diaphragm.[21,22,24]

IV. **ACCESSORY MUSCLE USE**

A. **The finding.** The only muscle used in normal breathing is the diaphragm, which contracts during inspiration. Normal expiration is a passive process that relies on the elastic recoil of the lungs.[25] The term "accessory muscle use," therefore, refers to the contraction of muscles other than the diaphragm during inspiration (usually the sternocleidomastoid and scalene muscles) or to the contraction of any muscle during expiration (primarily the abdominal oblique muscles). Accessory muscle use is a common finding in patients with chronic obstructive lung disease or respiratory muscle fatigue.

B. Pathogenesis. Contraction of the sternocleidomastoid and scalene muscles lifts the clavicle and first rib, which helps expand the thorax of distressed patients, especially those with chronic obstructive lung disease in whom the flattened diaphragm generates only meager inspiratory movements. Contraction of the abdominal oblique muscles assists ventilation in two ways. In patients with obstructed airways, the abdominal muscles help expel air across the obstructed airways; in patients with respiratory muscle fatigue (e.g., amyotrophic lateral sclerosis), the abdominal muscles characteristically contract right at the moment expiration ends to compress the respiratory system so that the early part of the subsequent inspiration can occur passively.[26]

C. Clinical significance. Accessory muscle use— defined as inspiratory contraction of the sternocleidomastoid and scalene muscles— is associated with severe obstructive disease.[17,19,27-29] Over 90% of patients hospitalized with acute exacerbations of chronic obstructive lung disease use accessory muscles, but by hospital day 5, less than half do.[30] In one study, patients whose clavicle lifted more than 5 mm during inspiration identified patients with more severe obstructive disease (mean FEV_1 0.6 L) than those whose clavicle moved smaller amounts (mean FEV_1 1.5 L, p <.001).[a][27]

V. INTENSITY OF BREATHING SOUNDS (INSPIRATORY "WHITE NOISE"; "NOISY BREATHING")

A. The finding. The breathing of normal persons is inaudible more than a few centimeters from the mouth, unless the person is sighing, panting, or gasping.[32] In three clinical settings, breathing sometimes becomes very noisy and is easily heard a distance from the bedside: in patients with lower airways obstruction, who may have audible *expiratory* wheezing (see Chapter 26), in patients with upper airway obstruction, who may have *inspiratory* stridor (see Chapter 26), and in patients with chronic bronchitis or asthma, who may have *inspiratory* "white noise."[32]

"White noise" is an acoustical term meaning that, unlike wheezing and stridor, the sound lacks a musical pitch and therefore resembles more the static of a radio tuned between stations. In patients with chronic bronchitis and asthma, the loud inspiratory white noise heard at the patient's bedside without the stethoscope often contrasts sharply with the quiet inspiratory sounds heard through the stethoscope during auscultation (see Chapter 26).

B. Pathogenesis. Inspiratory white noise results from air turbulence caused by narrowed central airways,[33] a conclusion based on the observation that the sounds diminish after the patient receives effective bronchodilator treatment

---

[a] FEV_1 is "forced expiratory volume in one second," which is a measure of ventilatory capacity. It is normally 3.0 to 3.8 L.[31] The FEV_1 is abnormally low in obstructive lung disease and restrictive lung disease, dyspnea first appearing in these conditions when the FEV_1 falls below 2.5 L. An FEV_1 less than 1.0 L in chronic obstructive lung disease indicates severe disease.

(which increases the patient's FEV_1) or breathes a mixture oxygen and helium (a gas mixture that reduces turbulence).[33] Inspiratory white noise is not a feature of emphysema, presumably because the inspiratory caliber of the central airways in these patients is normal.[33]

C. Clinical significance. Inspiratory white noise is a feature of chronic bronchitis and asthma, but not emphysema. The intensity of white noise in patients with asthma and chronic bronchitis correlates inversely with the patient's FEV_1 ($r = -0.60$ to -0.64).[33]

REFERENCES

1. Fischer DS, Singer DH, and Feldman SM. Clubbing, a review, with emphasis on hereditary acropachy, *Medicine* 43:459-479, 1964.
2. Hippocratic writings. In Lloyd GER, editor. Harmondsworth, Middlesex, England, 1978, Penguin Books, p. 212.
3. Pyke DA. Finger clubbing: validity as a physical sign, *Lancet* 2:352-354, 1954.
4. Waring WW and others. Quantitation of digital clubbing in children, *Am Rev Respir Dis* 104:166-174, 1971.
5. Bentley D, Moore A, and Shwachman H. Finger clubbing: a quantitative survey by analysis of the shadowgraph, *Lancet* 2:164-167, 1976.
6. Regan GM, Tagg B, and Thomson ML. Subjective assessment and objective measurement of finger clubbing, *Lancet* 1:530-532, 1967.
7. Bentley D and Cline J. Estimation of clubbing by analysis of shadowgraph, *Br Med J* 3:43, 1970.
8. Shamroth L. Personal experience, *South Afr Med J* 50:297-300, 1976.
9. Carroll DG. Curvature of the nails, clubbing of the fingers and hypertrophic pulmonary osteoarthropathy, *Trans Am Clin Climat Assoc* 83:198-208, 1971.
10. Coury C. Hippocratic fingers and hypertrophic osteoarthropathy: a study of 350 cases, *Br J Dis Chest* 54:202-209, 1960.
11. Hansen-Flaschen J and Nordberg J. Clubbing and hypertrophic osteoarthropathy, *Clin Chest Med* 8:287-298, 1987.

12. Shneerson JM. Digital clubbing and hypertrophic osteo-arthropathy: the underlying mechanisms, *Br J Dis Chest* 75:113-131, 1981.

13. Dickinson CJ. The aetiology of clubbing and hypertrophic osteoarthropathy, *Eur J Clin Invest* 23:330-338, 1993.

14. Pierce JA and Ebert RV. The barrel deformity of the chest, the senile lung and obstructive pulmonary emphysema, *Am J Med* 25:13-22, 1958.

15. Takahashi E and Atsumi H. Age differences in thoracic form as indicated by thoracic index, *Human Biol* 27:65-74, 1955.

16. Hurato A and others. Studies of total pulmonary capacity and its subdivisions. VI. Observations on cases of obstructive pulmonary emphysema, *J Clin Invest* 13:1027-1051, 1934.

17. Schneider IC and Anderson AE. Correlation of clinical signs with ventilatory function in obstructive lung disease, *Ann Intern Med* 62:477-485, 1965.

18. Ravid M and others. The "ruler sign": a semiquantitative physical sign of chronic obstructive pulmonary disease, *Israel J Med Sci* 24:10-12, 1988.

19. Fletcher CM. The clinical diagnosis of pulmonary emphysema: an experimental study, *Proc Roy Soc Med* 45:577-584, 1952.

20. Kilburn KH and Asmundsson T. Anteroposterior chest diameter in emphysema, *Arch Intern Med* 123:379-382, 1969.

21. Breslin EH. The pattern of respiratory muscle recruitment during pursed-lip breathing, *Chest* 101:75-78, 1992.

22. Thoman RL, Stoker GL, and Ross JC. The efficacy of pursed-lips breathing in patients with chronic obstructive pulmonary disease, *Am Rev Respir Dis* 93:100-106, 1966.

23. Mueller RE, Petty TL, and Filley GF. Ventilation and arterial blood gas changes induced by pursed lips breathing, *J Appl Physiol* 28:784-789, 1970.

24. Barach AL. Physiologic advantages of grunting, groaning, and pursed-lip breathing: adaptive symptoms related to the development of continuous positive pressure breathing, *Bull NY Acad Med* 49:666-673, 1973.

25. Goldman MD and others. Asynchronous thoracoabdominal movements in chronic airflow obstruction (CAO), *Adv Exp Med Biol* 393:95-100, 1995.

26. Grinman S and Whitelaw WA. Pattern of breathing in a case of generalized respiratory muscle weakness, *Chest* 84:770-772, 1983.

27. Anderson CL, Shankar PS, and Scott JH. Physiological significance of sternomastoid muscle contraction in chronic obstructive pulmonary disease, *Resp Care* 25:937-939, 1980.

28. Godfrey S and others. Clinical and physiological associations of some physical signs observed in patients with chronic airways obstruction, *Thorax* 25:285-287, 1970.

29. Stubbing DG and others. Some physical signs in patients with chronic airflow obstruction, *Am Rev Respir Dis* 125: 549-552, 1982.

30. O'Neill S and McCarthy DS. Postural relief of dyspnoea in severe chronic airflow limitation: relationship to respiratory muscle strength, *Thorax* 38:595-600, 1983.

31. Medical Section of the American Lung Association. Lung function testing: selection of reference values and interpretative strategies, *Am Rev Respir Dis* 144:1202-1218, 1991.

32. Forgacs P. The functional basis of pulmonary sounds, *Chest* 73:399-412, 1978.

33. Forgacs P, Nathoo AR, and Richardson HD. Breath sounds, *Thorax* 26:288-295, 1971.

CHAPTER 25

Palpation and Percussion of the Chest

PALPATION

I. INTRODUCTION. Palpation of the chest is limited because the bony rib cage hides many abnormalities of the underlying lungs. The traditional reasons to palpate the chest are to detect the following signs: (1) chest wall tenderness or masses, (2) pleural friction rubs, (3) bronchial fremitus, (4) abnormal respiratory excursion, and (5) asymmetric tactile fremitus. Bronchial fremitus is an inspiratory vibratory sensation felt in some patients with airway secretions. Respiratory excursion is assessed while the patient breathes in and out, either by simultaneously palpating symmetric areas of the chest or measuring the changing circumference with a tape measure. According to traditional teachings, chest excursion is reduced bilaterally in chronic airflow obstruction and neuromuscular disease (see Chapter 29) and unilaterally in pleural effusion and consolidation.

II. TACTILE FREMITUS

A. The finding. Tactile fremitus ("vocal fremitus") is the vibration felt by the clinician's hand resting on the chest wall of a patient who is speaking or singing.

B. Technique. To elicit the sign, the patient usually says "one-two-three" or "ninety-nine" repeatedly and evenly while the clinician compares symmetric areas of the chest. Some early German physical diagnosticians used the word *neun-und-neunzig* (German for "ninety-nine") to elicit vocal fremitus, prompting modern English-speaking authors to suggest that the "oy" sound is necessary to elicit the finding (e.g., "toy boat" or "Toyota," to mimic the vowel sound in the German word *neun-und-neunzig*). This is incorrect, however, and the early German diagnosticians just as often used other words, such as "one, one, one" (*eins, eins, eins*) and "one, two, three" (*eins, zwei, drei*),[1-3] or had their patients sing or scream to elicit the finding.[3]

C. Finding. Vocal fremitus is more prominent in men than women because men have lower-pitched voices, which conduct more easily through lung tissue than do higher-pitched voices (see Pathogenesis of Vocal Resonance in Chapter 26). Tactile fremitus, therefore, may be absent in some healthy persons, especially those with high-pitched or soft voices or those with thick chest walls (which insulate the hand from the vibrating lung). Consequently, only *asymmetric* tactile fremitus is an abnormal finding: According to traditional teachings, fremitus is asymmetrically diminished whenever air, fluid, or tumor pushes the lung away from the chest wall (*unilateral* pneumothorax, pleural effusion, neoplasm) and is asymmetrically increased when there is consolidation of the underlying lung (i.e., *unilateral* pneumonia).

The pathogenesis of tactile fremitus is discussed in Chapter 26 (see "vocal resonance").

PERCUSSION

I. INTRODUCTION. In 1761, after studying patients and cadavers at the Spanish Hospital in Vienna for

7 years, Leopold Auenbrugger published a 95-page booklet containing the first detailed description of chest percussion.[4] His work was largely ignored for half a century, until Corvisart (physician to Napoleon) translated it into French and taught the technique to his students, including Laennec, the subsequent inventor of the stethoscope.[5] The discovery of percussion was a major diagnostic advance because, for the first time, clinicians could reliably distinguish empyema from tuberculosis and other pneumonias.[5] Until the discovery of roentgen rays in 1895, percussion and auscultation were the only methods to investigate and define diseases of the lungs during the patient's life.

II. TECHNIQUE

A. Direct vs. indirect method. In the direct method, the percussion blow lands directly on the body wall (the method of Auenbrugger and Laennec). In the indirect method, the blow falls instead on an intervening substance, called a "pleximeter," placed against the body wall. Historically, pleximeters were made of ivory or wood, or a coin was used, although today most clinicians use the middle finger of their left hand.

B. Types of percussion. There are three ways to percuss the patient: (1) comparative percussion (the original method of Auenbrugger and Laennec), (2) topographic percussion (invented by Piorry of France in 1828),[6,7] and (3) auscultatory percussion (introduced by the Americans Camman and Clark in 1840).[5,8] Today, most clinicians use the indirect method with comparative and topographic percussion and the direct method with auscultatory percussion.

1. Comparative percussion. Comparative percussion identifies disease by comparing the right and left sides of the chest. Prominent dullness or unusual hyperresonance over one side indicates disease in that part.

Bilateral disease, by definition, is difficult to identify using comparative percussion.

2. **Topographic percussion.** Topographic percussion attributes any dullness in the chest or abdomen to airless intrathoracic tissue lying directly beneath the percussion blow. Topographic percussion differs from comparative percussion in implying the clinician can precisely outline the borders of underlying organs and then measure their span. The technique is still used today to measure excursion of the diaphragm (and to identify an enlarged heart or liver; see Chapters 32 and 45).

When using topographic percussion to determine diaphragm excursion, the clinician locates the point of transition between dullness and resonance on the lower posterior chest, first during full inspiration and then during full expiration. The diaphragm excursion is the vertical distance between these 2 points. The reported normal excursion of healthy persons ranges from 3 to 6 cm (for comparison, the corresponding excursion on the chest radiograph is about 5 to 7 cm in normal persons and 2 to 3 cm in patients with lung disease).[5,9,10]

3. **Auscultatory percussion.** Auscultatory percussion was introduced to further refine the goals of topographic percussion.[8] Instead of listening to sounds as they resonate off the chest into the surrounding room, the clinician using auscultatory percussion places the stethoscope on the body wall and listens through it to the sounds transmitted by nearby percussive blows.

Over the last 150 years, auscultatory percussion of the chest has repeatedly fallen out of favor and then resurfaced as a "new sign."[5] In the most recent version of auscultatory percussion of the chest, introduced in

1974, the clinician taps lightly over the manubrium and listens over the posterior part of the chest with the stethoscope.[11,12] Using this technique, the clinician should find identical sounds at corresponding locations of the two sides of the chest; a note of decreased intensity on one side supposedly indicates ipsilateral disease between the tapping finger and stethoscope.

The technique of using auscultatory percussion to detect pleural fluid, first developed in 1927,[13] is slightly different. The clinician places his stethoscope on the posterior chest of the seated patient, 3 cm below the twelfth rib and percusses the posterior chest from apex to base. At some point the normal dull note changes to an unusually loud note: if this occurs with strokes above the twelfth rib, the test is abnormal, indicating pleural fluid.[14]

C. The percussion blow

1. Force. Each percussion blow should strike the same part of the pleximeter with identical force, and the pleximeter finger should be applied with the same force and orientation when comparing right and left sides. Consistent technique is important because both the percussion force and the pleximeter govern the percussion sound produced. Lighter strokes produce sounds that are duller than those produced by stronger strokes. Lifting the pleximeter finger, even slightly, can transform a resonant note into a dull one.

Even though a consistent technique is important, the force and speed of percussion blows vary threefold among different clinicians,[15] which probably explains why interobserver agreement for topographic percussion is poor compared with that for other physical findings (see Chapter 3).

2. **Rapid withdrawal of plexor.** The traditional teaching is that the plexor finger should be promptly withdrawn after a blow, mimicking the action of a piano key striking a string. The only study of this found that clinicians could not distinguish the note created by a rapid withdrawal from one in which the plexor finger lightly rested on the pleximeter after the blow.[16]

III. THE FINDING

A. **Percussion sounds.** There are three percussion sounds—**tympany** (normally heard over the abdomen), **resonance** (heard over normal lung), and **dullness** (heard over the liver or thigh) (Table 25-1). Tympany differs from resonance and dullness because it contains vibrations of a dominant frequency, which allows the clinician to actually identify its musical pitch. Resonance and dullness, in contrast, are "noise" in an acoustical sense, consisting of a jumble of frequencies that prevent identification of a specific musical pitch. The three sound characteristics distinguishing resonance and dullness are intensity, duration, and frequency content: Resonance is louder and longer and contains more low-frequency energy.[5,17] Of these three sound characteristics, clinicians appreciate most easily that resonance is louder than dullness.

Some clinicians take advantage of resonance being louder than dullness, using a technique called threshold percussion, in which percussion blows are so light that dull areas produce no sound. As the blows move along the body wall with precisely the same amount of force, a note abruptly appears the moment the blow encounters a resonant area. An old adage in percussion, attributed to Weil, is that it is much easier to distinguish "something from nothing" than to distinguish "more from less."[5]

TABLE 25-1 The percussion sounds*

	TYMPANY	RESONANCE	DULLNESS
Sound pressure waveform			
Duration	>40 ms	≈15 ms	<3 ms
Frequency content	Dominant single frequency (200-600 Hz)	Assessed by the ear to have a low-frequency component, compared with dullness	Assessed by the ear to be high in frequency, compared with resonance

*Adapted from references 5 and 17, with permission. In the older literature, synonyms for resonance were "full," "clear," "distinct" sound; synonyms for dullness were "empty," "not distinct," "thigh" sound.

ms, Milliseconds.

B. **Sense of resistance.** All great teachers of percussion have emphasized that the tactile sense in the pleximeter finger provides as much information as the audible notes. Dull areas, according to these teachers, move less or offer more resistance than resonant areas (thus earning pleural effusion the descriptor "stony dullness"). Experiments using light-weight accelerometers taped to the pleximeter finger confirm that dull areas do move less than resonant areas.[18]

C. **Glossary of additional percussion terms.** Historically, the vocabulary of clinical percussion was diverse. Some of the more commonly used terms appear below.

   1. **Skodaic resonance.** Skodaic resonance is a hyperresonant note produced by percussion of the chest above a pleural effusion. The cause of this finding is unknown. Skodaic resonance was originally described by Josef Skoda,[19] a champion of topographic percussion and the first to apply the principles of physics to percussion.

   2. **Grocco's triangle.** Grocco's triangle is a right-angled triangle of dullness found over the posterior region of the chest *opposite* a large pleural effusion. The horizontal side of the triangle follows the diaphragm for several centimeters; the vertical side lies over the spinous processes but usually ends below the top level of the effusion.[5] This finding was originally described by Koranyi (Hungary, 1897) and later by Grocco (Italy, 1902) and Rauchfuss (Germany, 1903).

   3. **Metallic resonance ("amphoric resonance"; "coin test").** Metallic resonance is a pure tympanitic sound containing very high frequencies, found over large superficial pulmonary cavities or pneumothoraces.[19,20] Flicking the tense cheek while holding the mouth open mimics the sound. The

sound was best elicited with a hard plexor and pleximeter (e.g., two coins) and is best perceived through the stethoscope or with the examiner's ear near the patient's chest.[5]

4. **Krönig's isthmus.** Krönig's isthmus is a narrow band of resonance over each lung apex that lies between the dullness from the neck and the dullness from the shoulder muscles. Diseases of the lung apex, such as tuberculosis, supposedly reduced the width of the band.[5] Georg Krönig (Germany) described the finding in 1889.[21]

5. **Cracked-pot resonance.** Cracked-pot resonance is a percussion sound over superficial tubercular cavities, mimicked by pressing the palms together and hitting the back of one hand against the knee.[19,22] To detect the sound in patients, the clinician delivers a strong percussion blow and listens near the patient's open mouth.[2,23] Although the sound was traditionally attributed to the sudden efflux of air through bronchi communicating with a tubercular cavity, the only published pathologic study found no bronchial communication in 11 patients with this sound.[24]

IV. PATHOGENESIS
A. **Topographic percussion vs. cage resonance theory.** From the earliest days of percussion, two opposing theories have explained the genesis of percussion sounds: the "topographic percussion theory" and the "cage resonance theory." The topographic percussion theory argued that only the physical characteristics of the soft tissues directly beneath the percussion blow controlled whether resonance or dullness was produced. This theory emphasized that the body wall itself contributed little to the resulting sound but acted merely to convey the vibrations from the underlying tissues (much

like a diaphragm in a microphone transmits the sound vibrations imparted to it). A fundamental tenet of the topographic percussion theory was the "several centimeter rule," advanced by Weil in 1880,[25] which stated that the percussion stroke penetrated only the most superficial 4 to 6 cm of tissue, and only anatomic abnormalities in this layer influenced the sound produced.

In contrast, the cage resonance theory argued that the percussion sound reflected the ease with which the body wall vibrates, which in turn was influenced by many variables, including the strength of the stroke, the condition and state of the body wall, and the underlying organs. Advocates of the cage resonance theory argued that precise topographic percussion was impossible because underlying organs or disease could cause dullness to occur at distant sites.

The topographic percussion theory became very popular—largely through the persuasive efforts of renowned clinical teachers, including Piorry; Skoda; Mueller; and Mueller's pupil, Ralph Major, who wrote one of the most popular American physical diagnosis textbooks.[1] Nonetheless, the evidence cited to support this theory and the several centimeter rule was meager and of uncertain relevance[5]: it included only a few experiments with cadavers[25] and some sound recordings of exenterated lung slices as they were being percussed.[26]

In contrast, considerable evidence supports the cage resonance theory:

1. **Analysis of sound recordings.** The percussion sound contains more frequencies than can be explained by vibrations of just the area of the body wall percussed.[18,27-29] Areas of the body wall distant to the blow must also vibrate and contribute to the sound.

2. **Condition and state of the body wall.** External pressure on the chest—from a pil-

low, a stretcher, or an extra hand placed near the point of percussion—impedes chest wall motion and dampens the percussion note.[20,30]

Pressure against the inner wall of the chest of cadavers also causes dullness, even in areas of the body wall distant from where the pressure is applied.[20] The best clinical example of the distant effects of internal pressure is Grocco's triangle, a right-angled triangle of dullness found over the posterior region of the chest *opposite* a large pleural effusion (see above). Grocco's triangle proves that pressure on the chest wall at one point (e.g., from pleural fluid) may cause dullness at sites distant to that pressure (i.e., over the opposite chest). Even in patients without pleural fluid, external pressure on one side of the posterior chest from a hand or water bottle will produce Grocco's triangle on the opposite chest.[31,32]

Heavier patients have larger liver spans than patients who weigh less,[33] not because the livers of heavier patients are larger, but instead because the excess subcutaneous fat influences the cage resonance and dampens the vibrations, resulting in more dullness and larger spans.

3. **The strength of the percussion blow.** The strength of the blow influences whether resonance or dullness is produced, especially near areas of the body wall marking the transition between resonance and dullness. For example, in percussion of the liver, the span of the liver is about 3 cm smaller when using strong strokes than it is when using light strokes (see Chapter 45).[33-35] This occurs because the heavy stroke, when located near where the liver touches the body wall, more easily generates the vibrations neces-

sary for the resonant note, whereas the light stroke is insufficient until further removed. These findings contradict the assertion of topographic percussionists, who taught that stronger blows penetrated tissues more deeply than softer ones; if this were true, percussion of the liver with heavy strokes should produce a larger span than with light strokes (because heavier strokes would detect the dome of the liver, which is removed from the body wall).

B. Auscultatory percussion. The advocates of auscultatory percussion believe that sound waves travel directly from the tapping finger through the lung to the stethoscope and are altered along the way by diseased tissue. It is much more likely, however, that these sounds are conducted circumferentially in the chest wall, for several reasons: (1) The technique fails to detect the heart, which should render some notes of the left chest more dull if sound waves traveled directly to the stethoscope. (2) Sound recordings during auscultatory percussion are the same whether the patient breathes room air or a mixture of helium and oxygen.[36] Because sound characteristics depend on the gas density of the conducting medium, which is different for the two gas mixtures, it is unlikely sound travels through the lung. (3) The characteristics of the sound change during the Valsalva and Mueller maneuvers, which increase tension in the chest wall but do not alter the underlying lung.[36] (4) Contour maps reveal that the loudest sounds during auscultatory percussion appear over bony prominences, such as the scapula, indicating that the sound produced depends on the contour of the chest wall. The intervening lung contributes less to the sound heard because these sound maps do not change even when there is a large underlying tumor.[37]

V. CLINICAL SIGNIFICANCE

A. Comparative percussion.
Table 25-2 shows that asymmetric dullness is a helpful though infrequent finding, arguing for pneumonia in patients with fever and cough (LR = 3.0) and for underlying abnormalities on the chest radiograph of unselected patients (LR = 3.0). In these studies, percussion detected all large pleural effusions (sensitivity 100%), but very few consolidations (sensitivity 0% to 26%) and no intraparenchymal nodules or granulomata. The finding of normal percussion sounds is common in patients with significant lung disease and can never be used as a compelling argument against the presence of disease (all negative LRs are not significant, Table 25-2).

In chronic smokers, hyperresonance of the upper right anterior chest is a valuable finding arguing for chronic airflow obstruction (positive LR = 5.1; see Table 25-2).[46]

B. Topographic percussion of the diaphragm.
In patients with lung disease, clinicians usually overestimate the actual movements of the diaphragm and differ from the chest film by 1 to 3 cm.[9,47] The correlation between actual and percussed movements is poor in the only study of this finding (r = 0.14 to 0.42, not significant half the time).[9] Another study showed that a percussed diaphragm excursion of less than 2 cm is an infrequent and unreliable diagnostic sign of chronic obstructive lung disease (both LRs not significant).[46]

C. Auscultatory percussion.
Studies of auscultatory percussion have widely varying results, usually showing the technique has greater sensitivity than comparative percussion but also lower specificity. Overall, the pooled results show that this technique is an unreliable diagnostic sign (both positive and negative LRs not significant; see Table 25-2).

TABLE 25-2 Diagnostic accuracy of percussion of the chest*

Finding (ref)†	Sensitivity (%)	Specificity (%)	Positive LR	Negative LR
Comparative Percussion				
Percussion Dullness				
Detecting pneumonia in patients with fever and cough[38-42]	4-26	82-99	3.0	NS
Detecting any abnormality on chest radiograph[43-45]	8-15	94-98	3.0	NS
Hyperresonance				
Detecting chronic airflow obstruction[46]	33	94	5.1	NS
Topographic Percussion				
Diaphragm Excursion <2 cm				
Detecting chronic airflow obstruction[46]	13	98	NS	NS
Auscultatory Percussion				
Abnormal Dullness				
Detecting any abnormality on chest radiograph[43-45]	16-69	74-88	NS	NS
Detecting pleural fluid[14]	96	95	18.6	0.04

NS, Not significant.

*Diagnostic standard: For pneumonia or pleural effusion, infiltrate or effusion on chest radiograph; for chronic airflow obstruction, FEV₁ less than 60% predicted or the FEV₁/FVC ratio less than 0.6.

†Definition of findings: For hyperresonance, hyperresonance of the upper right anterior chest[46]; for abnormal dullness during auscultatory percussion for chest radiograph abnormalities, asymmetric dullness, with stethoscope on posterior chest and while directly percussing sternum anteriorly; for abnormal dullness during auscultatory percussion for pleural fluid, transition to unusually loud note above twelfth rib posteriorly in midclavicular line, with stethoscope 3 cm below twelfth rib and while directly percussing posterior chest from apex to base.[14]

Like conventional percussion, auscultatory percussion identifies almost all pleural effusions (sensitivity 96%; see Table 25-2).[14] The technique used in the study cited in Table 25-2 (see Section II-B-3 for definition) was specific for pleural fluid and resulted in few positive findings among patients with underlying lung masses, pneumonia, or other underlying diseases.

REFERENCES

1. Major R. *Physical diagnosis*, ed 3, Philadelphia, 1945, WB Saunders.
2. Sahli H. *A treatise on diagnostic methods of examination*, Philadelphia, 1911, WB Saunders.
3. Guttman P. A handbook of physical diagnosis: comprising the throat, thorax, and abdomen, New York: William Wood and Co.; 1880.
4. Auenbrugger L. On percussion of the chest (1761), a translation of Auenbrugger's original treatise entitled "Inventum novum ex percussione thoracis humani, ut signo abstrusos interni pectoris morbos detegendi" (facsimile edition by Johns Hopkins Press). Baltimore, 1936, The Johns Hopkins Press.
5. McGee S. Percussion and physical diagnosis: separating myth from science, *Disease-a-Month* 41:643-692, 1995.
6. Risse GB. Pierre A. Piorry (1794-1879): the French "master of percussion," *Chest* 60:484-488, 1971.
7. Sakula A. Pierre Adolphe Piorry (1794-1879): pioneer of percussion and pleximetry, *Thorax* 34:575-581, 1979.
8. Camman GP and Clark A. A new mode of ascertaining the dimensions, form, and condition of internal organs by percussion, *N Y J Med Surg* 3:62-96, 1840.
9. Williams TJ, Ahmad D, and Morgan WKC. A clinical and roentgenographic correlation of diaphragmatic movement, *Arch Intern Med* 141:878-880, 1981.
10. Young DA and Simon G. Certain movements measured on inspiration-expiration chest radiographs correlated with pulmonary function studies, *Clin Radiol* 23:37-41, 1972.
11. Guarino JR. Auscultatory percussion: a new aid in the examination of the chest, *J Kans Med Soc* 75:193-194, 1974.

12. Guarino JR. Auscultatory percussion of the chest, *Lancet* 1:1332-1334, 1980.

13. Webb GB. Auscultatory percussion in the diagnosis of pleural fluid, *JAMA* 88:99, 1927.

14. Guarino JR and Guarino JC. Auscultatory percussion: a simple method to detect pleural effusion, *J Gen Intern Med* 9:71-74, 1994.

15. Burger HC, Casteleyn G, and Jordan FLJ. How is percussion done? *Acta Med Scand* 142:106-112, 1952.

16. Coleman W. The alleged dullness over the apex of the normal right lung, *Am J Med Sci* 197:141-145, 1939.

17. Murray A and Neilson JMM. Diagnostic percussion sounds: 1. A qualitative analysis; 2. Computer-automated parameter measurement for quantitative analysis, *Med Biol Eng* 13:19-38, 1975.

18. Murray A and Neilson JMM. Diagnostic percussion: a study of chest-wall motion and the associated tactile sensation, *Med Biol Eng Comput* 16:269-278, 1978.

19. Skoda J. *Auscultation and percussion*, Philadelphia, 1854, Lindsay & Blakiston.

20. Mazoon JF. Die Theorie der Perkussion der Brust auf Grundlage directer Versuche und zahlreicher Beobachtungen, *Vierteljahrschrift Prakt Heilkd* 36:1-59, 1852.

21. Krönig G. Zur Topographie der Lungenspitzen und ihrer Perkussion, *Berl Klin Wochenschr* 26:809-812, 1889.

22. Barth M and Roger MH. *A manual of auscultation and percussion*, Philadelphia, 1866, Lindsay & Blakiston.

23. Cabot R. *Physical diagnosis of diseases of the chest*, New York, 1900, William Wood.

24. Walsh J. Necropsy findings under cracked-pot tympany, *Am Rev Tuberc* 18:202-204, 1928.

25. Weil A. Handbuch und Atlas der topographischen Perkussion, Leipzig, 1880, F.C.W. Vogel.

26. Martini P. Studien über Perkussion und Auskultation, *Dtsch Arch Klin Med* 139:65-98, 167-190, 257-284, 1922.

27. Bishop FW and others. Studies on pulmonary acoustics. IV. Notes on percussion and on forced vibrations, *Am Rev Tuberc Pulm Dis* 22:347-378, 1930.

28. Fahr G and Brandi B. Weitere Studien über Perkussion und Auskultation, *Dtsch Arch Klin Med* 164:1-33, 1929.

29. Metildi PF and others. Studies on pulmonary acoustics. III. The transmission of vibrations from percussion along ribs, *Am Rev Tuberc Pulm Dis* 21:711-744, 1930.

30. Gilbert VE. Detection of pneumonia by auscultation of the lungs in the lateral decubitus positions, *Am Rev Respir Dis* 140:1012-1016, 1989.

31. Turban K. Paralipomena der Tuberkuloseforschung, *Munch Med Wochschr* 74:1399-1404, 1927.

32. Hamburger F. Ueber die Oberflächenwirkung des Perkussionstosses, *Munch Med Wochenschr* 53:2283-2286, 1906.

33. Castell DO and others. Estimation of liver size by percussion in normal individuals, *Ann Intern Med* 70:1183-1189, 1969.

34. Sullivan S, Krasner N, and Williams R. The clinical estimation of liver size: A comparison of techniques and an analysis of the source of error, *Br Med J* 2:1042-1043, 1976.

35. Sapira JD and Williamson DL. How big is the normal liver? *Arch Intern Med* 139:971-973, 1979.

36. Bohadana AB and Kraman SS. Transmission of sound generated by sternal percussion, *J Appl Physiol* 66:273-277, 1989.

37. Bohadana AB, Patel R, and Kraman SS. Contour maps of auscultatory percussion in healthy subjects and patients with large intrapulmonary lesions, *Lung* 167:359-372, 1989.

38. Heckerling PS and others. Clinical prediction rule for pulmonary infiltrates, *Ann Intern Med* 113:664-670, 1990.

39. Melbye H and others. The diagnosis of adult pneumonia in general practice, *Scand J Prim Health Care*, 6:111-117, 1988.

40. Gennis P and others. Clinical criteria for the detection of pneumonia in adults: guidelines for ordering chest roentgenograms in the emergency department, *J Emerg Med* 7:263-268, 1989.

41. Melbye H and others. Diagnosis of pneumonia in adults in general practice, *Scand J Prim Health Care* 10:226-233, 1992.

42. Diehr P and others. Prediction of pneumonia in outpatients with acute cough—a statistical approach, *J Chron Dis* 37:215-225, 1984.

43. Nelson RS and others. Rapid clinical diagnosis of pulmonary abnormalities in HIV-seropositive patients by auscultatory percussion, *Chest* 105:402-407, 1994.

44. Bourke S and others. Percussion of the chest re-visited: a comparison of the diagnostic value of ausculatory and conventional chest percussion, *Ir J Med Sci* 158:82-84, 1989.

45. Bohadana AB, Coimbra FTV, and Santiago JRF. Detection of lung abnormalities by auscultatory percussion: a comparative study with conventional percussion, *Respiration* 50:218-225, 1986.

46. Badgett RG and others. Can moderate chronic obstructive pulmonary disease be diagnosed by historical and physical findings alone? *Am J Med* 94:188-196, 1993.
47. Cole MB and others. Bedside versus laboratory estimations of timed and total vital capacity and diaphragmatic height and movement, *Dis Chest* 38:519-521, 1970.

CHAPTER 26

Auscultation of the Lungs

The three categories of auscultatory findings of the lungs are breath sounds, vocal resonance (i.e., the sound of the patient's voice through the stethoscope), and adventitious sounds (i.e., sounds other than breath sounds or vocal resonance). Almost all of the findings discussed in this chapter were originally described in 1819 by Laennec, in his masterpiece *A Treatise on the Disease of the Chest.*[1]

I. BREATH SOUNDS
A. Finding
1. Vesicular vs. bronchial breath sounds.
There are two types of breath sounds: (1) vesicular breath sounds, which are normally heard over the posterior chest, and (2) bronchial breath sounds, which are normally heard over the trachea and right apex. These sounds are distinguished by their timing, intensity, and pitch (Table 26-1). Vesicular sounds are mostly inspiratory sounds that have a soft, breathy quality, which Laennec likened to the sound of leaves rustling in a gentle breeze. Bronchial sounds have a prominent expiratory component and much harsher quality, which sounds like air blow-

TABLE 26-1 Comparison of vesicular and bronchial breath sounds

	VESICULAR	BRONCHIAL
Timing*	Inspiration longer than expiration:	Expiration longer than inspiration:
Intensity	Soft, breathy	Loud, harsh, tubular
Pitch	Low (100 Hz)	High (300-400 Hz)
Location they normally are heard	Posterior bases	Trachea, right apex

Based on information from references 2 through 6.

*Bronchial breath sounds have a short gap between the inspiratory and expiratory sound; vesicular sounds do not.

ing forcibly through a tube (hence, they are sometimes called tubular breath sounds).

Bronchial breath sounds are abnormal when they occur over the posterior or lateral chest (especially the lower parts). According to traditional teachings, which in turn are based on postmortem examination, bronchial breath sounds occur in these locations only if solid, collapsed, or consolidated lung is contiguous with the chest wall and extends some distance toward the hilum.[7-9] The usual causes are pneumonia and pleural effusion (large pleural effusions presumably compress the underlying lung just enough to alter its acoustic properties).[10]

2. **Breath sound score.** One important feature of vesicular breath sounds is the sound's intensity, which can be graded using a scoring system developed by Pardee.[11] According to this system, the clinician listens sequentially to 6 locations on the patient's chest: bilaterally over the upper anterior portion of the chest, in the midaxillae, and at the posterior bases. At each site the clinician grades the *inspiratory* sound as absent (0 points), barely audible (1 point), faint but definitely heard (2 points), normal (3 points), or louder than normal (4 points). The patient's total score may range from 0 (absent breath sounds) to 24 (very loud breath sounds).

B. **Pathogenesis**
   1. **Vesicular sounds**
      a. **Origin.** The *inspiratory* component of vesicular breath sounds originates in the peripheral portions of the lung near where the stethoscope is placed. It does not represent simple filtration of tracheal sounds by the intervening inflated lung. The *expiratory* component of vesicular sounds probably originates in more prox-

imal, larger airways. Several lines of evidence support these statements:

(1) In experiments performed with sheep's and calf's lungs a century ago, Bullar kept the airways of both lungs patent, but rhythmically inflated only one of the two lungs using negative pressure.[12] He showed that vesicular sounds occurred only if the lung contiguous to the stethoscope filled with air; if it remained airless, it simply transmitted the upper airway bronchial sounds.

(2) The intensity of the inspiratory component of breath sounds, corrected for flow rate at the mouth, is roughly proportional to regional ventilation.[13]

(3) The inspiratory component of vesicular sounds remains the same as the stethoscope is moved progressively from the upper to lower posterior chest, although the expiratory component becomes softer.[14]

(4) Vesicular sounds contain low frequency components lacking in tracheal sounds, which cannot be reproduced in experiments interposing inflated lung between the trachea and stethoscope.[2-4]

b. Intensity. The intensity of vesicular sounds is proportional to the flow rate of air at the mouth, which in turn depends on the patient's effort and ventilatory capacity.[11,15,16] Breath sounds are thus louder if a normal person breathes hard after exercise and they are faint if obstructive lung disease diminishes flow rates.[17] Breath sounds are also reduced when air or fluid is interposed between the chest wall and lung, as in patients with pneumothorax or pleural effusion.

2. **Bronchial sounds.** Bronchial breath sounds originate in larger, proximal airways. They are normally heard over the right upper chest posteriorly but not over the left upper chest, because the trachea is contiguous with the right lung near the first thoracic vertebra but separated from the left lung by most of the mediastinum.[18] The glottis is not necessary to the sound, because bronchial sounds may occur in patients after laryngectomy or after intubation.[19] The pathogenesis of bronchial breath sounds in pneumonia and pleural effusion is discussed in Section II-B below.

C. **Clinical significance**

1. **Breath sound intensity.** A breath sound score of 9 or less is a compelling argument *for* chronic airflow obstruction (LR = 10.2; Table 26-2) and one more than 15 argues strongly *against* the diagnosis (LR = 0.1). The importance of developing some objective scoring system of breath sound intensity is demonstrated by two other studies relying just on general impressions of breath sound intensity: one study showed that reduced breath sounds argued strongly for obstructive lung disease (LR = 16.5),[26] whereas another showed the finding to have no significance.[27]

   The general impression of reduced breath sounds argues modestly for pneumonia in patients with fever and cough (LR = 2.3), and it argues for asthma if the finding appears during methacholine challenge testing (LR = 4.2).

2. **Bronchial breath sounds.** In patients with cough and fever, bronchial breath sounds argue for pneumonia (LR = 3.3), although the sign is infrequent (sensitivity 14%).

TABLE 26-2 Breath sounds and vocal resonance*

FINDING (REF)†	SENSITIVITY (%)	SPECIFICITY (%)	POSITIVE LR	NEGATIVE LR
Diminished Breath Sounds				
Detecting pneumonia in patients with cough and fever[20-23]	15-49	73-95	2.3	0.8
Detecting asthma during methacholine challenge testing[24]	78	81	4.2	0.3
Breath Sound Score				
Detecting chronic airflow obstruction[11,15]				
≤9	23-46	96-97	10.2	—
10-12	34-63	—	3.6	—
13-15	11-16	—	NS	—
>15	3-10	33-34	0.1	—
Bronchial Breath Sounds				
Detecting pneumonia in patients with cough and fever[20]	14	96	3.3	NS
Egophony				
Detecting pneumonia in patients with cough and fever[20,22,25]	4-16	96-99	4.1	NS

NS, Not significant.

*Diagnostic standard: For chronic airflow obstruction, FEV₁ <40% predicted (studies on breath sound intensity)[11,15] or FEV₁/FVC (%) ratio <0.6[26]; for pneumonia, infiltrate on chest radiograph; for asthma, 20% or greater fall in FEV₁ during methacholine challenge.

†Definition of findings: For breath sound score, see text.

II. VOCAL RESONANCE

A. The finding.
Vocal resonance refers to the sound of the patient's voice, heard through a stethoscope placed on the patient's chest. Normally, the voice sounds muffled, weak, and indistinct over most of the inferior and posterior chest, and words are unintelligible. Abnormal vocal resonance is usually classified as either bronchophony, pectoriloquy, or egophony, all terms originally introduced by Laennec.[1] Although these abnormalities have distinct definitions, the pathogenesis for all three is the same and all may appear simultaneously in the same patient. Bronchial breath sounds frequently accompany abnormal vocal resonance.

1. Bronchophony.
Bronchophony describes a voice that is much louder than normal, as

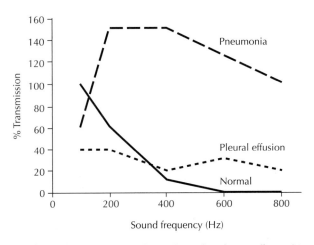

FIGURE 26-1 Transmission of sound to the chest wall. In this experiment, a speaker emitting pure musical tones of different frequencies was placed in the mouth of patients with normal lungs *(solid line)*, pneumonia *(long dashes)*, or massive pleural effusion *(short dashes)*. Microphones on the chest wall recorded the transmission of each frequency. (For purposes of comparison, "100% transmission" is the transmission of 100 Hz in normal persons.) (Adapted from reference 31.)

if the sounds were emitted directly into the stethoscope. The patient's words are not necessarily intelligible.

2. **Pectoriloquy.** Pectoriloquy implies that the patient's words are intelligible. Most clinicians test this by having the patient whisper words like "one-two-three"; intelligible whispered speech is called "whispered pectoriloquy."

3. **Egophony.** Egophony is a peculiar nasal quality to the sound of the patient's voice, which Laennec likened to the "bleating of a goat."[1] Clinicians usually elicit the finding by having the patient vocalize the vowel "EE" and then listening for the abnormal transformation of the sound into a loud nasal "AH" (the "AH" sound ranges from the "a" of the word *hat* to the "a" of the word *cart*; this finding is sometimes called "E-to-A" change).[a] Although all vowel sounds are altered by the lung (even healthy lung), what makes egophony distinctive is the intensity of the change and the suddenness with which it appears over a small area on *one* side of the chest.[30] Before concluding a patient has egophony, therefore, the clinician should confirm that a similar change of sound is absent over the identical location of the opposite chest.

B. **Pathogenesis.** Figure 26-1 depicts the transmission of sound from the larynx to the chest wall in normal persons and in those with pneumonia or pleural effusion. Normal lung behaves like a low-pass filter, which means it transmits

---

[a] The "E-to-A" change was simultaneously discovered in 1922 by Shibley[28] and Fröschel.[29] Shipley discovered the test while testing for pectoriloquy in Chinese patients. He asked the patients to say "one-two-three" in the local dialect ("ee-er-san"), and he noted that the long "EE" of "one" acquired a loud nasal "AH" quality over areas of pneumonia or effusion.[28]

low frequency sounds (100 to 200 Hz) easily but filters out high frequency sounds (>300 Hz), which include most upper airway sounds (e.g., bronchial breath sounds).[6,31-33] Consolidated lungs transmit all sound very well, both low and high frequencies. Large pleural effusions, but not small ones, reduce the transmission of frequencies below 200 to 300 Hz, but augment those more than 400 Hz.[6,10,31-33]

These observations explain why both pneumonia and large effusions cause abnormal vocal resonance and bronchial breath sounds, yet pneumonia increases tactile fremitus while effusion decreases it. Tactile fremitus consists of low frequency vibrations (100 to 200 Hz), explaining why it is more prominent over the chests of healthy men than healthy women (i.e., men's voices are lower pitched and therefore more likely to generate low frequency vibrations than women's) and why tactile fremitus progressively diminishes as a healthy person sings an ascending scale. According to Figure 26-1, pneumonia amplifies these low frequencies and thus increases tactile fremitus on the overlying chest wall. Large effusions, in contrast, reduce the transmission of low frequencies and thus diminish tactile fremitus.

Both pneumonia and large effusions transmit high frequencies much better than does healthy lung (see Figure 26-1), explaining why the high frequency bronchial breath sounds, which are poorly transmitted to the peripheral chest wall of healthy lungs, occur in both disorders. Most acoustic speech consists of frequencies less than 300 Hz, although understanding whispered speech requires the transmission of frequencies higher than 400 Hz, thus explaining why whispering pectoriloquy occurs in both pneumonia and large effusions. The sound "AH" contains more high frequency energy than the sound "EE," explaining how consolidated lung alters the "EE" by amplifying its small amount of high frequency energy and rendering it into a nasal "AH."[6,32]

C. Clinical significance. Abnormal vocal resonance has the same significance (and pathogenesis) as bronchial breath sounds. In patients with cough and fever, the finding of egophony argues *for* the diagnosis of pneumonia (LR = 4.1; see Table 26-2).

According to traditional teachings, an obstructed bronchus should diminish vocal resonance, although this teaching is probably incorrect, based on the more modern observations that some patients with egophony and pneumonia have obstructed bronchi from tumors[32] and on experiments showing that sound conducts down the substance of the porous lung itself to the chest wall, not down the airway ducts.[b34]

III. ADVENTITIOUS SOUNDS

A. Introduction. Adventitious sounds are all sounds heard during auscultation other than breath sounds or vocal resonance. The common adventitious sounds are crackles, rubs, wheezes, rhonchi, and stridor.

Adventitious sounds have the most ambiguous and confusing nomenclature in all of physical diagnosis, and studies show clinicians use up to 16 different terms in scientific publications to describe similar sounds.[35] This confusion stems from the earliest days of auscultation and the writings of Laennec, who, in the first edition of his treatise, identified five adventitious sounds but called them all "rales," distinguishing them further only by adding adjectives (e.g.,

---

[b] The acoustic characteristics of the transmitted sound are the same whether the patient breathes air or a mixture of oxygen and helium. If sound were conducted down the airways, its characteristics would change with different gas mixtures.[34]

"moist crepitus rale" for a crackling sound or "dry sibilus rale" for a whistling sound.[1,36] In later editions, Laennec substituted "rhonchus" for "rale" because he became worried that patients hearing "rale" would mistake it for the death rattle ("rale" means "rattle"). In 1831, a British editor introduced the Anglo-Saxon term "wheeze," again to refer to all lung sounds.[36] Finally, Robertson in 1957 proposed using "crackling sounds" for discontinuous sounds and "wheezes" for continuous, musical sounds, and suggested eliminating "rale" and "rhonchus" altogether.[37]

According to the American Thoracic Society, the recommended terms for lung sounds, based on their acoustic characteristics,[38] are "crackle" for discontinuous sounds and "wheeze" or "rhonchus" for continuous sounds (Table 26-3).

B. **The finding**

1. **Crackles.** Crackles are discontinuous sounds, resembling the sound produced by rubbing strands of hair together in front of the ear or by pulling apart strips of Velcro. There are **coarse crackles**, which are loud, low-pitched, and fewer in number per breath, and **fine crackles**, which are soft, higher-pitched, and greater in number per breath. Crackles that appear early during inspiration and do not continue beyond midinspiration are called **early inspiratory** crackles; those that continue into the second half of inspiration are called **late inspiratory** crackles.[41] Many American clinicians still use the word "rale" as a synonym for "crackle," although British clinicians more often use "crackle."[42,43]

The finding **posturally induced crackles**, which may have significance after myocardial infarction (see Clinical Significance below) indicates crackles that are present in the supine position but absent in the sitting

TABLE 26-3 Terminology for lung sounds

RECOMMENDED ATS TERM	ACOUSTIC CHARACTERISTICS	TERMS IN SOME TEXTBOOKS	BRITISH USAGE
Coarse crackle	Discontinuous sound: loud, low in pitch	Coarse rale	Crackle
Fine crackle	Discontinuous sound: soft, higher pitch, shorter duration	Fine rale	Crackle
Wheeze	Continuous sound: high-pitched, dominant frequency ≥400 Hz	Sibilant rhonchus	High-pitched wheeze
Rhonchus	Continuous sound: low-pitched, dominant frequency ≤200 Hz	Sonorous rhonchus	Low-pitched wheeze

Adapted from references 38-40.

ATS, American Thoracic Society.

position. To elicit the finding, the clinician listens to the lower chest wall near the posterior axillary line with the patient in three sequential positions: sitting, supine, and supine with legs elevated 30 degrees.[44] The clinician listens only after the patient has been in each position for 3 minutes. If crackles are absent when upright but appear either when supine or with legs elevated, the test is positive (i.e., the patient has "posturally induced crackles").

2. **Wheezes and rhonchi.** According to the American Thoracic Society, a wheeze is a high-pitched, continuous musical sound and a rhonchus is a low-pitched one (Table 26-3). This distinction may be superfluous because both sounds have the same pathophysiology and there is no proven clinical importance to separating them. The term "rhonchus" is probably best avoided, not only for these reasons but also because many use the term to refer to the coarse discontinuous sounds often heard in patients with airway secretions.[42]

3. **Stridor.** Stridor is a loud, musical sound of definite and constant pitch (usually about 400 Hz) that indicates upper airway obstruction.[33,40] It is identical to wheezing acoustically in every way except for two characteristics: (1) stridor is confined to inspiration, whereas wheezing is either confined entirely to expiration (30% to 60% of patients) or occurs during both expiration and inspiration (40% to 70% of patients)[45,46]; and (2) stridor is always louder over the neck, whereas wheezing is always louder over the chest.[46]

   In some patients with upper airway obstruction, stridor does not appear until the patient breathes rapidly through an open mouth.[47]

4. Pleural rub. Pleural rubs are loud grating or rubbing sounds associated with breathing that occur in patients with pleural disease. Sometimes, a pleural rub has a crackling character ("pleural crackling rub") and acoustically resembles the crackles heard in patients with parenchymal disease.[48,49] The timing of the crackling sound best distinguishes the pleural crackling rub from parenchymal crackles: the pleural crackling rub is predominately *expiratory* (i.e., 65% of crackling sound occurs during expiration), but parenchymal crackles are predominately *inspiratory* (i.e., only 10% of crackling sound occurs during expiration).[50]

5. Inspiratory squawk. The "squawk" is a short, late-inspiratory musical sound associated with parenchymal crackles in patients with interstitial lung disease.[51] It is best heard over the upper anterior chest when the patient is semirecumbent and breathing deeply. Because the sound is sometimes found in patients with bird-fancier's lung (a cause of hypersensitivity pneumonitis), the synonym "chirping rale" has been proposed.[52]

In patients with hypersensitivity pneumonitis, the squawk tends to be shorter, higher-pitched, and later in inspiration than the squawk of patients with diffuse pulmonary fibrosis.[51]

C. Pathogenesis

1. Crackles.[33,41,48,53,54] Crackles were initially attributed by Laennec and early auscultators to air bubbling through airway secretions. Although some crackles result from secretions, these promptly clear after the patient coughs. All remaining crackling sounds are felt to represent the sounds of distal airways, collapsed from the previous exhalation, as they abruptly open during inspiration. Several lines of evidence support this conclusion: (1) crackles are predominantly heard during inspiration, whereas air bubbling through secretions would cause both inspiratory and expiratory sounds; (2) the number of crackles has no relationship to the amount of sputum the patient produces (the disease having the most crackles, interstitial fibrosis, produces no or scant sputum)[55]; (3) crackles have a stereotypic pattern with each respiratory cycle (i.e., in a single patient at a single location on the chest, they are always early-, late-, or paninspiratory, and individual crackles occur at the same esophageal (transpulmonary) pressure in consecutive respiratory cycles[56]; and (4) crackles are loudest in the lower portions of the chest, even when the lung disease is distributed diffusely.

Course crackles are felt to originate in larger, more proximal airways than fine crackles, based on the observations that distinct patterns of coarse crackles (identified by their fingerprint of identical timing and number) radiate to a larger area of the chest wall than do distinct patterns of fine crackles.[57,58]

2. **Wheezes.** Wheezes are caused by vibrations of the opposing walls of narrowed airways.[48,53,59] They are not due to resonance of air in the airways (i.e., like the sound of a flute or pipe organ) because (1) if they were due to resonance of air in a hollow pipe, the length of pipe for some low-pitched wheezes would be several feet, far exceeding the length of human airways; (2) the pitch of a wheeze may change between inspiration and expiration; and (3) the pitch of the wheeze remains the same when inspired air is replaced with a gas mixture of oxygen and

helium (if due to resonance of air, the pitch should change).

D. Clinical significance

1. Crackles.
The crackles discussed below refer only to crackling sounds that persist after the patient coughs.

a. Normal persons. Crackles are rare in healthy persons during normal tidal breathing.[60,61] Fine crackling sounds, however, may appear in up to 60% of healthy persons, especially over the anterior chest, if the person first exhales as much as possible and breathes in from residual volume instead of functional residual capacity.[60,61]

b. Crackles and disease

(1) Presence of crackles. Table 26-4 indicates that the finding of crackles argues for pulmonary fibrosis in asbestos workers (LR = 5.9), for elevated left atrial pressure in patients with known heart disease (LR = 3.4), and for pneumonia in patients with cough and fever (LR = 2.0).

The frequency of crackles in interstitial lung disease depends on the etiology. Crackles are found in 100% of patients in idiopathic pulmonary fibrosis but only 5% to 20% of patients with fibrosis from sarcoidosis,[55,69] suggesting that the *absence* of crackles argues *against* the diagnosis of idiopathic fibrosis. The only finding from computed tomography that seems to predict crackles in interstitial fibrosis is the degree of subpleural fibrosis.[69]

After myocardial infarction, the finding of posturally induced crackles is associated with higher pulmo-

TABLE 26-4 Crackles and wheezes

Finding (ref)*	Sensitivity (%)	Specificity (%)	Positive LR	Negative LR
Crackles				
Detecting pulmonary fibrosis in asbestos workers[62]	81	86	5.9	0.2
Detecting elevated left atrial pressure in patients with cardiomyopathy[63-65]	19-64	82-94	3.4	NS
Detecting pneumonia in patients with cough and fever[20-23,25,66]	19-64	48-94	2.0	0.8
Early Inspiratory Crackles				
Detecting chronic airflow obstruction in patients with crackles[41,67]	25-77	97-98	14.6	NS
Detecting severe disease in patients with chronic airflow obstruction[41]	90	96	20.8	0.1
Unforced Wheezing				
Detecting chronic airflow obstruction[26,27,68]	13-56	86-99	6.0	NS
Wheezing During Methacholine Challenge Testing				
Detecting asthma[24]	44	93	6.0	0.6

NS, Not significant.

*Diagnostic standard: For pulmonary fibrosis, fibrosis on high resolution computed tomography; for elevated left atrial pressure, pulmonary capillary wedge pressure greater than 20 mm Hg[64] or 22 mm Hg[63]; for pneumonia, infiltrate on chest radiograph; for chronic airflow obstruction, $FEV_1/FVC < 0.6$[26], < 0.7[68], < 0.75[41], or less than lower 95% confidence interval for age, gender, and height[67]; for severe obstruction, FEV_1/FVC < 0.44[41]; and for asthma, 20% or greater fall in FEV_1 during methacholine challenge.[24]

nary capillary wedge pressures and worse survival.[44]

(2) *Characteristics   of   crackles.*[50,67,70-72]   Table 26-5 describes the characteristic number, timing, and type of crackles in common crackling disorders, such as pulmonary fibrosis, congestive heart failure, pneumonia, and chronic obstructive lung disease. The crackles of interstitial fibrosis are characteristically fine, have a large number of individual crackling sounds each inspiration (6 to 14), and persist to the end of inspiration (i.e., they are "late inspiratory"). Crackles of chronic airflow obstruction are coarse or fine, have the smallest number of crackling sounds (1 to 4), and are confined to the first half of inspiration ("early inspiratory"). The crackles of heart failure and pneumonia lie between these extremes; with treatment, the crackles of pneumonia become more fine and move more toward the end of inspiration.[71,72]

Table 26-4 indicates the finding of early inspiratory crackles argues strongly for chronic obstructive lung disease (LR = 14.6). Most patients with these crackles have severe obstruction (LR = 20.8; see Table 26-4).

2. Wheezes

a. Presence of wheezes. Table 26-4 indicates that the finding of unforced wheezing argues for the diagnosis of chronic obstructive lung disease (LR = 6.0). If wheezing appears during methacholine challenge testing, asthma is likely (LR = 6.0). The absence of wheezing in either setting is unhelpful.

TABLE 26-5 Characteristics of crackles in various disorders*

DIAGNOSIS	NUMBER OF CRACKLES PER INSPIRATION	TIMING OF CRACKLE	TYPE OF CRACKLE
Pulmonary fibrosis	6-14	Late inspiratory ($0.5 \rightarrow 0.9$)	Fine
Congestive heart failure	4-9	Late or paninspiratory ($0.4 \rightarrow 0.8$)	Coarse or fine
Pneumonia	3-7	Paninspiratory ($0.3 \rightarrow 0.7$)	Coarse
Chronic airflow obstruction	1-4	Early inspiratory ($0.3 \rightarrow 0.5$)	Coarse or fine

*Number of crackles is mean number of crackles plus or minus one standard deviation, after the patient first coughs to clear airway secretions. The descriptors early, late-, paninspiratory, coarse and fine are observations made by clinicians listening with the stethoscope; the numbers under timing refer to when crackles begin and end during a full inspiration (e.g., $0.5 \rightarrow 0.9$) means that crackles first appear at midinspiration (i.e., "0.5") and end when the patient has reached 90% of full inspiration (i.e., "0.9"). Based on references 50, 67, 70.

In contrast, the finding of *forced* wheezing lacks diagnostic value, since it can be produced by most healthy persons if they exhale forcibly enough.[68,73]

b. Characteristics of wheezing. The characteristics of wheezes are their length, pitch, and amplitude. Of these, only length and pitch vary with severity of obstruction. The longer the wheeze, the more severe the obstruction ($r = -0.89$ between the proportion of the respiratory cycle occupied by wheezing and the patient's FEV_1^c p <.001).[45,74,75] Higher-pitched wheezes indicate worse obstruction than lower-pitched ones, and effective bronchodilator therapy reduces the pitch of the patient's wheeze.[45,74]

The amplitude of the wheeze, however, does not reflect the severity of obstruction, primarily because many patients with severe obstruction have faint or no wheezes.[45,68,74,75] This finding supports the old adage that, in a patient with asthma, the quiet chest is not necessarily a favorable sign and may instead indicate the patient is tiring and unable to push air across the obstructed airways.

3. Stridor. In patients with tracheal stenosis after tracheostomy, stridor is a late finding, usually appearing after symptoms like dyspnea, irritative cough, or difficulty clearing throat.[47] Stridor indicates that the airway diameter is less than 5 mm.[47]

REFERENCES

1. Laennec RTH. *A treatise on the diseases of the chest* (facsimile edition by Classics of Medicine library), London, 1821, T & G Underwood.

---

^{c} See Chapter 24 for definition of FEV_1.

2. Hannon RR and Lyman RS. Studies on pulmonary acoustics. II. The transmission of tracheal sounds through freshly exenterated sheep's lung, *Am Rev Tuberc* 19:360-375, 1929.

3. Gavriely N, Palti Y, and Alroy G. Spectral characteristics of normal breath sounds, *J Appl Physiol* 50:307-314, 1981.

4. Gavriely N and others. Spectral characteristics of chest wall breath sounds in normal subjects, *Thorax* 50:1292-1300, 1995.

5. Cabot RC and Dodge HF. Frequency characteristics of heart and lung sounds, *JAMA* 84:1793-1795, 1925.

6. McKusick VA, Jenkins JT, and Webb GN. The acoustic basis of the chest examination: Studies by means of sound spectrography, *Am Rev Tuberc* 72:12-34, 1955.

7. Martini P and Mueller H. Studien über das Bronchialatmen, *Deut Archiv Klin Med* 143:159-172, 1923.

8. Skoda J. *Auscultation and percussion,* Philadelphia, 1854, Lindsay and Blakiston.

9. Flint A. *A manual of percussion and auscultation,* Philadelphia, 1876, Henry C. Lea.

10. Bernstein A and White FZ. Unusual physical findings in pleural effusion: Intrathoracic manometric studies, *Ann Intern Med* 37:733-738, 1952.

11. Pardee NE, Martin CJ, and Morgan EH. A test of the practical value of estimating breath sound intensity: breath sounds related to measured ventilatory function, *Chest* 70:341-344, 1976.

12. Bullar JF and Cantab MB. Experiments to determine the origin of the respiratory sounds, *Proc Roy Soc London Series B: Biolog Sci* 37:411-422, 1884.

13. Leblanc P, Macklem PT, and Ross WRD. Breath sounds and distribution of pulmonary ventilation, *Am Rev Respir Dis* 102:10-16, 1970.

14. Kraman SS. Determination of the site of production of respiratory sounds by subtraction phonopneumography, *Am Rev Respir Dis* 122:303-309, 1980.

15. Bohadana AB, Peslin R, and Uffholtz H. Breath sounds in the clinical assessment of airflow obstruction, *Thorax* 33:345-351, 1978.

16. Kraman SS. The relationship between airflow and lung sound amplitude in normal subjects, *Chest* 86:225-229, 1984.

17. Schreur HJW and others. Lung sound intensity in patients with emphysema and in normal subjects at standardised airflows, *Thorax* 47:674-679, 1992.

18. Kraman SS and Austrheim O. Comparison of lung sound and transmitted sound amplitude in normal men, *Am Rev Respir Dis* 128:451-454, 1983.

19. Fahr G. The acoustics of the bronchial breath sounds: application to phenomena of auscultation as heard in lobar pneumonia, *Arch Intern Med* 39:286-302, 1926.

20. Heckerling PS and others. Clinical prediction rule for pulmonary infiltrates, *Ann Intern Med* 113:664-670, 1990.

21. Melbye H and others. The diagnosis of adult pneumonia in general practice, *Scand J Prim Health Care* 6:111-117, 1988.

22. Gennis P and others. Clinical criteria for the detection of pneumonia in adults: guidelines for ordering chest roentgenograms in the emergency department, *J Emerg Med* 7:263-268, 1989.

23. Melbye H and others. Diagnosis of pneumonia in adults in general practice, *Scand J Prim Health Care* 10:226-233, 1992.

24. Purohit A and others. Lung auscultation in airway challenge testing, *Resp Med* 91:151-157, 1997.

25. Diehr P and others. Prediction of pneumonia in outpatients with acute cough—a statistical approach, *J Chron Dis* 37:215-225, 1984.

26. Badgett RG and others. Can moderate chronic obstructive pulmonary disease be diagnosed by historical and physical findings alone? *Am J Med* 94:188-196, 1993.

27. Holleman DR, Simel DL, and Goldberg JS. Diagnosis of obstructive airways disease from the clinical examination, *J Gen Intern Med* 8:63-68, 1993.

28. Shibley GS. A new auscultatory sign found in consolidation, or the collection of fluid, in pulmonary disease, *China Med J* 36:1-9, 1922.

29. Fröschels E and Stockert FG. Ueber ein neues Symptom bei Lungen- und Pleuraerkrankungen, *Wien Klin Wochenschr* 22:500-501, 1922.

30. Stokes W. *An introduction to the use of the stethoscope* (facsimile edition by the Classics of Cardiology Library), Edinburgh, 1825, Maclachlin and Stewart.

31. Buller AJ and Dornshorst AC. The physics of some pulmonary signs, *Lancet* 2:649-651, 1956.

32. Baughman RP and Loudon RG. Sound spectral analysis of voice-transmitted sound, *Am Rev Respir Dis* 134:167-169, 1986.

33. Forgacs P. The functional basis of pulmonary sounds, *Chest* 73:399-412, 1978.

34. Mahagnah M and Gavriely N. Gas density does not affect pulmonary acoustic transmission in normal men, *J Appl Physiol* 78:928-937, 1995.

35. Bunin NJ and Loudon RG. Lung sound terminology in case reports, *Chest* 76:690-692, 1979.

36. Andrews JL and Badger TL. Lung sounds through the ages: from Hippocrates to Laënnec to Osler, *JAMA* 241: 2625-2630, 1979.

37. Robertson AJ. Râles, rhonchi, and Laënnec, *Lancet* 2:417-423, 1957.

38. Murphy RLH, Holford SK, and Knowler WC. Visual lung-sound characterization by time-expanded wave-form analysis, *N Engl J Med* 296:968-971, 1977.

39. Cugel D and others. Updated nomenclature for membership reaction: reports from the ATS Ad Hoc Committee on Pulmonary Nomenclature, *ATS News* 3:5-6, 1977.

40. Loudon RG. The lung exam, *Clin Chest Med* 8:265-272, 1987.

41. Nath AR and Capel LH. Inspiratory crackles—early and late, *Thorax* 29:223-227, 1974.

42. Wilkins RL and others. Lung sound nomenclature survey, *Chest* 98:886-889, 1990.

43. Wilkins RL, Dexter JR, and Smith JR. Survey of adventitious lung sound terminology in case reports, *Chest* 85:523-525, 1984.

44. Deguchi F and others. Prognostic significance of posturally induced crackles: long-term follow-up of patients after recovery from acute myocardial infarction, *Chest* 103:1457-1462, 1993.

45. Shim CS and Williams MH. Relationship of wheezing to the severity of obstruction in asthma, *Arch Intern Med* 143:890-892, 1983.

46. Baughman RP and Loudon RG. Stridor: differentiation from asthma or upper airway noise, *Am Rev Respir Dis* 139:1407-1409, 1989.

47. Geffin B and others. Stenosis following tracheostomy for respiratory care, *JAMA* 216:1984-1988, 1971.

48. Forgacs P. Crackles and wheezes, *Lancet* 2:203-205, 1967.

49. Forgacs P. Lung sounds, *Br J Dis Chest* 63:1-12, 1969.

50. Al Jarad N and others. Lung crackle characteristics in patients with asbestosis, asbestos-related pleural disease and left ventricular failure using a time-expanded wave-form analysis: a comparative study, *Resp Med* 88:37-46, 1994.

51. Earis JE and others. The inspiratory "squawk" in extrinsic allergic alveolitis and other pulmonary fibroses, *Thorax* 37:923-926, 1982.

52. Reich JM. Chirping rales in bird-fancier's lung, *Chest* 104:326-327, 1993.

53. Forgacs P. The functional significance of clinical signs in diffuse airway obstruction, *Br J Dis Chest* 65:170-177, 1971.

54. Forgacs P. *Lung sounds,* London, 1978, Bailliere Tindall.

55. Epler GR, Carrington CB, and Gaensler EA. Crackles (rales) in the interstitial pulmonary diseases, *Chest* 73:333-339, 1978.

56. Nath AR and Capel LH. Inspiratory crackles and mechanical events of breathing, *Thorax* 29:695-698, 1974.

57. Murphy RLH. Discontinuous adventitious lung sounds, *Sem Respir Med* 6:210-219, 1985.

58. Loudon R and Murphy RLH. Lung sounds, *Am Rev Respir Dis* 130:663-673, 1984.

59. Gavriely N and others. Flutter in flow-limited collapsible tubes: a mechanism for generation of wheezes, *J Appl Physiol* 66:2251-2261, 1989.

60. Thacker RE and Kraman SS. The prevalence of auscultatory crackles in subjects without lung disease, *Chest* 81: 672-674, 1982.

61. Workum P and others. The prevalence and character of crackles (rales) in young women without significant lung disease, *Am Rev Respir Dis* 126:921-923, 1982.

62. Al Jarad N and others. Diagnosis of asbestosis by a time expanded wave form analysis, auscultation and high resolution computed tomography: a comparative study, *Thorax* 48:347-353, 1993.

63. Stevenson LW and Perloff JK. The limited reliability of physical signs for estimating hemodynamics in chronic heart failure, *JAMA* 261:884-888, 1989.

64. Chakko S and others. Clinical, radiographic, and hemodynamic correlations in chronic congestive heart failure: conflicting results may lead to inappropriate care, *Am J Med* 90:353-359, 1991.

65. Butman SM and others. Bedside cardiovascular examination in patients with severe chronic heart failure: importance of rest or inducible jugular venous distension, *J Am Coll Cardiol* 22:968-974, 1993.

66. Singal BM, Hedges JR, and Radack KL. Decision rules and clinical prediction of pneumonia: Evaluation of low-yield criteria, *Ann Emerg Med* 18:13-20, 1989.

67. Bettencourt PE and others. Clinical utility of chest auscultation in common pulmonary diseases, *Am J Respir Crit Care Med* 150:1291-1297, 1994.
68. Marini JJ and others. The significance of wheezing in chronic airflow obstruction, *Am Rev Respir Dis* 120:1069-1072, 1979.
69. Baughman RP and others. Crackles in interstitial lung disease: comparison of sarcoidosis and fibrosing alveolitis, *Chest* 100:96-101, 1991.
70. Piirila P and others. Crackles in patients with fibrosing alveolitis, bronchiectasis, COPD, and heart failure, *Chest* 99:1076-1083, 1991.
71. Piirila P. Changes in crackle characteristics during the clinical course of pneumonia, *Chest* 102:176-183, 1992.
72. Sovijarvi ARA, Piirila P, and Luukkonen R. Separation of pulmonary disorders with two-dimensional discriminant analysis of crackles, *Clin Physiol* 16:171-181, 1996.
73. King DK, Thompson BT, and Johnson DC. Wheezing on maximal forced exhalation in the diagnosis of atypical asthma: lack of sensitivity and specificity, *Ann Intern Med* 110:451-455, 1989.
74. Baughman RP and Loudon RG. Quantitation of wheezing in acute asthma, *Chest* 86:718-722, 1984.
75. Baughman RP and Loudon RG. Lung sound analysis for continuous evaluation of airflow obstruction in asthma, *Chest* 88:364-368, 1985.

CHAPTER 27

Ancillary Tests

I. FORCED EXPIRATORY TIME

A. Technique. To measure the forced expiratory time, the clinician places the stethoscope bell over the trachea of the patient in the suprasternal notch and asks the patient to take a deep breath and blow it all out as fast as possible.[1] Using a stopwatch, the duration of the audible expiratory sound is determined to the nearest half second.

Rosenblatt introduced this test in 1962 as a test of obstructive lung disease.[2]

B. Pathogenesis. The forced expiratory time should be prolonged in obstructive disease simply because, by definition, the ratio of FEV_1 to FVC (i.e., "forced expiratory volume in one second" divided by "forced vital capacity") is reduced in this disorder. Slower flow rates prolong expiratory times.

C. Clinical significance. Table 27-1 summarizes the accuracy of this finding, showing that a forced expiratory time less the 3 seconds is a compelling argument *against* obstructive disease (LR = 0.2, Table 27-1) and a time of 9 seconds or more argues *for* disease (LR = 4.8).

The forced expiratory time is a specific test for obstruction. Patients with restrictive lung disease, despite having reductions in the FEV_1 similar to those seen in obstructive lung disease,

TABLE 27-1 Ancillary tests

Finding (ref)	Sensitivity (%)	Specificity (%)	Positive LR	Negative LR
Forced Expiratory Time Detecting chronic airflow obstruction[1,3]				
<3 seconds	8-10	26-62	0.2	—
3-9 seconds	42-54	—	NS	—
≥9 seconds	36-50	86-98	4.8	—
Unable to Blow Out the Match (Snider Test)				
Detecting FEV_1 of ≤1.6 L[4,5]	62-90	91-93	9.6	0.2

NS, Not significant; FEV_1, forced expiratory volume in one second.

*Diagnostic standard: For chronic airflow obstruction, FEV_1/FVC less than 0.7.

usually have forced expiratory times of 4 seconds or less.[1,2]

II. BLOW-OUT-THE-MATCH TEST

A. Technique. The clinician lights a match and holds it 10 to 15 cm in front of the sitting patient, who then attempts to extinguish it by blowing as forcibly as possible. It is important that the patient hold the mouth open and not purse the lips. Inability to extinguish the burning match is the positive finding.

The "match test" was introduced by Snider in 1959, who reasoned that the ability to extinguish a match was related to the velocity of exhaled air.[4] The test is now often called the "Snider test."

B. Clinical significance. Table 27-1 indicates that a positive Snider test (i.e., unable to extinguish the match) is a compelling argument that the patient's FEV_1 is at least moderately reduced to 1.6 L or less (LR = 9.6, Table 27-1). Being able to extinguish the match argues against an FEV_1 this low (LR = 0.2). Unlike the forced expiratory time, the Snider test is abnormal in both obstructive and restrictive lung disease, which probably explains why the Snider test performs less well in studies using it as a specific sign of obstructive disease.[6]

REFERENCES

1. Lal S, Ferguson AD, and Campbell EJM. Forced expiratory time: a simple test for airways obstruction, *Br Med J* 1:814-817, 1964.
2. Rosenblatt G and Stein M. Clinical value of the forced expiratory time measured during auscultation, *N Engl J Med* 267:432-435, 1962.
3. Schapira RM and others. The value of the forced expiratory time in the physical diagnosis of obstructive airways disease, *JAMA* 270:731-736, 1993.

4. Snider TH and others. Simple bedside test of respiratory function, *JAMA* 170:1691-1692, 1959.
5. Marks A and Bocles J. The match test and its significance, *South Med J* 53:1211-1216, 1960.
6. Badgett RG and others. Can moderate chronic obstructive pulmonary disease be diagnosed by historical and physical findings alone? *Am J Med* 94:188-196, 1993.

PART SIX

Selected Pulmonary Disorders

CHAPTER 28

Pneumonia

I. **INTRODUCTION.** Like most of the pulmonary examination, the traditional findings of lobar pneumonia were described in 1819 by Laennec, who wrote that clinicians using his newly invented stethoscope could detect acute pneumonia "in every possible case."[1] According to traditional teachings, the earliest findings of pneumonia are crackles and diminished breath sounds, followed by dullness to percussion, increased tactile fremitus and vocal resonance, and bronchial breath sounds.[2]

II. **CLINICAL SIGNIFICANCE**

A. **Individual findings.** Table 28-1 reviews the findings from 4400 ambulatory patients presenting with acute fever, cough, sputum production, or dyspnea, all of whom underwent chest radiography (the diagnostic standard for pneumonia). In these patients, the findings arguing *for* pneumonia, in descending order of their positive LRs, were egophony (LR = 4.1), cachexia (LR = 4.0), bronchial breath sounds (LR = 3.3), percussion dullness (LR = 3.0), diminished breath sounds (LR = 2.3), abnormal mental status (LR = 2.2), temperature greater than 37.8° C (LR = 2.2), tachypnea (LR = 2.0), and crackles (LR = 2.0). The *absence* of sore throat (LR = 1.8) and *absence* of rhinorrhea (LR = 2.2) also

TABLE 28-1 Pneumonia*

FINDING (REF)†	SENSITIVITY (%)	SPECIFICITY (%)	POSITIVE LR	NEGATIVE LR
General Appearance				
Cachexia[3]	10	97	4.0	NS
Abnormal mental status[4,5]	13-14	92-95	2.2	NS
Vital Signs				
Temperature >37.8° C[3-7]	27-69	49-94	2.2	0.7
Respiratory rate >28/min[6]	36	82	2.0	0.8
Heart rate >100/min[3-6]	17-65	60-92	1.6	0.7
Lung Findings				
Percussion dullness[3-5,8,9]	4-26	82-99	3.0	NS
Diminished breath sounds[4,5,8,9]	15-49	73-95	2.3	0.8
Bronchial breath sounds[4]	14	96	3.3	NS

Egophony[3-5]	4-16	96-99	4.1	NS
Crackles[3-5,7-9]	19-64	48-94	2.0	0.8
Wheezing[4,5,7-9]	15-36	50-85	NS	NS
Diagnostic Score (Heckerling and others)[4,10]				
0 or 1 findings	7-29	33-65	0.3	—
2 or 3 findings	48-55	—	NS	—
4 or 5 findings	38-41	92-97	8.2	—

NS, Not significant.

*Diagnostic standard: For *pneumonia*, infiltrate on chest radiograph.

†*Definition of findings*: For Heckerling's diagnostic score, the clinician scores 1 point for each of the following 5 findings that are present: temperature >37.8° C, heart rate >100/min, crackles, diminished breath sounds, and *absence* of asthma.

argue *for* pneumonia among patients with acute cough.[3,8]

No finding argues convincingly *against* the diagnosis of pneumonia (i.e., no LR <0.5). In many studies, wheezing was found more often in patients *without* pneumonia, primarily because in these patients, the cause of the acute respiratory complaints was asthma, not pneumonia.[4,5,8,9]

B. Laennec vs. modern studies. There are three reasons why the studies in Table 28-1 contradict Laennec's assertion that physical diagnosis is the perfect diagnostic tool: (1) The diagnosis of pneumonia today includes patients with more mild disease than in Laennec's time, when the only available diagnostic standard was postmortem examination (i.e., his conclusions were drawn from patients with only the most severe disease). (2) Many traditional findings appear only after several days of illness, times when the modern clinician, already familiar with the chest radiograph, often examines patients in a more cursory fashion. In contrast, Laennec examined each of his patients diligently day after day, concluding that bronchial breath sounds and bronchophony usually appeared only after 1 to 3 days of hospitalization, and dullness to percussion appeared only after day 4.[1,11] (3) Antimicrobial medications probably alter the course of the physical findings. For example, in the preantibiotic era, fever usually lasted 7 days in patients with lobar pneumonia[12]; now, it usually lasts only 3 days.[13]

Even so, many great clinicians of the past tempered Laennec's enthusiasm and taught that auscultation was not a perfect diagnostic tool. Writing just 20 years after Laennec's treatise, Thomas Addison[a] stated it was high time "to

---

[a] Thomas Addison, the discoverer of adrenal insufficiency, was also a recognized master of percussion and auscultation.

strip the stethoscope of the extravagant and meretricious pretensions thrust upon it . . . and to state fairly what it will not, as well as what it will do . . . ."[14]

C. Combined findings. Combining findings improves the accuracy of bedside examination. One of the best models, validated in four different populations,[4,10] scores 1 point for each of the following five findings: (1) temperature >37.8° C, (2) heart rate greater than 100/min, (3) crackles, (4) diminished breath sounds, and (5) *absence* of asthma. Table 28-1 shows that a score of 4 or 5 argues compellingly *for* pneumonia (LR = 8.2), while a score of 0 or 1 argues *against* pneumonia (LR = 0.3), which, in some groups of patients, may lower the probability of pneumonia enough that a chest radiograph becomes unnecessary (e.g., in patients presenting to a community office with cough, in whom the probability of pneumonia is 10% or less, a score of 0 or 1 reduces the probability of pneumonia to 3% or less).[9]

D. Pneumonia and prognosis. In adult patients hospitalized because of pneumonia, several findings predict an increased risk of dying in the hospital (Table 28-2), although the most compelling ones are hypothermia (LR = 3.5) and hypotension (LR = 10.0). In contrast, finding a low oxygen saturation has little prognostic significance.[22]

Several prognostic scoring schemes that combine findings have been developed, one of the simplest of which is presented in Table 28-2.[17,23]

E. Hospital course. Among survivors of pneumonia, abnormalities of the vital signs—fever, tachycardia, tachypnea, and hypotension—usually become normal in about 2 or 3 days.[13] Once this occurs, subsequent clinical deterioration is rare, and fewer than 1% of patients will require subsequent intensive care, coronary care, or telemetry monitoring.[13]

TABLE 28-2 Pneumonia: predictors of hospital mortality

Finding (Ref)*	Sensitivity (%)	Specificity (%)	Positive LR	Negative LR
General Appearance				
Abnormal mental status[15,16]	48-65	70-80	2.3	0.6
Vital Signs				
Respiratory rate >30/min[16-19]	41-85	63-82	2.0	0.6
Systolic blood pressure <90 mm Hg[16,20,21]	11-35	97-99	10.0	NS
Heart rate >100/min[15]	45	78	2.1	NS
Hypothermia[16,21]	14-43	93	3.5	NS
Prognostic Score[17,18]				
2 or more: respiratory rate >30/min, diastolic blood pressure <60 mm Hg, and confusion	35-39	88-94	4.5	0.7
2 or more: respiratory rate >30/min, diastolic blood pressure <60 mm Hg, and BUN >20 mg/dl	70-88	79-84	4.2	0.3

NS, Not significant; *BUN*, blood urea nitrogen.

*Definition of findings: For *hypothermia*, body temperature <36.1° C[16] or <37.0° C[21]; for *BUN*, 20 mg/dl = 7 mmol/L.

REFERENCES

1. Laennec RTH. *A treatise on the diseases of the chest* (facsimile edition by Classics of Medicine library), London, 1821, T & G Underwood.

2. Cabot RC. Physical diagnosis, New York, 1926, William Wood and Co.

3. Diehr P and others. Prediction of pneumonia in outpatients with acute cough—a statistical approach, *J Chron Dis* 37:215-225, 1984.

4. Heckerling PS and others. Clinical prediction rule for pulmonary infiltrates, *Ann Intern Med* 113:664-670, 1990.

5. Gennis P and others. Clinical criteria for the detection of pneumonia in adults: Guidelines for ordering chest roentgenograms in the emergency department, *J Emerg Med* 7:263-268, 1989.

6. Heckerling PS. The need for chest roentgenograms in adults with acute respiratory illness: Clinical predictors, *Arch Intern Med* 146:1321-1324, 1986.

7. Singal BM, Hedges JR, and Radack KL. Decision rules and clinical prediction of pneumonia: evaluation of low-yield criteria, *Ann Emerg Med* 18:13-20, 1989.

8. Melbye H and others. Diagnosis of pneumonia in adults in general practice, *Scand J Prim Health Care* 10:226-233, 1992.

9. Melbye H and others. The diagnosis of adult pneumonia in general practice, *Scand J Prim Health Care* 6:111-117, 1988.

10. Emerman CL and others. Comparison of physician judgment and decision aids for ordering chest radiographs for pneumonia in outpatients, *Ann Emerg Med* 20:1215-1219, 1991.

11. Auenbrugger L. *On percussion of the chest (1761), being a translation of Auenbrugger's original treatise entitled "Inventum novum ex percussione thoracis humani, ut signo abstrusos interni pectoris morbos detegendi"* (facsimile edition by Johns Hopkins Press), Baltimore, 1936, The Johns Hopkins Press.

12. Sahli H. *A treatise on diagnostic methods of examination*, Philadelphia, 1911, WB Saunders.

13. Halm EA and others. Time to clinical stability in patients hospitalized with community-acquired pneumonia: Implications for practice guidelines, *JAMA* 279:1452-1457, 1998.

14. Addison T. The difficulties and fallacies attending physical diagnosis of diseases of the chest. In: Wilks, Daldy, eds. *A collection of the published writings of the late Thomas Addison* (facsimile edition by Classics of Medicine library). London, 1846, The New Sydenham Society, p. 242.

15. Starczewski AR and others. Clinical prognostic indices of fatality in elderly patients admitted to hospital with acute pneumonia, *Age Ageing* 17:181-186, 1988.

16. Conte HA and others. A prognostic rule for elderly patients admitted with community-acquired pneumonia, *Am J Med* 106:20-28, 1999.

17. Research Committee of the British Thoracic Society. Community-acquired pneumonia in adults in British hospitals in 1982-1983: a survey of aetiology, mortality, prognostic factors and outcome, *Q J Med* 62:195-220, 1987.

18. Farr BM, Sloman AJ, and Fisch MJ. Predicting death in patients hospitalized for community-acquired pneumonia, *Ann Intern Med* 115:428-436, 1991.

19. Brancati FL and others. Is pneumonia really the old man's friend? Two-year prognosis after community-acquired pneumonia, *Lancet* 342:30-33, 1993.

20. Fedullo AJ and Swinburne AJ. Relationship of patient age to clinical features and outcome for in-hospital treatment of pneumonia *J Gerontol* 40:29-33, 1985.

21. Allen SC. Lobar pneumonia in Northern Zambia: clinical study of 502 adult patients. *Thorax* 39:612-616, 1984.

22. Fine MJ and others. Prognosis of patients hospitalized with community-acquired pneumonia, *Am J Med* 88:5-1N-8N, 1990.

23. Fine MJ and others. A prediction rule to identify low-risk patients with community-acquired pneumonia, *N Engl J Med* 336:243-250, 1997.

CHAPTER 29

Chronic Obstructive Lung Disease

I. INTRODUCTION.

Although descriptions of emphysema date to autopsy reports from the 1600s, it was Laennec who in 1819 recorded the clinical features associated with the disease, including dyspnea, hyperresonance, faint breath sounds, and wheezes.[1] Over the last 200 years, others have embellished Laennec's description, but the principal bedside findings are the same. Writing in 1892, Osler stated that emphysema could be recognized "at a glance" from its characteristic features, including rounded shoulders; barrel chest; prominent epigastric cardiac impulse; hyperresonant chest; loss of cardiac, liver, and splenic dullness; enfeebled breath sounds; and prolonged expiration.[2]

In the 1920s, clinicians began to recognize that these traditional physical signs had shortcomings.[3] In 1927, Cabot wrote that only about 5% of patients with emphysema at autopsy were recognized during life and that, of patients diagnosed with emphysema during life, only 25% actually had it at autopsy.[4] Spirometry, invented in 1846 and used in many forms ("stethometers," "pneumatometers," "doppelstethograms") to supplement bedside diagnosis, gained favor because of these deficiencies and eventually became the favored diagnostic tool.[1]

This chapter compares the traditional physical signs with spirometry. As a general rule, the most accurate physical signs are also infrequent, occurring in fewer than 50% of affected patients, usually only those with the most severe disease.[5,6] For decades or longer, patients may harbor mild and moderate disease that is hidden from the eyes of the bedside examiner but is detectable by spirometry.

II. THE FINDINGS. Most of the traditional findings of chronic obstructive lung disease result from a hyperinflated chest and the great effort necessary to move air across obstructed airways. Some of these physical signs are discussed in other chapters: asynchronous breathing (Chapter 17); barrel chest, pursed lips breathing and accessory muscle use (Chapter 24); hyperresonance to percussion (Chapter 25); pulsus paradoxus (Chapter 13); diminished breath sounds and wheezing (Chapter 26), and prolonged forced expiratory times (Chapter 27).

Additional findings are discussed below.

A. Inspection

1. Inspiratory recession of supraclavicular fossa and intercostal spaces. Some patients with respiratory distress from obstructive lung disease have recession or indrawing of the soft tissues of the intercostal spaces and supraclavicular fossa. This finding is attributed to excess inspiratory resistance, which introduces a delay between the generation of large negative pleural pressures and subsequent increase in lung volume.[7]

2. Costal paradox ("Hoover's sign" or "costal margin paradox"). The costal paradox is an abnormal movement of the costal angle, which is the angle formed by both costal margins as they approach the xiphoid process on the anterior body wall. The clinician assesses costal movements by placing his hands on each costal margin and observing how the hands move with respect to each other as the patient breathes. In a normal person, inspiration causes the lateral aspects of the lower ribs to move outward, like the handle of a bucket, and the clinician's hands separate as the costal angle widens. In patients with the costal paradox, in contrast, the hyperinflated chest can expand no further and the flattened diaphragm instead pulls the costal margins and the clinician's hands together.

3. **Leaning forward on arms propped up on knees.**[8,9] Many patients with obstructive disease experience prompt relief of their dyspnea if they lean forward, which allows them to generate greater inspiratory force with fewer accessory muscles. This position probably diminishes dyspnea because it compresses the abdominal contents and pushes the diaphragm upward, helping restore the normal domed appearance necessary for efficient and strong inspiratory movements.

B. **Palpation: Tracheal length and tug.** According to traditional teachings, the distance between the thyroid cartilage and suprasternal notch ("tracheal length") is shorter than normal in obstructive lung disease, because the clavicles and sternum are positioned abnormally high (see Barrel Chest in Chapter 24). Patients with severe obstruction also have more forceful diaphragmatic contractions that, although ineffective in moving large amounts of air, do succeed in pulling the trachea abnormally downward during inspiration ("tracheal descent" or "tracheal tug").

III. CLINICAL SIGNIFICANCE
A. **Individual findings.** Table 29-1 shows that several findings argue strongly for the presence of obstructive lung disease: early inspiratory crackles (LR = 14.6), absence of cardiac dullness (LR = 11.8), a breath sound score of 9 or less (LR

TABLE 29-1 Chronic obstructive pulmonary disease*

FINDING (REF)†	SENSITIVITY (%)	SPECIFICITY (%)	POSITIVE LR	NEGATIVE LR
Palpation				
Subxiphoid cardiac impulse[5,6]	4-27	97-99	7.4	NS
Percussion				
Absent cardiac dullness left lower sternal border[5]	15	99	11.8	NS
Hyperresonance upper right anterior chest[5]	33	94	5.1	NS
Diaphragm excursion percussed <2 cm[5]	13	98	NS	NS
Auscultation				
Breath sound score[10,11]				
≤9	23-46	96-97	10.2	—
10-12	34-63	—	3.6	—
13-15	11-16	—	NS	—
>15	3-10	33-34	0.1	—
Early inspiratory crackles[12,13]	25-77	97-98	14.6	NS
Any unforced wheeze[5,6,14]	13-56	86-99	6.0	NS

Ancillary Tests

Forced expiratory time[15,16]

<3 seconds	8-10	26-62	0.2	—
3-9 seconds	42-54	—	NS	—
≥9 seconds	36-50	86-98	4.8	—

Combined Findings

Two out of the following three present: (1) smoked 70 pack-years or more; (2) self-reported history of chronic bronchitis or emphysema, (3) diminished breath sounds[5]	67	97	25.7	0.3

NS, Not significant.

*Diagnostic standards: For chronic obstructive lung disease, FEV$_1$/FVC ratio <0.6 to 0.7 (palpation, percussion, and combined findings), FEV$_1$/FVC <0.7 to 0.75 (crackles and forced expiratory time), or FEV$_1$ less than 40% predicted (breath sound score).

†Definition of finding: for breath sound score, see Chapter 26; for forced expiratory time, see Chapter 27.

= 10.2), a subxiphoid cardiac impulse (LR = 7.4), unforced wheezing (LR = 6.0), hyperresonance of the chest (LR = 5.1), and forced expiratory time of 9 seconds or more (LR = 4.8). Among patients with known obstructive lung disease, early inspiratory crackles also imply that the disease is severe (i.e., FEV_1/FVC <0.44; LR = 20.8).[13]

Only two findings argue convincingly *against* the diagnosis of obstructive disease: a breath sound score greater than 15 (LR = 0.1) and a forced expiratory time of 3 seconds or less (LR = 0.2).

The evidence supporting the chest wall signs of obstructive lung disease is meager (see also Barrel Chest in Chapter 24). One study showed that indrawing of the soft tissues correlated with severity of obstruction,[17] while another did not.[18] Only one study has shown a relationship between costal paradox and obstructive disease,[18] and three studies show no relationship whatsoever.[17,19,20] In 2 of 3 studies, the amount of tracheal descent correlated weakly with severity of obstruction ($r = 0.30$), although tracheal length did in only 1 of 3.[17,18,21]

The chest excursion of patients with obstructive disease (mean, 3 to 4 cm; measured as change in circumference between maximum inspiration and maximum expiration, using a tape measure at the level of the fourth intercostal space) is less than that of normal persons (mean, 6 to 7 cm), but the lower limit observed in normal persons (2 to 3 cm) makes it impossible to draw significant conclusions in a single person.[20,22]

B. Combined findings. Of the many successful diagnostic schemes that combine findings,[23] one of the simplest asks just three questions: (1) Has the patient smoked more than 70 pack-years? (2) Has the patient been previously diagnosed with chronic bronchitis or emphysema? and

(3) Are breath sounds diminished in intensity? Answering "yes" to two or three of these questions is a compelling argument for obstructive disease (LR = 25.7; see Table 29-1).

Although using the self-reported history of emphysema as a diagnostic indicator seems to be a circular argument, the specificity of this question is only 74%, which means that 26% of patients *without* obstructive lung disease actually remembered such a history. This question is more discriminatory than other symptoms (i.e., dyspnea, sputum production, age, or use of theophylline, steroids, inhalers, or home oxygen) and many other findings (i.e., hyperresonant chest, absence of cardiac dullness, and wheezes).[5]

REFERENCES

1. Rosenblatt MB. Emphysema in the nineteenth century, *Bull Hist Med* 43:533-552, 1969.
2. Osler W. *The principles and practice of medicine* (facsimile by Classics of Medicine library), Birmingham, 1892, Gryphon Editions.
3. Snider GL. Emphysema: the first two centuries—and beyond, *Am Rev Respir Dis* 146:1334-1344, 1992.
4. Cabot R. Physical diagnosis of diseases of the chest, New York, 1900, William Wood.
5. Badgett RG and others. Can moderate chronic obstructive pulmonary disease be diagnosed by historical and physical findings alone? *Am J Med* 94:188-196, 1993.
6. Holleman DR, Simel DL, and Goldberg JS. Diagnosis of obstructive airways disease from the clinical examination, *J Gen Intern Med* 8:63-68, 1993.
7. Stubbing DG. Physical signs in the evaluation of patients with chronic obstructive pulmonary disease, *Pract Cardiol* 10:114-120, 1984.
8. Sharp JT and others. Postural relief of dyspnea in severe chronic obstructive pulmonary disease, *Am Rev Respir Dis* 122:201-211, 1980.
9. O'Neill S and McCarthy DS. Postural relief of dyspnoea in severe chronic airflow limitation: relationship to respiratory muscle strength, *Thorax* 38:595-600, 1983.

10. Pardee NE, Martin CJ, and Morgan EH. A test of the practical value of estimating breath sound intensity: breath sounds related to measured ventilatory function, *Chest* 70:341-344, 1976.

11. Bohadana AB, Peslin R, and Uffholtz H. Breath sounds in the clinical assessment of airflow obstruction, *Thorax* 33:345-351, 1978.

12. Bettencourt PE and others. Clinical utility of chest auscultation in common pulmonary diseases, *Am J Respir Crit Care Med* 150:1291-1297, 1994.

13. Nath AR and Capel LH. Inspiratory crackles—early and late, *Thorax* 29:223-227, 1974.

14. Marini JJ and others. The significance of wheezing in chronic airflow obstruction, *Am Rev Respir Dis* 120:1069-1072, 1979.

15. Lal S, Ferguson AD, and Campbell EJM. Forced expiratory time: a simple test for airways obstruction, *Br Med J* 1:814-817, 1964.

16. Schapira RM and others. The value of the forced expiratory time in the physical diagnosis of obstructive airways disease, *JAMA* 270:731-736, 1993.

17. Godfrey S and others. Clinical and physiological associations of some physical signs observed in patients with chronic airways obstruction, *Thorax* 25:285-287, 1970.

18. Stubbing DG and others. Some physical signs in patients with chronic airflow obstruction, *Am Rev Respir Dis* 125:549-552, 1982.

19. Fletcher CM. The clinical diagnosis of pulmonary emphysema: an experimental study, *Proc Roy Soc Med* 45:577-584, 1952.

20. Schneider IC and Anderson AE. Correlation of clinical signs with ventilatory function in obstructive lung disease, *Ann Intern Med* 62:477-485, 1965.

21. Straus SE and others. The accuracy of patient history, wheezing, and laryngeal measurements in diagnosing obstructive airway disease, *JAMA* 283:1853-1857, 2000.

22. Pierce JA and Ebert RV. The barrel deformity of the chest, the senile lung and obstructive pulmonary emphysema, *Am J Med* 25:13-22, 1958.

23. Holleman DR and Simel DL. Does the clinical examination predict airflow limitation? *JAMA* 273:313-319, 1995.

CHAPTER 30

Pulmonary Embolism

I. INTRODUCTION. The diagnosis of pulmonary embolism is a difficult one that has frustrated clinicians for over a century. In up to half of hospitalized patients who die of pulmonary embolism, the diagnosis is not even considered.[1,2] Even when pulmonary embolism is suspected, however, clinicians have great difficulty making the diagnosis based just on bedside findings. Instead, they must rely on ventilation-perfusion scanning of the lung, reserving the bedside evaluation for determining whether further tests are necessary, especially when lung scanning is indeterminate.[3-7]

II. THE FINDINGS. Most patients with pulmonary embolism present with pleuritic chest pain or hemoptysis (65% of patients), isolated dyspnea (25% of patients), or syncope (5% to 10% of patients).[8] Syncope is more common (affecting 20% to 80% of patients) when pulmonary embolism is "massive," meaning that it obstructs more than half of the pulmonary circulation.[9-11]

Table 30-1 presents the findings of pulmonary embolism and their frequency. Other than tachycardia (heart rate >90/min), which affects 81% of patients, individual findings occur in only about 50% of patients or less. This includes the classic findings of tachypnea (sensitivity of 48% for respiratory rate >25/min), pleural rub (4% to 18%), a

TABLE 30-1 Pulmonary embolism

Physical Finding	Frequency (%)*
General Appearance	
Diaphoresis	11-36
Vital Signs	
Respiratory rate >25/min	48
Pulse rate >90/min	81
Temperature >38.5° C	7
Lung Examination	
Cyanosis	3-19
Accessory muscle use	17
Chest wall tenderness	11
Crackles	58
Pleural rub	4-18
Heart Examination	
Elevated neck veins	3
Loud pulmonary component (P_2) of second heart sound (S_2)	19-57
Third or fourth heart sound	6-34
Leg Examination	
Tender or swollen calf	15-52
Calf asymmetry of 1.5 cm or more	16

From 865 patients with pulmonary embolism documented by angiography, from references 3, 9, 10, 12, 13.

*Results are overall mean frequency or, if statistically heterogeneous, the range of values.

loud pulmonary component of S_2 (19% to 57%), and tender or swollen calf (15% to 52%). Up to 11% of patients with pulmonary emboli confirmed by angiography have chest wall tenderness, emphasizing that this sign is not diagnostic of costochondritis.[6,7,13] Hypoxemia (i.e., low Po_2) occurs in 74% to 81% of affected patients, and hypocapnia (i.e., low Pco_2) occurs in 51% to 70%.[3,14]

III. CLINICAL SIGNIFICANCE
   A. Individual findings. In large studies from centers having considerable experience with ve-

nous thromboembolism, only 1 of 5 patients suspected of pulmonary embolism actually has the diagnosis.[5,13] Table 30-2, which displays the diagnostic accuracy of individual clinical findings, explains why this is the case. Only a history of cancer (LR = 4.1) and the findings of calf pain or swelling (LR = 2.6) and tachycardia (LR = 2.5) argue *for* embolism; only a heart rate less than 90/min (LR = 0.3) argues *against* embolism. No other symptom, sign, or laboratory abnormality (excluding ventilation perfusion scanning), by itself, significantly discriminates between patients with pulmonary embolism and those without the disorder.[a] Since the stakes are high and misdiagnosis is potentially fatal, the careful clinician always has a low threshold for ordering lung scans.

B. Combining findings to determine clinical probability of embolism. Two studies have defined rules for estimating probability of embolism and then tested their accuracy in patients presenting with acute pleuritic chest pain, hemoptysis, or dyspnea (Tables 30-3 and 30-4).[3,5] In the scoring system by Hoellerich (Table 30-3), the clinician tallies up the patient's total number of points, based on findings that argue for pulmonary embolism (e.g., diagnosis of cancer, tachycardia, and leg pain, each of which adds points to the final score) and other findings arguing *against* pulmonary embolism (e.g., substernal chest pain and gallop, each of which deducts points from the final score). If the final score (which includes a correction factor of +8 that is added to all scores) is less than 11, the

Text continued on p. 394

---

[a] The following symptoms, signs, and laboratory abnormalities are just as frequent in patients with embolism as in those without it: dyspnea, pleuritic chest pain, substernal chest pain, hemoptysis, and syncope; fever, cyanosis, accessory muscle use, chest wall tenderness, rales, elevated neck veins, and gallop; hypocapnia, or a chest radiograph revealing infiltrate, pleural effusion, or elevated hemidiaphragm.

TABLE 30-2 Pulmonary embolism*

FINDING (REF)†	SENSITIVITY (%)	SPECIFICITY (%)	POSITIVE LR	NEGATIVE LR
Individual Findings				
Risk Factors				
Known cancer[3,13]	22-26	94-95	4.1	0.8
Physical Signs				
Heart rate >90/min[3]	81	55	1.8	0.3
Heart rate increased by 20 beats/min or more over previous rate[3]	41	84	2.5	NS
Respiratory rate >20/min[13]	75	55	1.7	0.5
Pleural friction rub[13]	14	91	NS	NS
Loud P_2[3]	19	84	NS	NS
Calf pain or swelling[3]	52	80	2.6	0.6
Laboratory Abnormalities				
Hypoxemia (Po_2 <80 mm Hg)[3,14]	74-81	24-29	NS	NS
Increased A-a gradient[14,15]	92-99	12-15	NS	NS

NS, Not significant.

Diagnostic standard: For pulmonary embolism, positive pulmonary angiogram.

†*Definition of findings:* For *increased A-a gradient,* alveolar-arterial Po_2 difference, in mm Hg, greater than [(the patient's age in years divided by 4) + 4] (if defined arbitrarily as >20 mm Hg, the likelihood ratios are still not significant).

TABLE 30-3 Probability of pulmonary embolism (Hoellerich)

Definition of Rule Finding*	Score
Patient Interview	
Age, <65 years	+3
Diagnosis of cancer	+4
Leg pain	+3
Substernal chest pain	−3
Physical Examination	
Heart rate >90/min	+4
Heart rate increase by >20/min	+4
S_3 or S_4 (new)	−4
Laboratory	
Positive lung scan	+5
Correction Factor	+8
Total Score	1-31

Accuracy of rule

Score	Sensitivity (%)	Specificity (%)	Positive LR
1-10 points	2	63-89	0.1
11-18 points	34-55	—	NS
19-23 points	30-48	—	3.7
24-31 points	16-20	99	17.3

From reference 3.

NS, Not significant.

*Definition of findings: For heart rate increase by >20/min, the patient's heart rate was compared with the baseline rate, determined from an average of 3 measurements made at least 1 week before the acute event, either earlier in the hospitalization or during outpatient clinic visits; for positive lung scan, the report indicated "definite" or "possible" pulmonary embolism. (These terms are no longer generally used; lung scanning in this study had a sensitivity of 0.52 and specificity of 0.82, which is between the accuracy of "high probability" and "intermediate probability" scan results from other studies.)[16]

TABLE 30-4 Probability of pulmonary embolism (Wells)

DEFINITION OF RULE

Step 1: Type of Presentation

	Definition
Typical	Two or more respiratory findings* and either (1) heart rate >90/min, (2) leg symptoms, (3) low-grade fever, or (4) chest radiograph compatible with pulmonary embolism
Atypical	Chest symptoms that do not meet criteria for "typical"
Severe	"Typical" presentation and either (1) syncope, (2) hypotension (systolic blood pressure <90 mm Hg), (3) severe hypoxemia (requiring oxygen supplementation >40%), or (4) acute cor pulmonale (elevated neck veins or $S_1Q_1T_3$ on electrocardiogram)

Step 2: Clinical probability, based on type of presentation, presence of risk factors and alternative diagnosis

ASSIGNED CLINICAL PROBABILITY	TYPE OF PRESENTATION	RISK FACTORS PRESENT?	ALTERNATIVE DIAGNOSIS LIKELY?
High	Severe	—	No
	Typical	Yes	No
	Typical	No	Yes
Low	Atypical	No	Yes
	Atypical	No	No
	Atypical	Yes	Yes
Moderate	All other combinations		

Accuracy of rule

Clinical probability	Sensitivity (%)	Specificity (%)	Positive LR
Low clinical probability	12	31	0.2
Moderate clinical probability	52	—	1.8
High clinical probability	37	98	17.1

From reference 5.

Definition of findings: For *respiratory findings*, dyspnea, pleuritic chest pain, chest pain that is nonretrosternal and nonpleuritic, arterial oxygen saturation less than 92% while breathing room air, hemoptysis, and pleural rub; for *risk factors*, known cancer; previous thromboembolism, strong family history for thromboembolic disease; or recent fracture, surgery, or immobilization.

probability of pulmonary embolism is low (LR = 0.1). If the score is 24 or more, the probability of pulmonary embolism is high (LR = 17.3).[b]

In the scoring system by Wells,[5] the clinician first identifies the type of presentation (top rows of Table 30-4) and then, depending on the associated risk factors and alternative diagnoses, determines the clinical probability as "low," "moderate," or "high" (middle rows of Table 30-4). The finding of "low clinical probability" argues *against* the diagnosis of pulmonary embolism (LR = 0.2); one of "high clinical probability" argues strongly *for* it (LR = 17.1).

Although both of these scoring systems are complicated and difficult to recall, they emphasize that clinical probability is high if the patient has typical signs (tachycardia, leg swelling) and risk factors (e.g., cancer, immobilization) and lacks an alternative diagnosis. Atypical presentations, the *absence* of risk factors, and the *presence* of an alternative diagnosis (e.g., angina, congestive heart failure) indicate the probability of embolism is low. If these estimates conflict with the results from lung scanning, further evaluation is indicated. In one study of patients with high probability scans but low clinical probability, only 33% actually had thromboembolism documented by subsequent ultrasonography, venography, and pulmonary angiography.[5] Similarly, in patients with nondiagnostic scans and high clinical probability, up to 47% actually had thromboembolism on further testing.[5]

---

[b] A disadvantage to this rule is that it includes the results from lung scanning, which may not be interpreted the same in all hospitals (see footnote to Table 30-3).

REFERENCES

1. Ryu JH, Olson EJ, and Pellikka PA. Clinical recognition of pulmonary embolism: Problem of unrecognized and asymptomatic cases, *Mayo Clin Proc* 73:873-879, 1998.

2. Morgenthaler TI and Ryu JH. Clinical characteristics of fatal pulmonary embolism in a referral hospital, *Mayo Clin Proc* 70:417-424, 1995.

3. Hoellerich VL and Wigton RS. Diagnosing pulmonary embolism using clinical findings. *Arch Intern Med* 146: 1699-1704, 1986.

4. Perrier A and others. Diagnosis of pulmonary embolism by a decision analysis-based strategy including clinical probability, D-dimer levels, and ultrasonography: a management study. *Arch Intern Med* 156:531-536, 1996.

5. Wells PS and others. Use of a clinical model for safe management of patients with suspected pulmonary embolism, *Ann Intern Med* 129:997-1005, 1998.

6. Hull RD and others. A noninvasive strategy for the treatment of patients with suspected pulmonary embolism, *Arch Intern Med* 154:289-297, 1994.

7. Hull RD and others. A new noninvasive management strategy for patients with suspected pulmonary embolism, *Arch Intern Med* 149:2549-2555, 1989.

8. Stein PD and Henry JW. Clinical characteristics of patients with acute pulmonary embolism stratified according to their presenting syndromes, *Chest* 112:974-979, 1997.

9. Stein PD, Willis PW, and DeMets DL. History and physical examination in acute pulmonary embolism in patients without preexisting cardiac or pulmonary disease, *Am J Cardiol* 47:218-223, 1981.

10. Bell WR, Simon TL, and DeMets DL. The clinical features of submassive and massive pulmonary emboli, *Am J Med* 62:355-360, 1977.

11. Sutton GC, Honey M, and Gibson RV. Clinical diagnosis of acute massive pulmonary embolism, *Lancet* 1:271-273, 1969.

12. Stein PD and others. Diagnosis of acute pulmonary embolism in the elderly, *J Am Coll Cardiol* 18:1542-1547, 1991.

13. Hull RD and others. Pulmonary embolism in outpatients with pleuritic chest pain, *Arch Intern Med* 148:838-844, 1988.

14. Stein PD and others. Arterial blood gas analysis in the assessment of suspected acute pulmonary embolism, *Chest* 109:78-81, 1996.

15. McFarlane MJ and Imperiale TF. Use of the alveolar-arterial oxygen gradient in the diagnosis of pulmonary embolism, *Am J Med* 96:57-62, 1994.
16. The PIOPED investigators. Value of the ventilation/perfusion scan in acute pulmonary embolism: results of the prospective investigation of pulmonary embolism diagnosis (PIOPED), *JAMA* 263:2753-2759, 1990.

PART SEVEN

The Heart

CHAPTER 31

Inspection of the Neck Veins

I. INTRODUCTION. Clinicians should inspect the neck veins (1) to detect elevated central venous pressure and (2) to detect specific abnormalities of the venous waveforms, which are characteristic of certain arrhythmias and some valvular, pericardial, and myocardial disorders.

Clinicians first associated conspicuous neck veins with heart disease about three centuries ago.[1,2] In the late 1800s, Sir James Mackenzie described venous waveforms of arrhythmias and various heart disorders, using a mechanical polygraph applied over the patient's neck or liver. His labels for the venous waveforms—A, C, and V waves—are still used today.[3,4] Clinicians began to estimate venous pressure at the bedside routinely in the 1920s, after the introduction of the glass manometer and after Starling's experiments linking venous pressure to cardiac output.[5]

II. VENOUS PRESSURE
   A. Definitions
   1. Central venous pressure. Central venous pressure (CVP) is mean vena caval or right atrial pressure, which, in the absence of tricuspid stenosis, equals right ventricular end-diastolic pressure. Disorders that in-

crease diastolic pressures of the right side of the heart—left heart disease, lung disease, primary pulmonary hypertension, and pulmonic stenosis—all increase the CVP and make the neck veins abnormally conspicuous. CVP is expressed in millimeters of mercury (mm Hg) or centimeters of water (cm H_2O) above atmospheric pressure (1.36 cm H_2O = 1.0 mm Hg).

Estimations of CVP are most helpful in patients with ascites or edema, in whom an elevated CVP indicates heart or lung disease and a normal CVP suggests alternative diagnoses, such as chronic liver disease. (Despite prevailing opinion, the CVP is normal in patients with liver disease; the edema in these patients results from hypoalbuminemia and the weight of ascites compressing veins to the legs.)[6-9]

2. **Physiologic zero point.** Physiologists have long assumed that a location in the cardiovascular system (presumed to be the right atrium in humans) tightly regulates venous pressure so that it remains the same even when the person changes position.[5,10-12] All measurements of CVP—whether by the clinician inspecting neck veins or by the catheter in intensive care units—attempt to identify the pressure at this zero point (e.g., if a manometer connected to a systemic vein supports a column of saline 8 cm above the zero point, with the top of the manometer open to atmosphere, the recorded pressure in that vein is 8 cm H_2O). Estimates of CVP are related to the zero point because interpretation of this value does not need to consider the hydrostatic effects of different patient positions, and any abnormal value thus indicates disease.

3. **External reference point.** Clinicians require some external reference point to reli-

ably locate the level of the zero point. Of the many such reference points that have been proposed over the last century,[5] only two are commonly used today: the sternal angle and the phlebostatic axis.

a. Sternal angle. In 1930, Sir Thomas Lewis, a pupil of Mackenzie, proposed a simple bedside method for measuring venous pressure designed to replace the manometer, which he found too burdensome for general use.[13] He observed that the top of the jugular veins of normal persons (and the top of the fluid in the manometer) always came to lie within 1 to 2 cm of vertical distance from the sternal angle, whether the person was supine, semi-upright, or upright (an observation since confirmed by others).[14] Neck veins whose top level is more than 3 cm above the sternal angle, according to Lewis, indicates that venous pressure is elevated.

Others have modified this method, stating that the CVP equals the vertical distance between the top of the neck veins and a point 5 cm below the sternal angle (Figure 31-1).[15] This variation is commonly called the "method of Lewis," even though Lewis never made such a claim.

b. Phlebostatic axis. The phlebostatic axis is the midpoint between the anterior and posterior surfaces of the chest at the level of the fourth intercostal space. This reference point, the most common landmark used in intensive care units and cardiac catheterization laboratories, was originally proposed in the 1940s, when studies showed that using it as the zero point minimized variation in venous pressure of normal persons as they changed position between 0 and 90 degrees.[11]

FIGURE 31-1 Measurement of venous pressure. The clinician should vary the patient's position until the top of the neck veins become visible. In this patient, who has normal CVP, the neck veins are fully distended when supine and completely collapsed when upright. A semiupright position, therefore, is used to estimate pressure. In this position, the top of the neck veins is 2 cm above the sternal angle, and according to the method of Lewis, the patient's CVP is 2 + 5 = 7 cm H_2O.

    c. Relative merits of sternal angle and phlebostatic axis. Obviously, the measurement of venous pressure is only as good as the reference point used. The phlebostatic axis locates a point in the right atrium several centimeters posterior to the point identified by the method of Lewis (i.e., the zero point using the phlebostatic axis is 9 to 10 cm posterior to the sternal angle; that using the method of Lewis is 5 cm below the sternal angle).[16,17] This means that clinicians using the phlebostatic axis will estimate the CVP to be several cm H_2O higher than those using the method of Lewis, even if these clinicians completely agree on the location of the neck veins.

The sternal angle is a better reference point for bedside examination, simply because clinicians can reproducibly locate it more easily than the phlebostatic axis. Even using flexible right-angle triangles and a standard patient position, intensive care nurses trying to locate a point similar to the phlebostatic axis disagreed by several centimeters in both horizontal and vertical directions.[18]

B. Elevated venous pressure

1. Technique. To measure the patient's venous pressure, the clinician should examine the veins on the right side of the patient's neck, because these veins have a direct route to the heart. Veins in the left side of the neck reach the heart by crossing the mediastinum, where the normal aorta may compress them, causing left jugular venous pressure to be sometimes elevated even when CVP and right venous pressure are normal.[19,20]

The patient should be positioned at whichever angle between the supine and upright position best reveals the top of the neck veins (see Figure 31-1). The top of the neck veins is indicated by the point above which the subcutaneous conduit of the external jugular vein disappears or above which the pulsating waveforms of the internal jugular wave become imperceptible.

2. External vs. internal jugular veins. Either the external or internal jugular veins may be used to estimate pressure, because measurements in both are similar.[21] Traditionally clinicians have been taught to use only the internal jugular vein because the external jugular vein contains valves which purportedly interfere with the development of a hydrostatic column necessary to measure pressure. This teaching is erroneous for two reasons: (1) The internal jugular vein also contains valves, a fact known to anatomists for centuries.[22,23] These valves are essential during cardiopulmonary resuscitation, preventing blood from flowing backward during chest compression.[24] (2) Valves in the jugular veins do not interfere with pressure measurements because flow is normally toward the heart. In fact, they probably act like a transducer membranes (e.g., the diaphragm of a speaker), which amplify right atrial pressure pulsations and make the venous waveforms easier to see.[22]

3. **Definition of elevated CVP.** After locating the top of the external or internal jugular veins, the clinician should measure vertical distance between the top of the veins and one of the external reference points discussed above. The venous pressure is abnormally elevated if (1) The top of the neck veins are >3 cm above the sternal angle, (2) The CVP exceeds 8 cm H_2O using the "method of Lewis" (i.e., >3 cm above the sternal angle + 5 cm), or (3) >12 cm H_2O using the phlebostatic axis.

C. **Bedside estimates of venous pressure vs. catheter measurements**

1. **Diagnostic accuracy.**[a] In studies employing a standardized reference point, bedside estimates of CVP were within 4 cm H_2O of catheter measurements 85% of the time.[21,28] According to these studies, the finding of an elevated CVP (i.e., top of neck veins >3 cm H_2O above sternal angle or > 8 cm H_2O using method of Lewis) is a strong argument *for* an

---

[a] Studies that test the diagnostic accuracy of bedside estimates of CVP are difficult to summarize because they often failed to standardize which external reference point was used.[25-27]

elevated catheter measurement (LR = 9.0; Table 31-1). If the clinician believes the CVP is normal, it almost certainly is less than 12 cm H_2O by catheter measurement (LR = 0.1; see Table 31-1), although some of these patients have catheter measurements that are mildly elevated, between 8 and 12 cm H_2O.[b]

This tendency to slightly underestimate measured values, which is explained further below, explains why estimates made during expiration are slightly more accurate than those made during inspiration: During expiration, the neck veins move upward in the neck, increasing the bedside estimate and minimizing the error.[21]

2. **Why clinicians underestimate measured values.** Of the many reasons why clinicians tend to underestimate measured values of CVP,[5] the most important one is that the vertical distance between the sternal angle and physiologic zero point varies as the patient shifts position (Figure 31-2). Catheter measurements of venous pressure are always made while the patient is lying supine, whether the venous pressure is high or low. Bedside estimates of venous pressure, however, must be made in the semiupright or upright positions if the venous pressure is high, because only these positions reveal the top of distended neck veins. Figure 31-2 shows that the semiupright position increases the vertical distance between the right atrium and sternal angle about 3 cm, compared with the supine position, which effectively lowers the bedside estimate by the same amount. The significance of this

---

[b] For purposes of comparison, "measured pressure" here is in cm H_2O using the method of Lewis. Most catheterization laboratories measure pressure in mm Hg using the phlebostatic axis as the reference point.

TABLE 31-1 Inspection of the neck veins*

Finding (ref)†	Sensitivity (%)	Specificity (%)	Positive LR	Negative LR
Elevated Venous Pressure at the Bedside				
Detecting measured CVP >8 cm H_2O[21,28]	47-92	93-96	9.0	NS
Detecting measured CVP >12 cm H_2O[21,28]	78-95	89-93	10.4	0.1
Detecting elevated left heart diastolic pressures[29-31]	10-58	96-97	3.9	NS
Detecting low left ventricular ejection fraction[32]	7	98	NS	NS
Predicting postoperative pulmonary edema[33,34]	19	98	11.3	NS
Predicting postoperative myocardial infarction or cardiac death[33,34]	17	98	9.4	NS
Positive Abdominojugular Test				
Detecting elevated left heart diastolic pressures[29,35,36]	55-84	83-98	8.0	0.3

CVP, Central venous pressure; *NS*, not significant.

*Diagnostic standards: For measured CVP, measurement by catheter in supine patient using method of Lewis[21,28]; for elevated left heart diastolic pressures, pulmonary capillary wedge pressure >15 mm Hg,[29,35,36] or left ventricular end diastolic pressure >15 mm Hg[30,31]; for low left ventricular ejection fraction, radionuclide left ventricular ejection fraction less than 0.53.[32]

†Definition of findings: For elevated venous pressure, bedside estimate >8 cm H_2O using method of Lewis,[21,28] >12 cm H_2O using phlebostatic axis,[33,34] or unknown method[29-32]; for positive abdominojugular test, see text.

FIGURE 31-2 Central venous pressure and position of patient. The top half of the figure shows the sagittal section of a 43-year-old man, just to the right of the midsternal line, demonstrating the relationship between the sternal angle, right atrium, and phlebostatic axis (indicated by the *black cross* in the posterior right atrium). The bottom half of the figure illustrates the changing vertical distance between the phlebostatic axis (solid horizontal line) and sternal angle in the supine (0 degrees), semiupright (45 degrees), and upright (90 degrees) positions. The venous pressure is the same in each position (14 cm above the phlebostatic axis), but the vertical distance between the sternal angle and the top of the neck veins changes in the different positions: the vertical distance is 5 cm in the supine and upright positions, but only 2 cm in the semiupright position. Using the method of Lewis (see text), therefore, the estimate of venous pressure from the semiupright position (7 cm = 2 + 5) is 3 cm *lower* than estimates from the supine or upright positions (10 cm = 5 + 5 cm). (Adapted from reference 5.)

is that patients with mildly elevated CVP by catheter measurements (8 to 12 cm), whose neck veins are interpretable only in more upright positions, may have bedside estimates that are normal (i.e., less than 8 cm H_2O).

In support of this, even catheter measurements using the sternal angle as reference point are about 3 cm lower when the patient is in the semiupright position than when the patient is supine.[38-40]

D. Clinical significance of elevated venous pressure

1. **Differential diagnosis of ascites and edema.** In patients with ascites and edema, an elevated venous pressure implies that the heart or pulmonary circulation is the problem; a normal venous pressure indicates another diagnosis is the cause.

2. **Elevated venous pressure and left heart disease.** Table 31-1 shows that in patients with symptoms of angina or dyspnea the finding of elevated venous pressure argues modestly for left heart disease and elevated left atrial pressure (LR = 3.9; see Table 31-1). The opposite finding (normal neck veins) provides no diagnostic information about left heart pressures (negative LR not significant; see Table 31-1). Finding a normal or elevated CVP does not help predict the patient's ejection fraction (both positive and negative LRs not significant; see Table 31-1), simply because venous pressure may increase for many reasons besides systolic dysfunction, such as diastolic dysfunction, valvular heart disease, pulmonary hypertension, and lung disease.

3. **Elevated venous pressure during preoperative consultation.** The finding of elevated venous pressure during preoperative consultation is a compelling finding predicting that the patient, without any intervening

diuresis or other treatment, will develop postoperative pulmonary edema (LR = 11.3; see Table 31-1) or myocardial infarction (LR = 9.4; see Table 31-1).

4. **Elevated venous pressure and pericardial disease.** Elevated venous pressure is a cardinal finding of cardiac tamponade (100% of cases) and constrictive pericarditis (98% of cases). Therefore, the absence of elevated neck veins is a conclusive argument against these diagnoses. In every patient with elevated neck veins, the clinician should search for other findings of tamponade (i.e., pulsus paradoxus; prominent x' descent but no y descent in venous waveforms) and constrictive pericariditis (pericardial knock, prominent x' and y descent in venous waveforms) (see Chapter 42).

5. **Unilateral elevation of venous pressure.** Distention of the left jugular veins with normal right jugular veins sometimes occurs because of kinking of the left innominate vein by a tortuous aorta.[19,20] In these patients the elevation often disappears after a deep inspiration.

   Persistent unilateral elevation of the neck veins usually indicates local obstruction by a mediastinal lesion, such as aortic aneurysm or intrathoracic goiter.[41]

III. ABDOMINOJUGULAR TEST

A. **The finding.** During the abdominojugular test, the clinician observes the neck veins while pressing firmly over the patient's midabdomen for 10 seconds, a maneuver that probably increases venous return by displacing splanchnic venous blood toward the heart.[36] The CVP of normal persons usually remains unchanged during this maneuver or rises for a beat or two before returning to normal or below normal.[28,35,36,42,43] If the CVP rises more than 4 cm

H_2O and remains elevated for the entire 10 seconds, the abdominojugular test is positive.[29,36] Most clinicians recognize the positive response by observing the neck veins at the moment the abdominal pressure is released, regarding a *fall* more than 4 cm as positive.

The earliest version of the abdominojugular test was the "hepatojugular reflux," introduced by Pasteur in 1885 as a pathognomonic sign of tricuspid regurgitation.[44] In 1898, Rondot discovered that patients with normal tricuspid valves could develop the sign, and by 1925, clinicians realized that pressure anywhere over the abdomen, not just over the liver, would elicit the sign.[42] Several investigators have contributed to the current definition of the abdominojugular test.[28,36,45]

B. Clinical significance. In patients presenting for cardiac catheterization (presumably because of chest pain or dyspnea), a positive abdominojugular test is an accurate sign of elevated left atrial pressure (i.e., 15 mm Hg or more, LR = 8.0; see Table 31-1). This is thus an important finding in patients with dyspnea, indicating that at least some of the dyspnea is due to disease in the left side of the heart. A negative abdominojugular test argues against the presence of left atrial hypertension (LR = 0.3; see Table 31-1).

IV. KUSSMAUL'S SIGN. Kussmaul's sign is the paradoxical elevation of CVP during inspiration. In healthy persons venous pressure falls during inspiration, because pressures in the right heart decrease as intrathoracic pressures fall. Kussmaul's sign is classically associated with constrictive pericarditis, but it occurs in only the minority of patients with constriction[46,47] and is found in other disorders such as severe heart failure,[47,48] pulmonary embolus,[49] and right ventricular infarction.[50-52]

V. PATHOGENESIS OF ELEVATED VENOUS PRESSURE, ABDOMINOJUGULAR TEST, AND KUSSMAUL'S SIGN.

The peripheral veins of normal persons are distensible vessels that contain about two thirds of the total blood volume and can accept or donate blood with relatively little change in pressure. In contrast, the peripheral veins of patients with heart failure are abnormally constricted from tissue edema and intense sympathetic stimulation, a change that reduces extremity blood volume and increases central blood volume. Because constricted veins are less compliant, the added central blood volume causes CVP to be abnormally increased.[5]

In addition to causing an elevated CVP, venoconstriction probably also contributes to the positive abdominojugular test and Kussmaul's sign, two signs that often occur together. Most patients with constrictive pericarditis and Kussmaul's sign also have a notably positive abdominojugular test; many patients with severe heart failure and a markedly positive abdominojugular test also have Kussmaul's sign.[47] The venous pressure of these patients, unlike that of healthy persons, is very susceptible to changes in venous return. Maneuvers that increase venous return—exercise, leg elevation, or abdominal pressure—increase the venous pressure of patients with the abdominojugular test and Kussmaul's sign, but not that of healthy persons.[5] Kussmaul's sign may be nothing more than an inspiratory abdominojugular test, the downward movement of the diaphragm compressing the abdomen and increasing venous return.[53]

Even so, an abnormal right ventricle probably also contributes to Kussmaul's sign, because all of the disorders associated with Kussmaul's sign are characterized by a right ventricle that is unable to accommodate more blood during inspiration (i.e., in constrictive pericarditis the normal ventricle is constrained by the diseased pericardium, and in severe heart failure, acute cor pulmonale, or right ventricular infarction, the dilated right ventricle is constrained by the normal pericardium). A right side of the heart thus constrained only exaggerates inspiratory increments of CVP, making Kussmaul's sign more prominent.[5]

VI. VENOUS WAVEFORMS

A. Identifying the internal jugular vein.
Venous waveforms are usually only conspicuous in the internal jugular vein, which lies under the sternocleidomastoid muscle and therefore becomes evident by causing pulsating movements of the soft tissues of the neck (i.e., it does not resemble a subcutaneous vein). Since the carotid artery also pulsates in the neck, the clinician must learn to distinguish the carotid artery from the internal jugular vein, using the principles outlined in Table 31-2.

Of the distinguishing features listed in Table 31-2, the most conspicuous one is the character of the movement. Venous pulsations have a prominent *inward* or *descending* movement, the outward one being slower and more diffuse. Arterial pulsations, in contrast, have a prominent *ascending* or *outward* movement, the inward one being slow and diffuse.

B. Components of venous waveforms.
Although venous pressure tracings reveal three positive and negative waves (Figure 31-3), the clinician at the bedside usually sees only two descents, a more prominent x' descent and a less prominent y descent (Figure 31-4). Figure 31-3 discusses the physiology of these waveforms.

C. Timing the x' and y descents.
The best way to identify the individual venous waveforms is to time their *descents*, by simultaneously listening to the heart tones or palpating the carotid pulsation (Figure 31-4).

1. Using heart tones. The x' descent ends just *before* S_2, as if it were a collapsing hill that

TABLE 31-2 Distinguishing internal jugular waveforms from carotid pulses

CHARACTERISTIC	INTERNAL JUGULAR VEIN	CAROTID ARTERY
Character of movement	Descending movement most prominent	Ascending movement most prominent
Number of pulsations per ventricular systole	Two, usually	One
Palpability of pulsations	Not palpable or only slight undulation	Easily palpable
Change with respiration	During inspiration, pulsations become more prominent but drop lower in neck	No change
Change with position	Pulsations lower in neck as patient sits up	No change
Change with abdominal pressure	Pulsations may temporarily become more prominent and move higher in neck	No change
Change with pressure applied to the neck just below pulsations	Pulsations become less prominent	No change

Based on references 54 to 57.

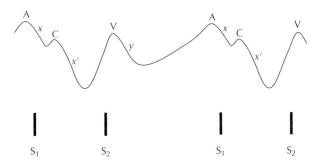

FIGURE 31-3 Venous waveforms on pressure tracings. There are three positive waves (A, C, and V) and three negative waves (x, x', and y descents). The A wave represents right atrial contraction; the x descent, right atrial relaxation. The C wave—named "C" because Mackenzie originally thought it was a carotid artifact—probably instead represents right ventricular contraction and closure of the tricuspid valve, which then bulges upward toward the neck veins.[58,59] The x' descent occurs because the floor of the right atrium (i.e., the A-V valve ring) moves downward, pulling away from the jugular veins, as the right ventricle contracts (physiologists call this movement the "descent of the base").[60] The V wave represents right atrial filling, which eventually overcomes the descent of the base and causes venous pressure to rise (most atrial filling normally occurs during ventricular systole, not diastole). The y descent begins the moment the tricuspid valve opens at the beginning of diastole, causing the atrium to empty into the ventricle and venous pressure to abruptly fall.

           slides into S_2 lying at the bottom. In contrast, the y descent begins just *after* S_2.

    2. Using the carotid artery. The x' descent is a systolic movement that coincides with the tap from the carotid pulsation. The y descent is a diastolic movement beginning after the carotid tap, with a delay roughly equivalent to the interval between the patient's S_1 and S_2.[56,61]

D. Clinical significance. The normal venous waveform has a prominent x' descent and a small or absent y descent; there are no abrupt outward movements.[61]

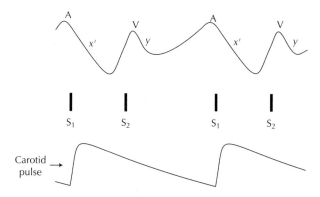

FIGURE 31-4 Venous waveform: What the clinician sees. Although tracings of venous waveforms display three positive and three negative waves (see Figure 31-3), the C wave is too small to see. Instead, the clinician sees two descents per cardiac cycle: the first represents merging of the x and x' descents and is usually referred to as the x' descent (i.e., "x-prime" descent). The second is the y descent, which is smaller than the x' descent in normal persons. The clinician identifies the descents by timing them with the heart tones or carotid pulsation (see text).

Abnormalities of the venous waveforms become conspicuous at the bedside for one of two reasons: (1) the descents are abnormal, or (2) there is a sudden outward movement in the neck veins.

1. **Abnormal descents.** There are three abnormal patterns: **(1) The "W" or "M" pattern** ($x' = y$ pattern). The y descent becomes unusually prominent, which, along with the normal x' descent, creates two prominent descents per systole and traces a "W" or "M" pattern in the soft tissues of the neck. **(2) The diminished x' descent pattern** ($x' < y$ pattern). The x' descent diminishes or disappears, making the y descent most prominent. This is the most common abnormal pattern, occurring both in atrial fibrillation (loss of A wave) and many different cardiomyopathies (more sluggish "descent of the base").

(3) **The absent y descent pattern.** This pattern is only relevant in patients with elevated venous pressure, because healthy persons with normal CVP also have a diminutive y descent.

The etiologies of each of these patterns are presented in Table 31-3.

2. **Abnormally prominent outward waves.** If the clinician detects an abnormally abrupt and conspicuous outward movement in the neck veins, he should determine if the outward movement begins just before S_1 (presystolic giant A waves) or after S_1 (tricuspid regurgitation and cannon A waves).

   a. **Giant A waves (abrupt presystolic outward waves).** Giant A waves have

TABLE 31-3 Venous waveforms

Finding	Etiology (ref)
Abnormal Descents	
"W" or "M" pattern ($x' = y$)	Constrictive pericarditis[55,62]*
	Atrial septal defect[63-65]
Diminished x' descent ($x' < y$)	Atrial fibrillation
	Cardiomyopathy[61]
	Mild tricuspid regurgitation
Absent y descent†	Cardiac tamponade[55]
	Tricuspid stenosis[66]
Abnormally Prominent Outward Waves	
Giant A wave (presystolic wave)	Pulmonary hypertension[55]
	Pulmonic stenosis[55]
	Tricuspid stenosis[66,67]
Systolic wave	Tricuspid regurgitation[68-70]
	Cannon A waves[55]

*The prominent y descent of constrictive pericarditis is sometimes called "Friedrich's diastolic collapse of the cervical veins" (after Nikolaus Friedrich, 1825-1882).

†If venous pressure is normal, the absence of a y descent is a normal finding; if venous pressure is elevated, however, the absence of the y descent is abnormal and suggests impaired early diastolic filling.

two requirements: (1) sinus rhythm and (2) some obstruction to right atrial or ventricular emptying, usually from pulmonary hypertension, pulmonic stenosis, or tricuspid stenosis.[54,55,67] Nonetheless, many patients with severe pulmonary hypertension lack this finding because their atria contract too feebly or at a time in the cardiac cycle when venous pressures are falling.[65,71]

Some patients with giant A waves have an accompanying abrupt presystolic sound that is heard with the stethoscope over the jugular veins.[72]

b. Systolic waves

(1) Tricuspid regurgitation.

In patients with tricuspid regurgitation and pulmonary hypertension, the neck veins are elevated (over 90% of patients) and consist of a single outward systolic movement that coincides with the carotid pulsation and collapses after S_2 (i.e., prominent y descent).[68-70] Some patients have an accompanying midsystolic clicking sound over the jugular veins.[73] Because the jugular valves often become incompetent in chronic tricuspid regurgitation, the arm and leg veins also may pulsate with each systolic regurgitant wave (see Chapter 41).

(2) Cannon A waves.

Cannon A waves represent an atrial contraction that occurs just after ventricular contraction, when the tricuspid valve is closed.[c] Instead of ejecting blood into the right ventricle, the contrac-

---

[c] The electrocardiographic correlate of the cannon A wave is a P wave (atrial contraction) falling between the QRS and T waves (ventricular systole).

tion forces blood upward into the jugular veins. Cannon A waves may be regular (i.e., with every arterial pulse) or intermittent.

(a) **Regular cannon A waves.** This finding occurs in many paroxysmal supraventricular tachycardias (fast heart rate) and junctional rhythms (normal heart rates), both of which have retrograde P waves buried within or just after the QRS complex.[55]

(b) **Intermittent cannon A waves.** If the arterial pulse is regular but cannon A waves are intermittent, only one mechanism is possible: atrioventricular dissociation (see Chapter 14). In patients with ventricular tachycardia, the finding of intermittently appearing cannon A waves detects atrioventricular dissociation with a sensitivity of 96%, specificity of 75%, positive LR of 3.8, and negative LR of 0.1[74] (see Chapter 14).

If the arterial pulse is irregular, intermittent cannon A waves have less importance because they commonly accompany ventricular premature contractions, and less commonly, atrial premature contractions (see Chapter 14).

REFERENCES

1. Lancisi GM. *De Aneurysmatibus (1745)*, New York, 1952, Macmillan Co.
2. Morgagni JB. *The seats and causes of diseases* (facsimile edition by Classics of Medicine library), London, 1769, Millar, Cadell, Johnson, and Payne.

3. Mackenzie J. *The study of the pulse: arterial, venous, and hepatic and of the movements of the heart* (facsimile by the Classics of Cardiology Library), Edinburgh, 1902, Young J. Pentland.

4. Mackenzie J. The venous and liver pulses, and the arrhythmic contraction of the cardiac cavities, *J Path Bacteriol* 2:84-154, 273-345, 1894.

5. McGee SR. Physical examination of venous pressure: a critical review, *Am Heart J* 136:10-18, 1998.

6. Hussey HH and Jeghers H. Practical considerations of venous pressure, *N Engl J Med* 237:776-782; 812-818, 1947.

7. Reynolds TB, Redeker AG, and Geller HM. Wedged hepatic venous pressure: a clinical evaluation, *Am J Med* 22:341-350, 1957.

8. Rössle M and others. The transjugular intrahepatic portosystemic stent-shunt procedure for variceal bleeding, *N Engl J Med* 330:165-171, 1994.

9. Reynolds TB and others. Comparison of wedged hepatic vein pressure with portal vein pressure in human subjects with cirrhosis, *J Clin Invest* 34:213-218, 1955.

10. Guyton AC and Greganti FP. A physiologic reference point for measuring circulatory pressures in the dog—particularly venous pressure, *Am J Physiol* 185:137-141, 1956.

11. Winsor T and Burch GE. Phlebostatic axis and phlebostatic level, reference levels for venous pressure measurements in man, *Proc Soc Exp Biol Med* 58:165-169, 1945.

12. Holt JP. The measurement of venous pressure in man eliminating the hydrostatic factor, *Am J Physiol* 130:635-641, 1940.

13. Lewis T. Early signs of cardiac failure of the congestive type, *Br Med J* 1:849-852, 1930.

14. Jaikaran SMN and Sagay E. Normal central venous pressure, *Br J Surg* 55:609-612, 1968.

15. Borst JGG and Molhuysen JA. Exact determination of the central venous pressure by a simple clinical method, *Lancet* 2:304-309, 1952.

16. Pedersen A and Husby J. Venous pressure measurement. I. Choice of zero level, *Acta Med Scand* 141:185-194, 1951.

17. Debrunner F and Buehler F. "Normal central venous pressure," significance of reference point and normal range, *Br Med J* 3:148-150, 1969.

18. Drake JJ. Locating the external reference point for central venous pressure determination, *Nurs Res* 23:475-482, 1974.

19. Sleight P. Unilateral elevation of the internal jugular pulse, *Br Heart J* 24:726-730, 1962.

20. Fred HL, Wukasch DC, and Petrany Z. Transient compression of the left innominate vein, *Circulation* 29:758-761, 1964.

21. Davison R and Cannon R. Estimation of central venous pressure by examination of jugular veins, *Am Heart J* 87:279-282, 1974.

22. Fisher J. Jugular venous valves and physical signs, *Chest* 85:685-686, 1984.

23. Fisher J and others. Determinants and clinical significance of jugular venous valve competence, *Circulation* 65:188-196, 1982.

24. Goetting MG and Paradis NA. Right atrial-jugular venous pressure gradients during CPR in children *Ann Emerg Med* 20:27-30, 1991.

25. Eisenberg PR, Jaffe AS, and Schuster DP. Clinical evaluation compared to pulmonary artery catheterization in the hemodynamic assessment of critically ill patients, *Crit Care Med* 12:549-553, 1984.

26. Connors AF, McCaffree DR, and Gray BA. Evaluation of right-heart catheterization in the critically ill patient without acute myocardial infarction, *N Engl J Med* 308:263-267, 1983.

27. Cook DJ. Clinical assessment of central venous pressure in the critically ill, *Am J Med Sci* 299:175-178, 1990.

28. Ducas J, Magder S, and McGregor M. Validity of the hepatojugular reflux as a clinical test for congestive heart failure, *Am J Cardiol* 52:1299-1303, 1983.

29. Butman SM and others. Bedside cardiovascular examination in patients with severe chronic heart failure: importance of rest or inducible jugular venous distension, *J Am Coll Cardiol* 22:968-974, 1993.

30. Zema MJ and others. Left ventricular dysfunction: bedside Valsalva manoeuvre, *Br Heart J* 44:560-569, 1980.

31. Harlan WR and others. Chronic congestive heart failure in coronary artery disease: clinical criteria, *Ann Intern Med* 86:133-138, 1977.

32. Gadsboll N and others. Interobserver agreement and accuracy of bedside estimation of right and left ventricular ejection fraction in acute myocardial infarction, *Am J Cardiol*, 63:1301-1307, 1989.

33. Goldman L and others. Multifactorial index of cardiac risk in noncardiac surgical procedures, *N Engl J Med* 297:845-850, 1977.

34. Goldman L and others. Cardiac risk factors and complications in non-cardiac surgery, *Medicine* 57:357-370, 1978.

35. Sochowski RA, Dubbin JD, and Naqvi SZ. Clinical and hemodynamic assessment of the hepatojugular reflux, *Am J Cardiol* 66:1002-1006, 1990.

36. Ewy GA. The abdominojugular test: technique and hemodynamic correlates, *Ann Intern Med* 109:456-460, 1988.

37. Gadsboll N and others. Symptoms and signs of heart failure in patients with myocardial infarction: reproducibility and relationship to chest x-ray, radionuclide ventriculography and right heart catheterization, *Eur Heart J* 10:1017-1028, 1989.

38. Haywood GA, Joy MD, and Camm AJ. Influence of posture and reference point on central venous pressure measurement, *Br Med J* 303:626-627, 1991.

39. Amoroso P and Greenwood RN. Posture and central venous pressure measurement in circulatory volume depletion, *Lancet* 2:258-260, 1989.

40. Haywood GA and Camm AJ. Posture and central venous pressure measurement in circulatory volume depletion, *Lancet* 2:555-556, 1989 (letter).

41. Klassen-Udding LM, van Lijf JH, and Napel HHT. Substernal goitre, deep venous thrombosis of the arm, and Pemberton's sign, *Neth J Med* 26:228-231, 1983.

42. Matthews MB. Hepatojugular reflux, *Lancet* 1:873-876, 1958.

43. Hitzig WM. Venous pressure curves in normal and abnormal circulatory states. I. Normal venous pressure curves and the negative "hepato-jugular reflux phenomenon," *J Mt Sinai Hosp* 12:309-334, 1945.

44. Pasteur W. Note on a new physical sign of tricuspid regurgitation, *Lancet* 2:524, 1885.

45. Constant J and Lippschutz EJ. The one-minute abdominal compression test or "the hepatojugular reflux," a useful bedside test, *Am Heart J* 67:701-708, 1964.

46. Lange RL and others. Diagnostic signs in compressive cardiac disorders: constrictive pericarditis, pericardial effusion, and tamponade, *Circulation* 33:763-777, 1966.

47. Hitzig WM. On mechanisms of inspiratory filling of the cervical veins and pulsus paradoxus in venous hypertension, *J Mt Sinai Hosp* 8:625-644, 1941.

48. Wood P. Chronic constrictive pericarditis, *Am J Cardiol* 7:48-61, 1961.

49. Burdine JA and Wallace JM. Pulsus paradoxus and Kussmaul's sign in massive pulmonary embolism, *Am J Cardiol* 15:413-415, 1965.

50. Cintron GB and others. Bedside recognition, incidence and clinical course of right ventricular infarction, *Am J Cardiol* 47:224-227, 1981.

51. Dell'Italia IJ, Starling MR, and O'Rourke RA. Physical examination for exclusion of hemodynamically important right ventricular infarction, *Ann Intern Med* 99:608-611, 1983.

52. Lorell B and others. Right ventricular infarction: clinical diagnosis and differentiation from cardiac tamponade and pericardial constriction, *Am J Cardiol* 43:465-471, 1979.

53. Meyer TE and others. Mechanism underlying Kussmaul's sign in chronic constrictive pericarditis, *Am J Cardiol* 64: 1069-1072, 1989.

54. Wood P. *Diseases of the heart and circulation,* ed 2, London, 1956, Eyre and Spottiswoode.

55. Benchimol A and Tippit HC. The clinical value of the jugular and hepatic pulses, *Prog Cardiovasc Dis* 10:159-186, 1967.

56. Constant J. *Bedside cardiology,* Boston, 1985, Little, Brown & Co.

57. Colman AL. *Clinical examination of the jugular venous pulse,* Springfield, 1966, Charles C. Thomas.

58. Rich LL and Tavel ME. The origin of the jugular C wave, *N Engl J Med* 284:1309-1311, 1971.

59. Bonner AJ and Tavel ME. The relationship of the jugular "C" wave to changing diastolic intervals, *Am Heart J* 84:441-445, 1972.

60. Constant J. The X prime descent in jugular contour nomenclature and recognition, *Am Heart J* 88:372-379, 1974.

61. Sivaciyan V and Ranganathan N. Transcutaneous Doppler jugular venous flow velocity recording: Clinical and hemodynamic correlates, *Circulation* 57:930-939, 1978.

62. El-Sherif A and El-Said G. Jugular, hepatic, and praecordial pulsations in constrictive pericarditis, *Br Heart J* 33: 305-312, 1971.

63. Tavel ME. The use of the jugular pulse in the diagnosis of atrial septal defect, *Dis Chest* 54:58-59, 1968.

64. Tavel ME and others. The jugular venous pulse in atrial septal defect, *Arch Intern Med* 121:524-529, 1968.

65. Hartman H. The jugular venous tracing, *Am Heart J* 59:698-717, 1960.

66. Wood P. An appreciation of mitral stenosis: Part 1. Clinical features. Part 2. Investigations and results, *Br Med J* 1:1051-1063, 1113-1124, 1954.

67. Puddu V. Rheumatic heart disease with normal rhythm and very large "a" waves in the jugular pulse, *Am Heart J* 41:708-717, 1951.

68. Salazar E and Levine HD. Rheumatic tricuspid regurgitation: the clinical spectrum, *Am J Med* 33:111-129, 1962.

69. Cha SD and Gooch AS. Diagnosis of tricuspid regurgitation, *Arch Intern Med* 143:1763-1768, 1983.

70. Lingamneni R and others. Tricuspid regurgitation: clinical and angiographic assessment. *Cath Cardiovasc Diag* 5:7-17, 1979.

71. Whitaker W. Clinical diagnosis of pulmonary hypertension in patients with mitral stenosis. *Q J Med* 23:105-112, 1954.

72. Dock W. Loud presystolic sounds over the jugular veins associated with high venous pressure, *Am J Med* 20:853-859, 1956.

73. Abinader EG. Systolic venous reflux sounds, *Am Heart J* 85:452-457, 1973.

74. Garratt CJ and others. Value of physical signs in the diagnosis of ventricular tachycardia. *Circulation* 90:3103-3107, 1994.

CHAPTER 32

Percussion of the Heart

I. INTRODUCTION. Percussion of the heart has its roots in the 1820s, when a student of Laennec, Pierre Piorry, enthusiastically introduced topographic percussion, a technique purportedly allowing clinicians to precisely outline the borders of the underlying organs, including the outline of the heart.[1-3] Although many of Piorry's claims seem extraordinary today—he declared, for example, that he could outline pulmonary cavities, the spleen, hydatid cysts, and even individual heart chambers—many of his innovations persist, including indirect percussion, the pleximeter (Piorry used an ivory plate, but most clinicians now use the left middle finger), and the current practice of using percussion to locate the border of the diaphragm on the posterior chest and the span of the liver on the anterior body wall.[4]

In 1899, only 4 years after the discovery of roentgen rays, Williams challenged the accuracy of cardiac percussion, showing that many patients with moderately large hearts (autopsy weight of 350 to 500 g) had normal findings during cardiac percussion.[5] Cardiac percussion suffered another setback in 1907, when Moritz published the composite outlines of cardiac dullness according to various authorities, showing that these authorities not only disagreed with each other but also with the true roentgenographic outline.[4,6] By the 1930s, many leading clinicians began to regard percussion of the heart as unreliable and often inaccurate.[4,7]

II. CLINICAL SIGNIFICANCE. Studies of cardiac percussion have several limitations, the most important of which is selectively enrolling only healthy patients lacking chest deformities or emphysema. Nonetheless, even these studies show that the percussed outline of the heart correlates only moderately with the true cardiac border. Whether the patient is supine or upright, the average error in locating the cardiac border is 1 to 2 cm (the standard deviation of this error is about 1 cm). The clinician usually overestimates the left border by placing it too far lateral and underestimates the right border by placing it too near the sternum (these errors tend to cancel each other if the study's endpoint is total transverse diameter of the heart).[8-11] In patients with emphysema, the errors are even greater.[12]

The traditional sign of an enlarged heart by percussion is cardiac dullness that extends too far laterally. The finding of cardiac dullness extending beyond the midclavicular line or more than 10.5 cm from the midsternal line argues modestly for an enlarged cardiothoracic ratio (LR = 2.4 to 2.5; Table 32-1). If cardiac dullness does *not* extend beyond these points, the patient probably does *not* have an enlarged cardiothoracic ratio (LR = 0.05 to 0.1; see Table 32-1). It is unlikely, however, that this information is clinically useful, since the cardiothoracic ratio has uncertain clinical significance.

TABLE 32-1 Percussion of the heart*

Finding (ref)	Sensitivity (%)	Specificity (%)	Positive LR	Negative LR
Dullness Extends More Than 10.5 cm from Midsternal Line, Patient Supine				
Detecting cardiothoracic ratio >0.5[13]	97	61	2.5	0.05
Detecting increased left ventricular end-diastolic volume[14]	94	32	1.4	NS
Dullness Extends Beyond Midclavicular Line, Patient Upright				
Detecting cardiothoracic ratio >0.5[8]	97	60	2.4	0.1

NS, Not significant.

*Diagnostic standards: Cardiothoracic ratio is maximal transverse diameter of heart on chest radiography divided by maximal transverse diameter of thoracic cage. Increased left ventricular end-diastolic volume is volume >186 ml by ultrafast computed tomography.[14]

REFERENCES

1. Buzzi A. Piorry on percussion of the heart, *Am J Cardiol* 5:703-705, 1960.

2. Risse GB. Pierre A. Piorry (1794-1879): The French "master of percussion," *Chest* 60:484-488, 1971.

3. Sakula A. Pierre Adolphe Piorry (1794-1879): pioneer of percussion and pleximetry, *Thorax* 34:575-581, 1979.

4. McGee S. Percussion and physical diagnosis: separating myth from science, *Disease-a-Month* 41:643-692, 1995.

5. Jarcho S. Percussion of the heart contrasted with roentgen examination (Williams, 1899), *Am J Cardiol* 23:845-849, 1969.

6. Moritz F. Einige Bemerkungen zur Frage der perkutorischen Darstellung der gesamten Vorderfläche des Herzens, *Dtsch Arch Klin Med* 88:276-285, 1907.

7. Parkinson J. Enlargement of the heart, *Lancet* 1:1337-1391, 1936.

8. Kurtz CM and White PD. The percussion of the heart borders and the roentgen ray shadow of the heart, *Am J Med Sci* 176:181-195, 1928.

9. Mainland D and Stewart CB. A comparison of percussion and radiography in locating the heart and superior mediastinal vessels, *Am Heart J* 15:515-527, 1938.

10. Karnegis JN and Kadri N. Accuracy of percussion of the left cardiac border, *Int J Cardiol* 37:361-364, 1992.

11. Stroud WD, Stroud MW, and Marshall DS. Measurement of the total transverse diameter of the heart by direct percussion, *Am Heart J* 35:780-786, 1948.

12. Dietlen H. Die Perkussion der wahren Herzgrenzen, *Dtsch Arch Klin Med* 88:286-301, 1906-1907.

13. Heckerling PS and others. Accuracy of precordial percussion in detecting cardiomegaly, *Am J Med* 91:328-334, 1991.

14. Heckerling PS and others. Accuracy and reproducibility of precordial percussion and palpation for detecting increased left ventricular end-diastolic volume and mass: a comparison of physical findings and ultrafast computed tomography of the heart, *JAMA* 270:1943-1948, 1993.

CHAPTER 33

Palpation of the Heart

I. **INTRODUCTION.** Much of the science of heart palpation is based on impulse cardiography and kinetocardiography, research tools from the 1960s that precisely timed normal and abnormal precordial movements and compared them with hemodynamic data and angiograms of the right and left ventricles. These precise and sensitive instruments could detect very small movements of the body wall, many of which are inconspicuous to the clinician's hand. Although this chapter refers to these studies to make certain points, only those movements easily palpable at the bedside are discussed.

Palpation of the heart is among the oldest physical examination techniques, having been recorded as early as 1550 B.C. by ancient Egyptian physicians (along with palpation of the peripheral pulses).[1] In the early nineteenth century, Jean-Nicolas Corvisart, personal physician to Napoleon and teacher of Laennec, was the first to correlate cardiac palpation with postmortem findings and point out the distinguishing features of right and left ventricular enlargement.[2-4] During animal experiments performed in 1830, James Hope proved that the cause of the apical impulse was ventricular contraction, which threw the heart up against the chest wall.[5]

II. TECHNIQUE. When palpating the chest, the clinician should describe the location, size, timing, and type of precordial movements.[6]

A. Patient position. The clinician should first palpate the heart when the patient is lying supine and again with the patient lying on his or her left side. The supine position is used to locate all precordial movements and to identify whether these movements are abnormally hyperkinetic, sustained, or retracting (see below). The left lateral decubitus position is used to measure the diameter of the apical impulse and to detect additional abnormal diastolic filling movements (i.e., palpable third or fourth heart sounds).[7]

Because the left lateral decubitus position distorts the systolic apical movement, including those of healthy subjects (i.e., up to half of healthy patients have "abnormal" sustained movements in the lateral decubitus position), only the supine position should be used to characterize the patient's outward systolic movement.[8]

B. Location of abnormal movements. Complete palpation of the heart includes four areas on the chest wall.[1,6,9-12]

1. Apex beat. The "apex beat" or "apical impulse" is the palpable cardiac impulse farthest away from the sternum and farthest down on the chest wall, usually caused by the left ventricle and located near the midclavicular line in the fifth intercostal space.

The clinician should also palpate the areas above and medial to the apex beat, where ventricular aneurysms sometimes become palpable.

2. Left lower sternal area (fourth intercostal space near left edge of sternum). Abnormal right ventricular and left atrial movements appear at this location.

3. **Left base (second intercostal space near the left sternum).** Abnormal pulmonary artery movements or a palpable P_2 appear at this location.

4. **Right base (second intercostal space near right edge of sternum) and sternoclavicular joint.** Movements from an ascending aortic aneurysm may become palpable here.

C. **Making precordial movements more conspicuous.** Two teaching techniques are often used to bring out precordial movements and make them easier to time and characterize. In the first technique, the clinician puts a dot of ink on the area of interest, whose direction and timing then become easy to see. In the second technique, the clinician holds a cotton-tipped applicator stick against the chest wall, with the wooden end of the stick just off the center of the area of interest (the stick should be several inches long). The stick becomes a lever and the pulsating chest wall a fulcrum, causing the free end of the stick to trace in the air a magnified replica of the precordial movement.

III. **THE FINDINGS.** Precordial movements are timed by simultaneously listening to the heart tones and noting the relationship between outward movements on the chest wall and the first and second heart sounds. There are four types of systolic movement: normal, hyperkinetic, sustained, and retracting.[1,6,9-11]

A. **Normal.** The normal systolic movement is a small outward movement that begins with S_1, ends by midsystole, and then retracts inward, returning to its original position long before S_2.

The normal apical impulse is caused by a brisk early systolic anterior motion of the anteroseptal wall of the left ventricle against the ribs.[13] Despite its name, the apex beat bears no consistent relationship to the anatomic apex of the left ventricle.[13] In the supine position, the apex beat is palpable in only 25% to 40% of adults.[14-17] In the lateral decubitus position, it is palpable in only about 50% of adults.[14,18] The apex beat is more likely to be palpable in patients who have less body fat and who weigh less.[19] Some studies show that the apical impulse is more likely to be present in women than men, but this difference disappears after controlling for the participants' weights.[16]

B. Hyperkinetic. The hyperkinetic (or "overacting" movement) is a movement identical in timing to the normal movement, although its amplitude is exaggerated. Distinguishing normal from hyperkinetic amplitude is a subjective process, even on precise tracings from impulse cardiography. This probably explains why the finding has minimal diagnostic value, appearing both in patients with volume overload of the left ventricle (e.g., aortic regurgitation, ventricular septal defect) and in some normal persons who have thin chests or increased cardiac output.

C. Sustained. The sustained movement is an abnormal outward movement that begins at S_1 but, unlike normal and hyperkinetic movements, extends to S_2 or even past it before beginning to descend to its original position. The amplitude of the sustained movement may be normal or increased. Sustained apical movements are always abnormal, indicating either pressure overload of the left ventricle (e.g., aortic stenosis), volume overload (e.g., aortic regurgitation, ventricular septal defect), a combination of pressure and volume overload (combined aortic stenosis and regurgitation), severe cardiomyopathy, or ventricular aneurysm.

D. Retracting. In the retracting movement, inward motion begins at S_1 and outward motion does not start until early diastole. Because retracting movements are sometimes identical to

normal movements in every characteristic except for timing, they are easily overlooked unless the clinician listens to the heart tones when
palpating the chest. Only two diagnoses cause
the retracting impulse, constrictive pericarditis
and severe tricuspid regurgitation.[1,8,11]

E. Heaves, lifts, and thrusts. The words
"heave" and "lift" sometimes refer to sustained
movements, and "thrust" to hyperkinetic ones,
but these terms, often used imprecisely, are best
avoided.[1,9-11]

IV. CLINICAL SIGNIFICANCE
A. Apex beat
1. **Location.** A traditional sign of an enlarged
heart is an abnormally displaced apical impulse, which means it is located lateral to
some external reference point. The three traditional reference points are (1) midclavicular line, (2) a set distance from the midsternal
line (the traditional upper limit of normal is
10 cm), and (3) nipple line.

Of these three landmarks, the midclavicular line is the best, as long as the clinician
locates it carefully by palpating the acromio-
clavicular and sternoclavicular joints and
marking the midpoint between them with a
ruler.[20,21] In the supine patient, an apical
impulse located outside the midclavicular
line argues that the heart is enlarged on the
chest radiograph (LR = 3.4; Table 33-1), that
the ejection fraction is depressed (LR =
5.7), and that the left ventricular end-
diastolic volume is increased (LR = 8.0).
Other studies confirm the relationship between displaced apical impulse and depressed ejection fraction.[27]

Using a point 10 cm from the midsternal
line to define the displaced impulse is not a
useful predictor of the enlarged heart (positive LR not significant, negative LR = 0.5; see

TABLE 33-1 Size and position of palpable apical impulse*

Finding (ref)†	Sensitivity (%)	Specificity (%)	Positive LR	Negative LR
Position of Apical Beat				
Supine Apical Impulse Lateral to MCL				
Detecting cardiothoracic ratio >0.5[17,19,22]	39-60	76-93	3.4	0.6
Detecting ejection fraction less than 50%[23,24]	24-31	93-98	5.7	0.8
Detecting increased left ventricular end-diastolic volume[25]	33	96	8.0	0.7
Detecting pulmonary capillary wedge pressure >12 mm Hg[25]	42	93	5.8	NS
Supine Apical Impulse Greater Than 10 cm from Midsternal Line				
Detecting cardiothoracic ratio >0.5[15,19,22]	61-80	28-97	NS	0.5
Size of Apical Beat				
Apical Beat Diameter 4 cm or More, in Left Lateral Decubitus Position at 45 Degrees				
Detecting increased left ventricular end-diastolic volume[18,26]	48-85	79-96	4.7	NS

MCL, Midclavicular line (see text for technique); *NS*, Not significant.

*Diagnostic standards: Cardiothoracic ratio is maximal transverse diameter of heart on chest radiography divided by maximal transverse diameter of thoracic cage. Increased left ventricular end-diastolic volume by echocardiography: >90 ml/m² [25], >138 ml² [26], or upper fifth percentile of normal measurements by age and body surface area.[18]

†Definition of findings: These data apply to all patients, whether or not an apical beat is palpable (i.e., if the apex beat is not palpable, the test is regarded as "negative"). The only exception is the data for "apical beat diameter," which applies only to patients who have a measurable apical beat in the left lateral decubitus position (i.e., apical beat diameter ≥4 cm = test positive; <4 cm = test negative; unable to measure diameter = unable to evaluate using these data).

Table 33-1), probably because the 10 cm threshold is set too low (the midclavicular line usually lies 10.5 to 11.5 cm from the midsternal line).[20] Finally, the nipple line is the least reliable of the three landmarks, bearing no consistent relationship to the apical impulse or to the size of the chest, even in men. The distance of the nipple line from the midsternum or midclavicular line varies greatly.[28]

2. **Diameter of the apical impulse.** As measured in the left lateral decubitus position at 45 degrees, an apical impulse with a diameter of 4 cm or more argues that the patient has a dilated heart (LR = 4.7 for increased left ventricular end-diastolic volume; see Table 33-1). Smaller thresholds (e.g., 3 cm) discriminate between dilated and normal hearts in some studies, but not others.[18,26]

3. **Abnormal movements**

   a. **Hyperkinetic apical movements.** The hyperkinetic apical movement is an important finding in one setting. In patients with mitral stenosis, left ventricular filling is impaired, causing the apical impulse to be normal or even reduced.[29] Therefore, if patients with the murmur of mitral stenosis also have a hyperkinetic apical impulse, an abnormality other than mitral stenosis also must be present, such as mitral regurgitation or aortic regurgitation (LR = 11.2; Table 33-2).

   b. **Sustained apical movements.** In patients with aortic flow murmurs, the finding of a sustained apical impulse argues that the murmur represents severe aortic stenosis (LR = 4.1; see Table 33-2). The sustained impulse is a less helpful finding in patients with the early diastolic murmur of aortic regurgitation (LR = 2.4 for significant regurgitation), but the finding

TABLE 33-2 Abnormal palpable movements*

Finding (ref)†	Sensitivity (%)	Specificity (%)	Positive LR	Negative LR
Hyperkinetic Apical Movement				
Detecting associated mitral regurgitation or aortic valve disease in patients with mitral stenosis[29]	74	93	11.2	0.3
Sustained Apical Movement				
Detecting severe aortic stenosis in patients with aortic flow murmurs[30]	78	81	4.1	0.3
Detecting moderate-to-severe aortic regurgitation in patients with basal early diastolic murmurs[31]	97	60	2.4	0.1
Sustained Left Lower Parasternal Movement				
Detecting right ventricular peak pressure of 50 mm Hg or more[32]	71	80	3.6	0.4
Palpable P$_2$				
Detecting pulmonary hypertension in patients with mitral stenosis[33]	96	73	3.6	0.05

*Diagnostic standards: For severe aortic stenosis and moderate-to-severe aortic regurgitation, see Tables in Chapters 39 and 40; for pulmonary hypertension, mean pulmonary artery pressure of 50 mm Hg or more.[33]

†Definition of findings: For abnormal apical movement "apical impulse heave or enlarged,"[31] "sustained,"[30] or "thrust";[29] for abnormal parasternal movement "movement extending to or past S$_2$";[32]; for palpable P$_2$ "palpable late systolic tap in second left intercostal space next to sternum, which frequently followed parasternal lift."[33]

of a normal or absent apical impulse (i.e., not sustained or hyperkinetic) in these patients argues strongly *against* moderate-to-severe aortic regurgitation (LR = 0.1; see Table 33-2).

In patients without murmurs, the sustained apical impulse is a sign of cardiomyopathy. In one study of consecutive patients on general medicine service, patients with a sustained apical impulse had a significantly lower ejection fraction (37%) than those with a normal or absent apical beat (49%).[27]

c. **Retracting apical impulse**

(1) *Constrictive pericarditis.* In up to 90% of patients with constrictive pericarditis, the apical impulse retracts during systole (sometimes accompanied by systolic retraction of the left parasternal area).[8,34] In these patients, the diseased pericardium prevents the normal outward systolic movement of the ventricles but allows rapid and prominent early diastolic filling of the ventricle. The prominent diastolic filling causes a palpable diastolic outward movement, which contributes to the overall impression that the apical impulse retracts during systole (see Chapter 42).

The first clinician to recognize the retracting apical impulse as a sign of "adhesive" pericarditis was Skoda in 1852.[35]

(2) *Tricuspid regurgitation.* In severe tricuspid regurgitation, a dilated right ventricle, occupying the apex, ejects blood into a dilated right atrium and liver, located nearer the sternum.[8] This causes a characteristic rocking motion, the apical area retracting in-

ward during systole and the lower left or right parasternal area moving outward during systole.[36]

B. Left lower parasternal movements. In normal persons, the clinician either palpates no movement or only a tiny inward one during systole at this location. Abnormal movements at this location are classified as "hyperkinetic" or "sustained," depending on their relationship to S_2.

1. Hyperkinetic movements. Hyperkinetic movements of the left lower parasternal area occur in up to 50% of patients with atrial septal defect, which causes volume overload of the right ventricle.[37] Nonetheless, this finding has limited diagnostic value without other findings of atrial septal defect—exaggerated y descent in the neck veins, wide and fixed S_2 splitting, and midsystolic murmur at the left second intercostal space (usually of grade 2/6)—because it is also sometimes found in patients without heart disease, such as those with thin chests, pectus excavatum, fever, or other high output states.[32,37]

2. Sustained movements. Sustained movements of the left lower sternal area may represent either an abnormal right ventricle (e.g., pressure overload from pulmonary hypertension or pulmonic stenosis or volume overload from atrial septal defect) or an enlarged left atrium (e.g., severe mitral regurgitation). Both right ventricular and left atrial parasternal movements are outward movements that begin to move inward only at S_2 or just after it and therefore are classified as "sustained"; they are distinguished by when the outward movement *begins.*

a. Right ventricle. Outward right ventricular movements begin at the first heart sound. If the clinician can exclude volume overload of the right ventricle and mitral regurgitation (both of which also cause parasternal movements), the finding of a sustained left parasternal movement is a modest sign of pulmonary hypertension. In patients with mitral stenosis, the duration of the sustained lower parasternal movement correlates well with pulmonary pressures.[29] In patients with a wide variety of valvular and congenital heart lesions (excluding mitral regurgitation), the sustained lower left parasternal movement is a modest discriminator between those with peak right ventricular pressures greater than 50 mm Hg and those with lower pressures (positive LR = 3.6, negative LR = 0.4; see Table 33-2). Up to 30% of patients with atrial septal defect, whether or not there is associated pulmonary hypertension, also have sustained lower left parasternal movements.[37]

b. Left atrium and mitral regurgitation.
In patients with severe mitral regurgitation, ventricular contraction forces blood backwards into a dilated left atrium, which lies on the posterior surface of the heart and acts like an expanding cushion to lift up the heart, including the left parasternal area. This sustained movement, most easily palpated in the fourth or fifth intercostal space near the sternum,[38,39] differs from those caused by the right ventricle, because outward movement begins in the second half of systole (it parallels the V wave on the left atrial pressure tracing).

In patients with isolated mitral regurgitation, the degree of the late systolic outward movement at the lower sternal edge correlates well with the severity of mitral regurgitation ($r = 0.93$, $p < .01$; the correlation is much worse if there is associated mitral stenosis, which may cause parasternal movements from pulmonary hypertension).[38,39] In pure mitral regurgitation, as in atrial septal defect, the parasternal movement has no relationship to right ventricular pressures.[40]

C. **Aneurysms.** In one study of consecutive patients with ventricular aneurysms identified by angiography, 33% had abnormal precordial movements.[41] Typical findings were (1) a double cardiac impulse, the first component representing the normal apical outward movement and the second the bulging of the aneurysm during peak ventricular pressures later in systole,[42,43] and (2) a sustained impulse that extended superiorly or medially from the usual location of the apical impulse.[41] If detectable by palpation, the aneurysm originates in the anterior wall or apex of the left ventricle; aneurysms originating from the inferior or lateral wall are too distant from the anterior chest wall to be detectable by palpation.[41]

D. **Diffuse precordial movements.** Diffuse outward movements of the entire precordium, from the apex to lower parasternal area, may result from (1) right ventricular enlargement (which dilates to occupy the apical area), (2) left ventricular enlargement (which rotates to occupy the lower parasternal area) or (3) biventricular enlargement.[11] Palpation alone cannot distinguish these different etiologies—even sensitive recordings from impulse cardiography or kinetocardiography could not do this—and the clinician must look to other findings to determine which chamber is most likely causing the diffuse movement.

E. **Right lower parasternal movements.** Abnormal systolic outward movements appear in the right lower parasternal area from tricuspid regurgitation (ejection of blood into the right atrium and liver, which lies under the right side of the sternum) or from mitral regurgitation (ejection of blood in a dilated left atrium).[11,36,44]

F. Palpable P$_2$. A palpable P$_2$ (i.e., the pulmonic component of second heart sound) is a sharp, brief snapping sensation felt over the left base, coincident with S$_2$. It is much briefer than other precordial movements. In patients with mitral stenosis, a palpable P$_2$ argues somewhat *for* the diagnosis of pulmonary hypertension (LR = 3.6 for mean pulmonary pressure >50 mm Hg). More importantly, the absence of a palpable P$_2$ in these patients argues strongly *against* a pulmonary pressure this high (LR = 0.05; see Table 33-2).

G. Palpable third and fourth heart sounds. Some patients with rapid early ventricular filling (e.g., mitral regurgitation) have a palpable early diastolic movement at the apex. Other patients with strong atrial contractions into stiff ventricles (e.g., hypertensive or ischemic heart disease) have palpable presystolic apical movements. These movements have the same significance as their audible counterparts, the third and fourth heart sound (S$_3$ and S$_4$) (see Chapter 36). They are usually called "palpable S$_3$" and "palpable S$_4$."

The S$_4$ is much more likely to be palpable than the S$_3$, and both are more likely to be felt when the patient is in the lateral decubitus position.[7,9,10] The palpable S$_4$ causes either a double outward impulse near S$_1$ (a common analogy is the "grace note" in music) or single outward movement, consisting of the palpable S$_4$ and apical beat together, which is distinguished from the apical beat alone because the outward movement begins slightly before S$_1$.[10,11]

REFERENCES

1. Basta LL and Bettinger JJ. The cardiac impulse: a new look at an old art, *Am Heart J* 97:96-111, 1979.

2. Stokes W. *An introduction to the use of the stethoscope* (facsimile edition by the Classics of Cardiology Library) Edinburgh, 1825, Maclachlin and Stewart.

3. Corvisart JN. *An essay on the organic diseases and lesions of the heart and great vessels* (facsimile edition by New York Academy of Medicine), Boston, 1812, Bradford and Read.

4. Willius FA and Dry TJ. A history of the heart and the circulation, Philadelphia, 1948, WB Saunders Co.

5. McCrady JD, Hoff HE, and Geddes LA. The contributions of the horse to knowledge of the heart and circulation: IV. James Hope and the heart sounds, *Conn Med* 30:126-131, 1966.

6. Feinstein AR and others. Glossary of cardiologic terms related to physical diagnosis and history. Part III. Anterior chest movements, *Dis Chest* 56:231-232, 1969.

7. Bethell HJN and Nixon PGF. Examination of the heart in supine and left lateral positions, *Br Heart J* 35:902-907, 1973.

8. Boicourt OW, Nagle RE, and Mounsey JPD. The clinical significance of systolic retraction of the apical impulse, *Br Heart J* 27:379-391, 1965.

9. Mounsey JPD. Inspection and palpation of the cardiac impulse, *Prog Cardiovasc Dis* 10:187-206, 1967.

10. Mounsey P. Praecordial pulsations in health and disease, *Postgrad Med J* 44:134-139, 1968.

11. Stapleton JF and Groves BM. Precordial palpation, *Am Heart J* 81:409-427, 1971.

12. Willis PW. Analysis of precordial movements, *Heart Dis Stroke* 2:284-289, 1993.

13. Deliyannis AA and others. The cardiac impulse and the motion of the heart, *Br Heart J* 26:396-411, 1964.

14. Heckerling PS and others. Accuracy and reproducibility of precordial percussion and palpation for detecting increased left ventricular end-diastolic volume and mass: a comparison of physical findings and ultrafast computed tomography of the heart, *JAMA* 270:1943-1948, 1993.

15. Heckerling PS and others. Accuracy of precordial percussion in detecting cardiomegaly, *Am J Med* 91:328-334, 1991.

16. Niehaus FW and Wright WD. Facts and fallacies about the normal apex beat, *Am Heart J* 30:604-609, 1945.

17. Mulkerrin E and others. The apex cardiac beat: not a reliable clinical sign in elderly patients, *Age Ageing* 20:304-306, 1991.

18. Dans AL and others. Evaluation of the reproducibility and accuracy of apex beat measurement in the detection of echocardiographic left ventricular dilation, *Can J Cardiol* 11:493-497, 1995.

19. O'Neill TW and others. Diagnostic value of the apex beat, *Lancet* 1:410-411, 1989.

20. Naylor CD, McCormack DG, and Sullivan SN. The midclavicular line: a wandering landmark, *Can Med Assoc J* 136:48-50, 1987.

21. Ryand DA. The midclavicular line: where is it? *Ann Intern Med* 69:329-330, 1968.

22. O'Neill TW and others. Diagnostic value of the apex beat, *Lancet* 2:499, 1989.

23. Gadsboll N and others. Interobserver agreement and accuracy of bedside estimation of right and left ventricular ejection fraction in acute myocardial infarction, *Am J Cardiol* 63:1301-1307, 1989.

24. Mattleman SJ and others. Reliability of bedside evaluation in determining left ventricular function: correlation with left ventricular ejection fraction determined by radionuclide ventriculography, *J Am Coll Cardiol* 1:417-420, 1983.

25. Gadsboll N and others. Symptoms and signs of heart failure in patients with myocardial infarction: reproducibility and relationship to chest x-ray, radionuclide ventriculography and right heart catheterization, *Eur Heart J* 10:1017-1028, 1989.

26. Eilen SD, Crawford MH, and O'Rourke RA. Accuracy of precordial palpation for detecting increased left ventricular volume, *Ann Intern Med* 99:628-630, 1983.

27. Eagle KA and others. Left ventricular ejection fraction: physician estimates compared with gated blood pool scan measurements, *Arch Intern Med* 148:882-885, 1988.

28. Kurtz CM and White PD. The percussion of the heart borders and the roentgen ray shadow of the heart, *Am J Med Sci* 176:181-195, 1928.

29. Wood P. An appreciation of mitral stenosis: Part 1. Clinical features. Part 2. Investigations and results, *Br Med J* 1:1051-1063, 1113-1124, 1954.

30. Forssell G, Jonasson R, and Orinius E. Identifying severe aortic valvular stenosis by bedside examination, *Acta Med Scand* 218:397-400, 1985.

31. Frank MJ and others. The clinical evaluation of aortic regurgitation, *Arch Intern Med* 116:357-365, 1965.

32. Gillam PMS, Deliyannis AA, and Mounsey JPD. The left parasternal impulse, *Br Heart J* 26:726-736, 1964.

33. Whitaker W. Clinical diagnosis of pulmonary hypertension in patients with mitral stenosis, *Q J Med* 23:105-112, 1954.

34. El-Sherif A and El-Said G. Jugular, hepatic, and praecordial pulsations in constrictive pericarditis, *Br Heart J* 33: 305-312, 1971.

35. Skoda J. *Auscultation and percussion,* Philadelphia, 1854 Lindsay and Blakiston.

36. Salazar E and Levine HD. Rheumatic tricuspid regurgitation: the clinical spectrum, *Am J Med* 33:111-129, 1962.

37. Fukumoto T and others. Right parasternal lift in atrial septal defect, *Am Heart J* 94:699-704, 1977.

38. James TM, Swatzell RH, and Eddleman EE. Hemodynamic significance of the precordial late systolic outward movement in mitral regurgitation, *Ala J Med Sci* 15:55-64, 1978.

39. Basta LL and others. The value of left parasternal impulse recordings in the assessment of mitral regurgitation, *Circulation* 48:1055-1065, 1973.

40. Manchester GH, Block P, and Gorlin R. Misleading signs in mitral insufficiency, *JAMA* 191:99-100, 1965.

41. Gorlin R, Klein MD, and Sullivan JM. Prospective correlative study of ventricular aneurysm: mechanistic concept and clinical recognition, *Am J Med* 42:512-531, 1967.

42. El-Sherif A, Saad Y, and El-Said G. Praecordial tracings of myocardial aneurysms, *Br Heart J* 31:357-364, 1969.

43. Eddleman EE and Langley JO. Paradoxical pulsation of the precordium in myocardial infarction and angina pectoris, *Am Heart J* 63:579-581, 1962.

44. El-Sherif N and El-Ramly Z. External left atrial pulse tracings in extreme left atrial dilation, *Am Heart J* 84:387-394, 1972.

CHAPTER 34

Auscultation of the Heart: General Principles

I. CHARACTERISTICS OF HEART SOUNDS AND MURMURS. Different heart sounds and murmurs are distinguished by four characteristics: (1) their timing (i.e., systolic, diastolic), (2) intensity (i.e., loud, soft), (3) duration (i.e., long or short), and (4) pitch (i.e., low or high frequency). A fifth characteristic, the sound's quality, is also sometimes included in descriptions of sounds (e.g., "musical," "whoop," "honk"). Almost all heart sounds contain a mixture of frequencies (i.e., they are not "musical" in the acoustical sense, but instead are "noise," like the static of a radio). Therefore, the descriptors "low frequency" and "high frequency" do not indicate that a sound has a pure musical tone of a certain low or high pitch, but instead that the bulk of the sound's energy is within the low or high range.

Although the human ear can hear sounds with frequencies from 20 to 20,000 cycles per second (Hz), the principle frequencies of heart sounds and murmurs are at the lower end of this range, from 20 to 500 Hz.[1,2] "Low frequency" sounds, therefore, are those whose dominant frequencies are below 100 Hz, such as third and fourth heart sounds and the diastolic murmur of mitral stenosis. These sounds are usually difficult to hear because the human ear perceives lower frequencies relatively less well than higher frequencies. The murmur containing the highest frequency sound is aortic regurgitation, whose dominant frequencies are about 400 Hz. The dominant frequencies of other sounds and murmurs are between 100 and 400 Hz.

II. THE STETHOSCOPE

A. Bell and diaphragm.
The stethoscope has two different heads to receive sound, the bell and the diaphragm. The bell is used to detect low frequency sounds; the diaphragm, high frequency sounds.

The traditional explanation that the bell selectively transmits low frequency sounds and the diaphragm selectively filters out low frequency sounds is probably incorrect. Actually, the bell transmits all frequencies well, but in some patients with high frequency murmurs (e.g., aortic regurgitation), any additional low frequency sound masks the high frequency sound and makes the murmur difficult to detect.[3] The diaphragm does not selectively filter out low frequency sounds, but instead attenuates all frequencies equally, thus dropping the barely audible low frequency ones below the threshold of human hearing.[3]

B. Performance of different stethoscope models.
Many studies have examined the acoustics of stethoscopes, but the clinical relevance of this research has never been formally tested. In general, these studies show that shallow bells transmit sound as well as deeper bells and that double tube stethoscopes are equivalent to single tube models.[3] The optimal internal bore of a stethoscope is somewhere between 1/8 and 3/16 of an inch because smaller bores diminish transmission of the higher frequency sounds.[1,4,5] Compared with shorter lengths of

stethoscope tubing, longer tubes also impair the conduction of high frequency sounds.[1]

Most modern stethoscopes, however, transmit sound equally well, the differences among various models for single frequencies being very small.[3] The most important source of poor acoustic performance is an air leak, which typically results from poor fitting ear pieces. Even a tiny air leak with a diameter of only 0.015 inch will diminish transmission of sound by as much as 20 dB,[a] particularly for those sounds below 100 Hz.[6]

III. USE OF THE STETHOSCOPE. Between the 1950s and late 1970s, cardiac auscultation was at its peak.[b] During this time cardiologists perfected their skills by routinely comparing the bedside findings to the patient's phonocardiogram, angiogram, and surgical findings, which allowed clinicians to make precise and accurate diagnoses from bedside findings alone. The principles of bedside diagnosis used by these clinicians are included elsewhere in this book. How these clinicians specifically used the stethoscope to examine the patient is presented below.

A. The room should be quiet. Many faint heart sounds and murmurs are inaudible unless there is complete silence in the room. The clinician should close the door to the examination room, turn off the television and radio, and ask that all conversation stop.

B. Varying pressure on the bell. To detect low frequency sounds, the bell should be applied to

---

[a] Decibels describe relative intensity (or loudness) on a logarithmic scale. A sound that is 20 dB louder than another sound is 10 times as loud as that sound.

[b] In the late 1970s, two events initiated the decline of cardiac auscultation: the widespread introduction of echocardiography and the decision by insurance companies to no longer reimburse phonocardiography.

the body wall with only enough pressure to create an air seal and exclude ambient noise. Excessive pressure with the bell stretches the skin, which then acts like a diaphragm and makes low frequency sounds more difficult to hear. By selectively varying the pressure on the stethoscope bell, the clinician can easily distinguish low from high frequency sounds: if a sound is audible with the bell using light pressure but disappears with firm pressure, it is a low frequency sound. This technique is frequently used to confirm that an early diastolic sound is indeed a third heart sound (i.e., third heart sounds are low frequency sounds, whereas other early diastolic sounds like the pericardial knock are high frequency sounds) and to distinguish the combined fourth and first heart sounds (S_4-S_1) from the split S_1 (the S_4 is a low frequency sound but the S_1 is not; firm pressure renders the S_4-S_1 into a single sound but does not affect the double sound of the split S_1).

C. **Patient position.** The clinician should listen to the patient's heart with the patient in three positions: supine, left lateral decubitus, and seated upright. The lateral decubitus position is best for detection of the third and fourth heart sounds and the diastolic murmur of mitral stenosis (to detect these sounds, the clinician places the bell lightly over the apical impulse or just medial to the apical impulse).[7] The seated upright position is necessary to further evaluate audible expiratory splitting of S_2 (see Chapter 35) and to detect some pericardial rubs and murmurs of aortic regurgitation (see Chapters 40 and 42).

D. **Order of examination.** Routine auscultation of the heart should include the right upper sternal area, the entire left sternal border, and the apex. Some cardiologists recommend proceeding from base to apex[2]; others from apex to base.[8] The diaphragm of the stethoscope should be applied to all areas, especially at the upper left sternal area to detect S_2 splitting and at all areas to detect other murmurs and sounds. After using the diaphragm to listen to the lower left sternal area and apex, the bell should also be applied to these areas to detect diastolic filling sounds (S_3 and S_4) and diastolic rumbling murmurs (e.g., mitral stenosis).

In selected patients, the clinician also should listen over the carotid arteries and axilla (in patients with systolic murmurs, to clarify radiation of murmur), the lower right sternal area (in patients with diastolic murmur of aortic regurgitation, to detect aortic root disease), the back (in young patients with hypertension, to detect the continuous murmur of coarctation), or other thoracic sites (in patients with central cyanosis, to detect the continuous murmur of pulmonary arteriovenous fistula).

E. Describing the location of sounds. When describing heart sounds and murmurs, the clinician should identify where on the chest wall the sound is loudest. Traditionally, the second right intercostal space next to the sternum is called the "aortic area" or "right base"; the second left intercostal space next to the sternum, the "pulmonary area" or "left base"; the fourth or fifth left parasternal space, the "tricuspid area" or "left lower sternal border"; and the most lateral point of the palpable cardiac impulse, the "mitral area" or "apex."

The terms "aortic area," "pulmonary area," "tricuspid area," and "mitral area" are ambiguous, however, and are best avoided. Many patients with aortic stenosis have murmurs loudest in the "mitral area," and many with mitral regurgitation have murmurs loudest in the "pulmonary" or "aortic area." A more precise way to describe the location of sounds is to use the apex and the parasternal areas as reference points, the parasternal location being further specified by the intercostal space (first, second, third, or lower sternal border) and whether it is the right or left edge of the sternum. For example, a sound might be loudest at the "apex," the "second left intercostal space" (i.e., next to the left sternal edge in the second intercostal space), or "between the apex and left lower sternal border."

F. **Technique of focusing.** The human brain has an uncanny ability to isolate and focus on one type of sensory information, by repressing awareness of all other sensations. A common example of this phenomenon is the person reading a book in a room in which a clock is ticking. The person can read long passages of the book without even hearing the clock but hears the ticking clock immediately after putting the book down. When listening to the heart, the clinician's attention is quickly drawn to the most prominent sounds, but this occurs at the expense of missing the fainter sounds. Therefore, to avoid missing these fainter sounds or subtle splitting, the clinician should concentrate sequentially on each part of the cardiac cycle, asking the following questions at each location: (1) Is S_1 soft or loud? (2) Is S_2 split and, if so, how is it split? (3) Are there any extra sounds or murmurs during systole? and (4) Are there any extra sounds or murmurs during diastole?

G. **Identifying systole and diastole.** Because all auscultatory findings are characterized by their timing, distinguishing systole from diastole accurately is essential. Three principles help the clinician distinguish these events.

1. **Systole is shorter than diastole.** If the heart rate is normal or slow, systole can be

easily distinguished from diastole because systole is much shorter. The normal cadence of the heart tones, therefore, is

lub dup   lub dup   lub dup   lub dup

(*lub* is S_1 and *dup* is S_2). When the heart rate accelerates, however, diastole shortens and, at a rate of 100 or more, the cadence of S_1 and S_2 resembles a "tic toc" rhythm:

lub dup lub dup lub dup lub dup lub dup

In these patients, other techniques are necessary to distinguish systole from diastole.

2. **Characteristics of the first and second heart sounds.** At the second left intercostal space, S_2 is generally louder, shorter, and sharper than S_1 (S_2 has more high frequency energy than S_1, which is why *dup*, a snappier sound than *lub*, is used to mimic S_2). If the timing of extra heart sounds and murmurs is confusing at the lower sternal edge or apex (as it often is in patients with fast heart rhythms), the clinician can return the stethoscope to the second left intercostal space, identify S_2 by its louder and sharper sound, and then inch slowly back to the area of interest, keeping track of S_2 along the way.

3. **Carotid impulse.** The palpable impulse from the carotid usually occurs just after S_1, which the clinician detects by simultaneously listening to the heart tones and palpating the carotid artery. In elderly patients with tachycardia, however, this rule is sometimes misleading because the carotid impulse seems to fall closer to S_2, although even in these patients the carotid impulse still falls between S_1 and S_2.

REFERENCES

1. Ongley PA and others. *Heart sounds and murmurs: a clinical and phonocardiographic study,* New York, 1960, Grune & Stratton.
2. Leatham A. *Auscultation of the heart and phonocardiography,* ed 2, Edinburgh, 1975, Churchill Livingstone.
3. Kindig JR and others. Acoustical performance of the stethoscope: a comparative analysis, *Am Heart J* 104:269-275, 1982.
4. Rappaport MB and Sprague HB. The effects of tubing bore on stethoscope efficiency, *Am Heart J* 42:605-609, 1951.
5. Ravin A and others. *Auscultation of the heart,* ed 3, Chicago, 1977, Year Book Medical Publishers, Inc.
6. Rappaport MB and Sprague HB. The effects of improper fitting of stethoscope to ears on auscultatory efficiency, *Am Heart J* 43:713-715, 1952.
7. Bethell HJN and Nixon PGF. Examination of the heart in supine and left lateral positions, *Br Heart J* 35:902-907, 1973.
8. Perloff JK. *Physical examination of the heart and circulation,* ed 1, Philadelphia, 1982, WB Saunders.

CHAPTER 35

The First and Second Heart Sounds

The first and second heart sounds (S_1 and S_2) define systole and diastole and therefore form the framework for analyzing all other auscultatory physical signs, including the third and fourth heart sounds, clicks and ejection sounds, knocks and opening snaps, and systolic and diastolic murmurs. In his classic treatise describing the discovery of the circulatory system, written in 1628, Harvey described both S_1 and S_2, comparing them to the gulping sound made by a horse drinking water.[1] The first person to state that S_1 and S_2 were the sounds of closing heart valves was Rouanet of France, who wrote in his 1832 M.D. thesis that S_1 occurred when the atrioventricular (i.e., mitral and tricuspid) valves closed, and S_2 occurred when the semilunar (i.e., aortic and pulmonic) valves closed.[2]

FIRST HEART SOUND (S_1)

I. THE FINDING. S_1 is heard well across the entire precordium, both with the bell and diaphragm of the stethoscope. It is usually loudest at or near the apex and contains more low frequency energy than does S_2, which explains why, when mimicking the sound, the term "lub" is used for S_1 and the sharper term "dup" for S_2.[a]

II. PATHOGENESIS

A. Cause of S_1. The precise cause of S_1 has been debated for decades. Although its two recordable components coincide with closure of the mitral and tricuspid valves, the force of valve closure alone is insufficient to generate sound.[4] Instead, their closure probably causes moving columns of blood to abruptly decelerate, which sets up vibrations in the chordae tendineae, ventricles, and blood as a unit (i.e., "cardiohemic" system).[4,5]

B. Intensity of S_1. The most important abnormalities of S_1 relate to its intensity: the sound can be abnormally loud, abnormally faint, or vary in intensity abnormally from beat to beat. The primary variables governing intensity of S_1 are strength of ventricular contraction and the position of the atrioventricular leaflets at the onset of ventricular systole.

1. **Ventricular contractility.** The stronger the ventricular contraction, the louder the S_1. Strong contractions, which have a high dP/dT (i.e., large increase in pressure with respect to time), intensify S_1 because the valves close with more force and generate more vibrations in the cardiohemic system.[6]

2. **Position of the valve leaflets at onset of ventricular systole.** If the mitral valve is wide open at the onset of ventricular systole, it will take longer to close completely than if it had been barely open. Even this small delay in closure intensifies S_1, because closure occurs on a later and steeper portion of the left ventricular pressure curve (i.e., the dP/dT is greater).[7]

---

[a] It was Williams in 1840 who invented the "lub dup" onomatopoeia.[3]

The PR interval is the main variable determining the position of the valves at the beginning of ventricular systole. If the PR interval is short, ventricular systole immediately follows atrial systole (i.e., the R wave immediately follows the P wave). Since atrial systole kicks the valve open, a short PR guarantees that the valve will be wide open at the onset of ventricular systole. In contrast, a long PR interval allows time for the cusps of the atrioventricular valves to float back together before ventricular systole occurs. Studies show that, with PR intervals less than 0.20 seconds, the intensity of S_1 varies inversely with the PR interval (the shorter the PR interval the louder the sound). With intervals greater than 0.20 seconds, S_1 is faint or absent.[7,8]

III. CLINICAL SIGNIFICANCE

A. Loud S_1. S_1 may be abnormally loud because of unusually vigorous ventricular contractions or because of delayed closure of the mitral valve.

1. Vigorous ventricular contractions. Vigorous contractions, such as those occurring from fever and sympathetic stimulation (e.g., β-adrenergic inhalers, thyrotoxicosis), increase dP/dT and intensify S_1.[6]

2. Delayed closure of the mitral valve

a. Prolapsed mitral valve. In patients with the murmur of mitral regurgitation, a loud S_1 is a clue to the diagnosis of early prolapse of the mitral valve (most patients with mitral regurgitation have a normal or soft S_1).[9,10] S_1 is loud in these patients because the prolapsing leaflets stop moving and tense later than normal, when dP/dT in the ventricle is greater.[9]

b. Mitral stenosis. Ninety percent of patients with pure uncomplicated mitral stenosis have a loud S_1.[11] Because the murmur of mitral stenosis is often difficult to hear, a traditional teaching is that clinicians should suspect the lesion in any patient with a loud, unexplained S_1 and listen carefully for the characteristic diastolic murmur with the patient lying on his left side.

Mitral stenosis delays closure of the mitral valve because the pressure gradient between the left atrium and left ventricle keeps the leaflets open until the moment of ventricular systole. After successful valvuloplasty, the loud S_1 becomes softer.[11]

 c. Left atrial myxoma. Many patients with left atrial myxoma (7 of 9 in one series) also have a loud S_1 because the tumor falling into the mitral orifice during diastole delays closure of the valve.[12]

B. Faint or absent S_1. S_1 is unusually faint if ventricular contractions are weak or if the mitral valve is already closed when ventricular systole occurs.

 1. Weak ventricular contractions (low dP/dT). Common examples of weak contractions causing a faint S_1 are myocardial infarction and left bundle branch block.[13]

 2. Early closure of the mitral valve. Common causes of early mitral closure causing the faint S_1 include the following:

  a. Long PR interval (>0.20 seconds). See Section II-B above.

  b. Acute aortic regurgitation. In patients with the murmur of aortic regurgitation, the faint or absent S_1 is an important clue that the regurgitation is acute (e.g., endocarditis) and not chronic. Patients with acute aortic regurgitation have much higher left ventricular end diastolic pressures than those with chronic regurgitation, because the acutely failing valve has not allowed time for the ventricle to enlarge, as it does to compensate for chronic regurgitation. The high pressures in the ventricle eventually exceed diastolic left atrial pressures, closing the mitral valve before ventricular systole and thus making S_1 faint or absent.[14]

C. Varying intensity of S_1. If the rhythm is *regular* but S_1 varies in intensity, the only possible explanation is that the PR interval is changing from beat to beat, which means the patient has atrioventricular dissociation. In contrast, in patients with *irregular* rhythms, changing intensity of S_1 has no diagnostic significance because ventricular filling and dP/dT—and therefore S_1 intensity—depend completely on cycle length.

In patients with pacer-induced regular rhythms, an S_1 that varies in intensity is compelling evidence for atrioventricular dissociation (LR = 24.4; Table 35-1). Presumably, the finding is also as accurate in patients with native rhythms. In patients with complete heart block, S_1 intensity is predictable, varying inversely with the PR interval for intervals less than 0.2 seconds, becoming inaudible for intervals between 0.2 and 0.5 seconds, and becoming louder again with intervals greater than 0.5 seconds (because the mitral valve reopens).[8]

D. Prominent splitting of S_1. Any delay in the closure of the tricuspid valve, the second component of S_1, accentuates splitting of S_1. This finding therefore occurs in patients with right bundle branch block or in left ventricular ectopic or paced beats, all of which delay the onset of right ventricular systole and also cause wide physiologic splitting of S_2 (see below).[5,20]

How to distinguish the split S_1 from other double sounds occurring around S_1, such as $S_4 + S_1$ and S_1 + ejection sound, is discussed in Chapter 36.

TABLE 35-1 The first and second heart sounds*

Finding (ref)†	Sensitivity (%)	Specificity (%)	Positive LR	Negative LR
First Heart Sound				
Varying Intensity S₁				
Detecting atrioventricular dissociation[15]	58	98	24.4	0.4
Second Heart Sound				
Fixed Wide Splitting				
Detecting atrial septal defect[16]	92	65	2.6	0.1
Paradoxic Splitting				
Detecting significant aortic stenosis[17]	50	79	NS	NS
Loud P₂				
Detecting pulmonary hypertension[18,19]	58-96	19-46	NS	NS
Palpable P₂				
Detecting pulmonary hypertension[18]	96	73	3.6	0.05

NS, Not significant.

*Diagnostic standard: For *atrioventricular dissociation*, ventricles were paced independently of atria; for *atrial septal defect*, right heart catheterization; for *significant aortic stenosis*, peak gradient >50 mm Hg; for *pulmonary hypertension*, mean pulmonary pressure of 50 mm Hg or more.

†Definition of findings: For *loud P₂*, splitting heard with loud second component[18] or S₂ louder at left second interspace than right second interspace[19]; the figures for fixed splitting of S₂ apply only to patients having audible expiratory splitting.

SECOND HEART SOUND (S₂)

I. INTRODUCTION. The most important diagnostic feature of S_2 is its "splitting," which refers to how the aortic and pulmonic components of S_2 vary in timing during the respiratory cycle. The intensity of S_2 has less diagnostic importance (this contrasts with S_1, in which intensity is more important than splitting). Splitting of S_2 was first recognized by Potain in 1865, and its importance to cardiac auscultation was described by Leatham in the 1950s, who called S_2 the "key to auscultation of the heart."[21,22] The correct explanation for normal splitting—increased "hangout" in the pulmonary circulation—was discovered in the 1970s.[23,24]

II. NORMAL SPLITTING OF S₂

A. The finding. In normal persons, the first component of S_2 is caused by closure of the aortic valve (A_2); the second, by closure of the pulmonic valve (P_2). During inspiration the interval separating A_2 and P_2 increases by about 20 to 30 milliseconds (ms) (Figure 35-1).[16,22,24]

Although the phonocardiogram almost always records both components of S_2, the human ear perceives them as a single sound *during expiration* in over 90% of normal persons.[25] In normal persons *during inspiration,* the human ear either perceives two components ("physiologic splitting," heard in 65% to 75% of normal adults; see Figure 35-1)[b] or still perceives a single component ("single S_2," heard in 25% to 35% of normal adults). The older the person,

---

[b] These two components are very close together, bordering the threshold of being perceived as a single sound. Harvey suggests mimicking the normal expiratory sound by striking a single knuckle against a tabletop and mimicking inspiratory physiologic splitting by striking two knuckles almost simultaneously.[26] Constant suggests mimicking inspiratory splitting by rolling the tongue as in a Spanish *dr* or *tr*, or saying "pa-da" as quickly and sharply as possible.[27]

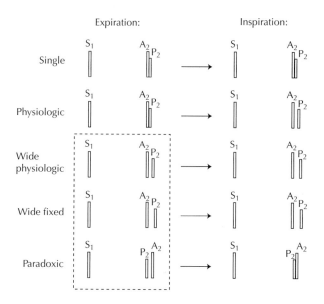

FIGURE 35-1 S_2 splitting. Splitting refers to the separation of the aortic component (A_2) and the pulmonic component (P_2) during expiration (*left column*) and inspiration (*right column*). There are two normal patterns ("single" and "physiologic") and three abnormal patterns ("wide physiologic," "wide fixed," and "paradoxic"). The dotted lines indicate that all three abnormal forms of splitting are distinguished by audible expiratory splitting. See text.

the more likely S_2 will be single instead of physiologic.[25,28]

In a minority of normal persons, expiratory splitting is heard in the supine position, although S_2 becomes single during expiration in these patients when they sit up.[29]

B. Location of sound. S_2 splitting is usually heard only in the second or third intercostal space, next to the left sternum.[28] It is sometimes heard at a slightly lower location, especially in patients with chronic pulmonary disease, and at a slightly higher location in those who are obese.[28] Splitting is not heard at other locations normally because P_2 is too faint.

C. Technique. It is important that the patient breathe regularly in and out when evaluating S_2 splitting because held inspiration or held expiration tends to make the two components drift apart, thus making it impossible to interpret the sound.[16]

D. Physiology of splitting. The normal delay in P_2 results from a "hangout" interval in the normal pulmonary circulation (it is not because right ventricular systole ends later than left ventricular systole; they actually end at the same moment). "Hangout" means that the pulmonary circulation offers so little resistance to blood flow that flow continues for a short period even after completion of right ventricular mechanical systole.[23,24] At the aortic valve, there is little hangout; flow ceases and the valve closes immediately after completion of left ventricular contraction.

A_2 and P_2 move apart during inspiration, primarily because inspiration delays P_2 even more. About half of the inspiratory augmentation of the A_2-P_2 interval is due to a further increase in the hangout interval in the pulmonary circulation. About 25% of inspiratory augmentation is due to lengthening of right ventricular systole (from increased filling of the right side of the heart during inspiration), and the remaining 25% is due to shortening of left ventricular systole (from a reduction of filling of the left side of the heart during inspiration).[24]

III. ABNORMAL SPLITTING OF S_2

A. The finding. There are three abnormalities of S_2 splitting (Figure 35-1):

   1. Wide physiologic splitting. Wide physiologic splitting means that splitting occurs during inspiration and expiration, although the A_2P_2 interval widens further during inspiration.

2. **Wide fixed splitting.** Wide fixed splitting means that splitting occurs during inspiration and expiration, but the A_2P_2 interval remains constant.

3. **Paradoxic splitting (also called "reversed splitting").** Paradoxic splitting means that audible expiratory splitting narrows or melds into a single sound during inspiration. Paradoxic splitting occurs because the order of the S_2 components has reversed: A_2 now follows P_2, and as P_2 is delayed during inspiration, the sounds move together.

B. **Screening for abnormal splitting of S_2.** Figure 35-1 reveals that all three abnormal second heart sounds—wide physiologic, fixed, and paradoxic—have audible splitting *during expiration* (dotted lines in Figure 35-1). Therefore, the best screening tool for the abnormal S_2 is audible expiratory splitting that persists when the patient sits up.[29-32]

C. **Clinical significance and pathogenesis.** Table 35-2 lists the common causes of abnormal S_2 splitting.

1. **Wide physiologic splitting.** Wide physiologic splitting may result from P_2 appearing too late or A_2 too early (Table 35-2).[16,30] The most common cause is right bundle branch block.

In pulmonic stenosis, the A_2P_2 interval correlates well with severity of stenosis (gauged by the right ventricular systolic pressure, $r = 0.87$, $p < .001$),[33] although in many patients the clinician must listen at the third interspace to hear splitting because the murmur is too loud at the second interspace.

In most patients with pulmonary hypertension, the normal "hangout" interval disappears and S_2 is single. S_2 becomes wide in these patients only if there is associated

TABLE 35-2 Abnormal S₂ splitting

SPLITTING AND PATHOGENESIS	ETIOLOGY
Wide Physiologic	
P_2 Late	
Electrical delay of RV systole	RBBB
	LV paced or ectopic beats
Prolongation of RV systole	Pulmonic stenosis
	Acute cor pulmonale
Increased hangout interval	Dilation of pulmonary artery
A_2 Early	
Shortening of LV systole	Mitral regurgitation
Wide and Fixed	
Increased hangout interval or prolongation of RV systole	Atrial septal defect
Prolongation of RV systole	Right ventricular failure
Paradoxic	
A_2 Late	
Electrical delay of LV systole	LBBB
	RV paced or ectopic beats
Prolongation of LV systole	Aortic stenosis
	Ischemic heart disease

LBBB, Left bundle branch block; *LV,* left ventricular; *RBBB,* right bundle branch block; *RV,* right ventricular; "RV systole" and "LV systole" refer to the duration of right and left ventricular contraction.

severe right ventricular dysfunction and prolonged right ventricular systole.[23,24,34] Most patients with pulmonary hypertension and a wide S₂ have either long-standing severe pulmonary hypertension[23,24,34] or massive pulmonary embolism (the wide S₂ of pulmonary embolism is temporary, usually lasting hours to days).[35]

2. **Wide and fixed splitting.** Patients with atrial septal defect have wide fixed splitting of S₂, although this is true only when their pulse is regular (if the patient has atrial fibrillation or frequent extrasystoles, the degree of splitting varies directly with the pre-

ceding cycle length).[22,36] The reason S_2 is wide is not the same in every patient: in some, hangout is increased; in others, right ventricular mechanical systole is prolonged.[36] S_2 is fixed because hangout remains constant during respiration[36] and because the presence of a common left and right atrial chamber interrupts the normal respiratory variation of right ventricular filling.[22]

In patients with audible expiratory splitting (and regular rhythm), the *absence* of fixed splitting argues strongly *against* the diagnosis of atrial septal defect (LR = 0.1; see Table 35-1), whereas the presence of fixed splitting increases the probability of atrial septal defect only modestly (LR = 2.6; see Table 35-1). Patients with false-positive results (i.e., fixed splitting without atrial septal defect) commonly have the combination of right ventricular failure and audible expiratory splitting from bundle branch block or some other cause.[16]

3. **Paradoxic splitting.** In elderly adults with aortic flow murmurs, the finding of paradoxic splitting does not significantly distinguish significant aortic stenosis from less severe disease (Table 35-1).

D. **S_2 splitting vs. other double sounds.**[32] Other double sounds that mimic S_2 splitting include the following (see also Chapter 37):

1. **S_2-opening snap.** In contrast to the split S_2, the S_2-opening snap interval is slightly wider, the opening snap is loudest at the apex, and the opening snap ushers in the diastolic rumble of mitral stenosis at the apex. Patients with S_2-opening snap often have a triple sound (split S_2 + opening snap) during inspiration at the upper sternal border.

2. **S_2-pericardial knock.** In contrast to the split S_2, the S_2-knock interval is slightly

wider, the pericardial knock is loudest at or near the apex, and the knock is always accompanied by elevated neck veins.

3. **S$_2$-third heart sound.** In contrast to the split S$_2$, the S$_2$-S$_3$ interval is 2 to 3 times wider, and S$_3$ is a low frequency sound heard best with the bell.

4. **Late systolic click-S$_2$.** Clicks are loudest at or near apex and are often multiple. Their timing changes with maneuvers (see Chapter 41).

IV. **INTENSITY OF S$_2$.** Despite traditional teachings, no evidence supports a loud P$_2$ as a sign of pulmonary hypertension. Whether defined as an S$_2$ that is louder at the left side of the upper sternum compared with the right side[19] or as a split S$_2$ with a louder second component,[18] the finding does not accurately discriminate patients with pulmonary hypertension from those without it (see Table 35-1). Even when A$_2$ and P$_2$ are precisely identified by phonocardiography (e.g., A$_2$ corresponds to aortic incisura on simultaneous aortic pressure tracing), the relative intensities of the two components do not correlate well with pulmonary pressure.[37] Another suggested sign of pulmonary hypertension is audible splitting at the apex, which is based on the observation that P$_2$ normally is not heard at the apex[25] and the assumption that splitting at this location therefore indicates P$_2$ is abnormally loud. But even this finding correlates better with the etiology of heart disease—it is common in atrial septal defect and primary pulmonary hypertension—than it does with pulmonary pressures.[34,37]

Nonetheless, the *palpable* S$_2$ does accurately detect pulmonary pressures of 50 mm Hg or more in patients with mitral stenosis (positive = LR 3.6, negative LR = 0.05; see Table 35-1). In this study, the palpable P$_2$ was defined as an abrupt tapping sensation coincident with S$_2$ at the second left intercostal space.

REFERENCES

1. Harvey W. *De Motu Cordis* (facsimile edition by Classics of Medicine library), London, 1928, Nonesuch.

2. McKusick VA. *Rouanet of Paris and New Orleans, Bull Hist Med* 32:137-151, 1958.

3. McCrady JD, Hoff HE, and Geddes LA. The contributions of the horse to knowledge of the heart and circulation: IV. James Hope and the heart sounds, *Conn Med* 30:126-131, 1966.

4. Luisada AA and Portaluppi F. The main heart sounds as vibrations of the cardiohemic system: Old controversy and new facts, *Am J Cardiol* 52:1133-1136, 1983.

5. Ronan JA. Cardiac auscultation: the first and second heart sounds, *Heart Dis Stroke* 1:113-116, 1992.

6. Sakamoto T and others. Hemodynamic determinants of the amplitude of the first heart sound, *Circ Res* 16:45-57, 1965.

7. Leech G and others. Mechanism of influence of PR interval on loudness of first heart sound, *Br Heart J* 43:138-142, 1980.

8. Burggraf GW and Craige E. The first heart sound in complete heart block: phono-echocardiographic correlations, *Circulation* 50:17-24, 1974.

9. Tei C and others. The correlates of an abnormal first heart sound in mitral-valve-prolapse syndrome, *N Engl J Med* 307:334-339, 1982.

10. Perloff JK and Harvey WP. Auscultatory and phonocardiographic manifestations of pure mitral regurgitation, *Prog Cardiovasc Dis* 5:172-194, 1962.

11. Wood P. An appreciation of mitral stenosis: Part 1. Clinical features. Part 2. Investigations and results, *Br Med J* 1:1051-1063, 1113-1124, 1954.

12. Gershlick AH and others. The loud first heart sound in left atrial myxoma, *Br Heart J* 52:403-407, 1984.

13. Stein PD, Sabbah HN, and Barr I. Intensity of heart sounds in the evaluation of patients following myocardial infarction, *Chest* 75:679-684, 1979.

14. Meadows WR and others. Premature mitral valve closure: a hemodynamic explanation for absence of the first sound in aortic insufficiency, *Circulation* 28:251-258, 1963.

15. Garratt CJ and others. Value of physical signs in the diagnosis of ventricular tachycardia. *Circulation* 90:3103-3107, 1994.

16. Perloff JK and Harvey WP. Mechanisms of fixed splitting of the second heart sound, *Circulation* 18:998-1009, 1958.

17. Aronow WS and Kronzon I. Correlation of prevalence and severity of valvular aortic stenosis determined by continuous-wave Doppler echocardiography with physical signs of aortic stenosis in patients aged 62 to 100 years with aortic systolic ejection murmurs, *Am J Cardiol* 60:399-401, 1987.

18. Whitaker W. Clinical diagnosis of pulmonary hypertension in patients with mitral stenosis, *Q J Med* 23:105-112, 1954.

19. Fowler NO and others. The clinical estimation of pulmonary hypertension accompanying mitral stenosis, *Am Heart J* 49:237-249, 1955.

20. Leatham A. *Auscultation of the heart and phonocardiography,* ed 2, Edinburgh, 1975, Churchill Livingstone.

21. Leatham A. The second heart sound: key to auscultation of the heart, *Acta Cardiol* 19:395-416, 1964.

22. Aygen MM and Braunwald E. The splitting of the second heart sound in normal subjects and in patients with congenital heart disease, *Circulation* 25:328-345, 1962.

23. Shaver JA and others. Sound pressure correlates of the second heart sound: an intracardiac sound study, *Circulation* 49:316-325, 1974.

24. Curtiss EI, Matthews RG, and Shaver JA. Mechanism of normal splitting of the second heart sound, *Circulation* 51:157-164, 1975.

25. Harris A and Sutton G. Second heart sound in normal subjects, *Br Heart J* 30:739-742, 1968.

26. Levine SA and Harvey WP. *Clinical auscultation of the heart,* Philadelphia, 1959, WB Saunders.

27. Constant J. *Bedside cardiology,* Boston, 1985, Little, Brown & Co.

28. Nelson WP and North RL. Splitting of the second heart sound in adults forty years and older, *Am J Med Sci* 234:805-807, 1967.

29. Breen WJ and Rekate AG. Effect of posture on splitting of the second heart sound, *JAMA* 173:1326-1328, 1960.

30. Shaver JA and O'Toole JD. The second heart sound: newer concepts. Part 1: Normal and wide physiologic splitting, *Mod Concept Cardiovasc Dis* 46:7-12, 1977.

31. Shaver JA and O'Toole JD. The second heart sound: newer concepts, Part 2: Paradoxical splitting and narrow physiological splitting, *Mod Concept Cardiovasc Dis* 46:13-16, 1977.

32. Adolph RJ and Fowler NO. The second heart sound: a screening test for heart disease, *Mod Concept Cardiovasc Dis* 39:91-96, 1970.

33. Leatham A and Weitzman D. Auscultatory and phonocardiographic signs of pulmonary stenosis, *Br Heart J* 19:303-317, 1957.

34. Perloff JK. Auscultatory and phonocardiographic manifestations of pulmonary hypertension, *Prog Cardiovasc Dis* 9:303-340, 1967.

35. Cobbs BW, Logue RB, and Dorney ER. The second heart sound in pulmonary embolism and pulmonary hypertension, *Am Heart J* 71:843-844, 1966.

36. O'Toole JD and others. The mechanism of splitting of the second heart sound in atrial septal defect, *Circulation* 56:1047-1053, 1977.

37. Sutton G, Harris A, and Leatham A. Second heart sound in pulmonary hypertension, *Br Heart J* 30:743-756, 1968.

CHAPTER 36

The Third and Fourth Heart Sounds

I. **INTRODUCTION.** Although the third and fourth heart sounds (S_3 and S_4) are both sounds that originate in the ventricle from rapid diastolic filling, they differ in timing and clinical significance. S_3 appears in early diastole and, if the patient is older that 40 years of age, the sound indicates severe systolic dysfunction or valvular regurgitation. In persons younger than 40 years of age, S_3 may be a normal finding (i.e., the "physiologic S_3").[1] S_4 appears in late diastole, immediately before S_1, indicating that the patient's ventricle is abnormally stiff from hypertrophy or fibrosis. If discovered in persons of any age, the S_4 is an abnormal finding.

In the late nineteenth century, the great French clinician Potain accurately described most features of S_3 and S_4, their pathogenesis, and their distinction from other double sounds such as the split S_1 or split S_2.[2] In his writings he called them "gallops," a term he attributed to his teacher Bouillard.[2,3]

II. **DEFINITIONS.** Several different terms have been used to describe these diastolic sounds.
   A. Gallop. A gallop is a triple rhythm with an extra sound in diastole (either an S_3, an S_4, or

their summation). The term refers only to pathologic sounds (i.e., it excludes physiologic S_3) and, despite its connotation, a patient may have a gallop whether the heart rate is fast or slow.[2,4]

B. Third heart sound (S_3). The third heart sound is sometimes called the "ventricular gallop" or "protodiastolic gallop."[2] It appears in early diastole, 120 to 180 ms after S_2.[5] To mimic the sound, the clinician should first establish the cadence of the normal S_1 (*lub*) and S_2 (*dup*):

lub   dup   lub   dup   lub   dup

and then add an early diastolic sound (*bub*)[a]:

lub   du bub   lub   du bub   lub   du bub

The overall cadence of the S_3 gallop (*lub du bub*) is similar to the cadence of the word "Kentucky."

C. Fourth heart sound (S_4). The fourth heart sound is sometimes called the "atrial gallop" or "presystolic gallop."[2] To mimic the sound, the clinician establishes the cadence of S_1 and S_2 (*lub dup*) and then adds a presystolic sound (*be*):

be lub   dup   be lub   dup   be lub   dup

The cadence of the S_4 gallop (*be lub dup*) is similar to the cadence of "Tennessee."

D. Summation gallop. The summation gallop is a loud gallop that occurs in patients with tachycardia. In fast heart rhythms, diastole shortens, causing the events that produce S_3 (rapid early diastolic filling) to coincide with those producing S_4 (atrial systole). The resulting sound sometimes is louder than the patient's S_1 or S_2.

---

[a] To pronounce the S_3 gallop with correct timing, the "p" of *dup* (S_2) must be dropped. In most patients the accent is on S_2 (*lub **du** bub*), although in others it falls on S_1 or S_3. The clinician can practice all 3 versions, always maintaining the same cadence, to become familiar with the varying sounds of S_3.

Not all gallop rhythms in patients with tachycardia are summation gallops. The only way to confirm the finding is to observe the patient after the heart rate slows. (In the past, slowing was often induced by carotid artery massage, although in elderly patients this is not recommended; see Chapter 14.) If slowing causes the gallop to disappear or evolve into two distinct but fainter sounds (i.e., S_3 and S_4), it was a genuine summation gallop. If the sound evolves instead into a single S_3 or single S_4, it was not a summation gallop.[4,6]

E. Quadruple rhythm. The quadruple rhythm consists of S_1, S_2, and both S_3 and S_4.[4] It is an uncommon finding, usually only evident in patients with slow heart rates. It is sometimes called the "train wheel" rhythm, because the sound resembles that produced by the two pairs of wheels from adjacent train cars as they cross the coupling of a railroad track.[3,6]

be lub   du bub   be lub   du bub   be lub   du bub

III. TECHNIQUE

A. Location of sound and use of stethoscope. S_3 and S_4 are both low frequency sounds (20 to 70 Hz), bordering on the threshold of hearing.[7] They therefore are best heard with the bell of the stethoscope, applied lightly to the body wall with only enough force to create an air seal.[2,5] Gallops that originate in the left ventricle are best heard with the bell over the apical impulse or just medial to it. They are sometimes only audible with the patient lying in the left lateral decubitus position.[8] Gallops from the right ventricle are best heard with the bell over the left lower sternal border or, in patients with chronic lung disease, the subxiphoid area.[2,5]

B. Right vs. left ventricular gallops. Aside from their different locations, other distinguishing features of right and left ventricular gallops are their response to respiration and association with other findings in the neck veins and precordium. Right ventricular gallops become louder during inspiration; left ventricular gallops become softer during inspiration.[9] The right ventricular S_4 may be associated with giant A waves in the neck veins and sometimes a loud presystolic jugular sound (see Chapter 31).[10] The left ventricular S_4 may be associated with a palpable presystolic movement of the apical impulse (see Chapter 33).

C. **Distinguishing the S_4-S_1 sound from other sounds.** Three combinations of heart sounds produce a double sound around S_1: (1) the S_4-S_1 sound, (2) the split S_1, and (3) the S_1-ejection sound. The following characteristics distinguish these sounds[9]:

1. **Use of the bell.** The S_4 is a low frequency sound, best heard with the bell. Firm pressure with the bell on the skin—which tends to remove low frequency sounds—will cause the S_4-S_1 combination to evolve into a single sound, in contrast to the split S_1 and the S_1-ejection sounds, which remain double.

2. **Location.** The S_4-S_1 sound is heard best at the apex, left lower sternal border, or subxiphoid area (see Section III-A above). The split S_1 is loudest from the apex to lower sternal border, but sometimes is also heard well over the upper left sternal area. The aortic ejection sound is heard from the apex to the upper right sternal border. The pulmonary ejection sound is restricted to the upper left sternal area.[11]

3. **Effect of respiration.** Although the S_4 may become louder (RV S_4) or softer (LV S_4) during inspiration, respiration does not affect the interval between S_4 and S_1. In contrast, the split S_1 interval varies with respiration in up to one third of patients.

Expiration makes the pulmonary ejection

sound louder.[11] The aortic ejection sound
does not vary with respiration.[12]

4. **Palpation.** Only the S_4-S_1 sound is accompanied by a presystolic apical impulse (see
Chapter 33). The intensity of the S_4 (i.e., by
auscultation) correlates moderately with the
amplitude of the presystolic impulse on
apexcardiography ($r = 0.46$, $p <.01$); similarly,
the palpability of the presystolic impulse
correlates roughly with the amplitude of S_4
on phonocardiography ($r = 0.52$, $p <.01$).[13]

IV. PATHOGENESIS

A. **Normal ventricular filling curves.** Filling of
the right and left ventricles during diastole is
divided into three distinct phases (Figure 36-1).
The first phase, the rapid filling phase, begins
immediately after the atrioventricular valves
open. During this phase, blood stored in the

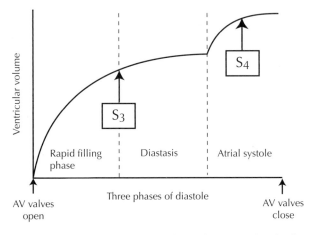

FIGURE 36-1 Timing of third and fourth heart sounds. The figure depicts the three phases of ventricular filling during diastole
(y-axis, ventricular volume; x-axis, time). The S_3 occurs at the
end of the rapid filling phase. The S_4 occurs during atrial systole.
AV, Atrioventricular.

atria rapidly empties into the ventricles. The second phase, the plateau phase (diastasis), begins at the moment the ventricles are unable to relax passively any further. Very little filling occurs during this phase. The third phase, atrial systole, begins with the atrial contraction, which expands the ventricle further just before the next S_1.

B. Ventricular filling and sound. Both S_3 and S_4 occur at those times during diastole when blood flow entering the ventricles temporarily stops, that is, the S_3 appears at the end of the rapid filling phase, and the S_4 toward the peak of atrial systole (Figure 36-1). Sounds become audible if the blood *decelerates abruptly* enough, which transmits sufficient energy to the ventricular walls and causes them to vibrate (an analogy is the tensing of a handkerchief between two hands: abrupt tensing produces sound whereas slow tensing is silent).[14-18] Two variables govern the suddenness of this deceleration and therefore whether a gallop becomes audible: (1) the flow rate during entry and (2) the stiffness of the ventricle. The greater the flow rate, the *louder* the sound. The stiffer the ventricle, the *higher the frequency* of the sound.[19] Since gallops consist of low frequencies that are difficult to hear (around 20 to 50 Hz), anything increasing its frequency content (i.e., stiff ventricles) makes the sound more likely to be heard.

Even though S_3 and S_4 both result from rapid flow rates into stiff ventricles, the diseases causing them differ completely.

C. The third heart sound (S_3). The S_3 gallop appears when early diastolic filling is exaggerated, which occurs in two types of cardiac disorders:

    1. Congestive heart failure. The most common cause of the S_3 gallop is congestive heart failure from systolic dysfunction. In these patients, the S_3 indicates that atrial pressure is abnormally high, an especially important finding in patients who are dyspneic, implying that heart disease is the principle cause of the shortness of breath. In addition to high atrial pressure, these patients typically have a dilated cardiomyopathy and low cardiac output.[20,21] Although both high atrial pressure (causing rapid flow rates) and cardiomyopathy (causing stiff ventricles) contribute to the sound, atrial pressure is the more important clinical variable because the sound disappears as soon as pressure falls after diuresis.

2. **Regurgitation and shunts.** Patients with valvular regurgitation or left-to-right cardiac shunts also may develop an S_3 gallop, whether or not atrial pressure is high, because these disorders all cause excess flow over the atrioventricular valves. Patients with mitral regurgitation, ventricular septal defect, or patent ductus arteriosus may develop a left ventricular S_3 from excess diastolic flow over the mitral valve into the left ventricle (in mitral regurgitation, the excess diastolic flow simply represents the diastolic return of the regurgitant flow). Patients with atrial septal defect may develop a right ventricular S_3 from excess flow over the tricuspid valve into the right ventricle.

D. **The fourth heart sound (S_4).** The S_4 gallop occurs in patients with hypertension, ischemic cardiomyopathy, hypertrophic cardiomyopathy, or aortic stenosis—all disorders characterized by ventricles stiffened from hypertrophy or fibrosis.[2,20-22] Patients with the sound must be in sinus rhythm and have strong atrial contractions, and most have normal atrial pressures, normal cardiac output, and normal ventricular chamber size. Unlike the S_3, the S_4 is a durable finding that does not wax and wane, although it does disappear if the patient develops atrial fibrillation (and loses the atrial kick).

E. **Summation gallop and quadruple rhythm.**
The summation gallop occurs because fast heart rates shorten diastole, primarily by eliminating the plateau phase (Figure 36-1), which brings the events causing S_3 close to those causing S_4. Diastolic filling is concentrated into a single moment, thus causing a very loud sound.

   The quadruple rhythm typically occurs in patients who have had a long-standing S_4 gallop from ischemic or hypertensive heart disease but who then develop cardiac decompensation, high filling pressures, and an S_3.[6]

F. **Physiologic S_3.** Persons younger than 40 years of age with normal hearts also may have an S_3 sound (i.e., physiologic S_3) because normal early filling can sometimes be so rapid that it ends abruptly and causes the ventricular walls to vibrate and produce sound. Compared with healthy persons lacking the sound, those with the physiologic S_3 are leaner and have more rapid early diastolic filling.[1] The physiologic S_3 disappears by age 40, because normal aging slows ventricular relaxation and shifts filling later in diastole, thus diminishing the rate of early diastolic filling and making the sound disappear.[23]

V. CLINICAL SIGNIFICANCE
A. The third heart sound
1. **Congestive heart failure.** Table 36-1 shows that the presence of the S_3 gallop is a significant finding indicating depressed ejection fraction (LR = 3.8 to 4.1; Table 36-1) and elevated left atrial pressures (LR = 5.7; see Table 36-1). Other studies confirm its value as a predictor of poor systolic function.[36] The *absence* of the S_3 gallop argues that the patient's ejection fraction is greater than 30% (i.e., negative LR for ejection fraction <30% is 0.3; see Table 36-1).

   In patients with a history of congestive

TABLE 36-1 Third and fourth heart sounds*

FINDING (REF)	SENSITIVITY (%)	SPECIFICITY (%)	POSITIVE LR	NEGATIVE LR
Third Heart Sound				
Detecting ejection fraction less than 0.5[24-26]	11-51	86-98	3.8	NS
Detecting ejection fraction less than 0.3[25,26]	68-78	80-88	4.1	0.3
Detecting elevated left heart filling pressures[27-29]	12-32	95-96	5.7	NS
Predicting postoperative pulmonary edema[30,31]	17	99	14.6	NS
Predicting postoperative myocardial infarction or cardiac death[30,31]	11	99	8.0	NS
Detecting moderate-to-severe mitral regurgitation, in patients with characteristic systolic murmur[32]	41	77	1.8	0.8
Fourth Heart Sound				
Predicting 5-year mortality in patients after myocardial infarction[33]	29	91	3.2	NS
Detecting elevated left heart filling pressures[28]	71	50	NS	NS
Detecting severe aortic stenosis[34,35]	29-50	57-63	NS	NS

NS, Not significant.

*Diagnostic standards: For ejection fraction, radionuclide left ventricular ejection fraction <0.5 or <0.3, as indicated above; for elevated left heart filling pressures, pulmonary capillary wedge pressure >12 mm Hg[27] or left ventricular end diastolic pressure >15 mm Hg[28,29]; for moderate-to-severe mitral regurgitation, visual assessment from angiogram[32]; for severe aortic stenosis, peak gradient >50 mm Hg[34] or valve area <0.75 cm^2.[35]

heart failure, the S_3 predicts responsiveness to digoxin[37] and overall mortality.[38]

2. **Valvular heart disease.** In patients with mitral regurgitation, the S_3 is a poor predictor of elevated filling pressure (LR not significant), depressed ejection fraction (LR = 1.9),[32] and even severity of regurgitation (LR only 1.8 for moderate-to-severe mitral regurgitation; see Table 36-1).

In contrast, the S_3 in patients with aortic stenosis or mixed aortic stenosis-regurgitation predicts depressed ejection fraction and elevated filling pressures just as well as it does in patients without valvular heart disease.[32]

3. **Preoperative consultation.** During preoperative consultation, the finding of S_3 is ominous, indicating that the patient, without any other intervention, has an increased risk of perioperative pulmonary edema (LR = 14.6) and myocardial infarction or cardiac death (LR = 8.0).[30]

B. **The fourth heart sound.** The finding of the S_4 gallop has less diagnostic value, simply because the disorders causing stiff ventricles are so diverse and because the S_4 does not predict the patient's hemodynamic findings. The finding does not predict ejection fraction, left heart filling pressures, or postoperative cardiac complications.[20,21,28,30,31] It also does not predict significant aortic stenosis in elderly patients with aortic flow murmurs, presumably because many patients with mild stenosis have the finding for other reasons, such as ischemic heart disease.[34,35]

Nonetheless, when detected 1 month after myocardial infarction, the S_4 is a modest predictor of 5-year cardiac mortality (LR = 3.2; see Table 36-1). Experienced auscultators in the past did show that clinical deterioration in patients with ischemic disease caused the S_4-S_1 interval to widen, which could be recognized at the bedside, but proper interpretation of this finding required knowledge of the patient's PR interval, thus limiting its utility.[39] In patients with chaotic heart rhythms, the finding of an S_4 excludes atrial fibrillation and suggests other diagnoses such as multifocal atrial tachycardia.

The S_4 is rare in patients with chronic mitral regurgitation, because the dilated atrium of these patients cannot contract strongly. Therefore, finding an S_4 gallop in a patient with mitral regurgitation is an important clue to the diagnosis of *acute* mitral regurgitation (e.g., ruptured chorda tendineae; see Chapter 41).[40-42]

REFERENCES

1. Kupari M and others. Prevalence and predictors of audible physiological third heart sound in a population sample aged 36 to 37 years, *Circulation* 89:1189-1195, 1994.
2. Craige E. Gallop rhythm, *Prog Cardiovasc Dis* 10:246-261, 1967.
3. Sloan AW. Cardiac gallop rhythm, *Medicine* 37:197-215, 1958.
4. Feinstein AR and others. Glossary of cardiologic terms related to physical diagnosis and history, *Am J Cardiol* 21:273-274, 1968.
5. Ronan JA. Cardiac auscultation: the third and fourth heart sounds, *Heart Dis Stroke* 1:267-270, 1992.
6. Harvey WP and Stapleton J. Clinical aspects of gallop rhythm with particular reference to diastolic gallop, *Circulation* 18:1017-1024, 1958.
7. Tavel ME. *Clinical phonocardiography and external pulse recording,* ed 4, Chicago, 1985, Year Book Publishers, Inc.
8. Bethell HJN and Nixon PGF. Examination of the heart in supine and left lateral positions, *Br Heart J* 35:902-907, 1973.
9. Fowler NO and Adolph RJ. Fourth sound gallop or split first sound? *Am J Cardiol* 30:441-444, 1972.
10. Dock W. Loud presystolic sounds over the jugular veins associated with high venous pressure, *Am J Med* 20:853-859, 1956.

11. Perloff JK. Auscultatory and phonocardiographic manifestations of pulmonary hypertension, *Prog Cardiovasc Dis* 9:303-340, 1967.

12. Leatham A. *Auscultation of the heart and phonocardiography,* ed 2, Edinburgh, 1975, Churchill Livingstone.

13. Jordan MD and others. Audibility of the fourth heart sound: relationship to presence of disease and examiner experience, *Arch Intern Med* 147:721-726, 1987.

14. Ozawa Y, Smith D, and Craige E. Origin of the third heart sound. I. Studies in dogs. *Circulation* 67:393-398, 1983.

15. Ozawa Y, Smith D, and Craige E. Origin of the third heart sound. II. Studies in human subjects. *Circulation* 67:399-404, 1983.

16. Kono T and others. Hemodynamic correlates of the third heart sound during the evolution of chronic heart failure, *J Am Coll Cardiol* 21:419-423, 1993.

17. Ishimitsu T and others. Origin of the third heart sound: comparison of ventricular wall dynamics in hyperdynamic and hypodynamic types, *J Am Coll Cardiol* 5:268-272, 1985.

18. Van de Werf F and others. Diastolic properties of the left ventricle in normal adults and in patients with third heart sounds, *Circulation* 69:1070-1078, 1984.

19. Glower DD and others. Mechanical correlates of the third heart sound, *J Am Coll Cardiol* 19:450-457, 1992.

20. Shah PM and others. Determinants of atrial (S4) and ventricular (S3) gallop sounds in primary myocardial disease, *N Engl J Med* 278:753-758, 1968.

21. Shah PM and Yu PN. Gallop rhythm: hemodynamic and clinical correlation, *Am Heart J* 78:823-828, 1969.

22. Homma S and others. Relationship of auscultatory fourth heart sound to the quantitated left atrial filling fraction, *Clin Cardiol* 14:671-674, 1991.

23. Van de Werf F and others. The mechanisms of disappearance of the physiologic third heart sound with age, *Circulation* 73:877-884, 1986.

24. Gadsboll N and others. Interobserver agreement and accuracy of bedside estimation of right and left ventricular ejection fraction in acute myocardial infarction, *Am J Cardiol* 63:1301-1307, 1989.

25. Mattleman SJ and others. Reliability of bedside evaluation in determining left ventricular function: correlation with left ventricular ejection fraction determined by radionuclide ventriculography, *J Am Coll Cardiol* 1:417-420, 1983.

26. Patel R, Bushnell DL, and Sobotka PA. Implications of an audible third heart sound in evaluating cardiac function, *West J Med* 158:606-609, 1993.

27. Gadsboll N and others. Symptoms and signs of heart failure in patients with myocardial infarction: reproducibility and relationship to chest x-ray, radionuclide ventriculography and right heart catheterization, *Eur Heart J* 10:1017-1028, 1989.

28. Zema MJ and others. Left ventricular dysfunction: bedside Valsalva manoevre, *Br Heart J* 44:560-569, 1980.

29. Harlan WR and others. Chronic congestive heart failure in coronary artery disease: clinical criteria, *Ann Intern Med* 86:133-138, 1977.

30. Goldman L and others. Multifactorial index of cardiac risk in noncardiac surgical procedures, *N Engl J Med* 297:845-850, 1977.

31. Goldman L and others. Cardiac risk factors and complications in non-cardiac surgery, *Medicine* 57:357-370, 1978.

32. Folland ED and others. Implications of third heart sounds in patients with valvular heart disease, *N Engl J Med* 327:458-462, 1992.

33. Ishikawa M and others. Prognostic significance of a clearly audible fourth heart sound detected a month after an acute myocardial infarction, *Am J Cardiol* 80:619-621, 1997.

34. Aronow WS and Kronzon I. Correlation of prevalence and severity of valvular aortic stenosis determined by continuous-wave Doppler echocardiography with physical signs of aortic stenosis in patients aged 62 to 100 years with aortic systolic ejection murmurs, *Am J Cardiol* 60:399-401, 1987.

35. Kavalier MA, Stewart J, and Tavel ME. The apical A wave versus the fourth heart sound in assessing the severity of aortic stenosis, *Circulation* 51:324-327, 1975.

36. Eagle KA and others. Left ventricular ejection fraction: physician estimates compared with gated blood pool scan measurements, *Arch Intern Med* 148:882-885, 1988.

37. Lee DCS and others. Heart failure in outpatients: a randomized trial of digoxin versus placebo, *N Engl J Med* 306:699-705, 1982.

38. Likoff MJ, Chandler SL, and Kay HR. Clinical determinants of mortality in chronic congestive heart failure secondary to idiopathic dilated or to ischemic cardiomyopathy, *Am J Cardiol* 59:634-638, 1987.

39. Barlow JB. Some observations on the atrial sound, *S Afr Med J* 34:887-892, 1960.
40. Cohen LS, Mason DT, and Braunwald E. Significance of an atrial gallop sound in mitral regurgitation: a clue to the diagnosis of rupture chordae tendineae, *Circulation* 35:112-118, 1967.
41. DePace NL, Nestico PF, and Morganroth J. Acute severe mitral regurgitation: pathophysiology, clinical recognition, and management, *Am J Med* 78:293-306, 1985.
42. Hultgren HN, Hancock EW, and Cohn KE. Auscultation in mitral and tricuspid valvular disease, *Prog Cardiovasc Dis* 10:298-322, 1968.

CHAPTER 37

Miscellaneous Heart Sounds

In addition to the first, second, third, and fourth heart sounds, several other discrete, short sounds may occur (Figure 37-1). These sounds include early systolic sounds (e.g., the aortic or pulmonary ejection sound), midsystolic or late systolic sounds (e.g., systolic click of mitral valve prolapse), early diastolic sounds (e.g., opening snap of mitral stenosis, pericardial knock of constrictive pericarditis, and tumor plop of atrial myxoma), and prosthetic valve sounds. All are high frequency sounds best heard with the diaphragm of the stethoscope.

EJECTION SOUNDS

I. THE FINDING AND PATHOGENESIS. The ejection sound is the most common early systolic sound. It results from abnormal sudden halting of the semilunar cusps as they open during early systole.[2,3] Patients with aortic ejection sounds typically have aortic stenosis, bicuspid aortic valves, or a dilated aortic root.[2,3] Those with pulmonary ejection sounds have pulmonary stenosis, pulmonary hypertension, or a dilated pulmonary trunk.[3,4]

Aortic and pulmonary ejection sounds are distinguished by their location, associated murmurs, and how they vary during respiration. An aortic

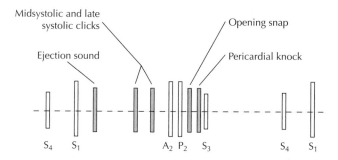

FIGURE 37-1 Miscellaneous heart sounds. The figure shows the timing of the miscellaneous systolic sounds (ejection sounds and mid-to-late systolic clicks) and diastolic sounds (opening snap and pericardial knock), in relation to the principle heart sounds (first, second, third, and fourth heart sounds). The tumor plop of atrial myxoma, not depicted in the figure, has variable timing, ranging from 80 ms after A_2 (i.e., timing of the opening snap) to 150 ms after A_2 (i.e., timing of the third heart sound).[1]

ejection sound is a loud high-frequency sound (often louder than S_1) best heard at the apex, although commonly also audible at the upper right sternal border.[5] It does not vary with respiration. Pulmonary ejection sounds are confined to the sternal edge at the second or third intercostal space; they often diminish in intensity during inspiration. Ejection sounds associated with aortic or pulmonic stenosis occur immediately before the onset of the systolic murmur.[5,6]

Chapter 36 describes how to distinguish ejection sounds from other double sounds around S_1, including the combination of S_4-S_1 and the split S_1.

II. CLINICAL SIGNIFICANCE. The primary importance of these sounds is their etiologic associations. In patients with aortic stenosis, the ejection sound implies that the stenosis is at the valvular level and that there is some mobility to the valve. Elderly patients with calcific aortic stenosis usually do not have ejection sounds because the calcific degeneration makes the valve leaflets inflexible. Children with noncalcific aortic stenosis, in contrast, usually have the ejection sound. In one consecutive series of 118 patients with aortic stenosis, the ejection sound was audible in 100% of patients with noncalcific valvular stenosis, in 32% with calcific valvular stenosis, and in none with subvalvular or supravalvular stenosis.[5]

MID-TO-LATE SYSTOLIC CLICKS

I. THE FINDING AND PATHOGENESIS. Mid-to-late systolic clicks occur in patients with mitral valve prolapse. These sounds, which are sometimes multiple, are caused by sudden deceleration of the billowing mitral leaflet as it prolapses backward into the left atrium during systole.[7] The click is loudest at the apex or left lower sternal border and is frequently associated with a late systolic murmur.[8]

The hallmark of the click of mitral valve prolapse (and also of the associated murmur) is that its timing shifts during maneuvers that change venous return. For example, the straining phase of the Valsalva maneuver or the squat-to-stand maneuver, both of which decrease venous return, cause the mitral leaflets to prolapse earlier in systole, thus shifting the click (and murmur) closer to S_1.[8,9]

Clicks have been heard by clinicians for over a century, although they were ascribed to pleuropericardial adhesions or other extracardiac causes[10] until the 1960s, when Barlow demonstrated the sound coincided with systolic prolapse of the posterior mitral leaflet.[11]

II. CLINICAL SIGNIFICANCE. The presence of the characteristic click or murmur alone is sufficient grounds for the diagnosis of mitral valve prolapse.[12,13] See Chapter 41 for further discussion of these findings.

OPENING SNAP

I. THE FINDING AND PATHOGENESIS. The open-
ing snap is an early diastolic sound heard in patients with mitral stenosis.[a] The sound occurs because the stenotic mitral leaflets (although fused, they are mobile) billow like a large sail into the ventricle during early diastole but then abruptly decelerate as they meet the limits of movement.[2,7] The abrupt deceleration causes a loud, medium-to-high frequency sound, which is then followed by the middiastolic rumbling murmur of mitral stenosis. The opening snap is best heard between the apex and left lower sternal border.

The clinician can mimic the sound of snap and murmur together by first setting up the cadence of S_1, S_2, and opening snap (RUP = S_1; bu = S_2; DUP = opening snap):

> RUP   bu DUP   RUP   bu DUP

and then adding the murmur:

> RUP   bu DUP~RRRRRRRR~RUP   bu DUP~RR~ ~RRRRR~RUP

In some patients the opening snap is so loud it is easily heard at the second left intercostal space, where it then mimics a widely split S_2. Careful attention to inspiration in these patients, however, may reveal a *triple* sound (split S_2 and opening snap) at this location, confirming the last sound to be the opening snap.

The opening snap of mitral stenosis was first described by Bouillard in 1835.[2]

II. CLINICAL SIGNIFICANCE. According to tradi-
tional teachings, the opening snap is inaudible in

---

[a] Patients with tricuspid stenosis also may have an opening snap, but all of these patients also have mitral stenosis and the mitral opening snap. Differentiating tricuspid and mitral opening snaps by auscultation alone is difficult.

patients with mitral stenosis whose valve leaflets have become so thickened and inflexible they cannot create sound.[7,14] Although mitral stenosis is sometimes silent, no systematic studies of this teaching could be found.

The interval between the A_2 component of S_2 and the opening snap (A_2-OS interval) has been used to gauge the severity of stenosis. Patients with more severe obstruction tend to have a narrower A_2-OS interval than those with milder disease. This occurs because the mitral valve opens when the pressure in the relaxing ventricle falls below the atrial pressure; the more severe the obstruction, the higher the atrial pressure and the sooner this crossover occurs. Nonetheless, determining the A_2-OS interval is primarily a phonocardiographic exercise, not an auscultatory one.[15] Furthermore, the A_2-OS interval also depends on variables other than severity of stenosis, such as ventricular relaxation time and heart rate, which further complicate interpreting it accurately at the bedside.[15]

The opening snap does indicate that the accompanying diastolic murmur represents mitral stenosis and not a flow rumble from increased flow over a nonstenotic valve (see Chapter 41 for discussion of flow rumbles).

PERICARDIAL KNOCK

The pericardial knock is a loud early diastolic sound heard in 28% to 94% of patients with constrictive pericarditis (see Chapter 42).[16-18] It is heard over a wide area between the apex and left lower sternal border. Compared with the third heart sound, the pericardial knock is a higher frequency sound (easily detected with the diaphragm of the stethoscope), appearing over a wider area of the precordium and occurring slightly earlier (although still later than the opening snap or widely split second heart sound).[17]

The pericardial knock results from the sudden deceleration of the filling ventricle as it meets the borders of the rigid pericardial sac.[17,18] In this way, it is similar to the third heart sound, although the more abrupt deceleration of constriction is what probably makes the pericardial knock higher-pitched and louder than the third heart sound (see Chapter 36).

TUMOR PLOP

The tumor plop, which may be heard in rare patients with atrial myxoma (only 1 of 9 patients in one series), is an early diastolic sound representing prolapse of the pedunculated tumor into the ventricle after the mitral (or tricuspid) valve opens.[19,20] Characteristically, the intensity and timing of the tumor plop vary between examinations: it may be as early as the timing of an opening snap or as late as that of the third heart sound.

PROSTHETIC HEART SOUNDS

I. **INTRODUCTION.** Abnormal prosthetic heart sounds may be the only clue explaining the patient's dyspnea, syncope, or chest pain. To recognize these abnormal sounds simply and quickly, the clinician must first understand the normal prosthetic heart sounds. This section focuses on rigid mechanical valves, such as caged-ball valves (Starr-Edwards), single tilting disc valves (Bjork-Shiley, Medtronic-Hall), and bileaflet tilting-disc valves (St. Jude Medical).[21-23]

II. **PRINCIPLES.** The important observations are (1) timing and intensity of opening and closing sounds, which typically have a clicking or metallic quality, and are often audible without a stethoscope, and (2) any associated murmurs. Any new or changing sound or murmur requires investigation.
   A. **Opening and closing sounds.** In patients with caged-ball valves, the opening sound is louder than the closing sound. In patients with tilting-disc valves (both single disc and bileaflet), the closing sounds are loud and the

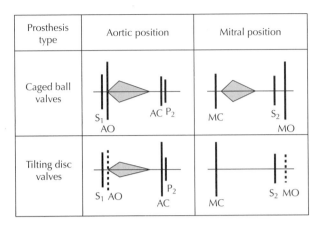

FIGURE 37-2 Prosthetic valve sounds. The normal findings of prosthetic valves, based on references.[21-23] *AC,* Closure sound of aortic prothesis; *AO,* opening sound of aortic prothesis; *MC,* closure sound of mitral prosthesis; *MO,* opening sound of mitral prosthesis; *P₂,* pulmonary component of second heart sound; *S₁,* first heart sound; *S₂,* second heart sound. See text.

opening sounds are only faint or inaudible (Figure 37-2).

1. Caged ball valves. In the aortic position, the caged ball valve produces a loud opening sound, which is an extra systolic sound occurring just after S_1 with timing identical to the aortic ejection sound (i.e., instead of just S_1 and S_2, *lub dup . . . lub dup,* the clinician hears *ledup dup . . . ledup dup*). Caged ball valves in the mitral position produce an extra diastolic sound when they open, with timing identical to that of the opening snap (i.e., instead of S_1 and S_2, *lub bup . . . lub bup,* it is *lub budup . . . lub budup*). These opening sounds should always be louder than the corresponding closing sound (i.e., closing sounds are coincident with S_2 in aortic prostheses and with S_1 in mitral prostheses). The finding of an inaudible or abnormally soft opening sound indicates something is interfering with excursion of the ball, such as thrombus.

2. **Tilting disc valves.** These valves produce distinct, metallic closing sounds coincident with S_1 (mitral position) or S_2 (aortic position). Patients whose closing sounds are abnormally quiet may have significant valve dysfunction.

B. **Murmurs.** In the aortic position, all rigid valves (caged ball and tilting disc) typically produce short midsystolic murmurs that are best heard at the base and sometimes radiate to the neck. Diastolic murmurs in these patients suggest perivalvular regurgitation and require investigation.[21-23]

In patients with rigid valves in the mitral position, any holosystolic murmur suggests perivalvular regurgitation and requires investigation. A normal finding in patients with the caged ball valve in the mitral position (but not tilting disc valves) is an early-to-midsystolic murmur at the left sternal border. This murmur does not indicate regurgitation but instead represents turbulence caused by the cage of the valve projecting into the left ventricular outflow tract.[21,23]

REFERENCES

1. Tavel ME. *Clinical phonocardiography and external pulse recording,* ed 4, Chicago, 1985, Year Book Publishers, Inc.

2. Leatham A. *Auscultation of the heart and phonocardiography,* ed 2, Edinburgh, 1975, Churchill Livingstone.

3. Perloff JK. The physiologic mechanisms of cardiac and vascular physical signs, *J Am Coll Cardiol,* 1:184-198, 1983.

4. Perloff JK. Auscultatory and phonocardiographic manifestations of pulmonary hypertension, *Prog Cardiovasc Dis* 9:303-340, 1967.

5. Hancock EW. The ejection sound in aortic stenosis, *Am J Med* 40:569-577, 1966.

6. Leatham A, Weitzman D. Auscultatory and phonocardiographic signs of pulmonary stenosis, *Br Heart J* 19:303-317, 1957.

7. Ronan JA. Cardiac auscultation: opening snaps, systolic clicks, and ejection sounds, *Heart Dis Stroke* 2:188-191, 1993.

8. Barlow JB and others. Late systolic murmurs and non-ejection ("mid-late") systolic clicks: an analysis of 90 patients, *Br Heart J* 30:203-218, 1968.

9. Fontana ME and others. Postural changes in left ventricular and mitral valvular dynamics in systolic click—late systolic murmur syndrome, *Circulation* 51:165-173, 1975.

10. Devereux RB and others. Mitral valve prolapse, *Circulation* 54:3-14, 1976.

11. Barlow JB and others. The significance of late systolic murmurs, *Am Heart J* 66:443-452, 1963.

12. Perloff JK and Child JS. Clinical and epidemiologic issues in mitral valve prolapse: overview and perspective, *Am Heart J* 113:1324-1332, 1987.

13. Perloff JK, Child JS, and Edwards JE. New guidelines for the clinical diagnosis of mitral valve prolapse, *Am J Cardiol* 57:1124-1129, 1986.

14. Wood P. An appreciation of mitral stenosis: Part 1. Clinical features. Part 2. Investigations and results, *Br Med J* 1:1051-1063, 1113-1124, 1954.

15. Hultgren HN, Hancock EW, and Cohn KE. Auscultation in mitral and tricuspid valvular disease, *Prog Cardiovasc Dis* 10:298-322, 1968.

16. Harvey WP. Auscultatory findings in diseases of the pericardium, *Am J Cardiol* 7:15-720, 1961.

17. Mounsey P. The early diastolic sound of constrictive pericarditis, *Br Heart J* 17:143-152, 1955.

18. Tyberg TI, Goodyer AVN, and Langou RA. Genesis of pericardial knock in constrictive pericarditis, *Am J Cardiol* 46:570-575, 1980.

19. Gershlick AH and others. The loud first heart sound in left atrial myxoma, *Br Heart J* 52:403-407, 1984.

20. Pitt A and others. Myxoma of the left atrium: Hemodynamic and phonocardiographic consequences of sudden tumor movement, *Circulation* 36:408-416, 1967.

21. Vongpatanasin W, Hillis LD, and Lange RA. Prosthetic heart valves, *N Engl J Med* 335:407-416, 1996.

22. Commerford PJ, Stevens JE, and Millar RS. Rumbles and prosthetic heart valves, *N Engl J Med* 336:1259-1260, 1997.

23. Smith ND, Raizada V, and Abrams J. Auscultation of the normally functioning prosthetic valve, *Ann Intern Med* 95:594-598, 1981.

CHAPTER 38

Heart Murmurs: General Principles

I. **INTRODUCTION.** Over the last 170 years, the understanding of the significance of heart murmurs has evolved in three distinct stages.[1] In the first stage, brilliant clinicians, like Hope, Steell, and Flint, attentively observed patients at the bedside, correlating the timing and quality of murmurs to the patients' clinical course and postmortem findings.[2] In the second stage, during the 1950s and 1960s, cardiac catheterization and phonocardiography helped clinicians understand the hemodynamics responsible for heart murmurs,[3,4] and the introduction of cardiac surgery increased the stakes of cardiac auscultation, stimulating clinicians to be as precise and accurate as possible. Finally, in the 1970s and 1980s, the introduction of echocardiography solved many of the remaining mysteries about murmurs, including the cause of ejection sounds in aortic stenosis and late systolic murmurs and clicks in mitral valve prolapse.

This chapter covers the principles of describing and diagnosing murmurs. Specific cardiac disorders and their associated murmurs are further discussed in Chapters 39 to 41.

II. **THE FINDINGS.** The important characteristics of heart murmurs are timing, intensity, frequency (or

491

"pitch," which is high, low, or a mixture of high and low frequencies), and location (both where the murmur is loudest and in which direction its sound travels, or "radiates").[5] The terms "rough," "rumbling," "blowing," "coarse," and "musical" are also sometimes used to describe the specific tonal quality of murmurs.

A. Timing. Murmurs are broadly classified as systolic, diastolic, and continuous (Table 38-1).[5] Systolic murmurs occur at any time from S_1 to S_2; diastolic murmurs occur at any time from S_2 to the next S_1. Continuous murmurs begin in systole but extend beyond S_2 into diastole, indicating they do not respect the confines of systole and diastole and thus do not arise within the four heart chambers. Despite their name, continuous murmurs do not necessarily occupy all of systole and diastole.

1. Systolic murmurs

   a. Etiology. There are two causes of systolic murmurs.

      (1) Abnormal flow over an outflow tract or semilunar valve (i.e., aortic or pulmonary valve). Such abnormal flow may occur for three reasons: (1) flow is obstructed (e.g., aortic stenosis, pulmonic stenosis, hypertrophic cardiomyopathy); (2) flow is normal, but the valve is abnormal without obstruction (e.g., aortic sclerosis); (3) flow is increased over a normal valve (e.g., atrial septal defect, flow murmurs of anemia, fever, pregnancy, and thyrotoxicosis).

      (2) Regurgitation from a ventricle into a low pressure chamber. Examples are mitral regurgitation (leak between left ventricle and left atrium), tricuspid regurgitation (leak between right ventricle and right atrium), and ventricular septal defect

TABLE 38-1 Classification of murmurs by timing and location

TIMING	ETIOLOGY	LOCATION WHERE LOUDEST
Systolic Murmurs		
Early systolic	Mitral regurgitation, acute	Apex or L base
	Tricuspid regurgitation, low pressure	LLSB
	Ventricular septal defect, small	LLSB
Midsystolic	Pulmonic stenosis	L base
	Atrial septal defect	L base
	Hypertrophic cardiomyopathy	LLSB
	Aortic stenosis	R base, LLSB, or apex
	Papillary muscle dysfunction*	Apex
Late systolic	Mitral valve prolapse	Apex
	Papillary muscle dysfunction*	Apex

apex, Point of apical impulse; *L base*, second left intercostal space next to sternum; *LLSB*, fourth and fifth left intercostal space next to sternum; *R base*, second right intercostal space next to sternum.

*Papillary muscle dysfunction is a form of mitral regurgitation that occurs in ischemic heart disease.

Continued

TABLE 38-1 Classification of murmurs by timing and location—cont'd

TIMING	ETIOLOGY	LOCATION WHERE LOUDEST
Systolic Murmurs—cont'd		
Holosystolic	Mitral regurgitation	Apex
	Ventricular septal defect	LLSB
	Tricuspid regurgitation, high pressure	LLSB, apex
	Aortic stenosis	R base, LLSB, or apex
Diastolic Murmurs		
Early diastolic	Aortic regurgitation	LLSB
	Pulmonary regurgitation, high pressure	L base
Middiastolic	Pulmonary regurgitation, low pressure	LLSB
Middiastolic, presystolic, or both	Mitral stenosis	Apex
	Tricuspid stenosis	LLSB
Continuous Murmurs		
	Patent ductus arteriosus	L base
	Arteriovenous fistula	Over fistula
	Venous hum	Above head of clavicle
	Mammary souffle†	Between breast and sternum
	Coarctation of the aorta	Over back

apex, Point of apical impulse; *L base,* second left intercostal space next to sternum; *LLSB,* fourth and fifth left intercostal space next to sternum; *R base,* second right intercostal space next to sternum.

†"Souffle" (Fr. sound or murmur) is pronounced "SOO-ful."

(leak between left and right ventricles).

b. Classification. In 1958, Leatham divided all systolic murmurs into "ejection murmurs" and "regurgitant murmurs," based entirely on their relationship to S_2.[3,4] According to his classification, ejection murmurs began after S_1, had a crescendo-decrescendo shape, and always ended before S_2.[a] Ejection murmurs represented abnormal flow across the aortic or pulmonic valve. In contrast, regurgitant murmurs (e.g., mitral and tricuspid regurgitation) began with S_1, had a plateau shape, and extended up to or even slightly past S_2, thus obliterating it.

Leatham's classification is no longer widely used, for the following reasons: (1) It relies entirely on phonocardiography and does not always correspond to what clinicians hear at the bedside.[6] (2) It depends entirely on the audibility of the aortic and pulmonary components of S_2, which are not always audible. (3) It assumes all "ejection" murmurs result from ejection over a semilunar valve, although experience has shown many are due to regurgitant lesions. (4) Its fundamental premise, that a murmur's intensity depends on pressure gradients, is not always true (e.g., the murmur of mitral valve prolapse is loudest during late systole, when gradients are decreasing).

Instead, systolic murmurs are now usually classified simply as "early sys-

---

[a] More precisely, ejection murmurs end before the S_2 component belonging to the same side of the heart generating the murmur. For example, the murmur of aortic stenosis ends before A_2; the murmur of pulmonic stenosis ends before P_2.

tolic," "midsystolic," "late systolic," or "holosystolic," based only on whether the murmurs obscure S_1, S_2, or both sounds.[1] Midsystolic murmurs obscure neither heart tone; holosystolic murmurs obscure both heart tones; early systolic murmurs obscure S_1 but preserve S_2; and late systolic murmurs obscure S_2 but preserve S_1.

2. Diastolic murmurs

a. Etiology.
There are two causes of diastolic murmurs: (1) abnormal backward flow across a leaking semilunar valve (e.g., aortic or pulmonic regurgitation) or (2) abnormal forward flow across an atrioventricular valve (e.g., mitral stenosis, tricuspid stenosis, and flow rumbles[b]).

b. Classification.
Diastolic murmurs are further classified as "early diastolic," "middiastolic," or "late diastolic" murmurs (the term "presystolic" murmur is synonymous with "late diastolic" murmur).

3. Continuous murmurs.
Continuous murmurs result from (1) abnormal connections between the aorta and pulmonary trunk (e.g., patent ductus arteriosus), (2) abnormal connections between arteries and veins (e.g., arteriovenous fistulas), (3) abnormal flow in veins (e.g., venous hum and mammary souffle), or (4) abnormal flow in arteries

---

[b] Flow rumbles are short low-frequency diastolic murmurs that result from increased flow over a nonobstructed atrioventricular valve. Atrial septal defects and tricuspid regurgitation may increase diastolic flow over the tricuspid valve, thus producing tricuspid flow rumbles (which resemble the murmur of tricuspid stenosis). Mitral regurgitation and ventricular septal defect may increase diastolic flow over the mitral valve, producing a mitral flow rumble (which resembles the murmur of mitral stenosis).

(e.g., coarctation of the aorta, renal artery stenosis).

B. Grading the intensity of murmurs. The intensity of murmurs is graded on a 1 to 6 scale, based on the work of Freeman and Levine, which was later modified by Constant and Lippschutz (their work is now collectively referred to as "Levine's grading system").[7-9] Although this system was devised for systolic murmurs, it now applies to all murmurs.

The six categories are as follows: **(1) Grade 1** murmurs are so faint they can be heard only with special effort. **(2) Grade 2** murmurs can be recognized readily after placing the stethoscope on the chest wall. **(3) Grade 3** murmurs are very loud. Murmurs of Grades 1 through 3 all lack thrills, which are palpable vibrations on the body wall resembling the purr of a cat. Grade 4 through 6 murmurs all have associated thrills. **(4) Grade 4** murmurs are very loud, although the stethoscope must be in complete contact with the skin to hear them. **(5) Grade 5** murmurs are very loud and still audible if only the edge of the stethoscope is in contact with the skin; they are not audible after complete removal of the stethoscope from the chest wall. **(6) Grade 6** murmurs are exceptionally loud and audible even when the stethoscope is just removed from the chest wall.

C. Timing and quality of murmurs: using onomatopoeia. Figure 38-1 presents traditional diagrams of various heart murmurs, which in turn are based on phonocardiographic tracings. Because murmurs are sounds, however, diagrams such as these often fail to convey the precise cadence and tonal qualities that distinguish murmurs. Throughout the history of cardiac auscultation, clinicians have used onomatopoeia to mimic heart sounds and murmurs, finding this to be an effective teaching

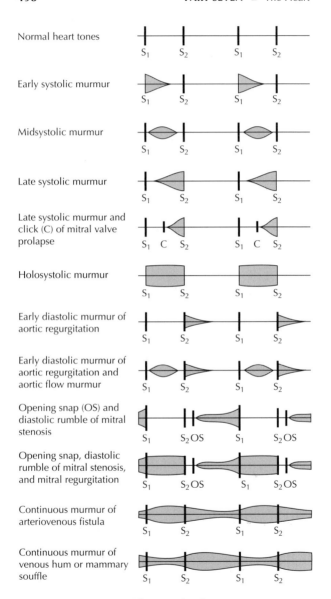

FIGURE 38-1 Diagrams of various murmurs.

tool allowing clinicians to rapidly recognize the patterns of different sounds.[2,10,11]

The system described here is based on the published work of Feinstein[12] and Adolph.[13-16] High-frequency murmurs are mimicked by sounds from the front of the mouth; low-frequency murmurs are mimicked by sounds from the back of the throat. The high-frequency murmur of mitral and tricuspid regurgitation is mimicked by saying "SHSHSHSH." The high-frequency murmur of aortic regurgitation is mimicked by blowing air out through slightly pursed lips, or whispering "PHEWEWEWEWEW" or "AHAHAHAHAH" (hence the "blowing" descriptor). The low-frequency murmurs of tricuspid or mitral stenosis are mimicked by the "RRRRR" portion of a growl (hence the "rumbling" descriptor). Murmurs containing a mixture of low and high frequencies, such as aortic stenosis, are mimicked by the sound made when clearing the throat (common descriptors are "coarse" or "harsh").

The clinician should first establish the normal cadence of S_1 and S_2 (*lub* is S_1 and *dup* is S_2):

lub dup   *lub dup*   *lub dup*

and then add the appropriate sound for the murmur at the appropriate time. For example, the high frequency late systolic murmur of mitral valve prolapse preserves S_1 but obscures S_2 (i.e., "dup is replaced by SHSHP):

lub SHSHP   *lub SHSHP*   *lub SHSHP*

Figure 38-2 describes how to mimic many other common murmurs using onomatopoeia.

By using onomatopoeia, clinicians can quickly learn the cadence of murmurs, which sometimes leads to rapid recognition of complicated sounds without first having to sort out the location of S_1 and S_2. For example, if ausculta-

Normal heart tones	**Lub**	**Dup**	**Lub**	**Dup**
	S_1	S_2	S_1	S_2

Normal heart tones **Lub** **Dup** **Lub** **Dup**
S_1 S_2 S_1 S_2

Early systolic murmur **L**SHSHSH **Dup** **L**SHSHSH **Dup**
S_1 S_2 S_1 S_2

Midsystolic murmur **Lub** SHSH **Dup** **Lub** SHSH **Dup**
S_1 S_2 S_1 S_2

Late systolic murmur **Lub** SHSH**P** **Lub** SHSH**P**
S_1 S_2 S_1 S_2

Late systolic murmur **Lub K**SHSH**P** **Lub K**SHSH**P**
and click (C) of mitral
valve prolapse S_1 C S_2 S_1 C S_2

Holosystolic murmur SHSHSHSHSH SHSHSHSHSH
S_1 S_2 S_1 S_2

Early diastolic murmur **Lub** **P**EWWwww **Lub** **P**EWWwww
of aortic regurgitation S_1 S_2 S_1 S_2

Early diastolic murmur **Lub** SHSH **P**EWWwww **Lub** SHSH **P**EWWwww
of aortic regurgitation
and aortic flow murmur S_1 S_2 S_1 S_2

Opening snap (OS) R**UP** bu **DUP**RRRRR**UP** bu **DUP**RRRRR**UP**
and diastolic rumble
of mitral stenosis S_1 S_2 OS S_1 S_2 OS

Opening snap, R**UP**SHSHSHS**P** **DUP**RRRRR**UP**SHSHSHS**P** **DUP**RRRRR**UP**
diastolic rumble of
mitral stenosis, and
mitral regurgitation S_1 S_2 OS S_1 S_2 OS

Continuous murmur of **Pu**SHSHSH**Pu**SHSHSHSHSH **Pu**SHSHSH**Pu**SHSHSHSHSH
arteriovenous fistula S_1 S_2 S_1 S_2

Continuous murmur of **Pu**SHSHSHS**Pu**SHSH**H**SHSH **Pu**SHSHSHS**Pu**SHSH**H**SHSH
venous hum or
mammary souffle S_1 S_2 S_1 S_2

FIGURE 38-2 Murmurs and onomatopoeia.

tion reveals a cadence consisting of a single murmur and no heart sounds

SHSHSHSH   SHSHSHSH   SHSHSHSH

the only possible diagnosis is a holosystolic murmur.

If instead auscultation reveals murmurs in systole and diastole, there are three possible causes: (1) a true continuous murmur, (2) a to-fro murmur, or (3) combined mitral stenosis and regurgitation. In true continuous murmurs, the cadence is uninterrupted by the cardiac cycles ("*SHSHSHSHSHSHSHSHSH*"). To-fro murmurs consist of two high frequency murmurs, one in systole and another in diastole ("*SHSHSHSHP PHEWEWEWEWEW*"). To-fro murmurs result from isolated severe aortic regurgitation (the diastolic component representing aortic regurgitation and the systolic one representing increased systolic flow over the aortic valve) or aortic regurgitation combined with another systolic murmur, such as aortic stenosis, mitral regurgitation, or ventricular septal defect. In combined mitral stenosis and regurgitation, a high frequency murmur is combined with a low frequency one ("PUSHSHSHSHP DUPRRRR RRRRUP").

III. CLINICAL SIGNIFICANCE

A. Detecting valvular heart disease.
Table 38-2 presents the diagnostic accuracy of murmurs. In this table, the "finding" refers to the characteristic murmur of that lesion (as described in Table 38-1 and Chapters 39 to 41). For example, the diagnostic accuracy of diastolic murmurs for aortic regurgitation refers not to just any diastolic murmur but instead to the finding of an early diastolic high frequency murmur along the lower sternal border. In these studies, trivial regurgitation (a common finding at echocardi-

TABLE 38-2 Murmurs and valvular heart disease*

Finding (ref)†	Sensitivity (%)	Specificity (%)	Positive LR	Negative LR
Abnormal Heart Examination				
Detecting any valvular heart disease[17]	70	98	38.3	0.3
Characteristic Systolic Murmur				
Detecting aortic stenosis[18]	96	71	3.3	0.1
Detecting mild mitral regurgitation or worse[19,20]	56-75	89-93	5.4	0.4
Detecting moderate-to-severe mitral regurgitation[19,20]	84-93	65-76	3.3	0.2
Detecting mild tricuspid regurgitation or worse[20]	23	98	14.6	0.8
Detecting moderate-to-severe tricuspid regurgitation[20]	62	94	10.1	0.4
Characteristic Diastolic Murmur				
Detecting mild aortic regurgitation or worse[20-27]	54-87	75-98	9.9	0.3
Detecting moderate-to-severe aortic regurgitation[20,25-27]	88-98	52-88	4.3	0.1
Detecting pulmonary regurgitation[20]	15	99	17.4	NS

NS, Not significant.

*Diagnostic standards: For all valvular lesions, Doppler echocardiography,[20,25,28] angiography,[19,21-23,26,27,29] or surgery.[18,24] Trivial regurgitation seen during echocardiography is classified as "absent regurgitation" (i.e., no disease).

†Definition of finding: For abnormal heart examination, see text; for all other murmurs, finding refers only to those murmurs characteristic in quality, location, and timing for that diagnosis. For example, the positive LR of 9.9 for aortic regurgitation refers to an early diastolic high-frequency blowing decrescendo murmur at the lower left sternal border, not any diastolic murmur.

ography of no clinical significance) was classified as "no regurgitation" (i.e., "no disease").

For three of the lesions in Table 38-2, the finding of the characteristic murmur is a conclusive argument that that lesion is present: tricuspid regurgitation (LR = 14.6; Table 38-2), aortic regurgitation (LR = 9.9), and pulmonary regurgitation (LR = 17.4). For two murmurs, aortic stenosis and mitral regurgitation, the positive LRs are less compelling (LR = 3.3 for aortic stenosis and LR = 5.4 for mitral regurgitation), primarily because these murmurs are often confused with each other and with other causes of systolic murmurs (see Section B below).

The *absence* of the characteristic murmur is a compelling argument *against* significant left-sided valvular lesions: aortic stenosis (negative LR = 0.1), moderate-to-severe mitral regurgitation (negative LR = 0.2), and moderate-to-severe aortic regurgitation (negative LR = 0.1). On the right side of the heart, however, the *absence* of the characteristic murmur does not exclude valvular disease (negative LR for moderate-to-severe tricuspid regurgitation is 0.4; the negative LR for pulmonary regurgitation is not significant), probably because right-sided pressures, which are lower than those on the left side, generate less turbulence and softer sounds. Many patients with *mild* mitral regurgitation or *mild* aortic regurgitation also lack murmurs.

B. Differential diagnosis of systolic murmurs. Systolic murmurs are common bedside findings, occurring in 5% to 52% of young adults and 29% to 60% of older persons.[35] Over 90% of younger adults and over half of older adults with systolic murmurs have a normal echocardiogram, which means the murmur is "innocent" or "functional."[35]

Therefore, in patients with systolic murmurs, the clinician should first address whether the murmur is functional or organic. If the murmur is organic, the clinician should then address which lesion is responsible. Once the cause of the organic murmur is determined, the clinician should then assess the severity of the lesion, a subject discussed further in Chapters 39 and 41.

1. **The functional murmur.** Functional murmurs are short, early, or midsystolic murmurs of grade 2/6 or less. They are well localized to the area of the left sternal border, and they diminish in intensity when the patient stands, sits up, or strains during the Valsalva maneuver. Patients with functional murmurs have normal neck veins, apical impulse, arterial pulse, and heart tones.

   In Table 38-2, "abnormal heart examination" refers to any murmur not meeting the definition of a functional murmur (i.e., the murmur is too long or loud, is heard away from the sternal border, intensifies during the Valsalva strain, or is associated with other abnormal cardiac findings). This definition of the abnormal murmur argues conclusively for valvular heart disease when the abnormal murmur is present (LR = 38.3). Murmurs meeting the criteria for functional murmurs argue *against* subsequently finding significant abnormalities on echocardiography (LR = 0.3).

2. **Identifying the cause of systolic murmurs.** The following comments apply only to patients with an abnormal systolic murmur (i.e., not meeting definition of functional murmur).

   a. **Timing and location.** Despite classic teachings, the timing and location of a systolic murmur often do not distinguish aortic stenosis from mitral regurgitation. For example, mitral regurgitation may be early systolic (acute mitral regurgitation), midsystolic (papillary muscle dysfunction), late systolic (mitral valve prolapse or papillary muscle dysfunction), or holosystolic (chronic valvular mitral regurgitation). Aortic stenosis may be midsystolic or, when S_2 is absent, holosystolic. Mitral regurgitation is classically heard at the apex, but it also may be loudest at the right base (aortic area), especially when the posterior leaflet is abnormal.[36,37] Aortic stenosis is usually loudest over the sternum and right base, but in many older patients with calcific aortic stenosis, the murmur is loudest at the apex, the traditional area for mitral regurgitation.[38,39]

Therefore, to distinguish these two systolic murmurs from each other and other murmurs, the clinician must rely on other characteristics. Of these, the most helpful are the murmur's response to irregular rhythms and maneuvers, its tonal quality, and its relationship to S_2.

b. **Changing cycle length.** One important clue to the etiology of a systolic murmur is how it changes in intensity with changing cycle lengths, as occur in the irregular pulse of atrial fibrillation or frequent premature beats. Mitral regurgitation remains the same loudness whether the beats are quick or delayed.[40] The intensity of aortic stenosis, in contrast, depends on cycle length: the longer the previous diastole (e.g., beat after a premature beat or after a pause in atrial fibrillation), the louder the murmur.[40,41]

Explaining why these two murmurs behave differently first requires an understanding of the physiology of the pause. The pause causes diastolic filling and contractility to be greater for the next beat than it would have been if the cycle had been quicker (contractility is increased because of Starling forces and, in the case of extrasystoles, postextrasystolic accentuation of contractility). The pause also reduces afterload for the next beat, because the aortic pressures have had more time to fall before the next ventricular systole. In aortic stenosis, all three of these changes—increased filling, increased contractility, and decreased afterload—promote greater flow across the stenotic valve after pauses than after quick beats, causing the murmur to become louder.[30] In mitral regurgitation, however, the stroke volume is divided between two paths: (1) blood flowing out the aorta or (2) into the left atrium. The reduced afterload promotes the extra filling from the pause to exit into the aorta, leaving the regurgitant volume the same as with quicker beats and making the intensity of the murmur independent of cycle length.

Another systolic murmur, that of hypertrophic cardiomyopathy, responds unpredictably to changing cycle lengths: the long pause may make the murmur louder, softer, and not change it at all.[41]

c. **Musical systolic murmurs.** Almost all musical systolic murmurs are due to mitral regurgitation (mitral valve prolapse or endocarditis) or tricuspid regurgitation (congestive heart failure).[42-45] Although they are called "musical," the sound resembles more a "honk" or "whoop." The pure musical tones emanate from vibrations of the chordae tendinae, vegetations, or portions of the atrioventricular leaflets themselves, all generated during ventricular contraction.

d. **Relationship to S$_2$.** Systolic murmurs from flow over semilunar valves must end before S_2, because S_2 marks cessation of forward flow. In contrast, regurgitant murmurs can extend past S_2, because the pressure gradient between the ventricle and the low pressure chamber may persist after S_2 (e.g., mitral regurgitation may persist until the early diastolic mitral opening).

This relationship to S_2, part of Leatham's original classification of systolic murmurs (see Section II-A-1-b above), is still useful during auscultation, as long as the clinician is certain S_2 is audible somewhere on the chest. For example, in a patient with a long holosystolic murmur at the apex (*"SHSHSH......SHSHSH.......SHSHSH"*), the clinician should return to the left second intercostal space to search for S_2. If S_2 is present (*"SHSHSH dup...SHSHSH dup"*), the clinician can conclude that the murmur at the apex is obliterating S_2 and thus represents regurgitation.[15,39] On the other hand, if the clinician still cannot hear S_2 at the left second intercostal space, the finding is unhelpful: S_2 could be inaudible either because the murmur is regurgitant or because S_2 has disappeared for some other reason (i.e., the aortic valve is inflexible from calcific aortic stenosis and does not make a sound).

e. **Maneuvers.** Several maneuvers help differentiate systolic murmurs (Table 38-3). They are classified into respiratory maneuvers, maneuvers that change venous return (e.g., Valsalva maneuver, squatting to standing, standing to squatting, passive leg elevation), and maneuvers that primarily change systemic vascular resistance (isometric hand grip, transient arterial occlusion, and inhalation of amyl nitrite).

TABLE 38-3 Maneuvers and heart murmurs

MANEUVER*	TECHNIQUE	WHEN TO NOTE CHANGE IN MURMUR
Normal respiration	The patient breathes normally in and out	During inspiration and expiration
Maneuvers Affecting Venous Return		
Valsalva maneuver (↓ venous return)	The patient exhales against closed glottis for 20 seconds	At end of the strain phase (i.e., at 20 seconds)
Squatting to standing (↓ venous return)	The patient squats for at least 30 seconds and then rapidly stands up	Immediately after standing
Standing to squatting (↑ venous return)	The patient squats rapidly from the standing position, while breathing normally to avoid a Valsalva maneuver	Immediately after squatting
Passive leg elevation (↑ venous return)	The patient's legs are passively elevated to 45 degrees while the patient is supine	15 to 20 seconds after leg elevation

Maneuvers Affecting Systemic Vascular Resistance

Isometric handgrip exercise (↑ afterload)	The patient uses one hand to squeeze the examiner's index and middle fingers together tightly†	After one minute of maximal contraction
Transient arterial occlusion (↑ afterload)	The examiner places blood pressure cuffs around both upper arms of patient and inflates them to pressures above the patient's systolic blood pressure	20 seconds after cuff inflation
Amyl nitrite (↓ afterload)	The patient takes 3 rapid, deep breaths from a broken amyl nitrite capsule	15 to 30 seconds after inhalation

From information cited in references 30 to 34.

*Arrows indicated how maneuver affects venous return or systemic vascular resistance. The squatting-to-standing maneuver also decreases systemic vascular resistance, and amyl nitrite also diminishes pulmonary vascular resistance a small amount

†In clinical studies, a hand dynamometer was used to confirm that at least 75% of maximal hand grip strength was sustained for 1 minute.[33]

(1) ***Respiration.*** Inspiration increases venous return to the right side of the heart and decreases it to the left side of the heart.[c] Therefore murmurs that intensify during inspiration characteristically originate in the right side of the heart (e.g., tricuspid regurgitation or pulmonic stenosis; LR = 7.8; Table 38-4). Murmurs that become *softer* during inspiration are most likely *not* right-sided murmurs (LR = 0.2; see Table 38-4).

Before interpreting the test, the clinician should be certain the patient is breathing evenly in and out, because breath holding during inhalation or exhalation makes interpretation impossible. To help direct the patient's breathing, the clinician can move his arm slowly up and down and ask the patient to breathe in when the arm is going up and out when it is going down.

Inspiratory intensification of the murmur of tricuspid regurgitation was originally described by Rivero-Carvallo in 1946 (the sign is sometimes called "Carvallo's sign").[50]

(2) ***Maneuvers changing venous return.*** Venous return to the heart *decreases* during the straining phase of the Valsalva maneuver and the squatting-to-standing maneuver. Venous return *increases* during passive

---

[c] This occurs because pressures in the right side of the heart diminish with intrathoracic pressures during inspiration, increasing the pressure gradient between the right side of the heart and systemic veins and causing filling to increase to the right side of the heart. In contrast, inspiration increases the capacitance of pulmonary veins, thus reducing flow to the left side of the heart during inspiration.

TABLE 38-4 Systolic murmurs and maneuvers*

FINDING (REF)†	SENSITIVITY (%)	SPECIFICITY (%)	POSITIVE LR	NEGATIVE LR
Respiration				
Louder During Inspiration				
Detecting right-sided murmurs (tricuspid regurgitation or pulmonic stenosis)[32,46]	78-95	87-97	7.8	0.2
Changing Venous Return				
Louder with Valsalva Strain				
Detecting hypertrophic cardiomyopathy[32]	70	95	14.0	0.3
Louder with Squatting-to-Standing				
Detecting hypertrophic cardiomyopathy[32]	95	84	6.0	0.1
Softer with Standing-to-Squatting				
Detecting hypertrophic cardiomyopathy[32,47]	88-95	84-97	7.6	0.1
Softer with Passive Leg Elevation				
Detecting hypertrophic cardiomyopathy[32]	90	90	9.0	0.1

*Diagnostic standards: Doppler echocardiography or angiography.

†Definition of finding: See text.

Continued

TABLE 38-4 Systolic murmurs and maneuvers*—cont'd

Finding (ref)†	Sensitivity (%)	Specificity (%)	Positive LR	Negative LR
Changing Systemic Vascular Resistance (Afterload)				
Softer with Isometric Hand Grip				
Detecting hypertrophic cardiomyopathy[32]	90	75	3.6	0.1
Louder with Isometric Hand Grip				
Detecting mitral regurgitation or ventricular septal defect[32,33]	70-76	78-93	5.8	0.3
Louder with Transient Arterial Occlusion				
Detecting mitral regurgitation or ventricular septal defect[32]	79	98	48.7	0.2
Softer with Amyl Nitrite Inhalation				
Detecting mitral regurgitation or ventricular septal defect[32,33,48,49]	41-95	89-95	10.5	0.2

**Diagnostic standards:* Doppler echocardiography or angiography.

†*Definition of finding:* See text; for amyl nitrite inhalation, the test was interpretable only if it induced tachycardia.

leg elevation and the standing-to-squatting maneuver (see Table 38-3 for definitions).

These maneuvers are most useful in identifying hypertrophic cardiomyopathy, which, unlike most systolic murmurs, intensifies with decreased venous return and becomes softer with increased venous return. This paradoxical response occurs because the murmur is caused by obstruction in the outflow tract, below the aortic valve and between the anterior leaflet of the mitral valve and the hypertrophied interventricular septum. Decreased venous return brings the mitral leaflet and septum closer together and aggravates the obstruction; increased return moves them apart and relieves the obstruction.

All four venous return maneuvers are useful in diagnosing hypertrophic cardiomyopathy (LR = 6.0 to 14.0; Table 38-4), although the most compelling argument is a systolic murmur that intensifies during the Valsalva strain (positive LR = 14.0; see Table 38-4). For three of the maneuvers (squatting-to-standing, standing-to-squatting, passive leg elevation), the *absence* of the response characteristic of hypertrophic cardiomyopathy is a compelling argument *against* the diagnosis (LR = 0.1; see Table 38-4). Of these four maneuvers, only passive leg elevation can be easily performed in patients who are frail.

One other systolic murmur, mitral valve prolapse, may intensify during squatting-to-standing, although it does *not* become louder during Valsalva strain. This paradoxical finding is discussed further in Chapter 41, but is presented now to explain why the specificity for Valsalva strain (95%) is slightly higher than that for squatting-to-standing (84%).

(3) Maneuvers changing systemic vascular resistance (or "afterload"). Before employing maneuvers that change afterload in diagnosing systolic murmurs, the clinician has already addressed the possibility of right-sided murmurs (respiratory maneuver) and hypertrophic cardiomyopathy (venous return maneuvers). The primary remaining diagnostic possibilities are murmurs generated by flow over the aortic valve (e.g., aortic stenosis, aortic sclerosis) and murmurs from left-sided regurgitant lesions (e.g., mitral regurgitation, ventricular septal defect).

Changing afterload is most useful in distinguishing these last two groups of lesions. The murmurs of mitral regurgitation and ventricular septal defect intensify with increased afterload because blood leaving the ventricle, having two paths to potentially follow, encounters more resistance in the aorta and therefore flows more readily through the regurgitant lesion. Similarly, these murmurs become softer when afterload is decreased, because enhanced aortic flow reduces the regurgitant volume.

The common techniques of manipulating afterload at the bedside are isometric hand grip and transient arterial occlusion (Table 38-3), both of which increase afterload. The finding of a systolic murmur that intensifies with either maneuver is a strong argument the murmur represents mitral regurgitation or ventricular septal defect (LR = 5.8 and 48.7; see Table 38-4). Another maneuver that reduces afterload, amyl nitrite inhalation, was used commonly 30 to 40 years ago but is rarely used today.

REFERENCES

1. Perloff JK. The physiologic mechanisms of cardiac and vascular physical signs, *J Am Coll Cardiol* 1:184-198, 1983.
2. Flint A. On cardiac murmurs, *Am J Med Sci* 44:29-54, 1862.
3. Leatham A. *Auscultation of the heart and phonocardiography,* ed 2, Edinburgh, 1975, Churchill Livingstone.
4. Leatham AM. Systolic murmurs, *Circulation* 17:601-611, 1958.
5. Soffer A and others. Glossary of cardiologic terms related to physical diagnosis and history, *Am J Cardiol* 20:285-286, 1967.
6. Tavel ME. Classification of systolic murmurs: still in search of a consensus, *Am Heart J* 134:330-336, 1997.
7. Freeman AR and Levine SA. The clinical significance of the systolic murmur: a study of 1000 consecutive "noncardiac" cases, *Ann Intern Med* 6:1371-1385, 1933.
8. Levine SA. Notes on the gradation of the intensity of cardiac murmurs, *JAMA* 177:261, 1961.
9. Constant J and Lippschutz EJ. Diagramming and grading heart sounds and murmurs, *Am Heart J* 70:326-332, 1965.
10. Willius FA and Dry TJ. *A history of the heart and the circulation,* Philadelphia, 1948, WB Saunders Co.
11. Vaslef SN. Early descriptions of aortic valve stenosis, *Am Heart J* 125:1465-1474, 1993.
12. Feinstein AR. Acoustic distinctions in cardiac auscultation: with emphasis on cardiophonetics, synecphonesis, the analysis of cadence, and problems of hydraulic distortion, *Arch Intern Med* 121:209-224, 1968.
13. Adolph RJ. The value of bedside examination in an era of high technology—Part 1, *Heart Dis Stroke* 3:128-131, 1994.

14. Adolph RJ. The value of bedside examination in an era of high technology—Part 2, *Heart Dis Stroke* 3:188-190, 1994.

15. Adolph RJ. The value of bedside examination in an era of high technology—Part 3, *Heart Dis Stroke* 3:236-239, 1994.

16. Adolph RJ. The value of bedside examination in an era of high technology—Part 4, *Heart Dis Stroke* 3:312-315, 1994.

17. Roldan CA, Shively BK, and Crawford MH. Value of the cardiovascular physical examination for detecting valvular heart disease in asymptomatic subjects, *Am J Cardiol* 77: 1327-1331, 1996.

18. Aronow WS, Schwartz KS, and Koenigsberg M. Correlation of aortic cuspal and aortic root disease with aortic systolic ejection murmurs and with mitral anular calcium in persons older than 62 years in a long-term health care facility, *Am J Cardiol* 58:651-652, 1986.

19. Meyers DG and others. Duplex pulsed Doppler echocardiography in mitral regurgitation, *J Clin Ultrasound* 14:117-121, 1986.

20. Rahko PS. Prevalence of regurgitant murmurs in patients with valvular regurgitation detected by Doppler echocardiography, *Ann Intern Med* 111:466-472, 1989.

21. Linhart JW. Aortic regurgitation: clinical, hemodynamic, surgical, and angiographic correlations, *Ann Thor Surg* 11:27-37, 1971.

22. Meyers DG and others. Diagnosis of aortic insufficiency: comparison of auscultation and M-mode echocardiography to angiography, *South Med J* 75:1192-1194, 1982.

23. Meyers DG, Olson TS, and Hansen DA. Auscultation, M-mode, echocardiography and pulsed Doppler echocardiography compared with angiography for diagnosis of chronic aortic regurgitation, *Am J Cardiol* 56:811-812, 1985.

24. Cohn LH and others. Preoperative assessment of aortic regurgitation in patients with mitral valve disease, *Am J Cardiol* 19:177-182, 1967.

25. Aronow WS and Kronzon I. Correlation of prevalence and severity of aortic regurgitation detected by pulsed Doppler echocardiography with the murmur of aortic regurgitation in elderly patients in a long-term health care facility, *Am J Cardiol* 63:128-129, 1989.

26. Dittmann H, Karsch KR, and Seipel L. Diagnosis and quantification of aortic regurgitation by pulsed Doppler echocardiography in patients with mitral valve disease, *Eur Heart J* 8(suppl C):53-57, 1987.

27. Grayburn PA and others. Detection of aortic insufficiency by standard echocardiography, pulsed Doppler echocardiography, and auscultation: a comparison of accuracies, *Ann Intern Med* 104:599-605, 1986.

28. Desjardins VA and others. Intensity of murmurs correlates with severity of valvular regurgitation, *Am J Med* 100:149-156, 1996.

29. Frank MJ and others. The clinical evaluation of aortic regurgitation, *Arch Intern Med* 116:357-365, 1965.

30. Karliner JS and others. Haemodynamic explanation of why the murmur of mitral regurgitation is independent of cycle length, *Br Heart J* 35:397-401, 1973.

31. Lembo NJ and others. Diagnosis of left-sided regurgitant murmurs by transient arterial occlusion: a new maneuver using blood pressure cuffs, *Ann Intern Med* 105:368-370, 1986.

32. Lembo NJ and others. Bedside diagnosis of systolic murmurs, *N Engl J Med* 318:1572-1578, 1988.

33. McCraw DB and others. Response of heart murmur intensity to isometric (handgrip) exercise, *Br Heart J* 34:605-610, 1972.

34. Rothman A and Goldberger AL. Aids to cardiac auscultation, *Ann Intern Med* 99:346-353, 1983.

35. Etchells E, Bell C, and Robb K. Does this patient have an abnormal systolic murmur? *JAMA* 277:564-571, 1997.

36. Antman EM, Angoff GH, and Sloss LJ. Demonstration of the mechanism by which mitral regurgitation mimics aortic stenosis, *Am J Cardiol* 42:1044-1048, 1978.

37. Perloff JK and Harvey WP. Auscultatory and phonocardiographic manifestations of pure mitral regurgitation, *Prog Cardiovasc Dis* 5:172-194, 1962.

38. Roberts WC, Perloff JK, Costantino T. Severe valvular aortic stenosis in patients over 65 years of age: a clinicopathologic study, *Am J Cardiol* 27:497-506, 1971.

39. Burch GE and Phillips JH. Murmurs of aortic stenosis and mitral insufficiency masquerading as one another, *Am Heart J* 66:439-442, 1963.

40. Henke RP, March HW, and Hultgren HN. An aid to identification of the murmur of aortic stenosis with atypical localization, *Am Heart J* 60:354-363, 1960.

41. Kramer DS, French WJ, and Criley JM. The postextrasystolic murmur response to gradient in hypertrophic cardiomyopathy, *Ann Intern Med* 104:772-776, 1986.

42. Sheikh MU and others. Musical murmurs: clinical implications, long-term prognosis, and echo-phonocardiographic features, *Am Heart J* 108:377-386, 1984.

43. Upshaw CB. Precordial honk due to tricuspid regurgitation, *Am J Cardiol* 35:85-88, 1975.

44. Rackley CE and others. The precordial honk, *Am J Cardiol* 17:509-515, 1966.

45. Keenan TJ and Schwartz MJ. Tricuspid whoop, *Am J Cardiol* 31:642-645, 1973.

46. Maisel AS and others. The murmur of papillary muscle dysfunction in acute myocardial infarction: clinical features and prognostic implications, *Am Heart J* 112:705-711, 1986.

47. Nellen M and others. Effects of prompt squatting on the systolic murmur in idiopathic hypertrophic obstructive cardiomyopathy, *Br Med J* 3:140-143, 1967.

48. Luisada AA and Madoery RJ. Functional tests as an aid to cardiac auscultation, *Med Clin North Am* 50:73-89, 1966.

49. Barlow J and Shillingford J. The use of amyl nitrite in differentiating mitral and aortic systolic murmurs, *Br Heart J* 20:162-166, 1958.

50. Vitums VC, Gooch AS, and Evans JM. Bedside maneuvers to augment the murmur of tricuspid regurgitation, *Med Ann DC* 38:533-542, 1969.

PART EIGHT

Selected Cardiac Disorders

CHAPTER 39

Aortic Stenosis

I. **INTRODUCTION.** Aortic stenosis is any disorder of the aortic valve that obstructs the ejection of blood from the left ventricle into the aorta. Its characteristic findings are a systolic murmur, abnormal carotid pulse, and sustained apical impulse.

   The pathology of aortic stenosis was recognized in the 1600s, but it was James Hope who in 1832 first clearly described the characteristic murmur.[1,2]

II. **THE FINDINGS**

   A. **The murmur.** The murmur of aortic stenosis is midsystolic or holosystolic. It is loudest at the right second intercostal space, left sternal border, or apex, and it characteristically radiates into the neck, especially on the right side. In calcific aortic stenosis, the most common etiology of aortic stenosis today, the murmur at the upper sternal borders contains both high and low frequency vibrations, which gives it a harsh or rough sound, like that of clearing the throat. At the apex, in contrast, the murmur of calcific aortic stenosis often contains a narrow band of high frequency sound, thus making it sound like mitral regurgitation. This harmonic distortion of sound—the loss of low frequency components of the murmur when the stethoscope is moved upstream—is called the "Gallavardin phenomenon."[3]

B. **Associated cardiac signs.** Other traditional findings of severe aortic stenosis are (1) a carotid pulse that is abnormally small in volume and delayed ("pulsus parvus et tardus"); (2) a palpable apical impulse that is abnormally sustained (see Chapter 33 for definition of sustained impulse); and (3) reduced intensity of the second heart sound, which occurs because the inflexible aortic leaflets close with less force than normal. Another traditional finding is a prominent A wave in the neck veins (i.e., the "Bernheim phenomenon"), although this wave is more often seen on pressure tracings than at the bedside. Its mechanism is still disputed.[4]

III. CLINICAL SIGNIFICANCE

A. **Detecting aortic stenosis.** Although the *presence* of a characteristic aortic systolic murmur, anywhere from the base to apex, argues modestly *for* aortic stenosis (likelihood ratio [LR] = 3.3; see Table 38-2 in Chapter 38),[5] the *absence* of a systolic murmur argues strongly *against* the diagnosis (LR = 0.1). The presence of the characteristic murmur, by itself, is less compelling, simply because this murmur is often confused with systolic murmurs from other valvular lesions. Chapter 38 discusses the differential diagnosis of systolic murmurs, and how the clinician—by observing the second heart sound, quality of the murmur, and how the murmur responds to irregular heart beats and different maneuvers—can be more confident a systolic murmur indeed represents aortic stenosis or sclerosis.

B. **Severity of aortic stenosis.** Once the clinician is confident the murmur is an aortic flow murmur (i.e., aortic stenosis or aortic sclerosis), he must decide whether the patient has significant aortic stenosis. Significant aortic stenosis refers to those lesions with such severe obstruction that, if the patient has symptoms of angina, syncope, or dyspnea, valvular replacement is indicated (see footnotes to Table 39-1 for diagnostic standards used).

Many of the traditional teachings about aortic stenosis were first described at a time when congenital and rheumatic disease were more common than they are today. Since the primary cause of aortic stenosis today is calcific aortic stenosis, some of these teachings may not be as relevant as they were in the past. In comparison to congenital and rheumatic disease, calcific aortic stenosis affects older patients, who commonly have aortic flow murmurs *without* stenosis (i.e., aortic sclerosis) and who often have ischemic heart disease, a disorder complicating the bedside evaluation because patients then have two possible explanations (i.e., severe aortic stenosis or ischemic heart disease) for symptoms of angina or dyspnea.

The patients whose clinical signs are summarized in Table 39-1 (over 1000 patients in all) were all elderly (mean age 66 years) with aortic ejection murmurs (largely calcific aortic stenosis and sclerosis). Although some had mild aortic regurgitation, other significant valvular disease was excluded from most of these studies.

1. **Individual findings.** The following findings, in descending order of diagnostic accuracy (see Table 39-1), distinguish severe aortic stenosis from other causes of aortic flow murmurs (i.e., aortic sclerosis and mild-to-moderate aortic stenosis): absent A_2 (LR = 4.5), late peaking murmur (LR = 4.4), sustained apical impulse (LR = 4.1), prolonged murmur (LR = 3.9), delayed carotid artery upstroke ("pulsus tardus," LR = 3.7), apical-carotid delay (i.e., a palpable delay between the apical impulse and carotid impulse, LR = 2.6), brachioradial delay (i.e., palpable delay between the brachial and radial artery pulses, LR = 2.5), and reduced carotid artery volume (i.e., "pulsus parvus," LR = 2.3).

TABLE 39-1 Characteristics of severe aortic stenosis*

FINDING (REF)†	SENSITIVITY	SPECIFICITY	POSITIVE LR	NEGATIVE LR
Arterial Pulse				
Delayed carotid artery upstroke[6-9]	31-90	68-93	3.7	0.4
Reduced carotid artery volume[7,8]	74-80	65-67	2.3	0.3
Brachioradial delay[10]	97	62	2.5	0.04
Apical Impulse				
Sustained apical impulse[7]	78	81	4.1	0.3
Apical-carotid delay[11]	97	63	2.6	0.05

Heart Tones				
Absent A$_2$[6,12]	18-20	96-98	4.5	NS
Absent or diminished A$_2$[6,8,9,12]	44-90	76-98	3.6	0.4
S$_4$ gallop[9,13]	29-50	57-63	NS	NS
Murmur				
Late peaking[6,7,9]	83-90	72-88	4.4	0.2
Prolonged duration[6,9]	83-90	72-84	3.9	0.2
Loudest over aortic area[8,9]	58-75	41-73	1.8	0.6
Murmur transmits to neck[8,9]	90-98	22-36	1.4	0.1

NS, Not significant.

*Diagnostic standard: For severe aortic stenosis, aortic valve area <0.75 cm^2[10,12] <0.8 cm^2[8,11] <0.9 cm^2[7]; peak gradient >50 mm Hg[8,9], or peak velocity of aortic flow >3.6 m/sec.[6]

†Definition of findings: For late peaking murmur, murmur peaks at midsystole or beyond; for aortic area, second right intercostal space.

The findings that best argue *against* the diagnosis of severe aortic stenosis are (see Table 39-1): the absence of brachioradial delay (LR = 0.04), absence of an apical carotid delay (LR = 0.05), absence of transmission of the murmur to the neck (LR = 0.1), peaking of murmur in early systole (LR = 0.2), and short duration of the murmur (LR = 0.2). Brachioradial delay and apical-carotid delay were each investigated in only one study and therefore require confirmation by others.

Two additional bedside findings are the chest radiograph and electrocardiogram. On the chest radiograph, calcification of the aortic valve detects severe stenosis with a sensitivity of 31% to 81%, specificity of 63% to 96%, positive LR of 3.9 and negative LR of 0.5.[8,12,14,15] Left ventricular hypertrophy on the electrocardiogram detects severe stenosis with a sensitivity of 49% to 94%, specificity of 57% to 86%, positive LR of 2.1 and negative LR of 0.5.[6,8,11,12,14,15]

The following findings are not helpful in identifying patients with severe aortic stenosis: narrow pulse pressure,[16] fourth heart sound,[9,12] third heart sound,[12] reversed splitting of the second heart sound,[9] aortic ejection click,[9] and intensity of the murmur.[15]

2. **Why positive LRs are so low.** The highest positive LR for the findings listed in Table 39-1 is 4.5 (i.e., the absent A_2). In general, positive LRs are low when patients *without* disease also have the physical finding (i.e., specificity is low and there are many *false-positive* results). The cause of false-positive results in the studies of aortic stenosis is principally *moderate* aortic stenosis (defined as aortic valve area between 0.8 and 1.2 cm^2 or peak gradient 25 to 50 mm Hg).

Therefore, if "disease" is instead defined as "combined moderate-to-severe aortic stenosis," the positive likelihood ratios improve dramatically, especially for delayed carotid upstroke (positive LR = 13.1, negative LR = 0.5), A_2 reduced or absent (positive LR = 10.7, negative LR = 0.4), prolonged duration of murmur (positive LR = 29.5, negative LR = 0.3), and late peaking murmur (positive LR = 29.5, negative LR = 0.3).[6,9,17]

This means that the clinician examining patients with aortic flow murmurs can easily distinguish patients with moderate-to-severe aortic stenosis from those with mild aortic stenosis and aortic sclerosis, but has greater difficulty distinguishing severe stenosis from those with moderate stenosis.

3. **Combined findings.** One study has validated the use of combined findings in the diagnosis of aortic stenosis.[8] According to this diagnostic scheme, the clinician evaluates 5 bedside findings and assigns the following points: delayed carotid upstroke (3 points), diminished carotid volume (2 points), murmur loudest at right upper sternal border (2 points), single/absent second heart sound (3 points), and calcification of the aortic valve on chest radiography (4 points).

This diagnostic scheme distinguishes moderate-to-severe aortic stenosis from other causes of aortic flow murmurs. The probability of moderate-to-severe aortic stenosis is low with 0 to 6 points (LR = 0.2) and high with 10 to 14 points (LR = 10.6). Scores from 7 to 9 points are not helpful (LR not significant).

REFERENCES

1. Vaslef SN. Early descriptions of aortic valve stenosis, *Am Heart J* 125:1465-1474, 1993.

2. Willius FA and Dry TJ. *A history of the heart and the circulation,* Philadelphia, 1948, WB Saunders Co.

3. Roberts WC, Perloff JK, and Costantino T. Severe valvular aortic stenosis in patients over 65 years of age: a clinico-pathologic study, *Am J Cardiol* 27:497-506, 1971.

4. Henein MY and others. Bernheim "a" wave: obstructed right ventricular inflow or atrial cross talk? *Br Heart J* 69:409-413, 1993.

5. Aronow WS, Schwartz KS, and Koenigsberg M. Correlation of aortic cuspal and aortic root disease with aortic systolic ejection murmurs and with mitral anular calcium in persons older than 62 years in a long-term health care facility, *Am J Cardiol* 58:651-652, 1986.

6. Aronow WS and Kronzon I. Prevalence and severity of valvular aortic stenosis determined by Doppler echocardiography and its association with echocardiographic and electrocardiographic left ventricular hypertrophy and physical signs of aortic stenosis in elderly patients, *Am J Cardiol* 67:776-777, 1991.

7. Forssell G, Jonasson R, and Orinius E. Identifying severe aortic valvular stenosis by bedside examination, *Acta Med Scand* 218:397-400, 1985.

8. Hoagland PM and others. Value of noninvasive testing in adults with suspected aortic stenosis, *Am J Med* 80:1041-1050, 1986.

9. Aronow WS and Kronzon I. Correlation of prevalence and severity of valvular aortic stenosis determined by continuous-wave doppler echocardiography with physical signs of aortic stenosis in patients aged 62 to 100 years with aortic systolic ejection murmurs, *Am J Cardiol* 60:399-401, 1987.

10. Leach RM and McBrien DJ. Brachioradial delay: a new clinical indicator of the severity of aortic stenosis, *Lancet* 335:1199-1201, 1990.

11. Chun PKC and Dunn BE. Clinical clue of severe aortic stenosis: simultaneous palpation of the carotid and apical impulses, *Arch Intern Med* 142:2284-2288, 1982.

12. Nakamura T and others. Noninvasive evaluation of the severity of aortic stenosis in adult patients, *Am Heart J* 107:959-966, 1984.

13. Kavalier MA, Stewart J, and Tavel ME. The apical A wave versus the fourth heart sound in assessing the severity of aortic stenosis, *Circulation* 51:324-327, 1975.

14. Nitta M and others. Noninvasive evaluation of the severity of aortic stenosis in adults, *Chest* 91:682-687, 1987.

15. Danielsen R, Nordrehaug JE, and Vik-Mo H. Clinical and haemodynamic features in relation to severity of aortic stenosis in adults, *Eur Heart J* 12:791-795, 1991.

16. Hancock EW and Abelmann WH. A clinical study of the brachial arterial pulse form: with special reference to the diagnosis of aortic valvular disease, *Circulation* 16:572-581, 1957.

17. Etchells E and others. A bedside clinical prediction rule for detecting moderate or severe aortic stenosis, *J Gen Intern Med* 13:699-704, 1998.

CHAPTER 40

Aortic Regurgitation

I. **INTRODUCTION.** The principal problem in aortic regurgitation is defective closure of the aortic valve, which allows blood to return from the aorta to the left ventricle during diastole. In patients with significant chronic regurgitation, the traditional physical findings are a diastolic murmur, dilated apical impulse, and abnormally forceful and collapsing arterial pulses (pulsus celer).

In the 1700s, clinicians associated the postmortem finding of damaged aortic valves with hearts "larger than that of an ordinary ox" (the origin of the phrase "cor bovinum") and the finding during life of "violently throbbing" carotid arteries. In 1832, Sir Dominic John Corrigan, a Dublin surgeon, taught clinicians how to diagnose the disease during life, by emphasizing the importance of these dramatic arterial pulsations and the associated diastolic murmur.[1,2]

II. **THE FINDINGS**
   A. **The murmur(s).** Severe aortic regurgitation may cause three distinct murmurs: (1) the early diastolic murmur of aortic regurgitation, (2) a systolic aortic flow murmur, and (3) the apical diastolic rumble of the Austin Flint murmur.
      1. **Early diastolic murmur of regurgitation.** The most important physical sign of aortic regurgitation is the early diastolic murmur,

which is blowing, high-frequency, and decrescendo in shape (**Lub** **P**EWWWwwww, see Chapter 38). The murmur may occupy all of diastole or just its early part.[3] Pressing firmly against the chest wall with the diaphragm of the stethoscope brings out the murmur, which is usually loudest in the left parasternal area at the third or fourth intercostal space. In some patients, the murmur is only audible when the patient sits up, leans forward, and holds his breath in exhalation.

2. **Systolic aortic flow murmur.** Severe aortic regurgitation also produces a short systolic aortic flow murmur, which results from ejection over the aortic valve of the large stroke volume characteristic of the disease. The combination of this murmur and the early diastolic one causes a characteristic "to-fro" sound near the sternum (**Lub** SHSHSH **P**EWWWwwww, see Chapter 38). This systolic murmur may superficially resemble that of aortic stenosis, although the flow murmur of pure regurgitation is shorter and associated with the peripheral pulse findings of severe regurgitation (see below).

3. **Apical diastolic rumble: Austin Flint murmur**

   a. **Definition.** The Austin Flint murmur is a diastolic rumbling murmur heard at the apex in patients with severe aortic regurgitation, which resembles mitral stenosis even though the mitral valve is completely normal. It was first described by the American physician Austin Flint in 1862.[4]

   The Austin Flint murmur is found in up to 60% of patients with moderate or severe aortic regurgitation but is rarely heard in mild aortic regurgitation.[5,6] Austin Flint called his murmur "presystolic," but by this he meant it was loudest before S_1 and thus different from the murmur of aortic regurgitation, which began immediately after S_2 and tapered off during diastole. About half of Austin Flint murmurs have two diastolic components (middiastolic and presystolic), whereas the other half have just a presystolic component.[6,7]

b. Pathogenesis. The cause of the Austin Flint murmur is still debated. Although all hypotheses assume the murmur depends on a strong regurgitant stream of blood being directed back toward the left ventricle during diastole, these hypotheses differ in how this regurgitant stream causes an apical rumbling sound. Proposed mechanisms include fluttering of the anterior leaflet of the mitral valve, premature closure of the mitral valve from elevated left ventricular end-diastolic pressure, collision of the regurgitant stream with the anterior mitral leaflet, ventricular vibrations caused by the regurgitant stream itself, and harmonic distortion of the aortic regurgitant murmur.[6,8,9]

B. Water hammer pulse and increased pulse pressure. Because of the large stroke volume and diastolic emptying of aortic blood into the left ventricle (i.e., "aortic runoff"), the arterial pulse wave of aortic regurgitation rises suddenly and collapses abruptly. This abnormality has many names, although the most common ones are "collapsing pulse," "Corrigan pulse," or the "water hammer pulse."[a] In most patients with aortic regurgitation, the collapsing pulse

---

[a] Corrigan actually emphasized the exaggerated *visible* pulsations of aortic regurgitation, not the palpable ones. The term "water hammer pulse" was coined by Sir Thomas Watson in 1836, who likened the pulse to a Victorian toy called a water-hammer, which imparted to a child's hands the same sensation of a collapsing pulse of aortic regurgitation.[2]

becomes more prominent as the examiner elevates the patient's wrist.[10,11] This occurs because elevation of the arm with respect to the heart reduces the diastolic pressure in that arm, causing the vessel to collapse more completely with each beat. (The pounding sensation of the water-hammer pulse is identical to the sensation felt by the examiner when palpating a person's blood pressure, with the cuff pressure just above the person's diastolic pressure; see Chapter 15).

C. **Abnormal pulsations of other structures: The aortic regurgitation eponyms.** The large stroke volume and aortic runoff of aortic regurgitation often induce pulsations in other parts of the body, which has generated many eponyms of what is fundamentally a single physical finding (the number of eponyms for aortic regurgitation rivals those of some neurologic reflexes).[1,12,13] These various bobbings include (1) abnormally conspicuous capillary pulsation, best elicited by blanching a portion of the nail and then observing the pulsating border between the white and red color (Quincke's capillary pulsations, 1868, although Heinrich Quincke should be known instead for inventing the lumbar puncture); (2) anterior-posterior bobbing of the head, synchronous with the arterial pulsations (de Musset's sign, named after the French poet Alfred de Musset, who was afflicted with aortic regurgitation)[14]; (3) alternate blanching and flushing of the forehead and face (Lighthouse sign) (4) pulsations of organs or their parts, including the uvula (Müller's sign; 1899), retinal arteries (Becker's sign), larynx (Oliver-Cardavelli's sign), spleen (Sailer's sign, 1928),[15] and cervix (Dennison's sign).[b16]

---

[b] The eponym does not necessarily indicate priority: Sailor gave credit for the pulsating spleen to Tulp of the 1600s,[15] and Dennison gave credit for the pulsating cervix to Shelly, one of his house officers.[16]

In many of the original descriptions of these eponymic findings, the sign was presented simply as an interesting observation, not one of particular diagnostic value.

D. Hill's test. In 1909, Leonard Hill of Britain observed that patients with severe aortic regurgitation often have a systolic pressure in the foot that is much greater than a simultaneously measured systolic pressure in the arm.[17,18] "Hill's test" specifically refers to the systolic pressure of the foot minus that of the arm. The correct technique for measuring the pressure in the foot is to wrap the arm cuff around the patient's calf and to measure the systolic pressure in the dorsalis pedis and posterior tibial arteries by palpation. The higher of these two pressures is the "foot pressure."

E. Auscultation over arteries. Two auscultatory findings may appear over the peripheral arteries of patients with aortic regurgitation: pistol shot sounds and Duroziez's murmur (or Duroziez's sign).

1. Pistol shot sound

   a. Definition. Pistol shot sounds are short, loud, snapping sounds with each pulse, heard over the femoral, brachial, or radial arteries. They are identical in quality to the Korotkoff sounds heard when measuring blood pressure. Pistol shot sounds are heard with only *light* pressure of the stethoscope and, like the water hammer pulse, may first appear only after elevation of the patient's arm.[11]

   Pistol shot sounds were first described by Traube in 1872.[19]

   b. Pathogenesis. Pistol shot sounds occur because of sudden expansion and tensing of the walls of the vessels during systole. Consequently, they are not only associated with the collapsing pulses of aortic regurgitation but also are inducible in normal individuals by administering intravenous vasodilator medications.[20] The sounds are analogous to the loud, snapping notes heard when a sail or parachute suddenly fills with wind.[21] The quicker the vessel dilates, the louder the note, and in patients with aortic regurgitation, the intensity of the pistol-shot sound correlates with the height of the pulse pressure[22] and the change in pressure over time (dP/dt) of the pulse.[20]

2. Duroziez's murmur or sign.[12,19,23-26]

a. Definition.

Duroziez's sign is a *double* to-fro murmur heard over the brachial or femoral artery. It is heard only with *firm* pressure from the stethoscope. For Duroziez's sign to be positive, both a systolic and diastolic murmur must be present (many normal persons develop systolic murmurs with pressure on the stethoscope). The diastolic component often becomes louder with pressure applied distal to the stethoscope.

Although some claim Duroziez's murmur also may occur in normal individuals who have increased flow because of fever, anemia, or peripheral vasodilation,[23] the vascular sound produced in these conditions does not have the characteristic "to-fro" sound of Duroziez's murmur, but instead resembles the continuous murmur of an arteriovenous fistula (**Pu**SHSHSHSH**Pu**SHSHSHSHSHSH).[25]

Duroziez described his "double intermittent murmur" in 1861.[19,27]

b. Pathogenesis.

The diastolic component of Duroziez's sign results from the blood actually reversing directions in the artery during diastole.[24,25]

III. CLINICAL SIGNIFICANCE

A. Detecting aortic insufficiency.
The presence of the characteristic early diastolic murmur of aortic insufficiency argues strongly that an aortic leak is actually present (LR = 9.9; Table 40-1). Although some patients with mild regurgitation have no murmur, the *absence* of the characteristic murmur does argue strongly *against* the presence of moderate-to-severe aortic regurgitation (LR = 0.1; see Table 40-1).

B. Distinguishing aortic valve disease from aortic root disease.
The early diastolic murmur of aortic regurgitation is usually loudest in the left parasternal area. In some patients, the murmur may be loudest to the right of the sternum, which suggests an eccentric regurgitant stream from dilation of the aortic root (e.g., Marfan syndrome, aortic dissection, syphilitic aortitis) or damage to a single aortic cusp (e.g., endocarditis). The presence of this sign, introduced by Harvey in 1963,[37] argues strongly for a dilated root or endocarditis (LR = 8.2; see Table 40-1); its absence is diagnostically less helpful (LR = 0.7).[c]

C. Distinguishing aortic regurgitation from pulmonary regurgitation.
Distinguishing aortic from pulmonary regurgitation was particularly relevant in patients with rheumatic mitral stenosis, who often had associated aortic valve disease but who also could develop pulmonary hypertension and the early diastolic murmur of pulmonary insufficiency (i.e., the Graham Steell murmur).

In patients with mitral stenosis who also have an early diastolic murmur of regurgitation heard next to the sternum, the additional lesion

---

[c] The diagnostic accuracy of "Harvey's sign" is based on patients from the 1960s, when most patients had rheumatic valvular disease or syphilitic root disease. Whether it is as accurate today is unknown.

TABLE 40-1 Aortic regurgitation*

FINDING (REF)	SENSITIVITY (%)	SPECIFICITY (%)	POSITIVE LR	NEGATIVE LR
Characteristic Diastolic Murmur				
Detecting mild aortic regurgitation or worse[28-35]	54-87	75-98	9.9	0.3
Detecting moderate-to-severe aortic regurgitation[32-35]	88-98	52-88	4.3	0.1
Early Diastolic Murmur Loudest on Right Side of Sternum				
Detecting dilated aortic root or endocarditis[3]	29	96	8.2	0.7
Early Diastolic Murmur Softer with Amyl Nitrite Inhalation				
Detecting aortic regurgitation (vs. Graham Steell murmur)[36]	95	83	NS	0.1

NS, Not significant.

Diagnostic standard: For moderate-to-severe aortic regurgitation, see Table 40-2.

is aortic regurgitation at least 80% of the time. Aortic regurgitation is the most common correct diagnosis even when there are no peripheral pulse findings of aortic regurgitation and the patient shows signs of severe pulmonary hypertension.[28,38,39] In the past, reducing afterload with amyl nitrite inhalation was used to distinguish aortic from pulmonary regurgitation, since amyl nitrite should diminish the intensity of the aortic regurgitation murmur (i.e., less regurgitant flow) but not affect the pulmonary regurgitation murmur. The finding of an early diastolic murmur that instead becomes louder or does not change after amyl nitrite inhalation argues strongly *against* aortic regurgitation (LR = 0.1; see Table 40-1).

D. Severity of aortic regurgitation. This section applies only to patients with the characteristic early diastolic murmur of chronic aortic regurgitation (Table 40-2). It does not apply to acute aortic regurgitation (see Section E below). Many of the patients enrolled in the studies also had additional murmurs of aortic stenosis or mitral regurgitation.

   1. The diastolic murmur. The louder the murmur, the more severe the aortic regurgitation ($r = 0.67$).[40] Murmurs of grade 3 or more indicate moderate-to-severe aortic regurgitation (LR = 8.2; see Table 40-2).

   2. Blood pressure. Two findings arguing strongly *for* moderate-to-severe regurgitation are a diastolic blood pressure of 50 mm Hg or less (LR = 19.3; see Table 40-2) and a pulse pressure of 80 mm Hg or more (LR = 10.9; see Table 40-2). Two findings arguing *against* significant regurgitation are a diastolic blood pressure more than 70 mm Hg (LR = 0.2) and a pulse pressure less than 60 mm Hg (LR = 0.3). These signs have no diagnostic value when applied to other patients lacking the characteristic murmur of aortic regurgitation.[31]

TABLE 40-2 Characteristics of moderate-to-severe aortic regurgitation*

Finding (ref)†	Sensitivity (%)	Specificity (%)	Positive LR	Negative LR
Diastolic Murmur				
Murmur grade at least 3 or greater[31,40]	30-61	86-98	8.2	0.6
Blood Pressure				
Diastolic blood pressure[28,41]				
>70 mm Hg	8-21	32-55	0.2	—
51-70 mm Hg	42-50	—	NS	—
≤50 mm Hg	30-50	98	19.3	—
Pulse pressure[41]				
<60 mm Hg	21	32	0.3	—
60-79 mm Hg	21	—	NS	—
≥80 mm Hg	57	95	10.9	—

NS, Not significant.

*Diagnostic Standards: For moderate-to-severe regurgitation, regurgitation was either 3+ (moderate) or 4+ (severe) on a 0 to 4+ scale, using angiography,[28-30,34,35,41] Doppler echocardiography,[32,33,40] or surgery.[31] Trivial regurgitation on echocardiography was classified as "absent regurgitation."

†Definition of findings: See text.

Continued

TABLE 40-2 Characteristics of moderate-to-severe aortic regurgitation*—cont'd

Finding (ref)†	Sensitivity (%)	Specificity (%)	Positive LR	Negative LR
Hill's Test				
Hill's test[41]				
<40 mm Hg	29	13	0.3	—
40-59 mm Hg	29	—	NS	—
≥60 mm Hg	42	98	17.3	—
Other Signs				
Enlarged or sustained apical impulse[41]	97	60	2.4	0.1
Duroziez's sign, femoral pistol shot, water hammer pulse[25,41]	37-55	63-98	NS	0.7

3. **Hill's test.** If the abnormal response in Hill's test is defined as a foot-arm blood pressure difference of 60 mm Hg or more, the positive test argues strongly for significant regurgitation (LR = 17.3; see Table 40-2).

Some doubt Hill's test is accurate, citing experiments that show the intraarterial pressure in the *femoral arteries* of patients with aortic regurgitation to be identical to that of the brachial arteries.[42,43] Hill's test, however, measures the pressure of the pedal arteries, not the femoral arteries. It is possible that the systolic pressure is augmented in the foot, which is near the point of reflection of the abnormal pulse waveform.

4. **Other signs.** The *absence* of an enlarged or sustained apical impulse argues *against* moderate-to-severe regurgitation (LR = 0.1; see Table 40-2).

In patients with pure aortic regurgitation, the finding of a third heart sound does not predict the severity of regurgitation, ejection fraction, or left atrial pressure.[44,45] Duroziez's sign, femoral pistol shots, and the water hammer pulse are unreliable signs of the severity of regurgitation.

E. **Acute aortic regurgitation.** Compared with chronic aortic regurgitation, acute aortic regurgitation (e.g., from endocarditis or acute aortic dissection) causes a much shorter murmur, faster pulse rate (108/min vs. 71/min, mean values), smaller pulse pressure (55 mm Hg vs. 105 mm Hg), and lower systolic blood pressures (110 mm Hg vs. 155 mm Hg).[46] The murmur of acute aortic regurgitation is shorter because the combination of low arterial pressure and very high ventricular filling pressure eliminates the pressure gradient causing regurgitation by mid-diastole.[46] The first heart sound is faint or absent in acute aortic regurgitation because of premature closure of the mitral valve (see Chapter 35).[47] In patients with aortic regurgitation from endocarditis, an associated pericardial rub often indicates extravalvular extension of the infection.[46]

F. Distinguishing the Austin Flint murmur from mitral stenosis. Based on an older analysis of 400 patients with severe aortic regurgitation, many of whom also had apical diastolic rumbles, the following findings argue for mitral stenosis: atrial fibrillation, a loud S_1, no S_3, and an opening snap. The findings arguing that the apical rumble is more likely the Austin Flint murmur are sinus rhythm, a faint S_1, an S_3, and no opening snap.[48] In addition, inhalation of amyl nitrite, which reduces systemic vascular resistance, makes the Austin Flint murmur (and the aortic regurgitation murmur) softer but the apical rumble of true mitral stenosis louder.[49]

REFERENCES

1. Vaslef SN and Roberts WC. Early descriptions of aortic regurgitation, *Am Heart J* 125:1475-1483, 1993.
2. Dock G. I. Dominic John Corrigan: his place in the development of our knowledge of cardiac disease. II. The water-hammer pulse, *Ann Med Hist* 6:381-395, 1934.
3. Sakamoto T and others. The point of maximum intensity of aortic diastolic regurgitant murmur, with special emphasis to the "right-sided aortic diastolic murmur," *Jap Heart J* 9:117-133, 1968.
4. Flint A. On cardiac murmurs, *Am J Med Sci* 44:29-54, 1862.
5. Lee D and others. Reappraisal of cardiac murmurs related to aortic regurgitation, *Chin Med J (Taipei)* 56:152-158, 1995.
6. Rahko PS. Doppler and echocardiographic characteristics of patients having an Austin Flint murmur, *Circulation* 83:1940-1950, 1991.
7. Fortuin NJ and Craige E. On the mechanism of the Austin Flint murmur, *Circulation* 45:558-570, 1972.
8. Feinstein AR. Acoustic distinctions in cardiac auscultation: with emphasis on cardiophonetics, synecphonesis, the analysis of cadence, and problems of hydraulic distortion, *Arch Intern Med* 121:209-224, 1968.

9. Emi S and others. Genesis of the Austin Flint murmur: relation to mitral inflow and aortic regurgitant flow dynamics, *J Am Coll Cardiol* 21:1399-1405, 1993.

10. Warnes CA, Harris PC, and Fritts HW. Effect of elevating the wrist on the radial pulse in aortic regurgitation: Corrigan revisited, *Am J Cardiol* 51:1551-1553, 1983.

11. Palfrey FW. Auscultation of the Corrigan or water-hammer pulse, *N Engl J Med* 247:771-772, 1952.

12. Sapira JD. Quincke, de Musset, Duroziez, and Hill: some aortic regurgitations, *South Med J* 74:459-467, 1981.

13. Kishan CV and Talley JD. Hill's sign: a non-invasive clue of the severity of chronic aortic regurgitation, *J Ark Med Soc* 95:501-502, 1999.

14. Delpeuch A. Le signe de Musset: secousses rhythmées de la téte chez les aortiques, *Presse Méd* 8:237-238, 1900.

15. Sailer J. Pulsating spleen in aortic insufficiency, *Am Heart J* 3:447-453, 1928.

16. Dennison AD. Aortic regurgitation: multiple eponyms, physical signs and etiologies, *J Ind State Med Assoc* 52:1283-1289, 1959.

17. Hill L. The measurement of systolic blood pressure in man, *Heart* 1:73-82, 1909.

18. Hill L and Rowlands RA. Systolic blood pressure: (1) In change of posture. (2) In cases of aortic regurgitation, *Heart* 3:219-232, 1911.

19. Luisada AA. On the pathogenesis of the signs of Traube and Duroziez in aortic insufficiency, *Am Heart J* 26:721-736, 1943.

20. Lange RL and Hecht HH. Genesis of pistol-shot and Korotkoff sounds, *Circulation* 18:975-978, 1958.

21. McGee SR and Adcox M. Unilateral femoral pistol-shot sounds: a clue to aortic dissection, *West J Med* 162:547-548, 1995.

22. Boudoulas H and others. Mechanisms of pistol shot sounds in aortic regurgitation, *Acta Cardiologica* 46:139-145, 1991.

23. Blumgart HL and Erstene AC. Two mechanisms in the production of Duroziez's sign: their diagnostic significance and a clinical test for differentiating between them, *JAMA* 100:173-177, 1933.

24. Rowe GG and others. The mechanism of the production of Duroziez's murmur, *N Engl J Med* 272:1207-1210, 1965.

25. Folts JD, Young WP, and Rowe GG. A study of Duroziez's murmur of aortic insufficiency in man utilizing an electromagnetic flowmeter, *Circulation* 38:426-431, 1968.

26. MacAlpin RN and Kattus AA. Brachial-artery bruits in aortic-valve disease and hypertrophic subaortic stenosis, *N Engl J Med* 273:1012-1018, 1965.

27. Willius FA and Keys TE. *Classics of cardiology: a collection of classic works on the heart and circulation with comprehensive biographic accounts of the authors.* New York, 1941, Henry Schuman, Inc.

28. Linhart JW. Aortic regurgitation: clinical, hemodynamic, surgical, and angiographic correlations, *Ann Thorac Surg* 11:27-37, 1971.

29. Meyers DG and others. Diagnosis of aortic insufficiency: comparison of auscultation and M-mode echocardiography to angiography, *South Med J* 75:1192-1194, 1982.

30. Meyers DG, Olson TS, and Hansen DA. Auscultation, M-mode, echocardiography and pulsed Doppler echocardiography compared with angiography for diagnosis of chronic aortic regurgitation, *Am J Cardiol* 56:810-811, 1985.

31. Cohn LH and others. Preoperative assessment of aortic regurgitation in patients with mitral valve disease, *Am J Cardiol* 19:177-182, 1967.

32. Rahko PS. Prevalence of regurgitant murmurs in patients with valvular regurgitation detected by Doppler echocardiography, *Ann Intern Med* 111:466-472, 1989.

33. Aronow WS and Kronzon I. Correlation of prevalence and severity of aortic regurgitation detected by pulsed Doppler echocardiography with the murmur of aortic regurgitation in elderly patients in a long-term health care facility, *Am J Cardiol* 63:128-129, 1989.

34. Dittmann H, Karsch KR, and Seipel L. Diagnosis and quantification of aortic regurgitation by pulsed Doppler echocardiography in patients with mitral valve disease, *Eur Heart J* 8(suppl C):53-57, 1987.

35. Grayburn PA and others. Detection of aortic insufficiency by standard echocardiography, pulsed Doppler echocardiography, and auscultation: a comparison of accuracies, *Ann Intern Med* 104:599-605, 1986.

36. Luisada AA and Madoery RJ. Functional tests as an aid to cardiac auscultation, *Med Clin North Am* 50:73-89, 1966.

37. Harvey WP, Corrado MA, and Perloff JK. "Right-sided" murmurs of aortic insufficiency (diastolic murmurs better heard to the right of the sternum rather than to the left), *Am J Med Sci* 245:533-543, 1963.

38. Cohn KE and Hultgren HN. The Graham Steell murmur re-evaluated, *N Engl J Med* 274:486-489, 1966.

39. Runco V and others. The Graham Steell murmur versus aortic regurgitation in rheumatic heart disease: results of aortic valvulography, *Am J Med* 31:71-80, 1961.

40. Desjardins VA and others. Intensity of murmurs correlates with severity of valvular regurgitation, *Am J Med* 100:149-156, 1996.

41. Frank MJ and others. The clinical evaluation of aortic regurgitation, *Arch Intern Med* 116:357-365, 1965.

42. Pascarelli EF, Bertrand CA, and Lopez M. Comparison of arm and leg blood pressure in aortic insufficiency: an appraisal of Hill's sign, *Br Med J* 2:73-75, 1965.

43. Kutryk M and Fitchett D. Hills sign in aortic regurgitation: enhanced pressure wave transmission or artefact? *Can J Cardiol* 13:237-240, 1997.

44. Abdulla AM and others. Clinical significance and hemodynamic correlates of the third heart sound gallop in aortic regurgitation: a guide to optimal timing of cardiac catheterization, *Circulation* 64:464-471, 1981.

45. Folland ED and others. Implications of third heart sounds in patients with valvular heart disease, *N Engl J Med* 327:458-462, 1992.

46. Mann T and others. Assessing the hemodynamic severity of acute aortic regurgitation due to infective endocarditis, *N Engl J Med* 293:108-113, 1975.

47. Meadows WR and others. Premature mitral valve closure: a hemodynamic explanation for absence of the first sound in aortic insufficiency, *Circulation* 28:251-258, 1963.

48. Segal JP, Harvey WP, and Corrado MA. The Austin Flint murmur: its differentiation from the murmur of rheumatic mitral stenosis, *Circulation* 18:1025-1033, 1958.

49. Nasser W and others. Austin-Flint murmur versus the murmur of organic mitral stenosis, *N Engl J Med* 275:1007-1009, 1966.

CHAPTER 41

Miscellaneous Heart Murmurs

HYPERTROPHIC CARDIOMYOPATHY

I. THE MURMUR. The murmur of hypertrophic cardiomyopathy is usually midsystolic, harsh in quality, and loudest at the lower left sternal border or between the lower left sternal border and apex.[1] The murmur may obliterate the second heart sound and become late systolic, especially if mitral regurgitation is associated. The intensity of the murmur behaves in distinctive ways during maneuvers altering venous return to the heart (see Chapter 38).

II. ASSOCIATED FINDINGS. The palpable apex beat may be sustained and the arterial pulse hyperkinetic (see Chapters 13 and 33). Although pulsus bisferiens has been described in hypertrophic cardiomyopathy,[2] this refers to a finding on intraarterial pressure tracings, not a palpable finding at the bedside.[3] The second heart sound is usually single or physiologically split, although in 10% splitting is paradoxic or reversed.[1] Over half of patients have audible fourth heart sound.[1]

MITRAL REGURGITATION

I. THE FINDING

A. The murmur. The murmur of chronic mitral regurgitation is usually holosystolic, high in frequency, and loudest at the apex.[4] It radiates to the axilla and inferior angle of the left scapula, although in some patients with isolated incompetence of the medial portion of the posterior leaflet, the murmur radiates instead to the right base and even into the neck, thus mimicking aortic stenosis.[4,5]

In 1832, James Hope was the first to describe the apical systolic murmur of mitral regurgitation.[4,6]

B. Associated findings. In chronic mitral regurgitation, the intensity of S_1 is normal 75% of the time, loud 12% of the time, and soft 12% of the time. In 50% of patients, S_2 splitting is wide and physiologic.[4] An associated S_3 is common, appearing in 89% with severe regurgitation. S_4 is rare.

Associated cardiac findings are an enlarged, laterally displaced palpable apical movement,[7] a palpable lower parasternal movement from an enlarged left atrium (see Chapter 33),[8] and a hyperkinetic arterial pulse (see Chapter 13).[9] Neck veins are normal unless the patient has decompensated heart failure.

II. CLINICAL SIGNIFICANCE

A. Detecting mitral regurgitation. The presence of the characteristic murmur of mitral regurgitation argues that regurgitation is present, at least to a mild degree (LR = 5.4; see Chapter 38). Although 25% to 50% of patients with *mild* regurgitation lack a murmur, the absence of the characteristic murmur does argues against the presence of *moderate-to-severe* mitral regurgitation (LR = 0.2; see Chapter 38).

B. Severity of mitral regurgitation

1. The murmur. In a very general way, the intensity of the murmur of mitral regurgitation correlates with the severity of regurgitation, especially for rheumatic mitral regurgitation ($r = 0.67$) but less so for ischemic or functional[a] mitral regurgitation ($r = 0.45$).[10-12] A murmur of grade 3 intensity or louder argues moderately for severe mitral regurgitation (LR = 4.4; see Table 41-1).

2. Other findings. Patients with severe mitral regurgitation may have a late systolic, sustained left lower parasternal impulse from a dilated left atrium. (Chapter 33 discusses how to distinguish this impulse from a right ventricular one.) The degree of this movement correlates well with severity of regurgitation ($r = 0.93$, $p < .01$), as long as the patient does not have associated mitral stenosis (the presence of mitral stenosis confounds analyzing the parasternal impulse of patients with mitral regurgitation because the impulse could be due to either a large left atrium from severe regurgitation or a hypertensive right ventricle from mitral stenosis).[8,15]

The third heart sound is only a weak discriminator between significant mitral regurgitation and less severe disease (positive LR = 1.8, negative LR = 0.8; see Table 41-1).

C. Distinguishing acute from chronic mitral regurgitation.
The physical signs of acute and chronic mitral regurgitation differ in several ways: in acute lesions, the patient is acutely ill with elevated neck veins and signs of pulmonary edema: in chronic lesions, these signs may

---

[a] Functional mitral regurgitation implies that the primary problem is cardiomyopathy, which dilates the atrioventricular ring and renders the valve incompetent. Because of their low ejection fraction, these patients often tolerate valve replacement poorly.

TABLE 41-1 Severity of mitral and tricuspid regurgitation*

Finding (ref)	Sensitivity (%)	Specificity (%)	Positive LR	Negative LR
Mitral Regurgitation				
Systolic Murmur Grade 3 or Louder				
Detecting moderate-to-severe mitral regurgitation, in patients with characteristic systolic murmur[12]	85	81	4.4	0.2
Third Heart Sound				
Detecting moderate-to-severe mitral regurgitation, in patients with characteristic systolic murmur[13]	41	77	1.8	0.8
Tricuspid Regurgitation				
Pulsatile Liver				
Detecting moderate-to-severe tricuspid regurgitation, in patients with characteristic systolic murmur[14]	30	92	3.9	NS
Systolic Regurgitant Wave in Neck Veins				
Detecting moderate-to-severe tricuspid regurgitation, in patients with characteristic systolic murmur[14]	51	66	NS	NS

NS, Not significant.

*Diagnostic standard: For *moderate-to-severe mitral regurgitation,* regurgitant fraction >40% by Doppler echocardiography[12] or as assessed visually from angiogram[13]; for *moderate-to-severe tricuspid regurgitation,* 3+ or 4+ by angiography.[14]

be absent. In acute lesions the pulse is rapid and regular; in chronic lesions, it may be slow and commonly is irregular (from atrial fibrillation).[16] In acute lesions, the murmur may be very short, confined just to early systole (40% of patients in one series), because the left atrial pressures are so high they equal ventricular pressures by mid-to-late systole, thus eliminating the regurgitation gradient.[17,18] In chronic lesions, the murmur is holosystolic, late systolic, or midsystolic, but not early systolic. In acute lesions, the fourth heart sound is common (80% in one series); in chronic lesions, the fourth heart sound is rare because there is either no atrial contraction (i.e., atrial fibrillation) or the atrium is so dilated it cannot contract strongly.[10,16,19]

D. Papillary muscle dysfunction. Papillary muscle dysfunction refers to the murmur of mitral regurgitation that develops in the setting of myocardial ischemia. The murmur, which is usually transient, may be holosystolic, midsystolic, or late systolic. It appears in up to 20% of patients with myocardial infarction,[20] in whom it is associated with a higher incidence of persistent chest pain in the intensive care unit (45% vs. 26% without murmur) and a higher 1-year mortality (18% vs. 10%).[20]

MITRAL VALVE PROLAPSE

I. INTRODUCTION. Mitral valve prolapse describes an abnormal posterosuperior movement of the mitral valve leaflets into the left atrium after they close at the beginning of systole. It is an important cause of mitral regurgitation and the physical findings of late systolic murmurs and mid-to-late systolic clicks.[21-23]

At the beginning of the twentieth century, most clinicians believed that all late systolic murmurs were benign and that late systolic clicks were generated outside of the heart.[21,22] In 1963, Barlow performed angiograms in several patients with late systolic murmurs and proved the cause of the murmur was mitral prolapse and regurgitation.[24]

II. THE FINDINGS

A. The murmur. The murmur of mitral valve prolapse is loudest at the apex and is sometimes musical (see Chapter 38). It is characteristically late systolic because the mitral leaflets are well supported by their chordae tendineae and competent during early systole, but lose this support as the ventricle becomes smaller during late systole. The leaflets then buckle backwards toward the left atrium and create a regurgitant leak.[21-23]

B. The clicks. The clicks of mitral valve prolapse occur during mid-to-late systole and are loudest at the apex or left lower sternal border.[21] They are sometimes multiple. In patients with both a click and a murmur, the click introduces the murmur 65% of the time and occurs just after the beginning of the murmur 35% of the time.[21] Sudden deceleration of the billowing mitral leaflet, as it prolapses into the left atrial cavity, causes the sound, thus resembling the sound produced by a parachute or sail that suddenly tenses as it fills with wind.[25]

C. Response of murmurs and clicks to maneuvers. Bedside maneuvers that alter venous return or afterload (i.e., systemic vascular resistance) change both the timing of the clicks and murmurs and the intensity of the murmur, although they affect timing and intensity independently.

The *timing* of clicks and murmurs depends on the venous return to the heart. Reductions in venous return—by straining during the Valsalva maneuver or moving from squatting-to-standing—cause the ventricular chamber to become smaller and the mitral leaflets to prolapse earlier during systole, thus moving the click closer to S_1 and making the murmur longer.[21,23]

In contrast, the *intensity* of the murmur depends more on afterload, and in this way the response resembles that of chronic mitral regurgitation (see Chapter 38). As afterload is reduced with amyl nitrite inhalation, the murmur of mitral valve prolapse becomes fainter.[21] The Valsalva strain usually makes the murmur *softer*, whereas squatting-to-standing makes it *louder*, perhaps because the Valsalva strain causes more hypotension (and a greater fall in systemic vascular resistance) than does standing.[b,21]

III. CLINICAL SIGNIFICANCE

A. Detection of mitral valve prolapse.

The accuracy of bedside examination for mitral valve prolapse cannot be addressed, simply because auscultatory criteria alone are sufficient for diagnosis.[26,27] The criteria for diagnosing mitral valve prolapse are the reproducible finding in a young patient of a mid-to-late systolic click or late systolic murmur at or near the apex. These sounds should shift their timing with respect to S_1 and S_2 in response to the Valsalva and squatting-to-standing maneuvers (see Section II-C above). These criteria require the patient to be young to avoid confusion with papillary muscle dysfunction, which is a common cause of late systolic murmurs in older patients.[26] The click should be mobile and occur in mid-to-late systole to eliminate confusion with other short systolic sounds, such as the split S_1 and the aortic ejection sound (Chapters 36 and 37 further discuss the differentiation of these sounds).[26,27]

---

[b] Mitral valve prolapse is therefore an important cause of the false-positive result when using the squatting-to-standing maneuver to diagnose obstructive cardiomyopathy (see Chapter 38).

B. Risk of significant mitral regurgitation.
The risk of significant mitral regurgitation in mitral valve prolapse is low. In one study of 291 patients with a click or murmur presenting to a cardiologist (which biases selection towards more severe cases), none of the patients with an isolated click developed significant mitral regurgitation over 8 years of follow-up, and only 3% of those with murmurs ever required mitral valve replacement.[28]

TRICUSPID REGURGITATION

I. THE FINDINGS. The physical findings of tricuspid regurgitation depend on the patient's pulmonary pressure, which may be high ("high pressure" tricuspid regurgitation) or normal ("low pressure" tricuspid regurgitation). High pressure tricuspid regurgitation is commonly due to left-sided heart disease; low pressure tricuspid regurgitation commonly results from endocarditis of the tricuspid valve.

A. The murmur. Whether pulmonary pressures are high or low, the murmur of tricuspid regurgitation is typically loudest at the lower left sternal border, becomes louder during inspiration, and may radiate below the xiphoid process.[29]

1. "High-pressure" tricuspid regurgitation. The murmur of high-pressure tricuspid regurgitation is holosystolic because the elevated right ventricular pressures exceed right atrial pressures throughout systole. The murmur becomes louder during inspiration (Carvallo's sign) in 75% of patients and during manual pressure over the liver in 60% of patients.[14,30-34]

In some patients with high-pressure tricuspid regurgitation, the murmur is loudest at the apex because the enlarged right ventricle has replaced the normal position of the left ventricle. At this location, the resulting holosystolic apical murmur resembles mitral regurgitation, which, in the 1950s, led to the significant bedside error of misdiagnosing mitral regurgitation in some patients with mitral stenosis, thus inappropriately denying them valvuloplasty (a procedure contraindicated with severe mitral regurgitation).[35] Clues that help the clinician correctly recognize the apical holosystolic murmur as tricuspid regurgitation are the associated findings of an identical murmur at the lower sternal border, inspiratory augmentation of the murmur, elevated neck veins and pulsatile liver.[35]

2. **Low-pressure tricuspid regurgitation.** If pulmonary and right ventricular pressures are normal, the murmur of tricuspid regurgitation is confined to early systole because by midsystole right atrial and right ventricular pressure are the same, thus eliminating the gradient causing the murmur.[36]

B. Other findings

1. **High pressure tricuspid regurgitation.** Other important cardiac findings are elevated neck veins (over 90% of patients), a systolic regurgitant wave in the neck veins (51% to 83% of patients), and systolic retraction of the apical impulse (22% of patients).[14,31,33] Thirty to 91% of patients have a pulsatile liver, and 90% have edema, ascites, or both.[14,29,31,33]

2. **Low pressure tricuspid regurgitation.** In these patients, the neck veins and apical impulse are normal, and there is no edema, pulsatile liver, or ascites.

C. Estimating venous pressure in tricuspid regurgitation. Estimates of venous pressure are useful because they indicate right ventricular *diastolic* pressures (or filling pressures), which provide important clues to the etiology of ascites and edema (see Chapter 31). In tricuspid regurgitation, however, the neck veins characteristically reveal a large *systolic* wave, raising the question of whether these bedside estimates of venous pressure still reliably indicate the right heart filling pressures.

In patients with tricuspid regurgitation (and no tricuspid stenosis), catheter measurements of the *mean* pressure in the right atrium correlate closely with right ventricular end diastolic pressure ($r = 0.94$, $p < .001$, slope 1.0).[31] Mean atrial pressure is estimated at the bedside by identifying which patient position brings out the regurgitant waves. If the regurgitant waves are visible when the patient is supine, then the diastolic pressure in the veins must be very low (i.e., the waves collapse and become visible because the diastolic venous pressure is below the level of the sternum, or very low). The mean atrial pressure (i.e., central venous pressure) in these patients is probably normal. On the other hand, if the regurgitant waves are only visible in the upright position, the diastolic pressure in the veins must be high (otherwise the neck veins would collapse and be visible in lower positions). The mean atrial and central venous pressure of these patients is probably high.

For the 15% to 30% of patients with severe tricuspid regurgitation who lack conspicuous systolic waves in the neck veins, the clinician should estimate venous pressure in the usual way (see Chapter 31).

II. CLINICAL SIGNIFICANCE

A. Detecting tricuspid regurgitation. The presence of the characteristic systolic murmur of tricuspid regurgitation is a strong argument that some degree of tricuspid regurgitation is present (LR = 14.6; see Chapter 38). Many patients with tricuspid regurgitation, however, lack a murmur, which means that the *absence* of a

murmur has less diagnostic significance (negative LR is 0.8 for detecting mild regurgitation or worse and 0.4 for detecting moderate-to-severe regurgitation, Chapter 38).

B. Severity of tricuspid regurgitation. In patients with the murmur of tricuspid regurgitation, the finding of a pulsatile liver argues for moderate-to-severe regurgitation (LR = 3.9; see Table 41-1). Its absence is not helpful. The presence or absence of the systolic wave in the neck veins does not indicate severity because many patients with mild tricuspid regurgitation have a systolic wave when supine, and many with severe regurgitation have such high diastolic pressures in the neck veins that the veins do not collapse (and the wave is not visible) even after the patient sits up.

PULMONIC REGURGITATION

I. THE FINDING. The murmur of pulmonic regurgitation is a diastolic murmur heard best at the second or third left intercostal space. Its timing and frequency depend on pulmonary pressures.

A. High pressure pulmonic regurgitation. Sustained pulmonary hypertension may cause the pulmonic valve to become incompetent, producing an early diastolic, high-frequency murmur at the second left intercostal space. The murmur begins immediately with a loud S_2, and most patients have elevated neck veins and other auscultatory findings of pulmonary hypertension, such as the pulmonary ejection sound, abnormal S_2 splitting, and right ventricular gallops (see Chapters 35 to 37).[37] Chapter 40 discusses how to distinguish this murmur from that of aortic regurgitation.

The high pressure pulmonic regurgitation murmur was first described by the British clinician Graham Steell in 1888[38] and is often called the "Graham Steell" murmur.

B. **Low pressure pulmonic regurgitation.**
When pulmonary pressures are normal, pulmonic regurgitation represents primary valvular disease (e.g., endocarditis). This murmur is middiastolic and contains a mixture of low and high frequency sound. It begins with a short delay after S_2.[36]

II. CLINICAL SIGNIFICANCE

A. **Detecting pulmonic regurgitation.** Although the presence of the characteristic murmur is diagnostic (LR = 17.4; see Chapter 38), the absence of the murmur is unhelpful (LR not significant; see Chapter 38).

B. **Hemodialysis patients.** A common cause of an early diastolic murmur at the sternal border in patients with end-stage renal disease is pulmonic regurgitation.[39] This murmur presumably occurs because of volume overload, because it is loudest immediately before dialysis and often disappears just after dialysis.

MITRAL STENOSIS

I. THE FINDINGS

A. **The murmur.** Mitral stenosis causes a low-frequency, rumbling middiastolic murmur, which is usually heard with the bell lightly applied to the apex, often only after the patient has turned to the left lateral decubitus position. The murmur peaks during middiastole and again immediately before the first heart sound ("presystolic accentuation"). The middiastolic peak occurs because the mitral leaflets move backward toward the left atrium at this time, narrowing the mitral orifice and causing more turbulence (an analogy is the difficulty whistling with the mouth open).[40,41] The importance of these movements to the sound may explain why some patients with severe calcific mitral stenosis and inflexible leaflets have no murmur.[41]

The traditional explanation for presystolic accentuation is atrial systole, but this is probably incorrect, because presystolic accentuation also occurs in patients with atrial fibrillation.[42] Instead, there is some evidence that presystolic accentuation is actually caused by *ventricular* contraction: The crescendo sound occurs because the closing movement of the mitral leaflets, induced by ventricular systole, occurs when a pressure gradient is still maintaining forward flow across the valve. The sound continues and crescendos up until the moment the valves completely close, at the first heart sound (therefore, the "presystolic" accentuation is not presystolic at all, but instead is systolic).[40-42]

Because the sound vibrations of mitral stenosis border on the threshold of human hearing, this murmur is indistinct and the most difficult to detect, as reflected in metaphors used to describe the sound: "the faint sound of distant thunder," "the rumbling sound of a ball rolling down a bowling alley," and "the absence of silence."[43]

B. **Other cardiac findings.** Other cardiac findings in mitral stenosis include an irregular pulse (atrial fibrillation); a loud first heart sound; opening snap (early diastolic sound); and associated findings of pulmonary hypertension, including elevated neck veins with an exaggerated A wave, right ventricular parasternal impulse, and a palpable P_2 (see Chapters 31, 33, and 35).[9] The palpable apical impulse is small or absent because of obstruction of blood flow into the left ventricle.[9]

II. CLINICAL SIGNIFICANCE
A. **The murmur.** Not all apical diastolic rumbles are due to mitral stenosis, which has become a rare diagnosis in developed countries. Other

causes of this murmur include mitral annular calcification, the Austin-Flint murmur, atrial myxoma, and increased flow over a nonobstructed mitral valve from mitral regurgitation, ventricular septal defect, or high output states (see Chapter 36). In one study of 529 elderly patients living in the United States, an apical diastolic rumble detected *mitral annular calcification* on echocardiography with a sensitivity of 10%, specificity of 99%, and positive LR of 7.5 (90% of patients with this murmur had *no* mitral stenosis).[44]

B. **Other cardiac findings.** In patients with mitral stenosis, the apical impulse should be absent or small and the arterial pulse should be normal or reduced. Consequently, the finding of a hyperkinetic apical movement in patients with mitral stenosis suggests additional mitral or aortic regurgitation (LR = 11.2; see Table 41-2), and the finding of a hyperkinetic arterial pulse strongly suggests additional mitral regurgitation (LR = 14.2; see Table 41-2).

ARTERIOVENOUS FISTULAE: THE HEMODIALYSIS FISTULA

The hemodialysis fistula provides a good example of the continuous murmur typical of arteriovenous fistulae: it is a high-frequency murmur, persisting throughout systole and diastole but peaking during late systole ("**Pu**SHSHSHSH**Pu**SHSHSHSHSHSH"; venous hums, in contrast peak during diastole; see Chapter 38). Moving the stethoscope progressively away from the fistula and toward the heart makes the diastolic component of the murmur fainter until only a systolic murmur remains.[46]

The importance of this murmur is that its systolic remnants are transmitted to the upper sternal border, where they can be mistaken for cardiac murmurs unless the clinician traces them to the fistula.[46]

TABLE 41-2 Other cardiac findings in mitral stenosis*

FINDING (REF)†	SENSITIVITY (%)	SPECIFICITY (%)	POSITIVE LR	NEGATIVE LR
Graham Steell Murmur Detecting pulmonary hypertension[45]	69	83	4.2	0.4
Hyperkinetic Apical Movement Detecting associated mitral regurgitation or aortic valve disease[9]	74	93	11.2	0.3
Hyperkinetic Arterial Pulse Detecting associated mitral regurgitation[9]	71	95	14.2	0.3

*Diagnostic standard: For pulmonary hypertension, mean pulmonary pressure >50 mm Hg.[45]

†Definition of findings: For Graham Steell murmur, early diastolic decrescendo murmur of high pressure pulmonic regurgitation at second left intercostal space; for hyperkinetic apical movement, apical "thrust"[9] (see Chapter 33); for hyperkinetic pulse, arterial pulse strikes fingers abruptly and strongly (see Chapter 13).

REFERENCES

1. Tucker RBK and others. Auscultatory features of hypertrophic obstructive cardiomyopathy: a study of 90 patients, *S Afr Med J* 49:179-186, 1975.

2. Frank S and Braunwald E. Idiopathic hypertrophic subaortic stenosis: clinical analysis of 126 patients with emphasis on the natural history, *Circulation* 37:759-788, 1968.

3. Perloff JK. Clinical recognition of aortic stenosis: the physical signs and differential diagnosis of the various forms of obstruction to left ventricular outflow, *Prog Cardiovasc Dis* 10:323-352, 1968.

4. Perloff JK and Harvey WP. Auscultatory and phonocardiographic manifestations of pure mitral regurgitation, *Prog Cardiovasc Dis* 5:172-194, 1962.

5. Antman EM, Angoff GH, and Sloss LJ. Demonstration of the mechanism by which mitral regurgitation mimics aortic stenosis, *Am J Cardiol* 42:1044-1048, 1978.

6. Willius FA and Dry TJ. *A history of the heart and the circulation,* Philadelphia, 1948, WB Saunders Co.

7. Sutton GC, Craige E, and Grizzle JE. Quantitation of precordial movement: II. Mitral regurgitation, *Circulation* 35:483-491, 1967.

8. Basta LL and others. The value of left parasternal impulse recordings in the assessment of mitral regurgitation, *Circulation* 48:1055-1065, 1973.

9. Wood P. An appreciation of mitral stenosis: Part 1. Clinical features. Part 2. Investigations and results, *Br Med J* 1:1051-1063, 1113-1124, 1954.

10. Hultgren HN, Hancock EW, and Cohn KE. Auscultation in mitral and tricuspid valvular disease, *Prog Cardiovasc Dis* 10:298-322, 1968.

11. Rahko PS. Prevalence of regurgitant murmurs in patients with valvular regurgitation detected by Doppler echocardiography, *Ann Intern Med* 111:466-472, 1989.

12. Desjardins VA and others. Intensity of murmurs correlates with severity of valvular regurgitation, *Am J Med* 100:149-156, 1996.

13. Folland ED and others. Implications of third heart sounds in patients with valvular heart disease, *N Engl J Med* 327:458-462, 1992.

14. Cha SD and Gooch AS. Diagnosis of tricuspid regurgitation, *Arch Intern Med* 143:1763-1768, 1983.

15. James TM, Swatzell RH, and Eddleman EE. Hemodynamic significance of the precordial late systolic outward movement in mitral regurgitation, *Ala J Med Sci* 15:55-64, 1978.

16. DePace NL, Nestico PF, and Morganroth J. Acute severe mitral regurgitation: pathophysiology, clinical recognition, and management, *Am J Med* 78:293-306, 1985.

17. Friedman AW and Stein L. Pitfalls in bedside diagnosis of severe acute mitral regurgitation: clinical and hemodynamic features, *Chest* 78:436-441, 1980.

18. Sutton GC and Craige E. Clinical signs of severe acute mitral regurgitation, *Am J Cardiol* 20:141-144, 1967.

19. Cohen LS, Mason DT, and Braunwald E. Significance of an atrial gallop sound in mitral regurgitation: a clue to the diagnosis of rupture chordae tendineae, *Circulation* 35:112-118, 1967.

20. Maisel AS and others. The murmur of papillary muscle dysfunction in acute myocardial infarction: Clinical features and prognostic implications, *Am Heart J* 112:705-711, 1986.

21. Barlow JB and others. Late systolic murmurs and non-ejection ("mid-late") systolic clicks: an analysis of 90 patients, *Br Heart J* 30:203-218, 1968.

22. Devereux RB and others. Mitral valve prolapse, *Circulation* 54:3-14, 1976.

23. Fontana ME and others. Postural changes in left ventricular and mitral valvular dynamics in systolic click—late systolic murmur syndrome, *Circulation* 51:165-173, 1975.

24. Barlow JB and others. The significance of late systolic murmurs, *Am Heart J* 66:443-452, 1963.

25. Ronan JA. Cardiac auscultation: opening snaps, systolic clicks, and ejection sounds, *Heart Dis Stroke* 2:188-191, 1993.

26. Perloff JK and Child JS. Clinical and epidemiologic issues in mitral valve prolapse: overview and perspective, *Am Heart J* 113:1324-1332, 1987.

27. Perloff JK, Child JS, and Edwards JE. New guidelines for the clinical diagnosis of mitral valve prolapse, *Am J Cardiol* 57:1124-1129, 1986.

28. Tofler OB and H. TG. Use of auscultation to follow patients with mitral systolic clicks and murmurs, *Am J Cardiol* 66:1355-1358, 1990.

29. Müller O and Shillingford J. Tricuspid incompetence, *Br Heart J* 16:195-207, 1954.

30. Gooch AS, Cha SD, and Maranhao V. The use of the hepatic pressure maneuver to identify the murmur of tricuspid regurgitation, *Clin Cardiol* 6:277-280, 1983.

31. Salazar E and Levine HD. Rheumatic tricuspid regurgitation: the clinical spectrum, *Am J Med* 33:111-129, 1962.

32. Maisel AS, Atwood JE, and Goldberger AL. Hepatojugular reflux: useful in the bedside diagnosis of tricuspid regurgitation, *Ann Intern Med* 101:781-782, 1984.

33. Lingamneni R and others. Tricuspid regurgitation: clinical and angiographic assessment, *Cath Cardiovasc Diag* 5:7-17, 1979.

34. Vitums VC, Gooch AS, and Evans JM. Bedside maneuvers to augment the murmur of tricuspid regurgitation, *Med Ann DC* 38:533-542, 1969.

35. Schilder DP and Harvey WP. Confusion of tricuspid incompetence with mitral insufficiency—a pitfall in the selection of patients for mitral surgery, *Am Heart J* 54:352-367, 1957.

36. Perloff JK. The physiologic mechanisms of cardiac and vascular physical signs, *J Am Coll Cardiol* 1:184-198, 1983.

37. Perloff JK. Auscultatory and phonocardiographic manifestations of pulmonary hypertension, *Prog Cardiovasc Dis* 9:303-340, 1967.

38. Willius FA and Keys TE. *Classics of cardiology: a collection of classic works on the heart and circulation with comprehensive biographic accounts of the authors,* New York, 1941, Henry Schuman, Inc.

39. Perez JE, Smith CA, and Meltzer VN. Pulmonic valve insufficiency: a common cause of transient diastolic murmurs in renal failure, *Ann Intern Med* 103:497-502, 1985.

40. Fortuin NJ and Craige E. Echocardiographic studies of genesis of mitral diastolic murmurs, *Br Heart J* 35:75-81, 1973.

41. Toutouzas P and others. Mechanism of diastolic rumble and presystolic murmur in mitral stenosis, *Br Heart J* 36:1096-1105, 1974.

42. Criley JM and Hermer AJ. The crescendo presystolic murmur of mitral stenosis with atrial fibrillation, *N Engl J Med* 285:1284-1287, 1971.

43. Constant J. *Bedside cardiology,* Boston, 1985, Little, Brown & Co.

44. Aronow WS, Schwartz KS, and Koenigsberg M. Correlation of murmurs of mitral stenosis and mitral regurgitation with presence or absence of mitral anular calcium in persons older than 62 years in a long-term health care facility, *Am J Cardiol* 59:181-182, 1987.

45. Whitaker W. Clinical diagnosis of pulmonary hypertension in patients with mitral stenosis, *Q J Med* 23:105-112, 1954.

46. Rault R. Transmitted murmurs in patients undergoing hemodialysis, *Arch Intern Med* 149:1392-1393, 1989.

CHAPTER 42

Disorders of the Pericardium

PERICARDITIS AND THE PERICARDIAL RUB

I. INTRODUCTION. The pericardial rub is a physical sign of pericarditis, or inflammation of the pericardium, which is caused by a wide variety of disorders, including infections, connective tissue diseases, myocardial infarction, neoplasia, uremia, and trauma.

In the 1820s, shortly after the introduction of the stethoscope, Collin first described the pericardial rub, as a sound "similar to that of the crackling of new leather."[1]

II. THE FINDING. Pericardial rubs are grating, scratching, or creaking sounds that are loudest near the left sternal border and are most apparent when the patient is sitting upright, leaning forward, and holding his or her breath in deep expiration.[2,3] They resemble the sound of two pieces of sandpaper being rubbed together. Compared with heart murmurs, the pericardial rub has more high frequency energy and sounds closer to the ear.[2] Rubs often become louder during inspiration, and up to one fourth are palpable.[3]

In about 50% of patients, the rub has three components per cardiac cycle—one during ventricular systole and two during diastole (middiastole and atrial systole).[a] In about one third of patients, only two components are heard (usually the atrial and ventricular systolic rub), and in the remaining 15%, only a single-component ventricular systolic rub is heard.[3]

III. CLINICAL SIGNIFICANCE

A. The rub and pericarditis. Because the diagnosis of pericarditis relies on bedside criteria, one of which is the rub, the diagnostic accuracy of the rub cannot be assessed. The other two criteria for pericarditis are the characteristic pericardial chest pain (precordial pleuritic pain radiating to the trapezius ridge, which is relieved sitting up) and the characteristic electrocardiographic changes (diffuse concave ST elevation, PR segment depression, absence of Q waves).[4] Most clinical studies of pericarditis require two of these three criteria. Echocardiography is not a criteria for pericarditis because only half of patients with pericarditis have detectable pericardial effusions.[4]

B. The rub and pericardial effusion. Although the pericardial rub suggests the rubbing together of contiguous pericardial surfaces, the sound often persists after accumulation of significant pericardial effusions.[3] The rub is heard, for example, in up to one fourth of patients with cardiac tamponade (see below). Therefore, the *presence* of the rub cannot be used to argue *against* the development of pericardial effusion.

C. The rub and neoplastic disease. In patients with known cancer, who subsequently develop pericardial disease, the presence of a rub argues that the pericarditis is idiopathic or radiation-induced, not neoplastic pericarditis (sensitivity

---

[a] These three components represent the three moments in the cardiac cycle when the ventricle is moving the most.

62%, specificity 89%, positive LR = 5.5, negative LR = 0.4).[5]

D. The rub and myocardial infarction. A pericardial rub is found in 5% to 20% of patients with acute myocardial infarction, usually appearing between hospital days 1 to 3.[6-9] Compared with patients who do not develop rubs, patients with rubs have significantly larger myocardial infarctions; lower ejection fractions; more extensive coronary artery disease; and more complications, including congestive heart failure and atrial arrhythmias.[6,8,9] In these patients, however, tamponade is rare.

CARDIAC TAMPONADE

I. INTRODUCTION. Cardiac tamponade is present when a pericardial effusion has become so large and tense that intrapericardial pressures exceed the normal filling (i.e., diastolic) pressures of the heart, thus impairing diastolic filling of the heart and reducing cardiac output.

The history of diagnosing tamponade illustrates well the tension that sometimes exists between older diagnostic standards based on physical signs and newer ones based on clinical imaging. For example, early descriptions of tamponade, which were based on catastrophic acute intrapericardial hemorrhage, emphasized hypotension; elevated neck veins; and the small, quiet heart as diagnostic findings ("Beck's triad").[10,11] Later, after it became obvious that many medical patients with tamponade had normal blood pressure and loud heart tones, the definition of tamponade shifted to emphasize large pericardial effusions, elevated neck veins, pulsus paradoxus, and relief of symptoms and signs after pericardiocentesis.[12] Finally, in the 1980s, several echocardiographic criteria for tamponade were introduced,[11,13] although studies have subsequently shown that relying solely on these criteria sometimes identifies patients who fail to improve symptomatically or physiologically after pericardiocentesis.[14]

Therefore, the diagnosis of tamponade should not rely solely on the echocardiographic report but requires synthesis of all the findings, emphasizing especially the ones from physical diagnosis—elevated neck veins, tachycardia, and pulsus paradoxus.[15]

II. THE FINDINGS. Table 42-1 presents the physical signs observed in several studies of patients with

TABLE 42-1 Cardiac tamponade*

Physical Finding†	Frequency (%)‡
Neck Veins	
Elevated neck veins	100
Kussmaul's sign	0
Arterial Pulse	
Tachycardia (>100 beats/min)	81-100
Blood Pressure	
Systolic blood pressure >100 mm Hg	58-100
Pulsus paradoxus >10 mm Hg	98
Pulsus paradoxus >20 mm Hg	78
Pulsus paradoxus >30 mm Hg	49
Pulsus paradoxus >40 mm Hg	38
Total paradox	23
Auscultation of Heart	
Diminished heart tones	36-84
Pericardial rub	27
Other	
Hepatomegaly	58
Edema	27

Data from 121 patients from references 12 and 16 to 19.

*Diagnostic Standard: For *tamponade,* cardiac output that improved after drainage of pericardial effusion.

†Definition of finding: For *total paradox,* palpable pulse disappears completely during inspiration.

‡Results are overall mean frequency or, if statistically heterogenous, the range of values.

proven cardiac tamponade, most of whom presented with shortness of breath.[12,19] The definition and pathogenesis of elevated neck veins and pulsus paradoxus are discussed in Chapters 13 and 31.

The three key findings of tamponade are elevated neck veins (100% of patients), tachycardia (81 to 100% of patients), and pulsus paradoxus greater than 10 mm Hg (98% of patients). In patients with pericardial effusions, the finding of pulsus paradoxus >12 mm Hg detects tamponade with a sensitivity of 98%, specificity of 83%, positive LR of 5.9, and negative LR of 0.03 (see Chapter 13).[20]

Cardiac tamponade is one of the few causes of elevated neck veins with absent y descent (see Chapter 31). This finding contrasts sharply with the exaggerated y descent of constrictive pericarditis (see below).

CONSTRICTIVE PERICARDITIS

I. INTRODUCTION. Constrictive pericarditis is present when calcification or fibrosis of the pericardium impairs diastolic filling, which then elevates venous pressure and reduces cardiac output.

II. THE FINDINGS. Table 42-2 presents the physical signs of patients with constrictive pericarditis, most of whom presented with edema, abdominal swelling, and dyspnea.[25,26,28] The key physical findings are elevated neck veins (98%), prominent y descent in venous waveform (57% to 94%), pericardial knock (28% to 94%), and hepatomegaly (87% to 100%).

   A. Neck veins (see also Chapter 31). In addition to the elevated venous pressure, the venous waveform displays an unusually prominent y descent, which combined with an exaggerated x' descent creates two conspicuous dips per cardiac cycle, making the waveform appear to trace an "M" or "W" with each arterial pulse ("Friedrich's sign," see Chapter 31). Sometimes these movements are transmitted to the liver,

TABLE 42-2 Constrictive pericarditis*

PHYSICAL FINDING	FREQUENCY (%)†
Neck Veins	
Elevated neck veins	98
Prominent y descent (Friedrich's sign)	57-94
Kussmaul's sign	50
Arterial Pulse	
Irregularly irregular (atrial fibrillation)	36-70
Blood Pressure	
Pulsus paradoxus >10 mm Hg	17-43
Auscultation of Heart	
Pericardial knock	28-94
Pericardial rub	4
Other	
Hepatomegaly	87-100
Edema	63
Ascites	53-89

Data from 181 patients from references 16 and 21 to 27.

*Diagnostic standard: For constrictive pericarditis, surgical and postmortem findings,[16,21,22,25] sometimes in combination with hemodynamic findings.[23,24,26,27]

†Results are overall mean frequency or, if statistically heterogenous, the range of values.

causing it to pulsate inward twice with each cardiac cycle.[29]

The prominent y descent occurs because diastolic filling is only impaired during the last two thirds of diastole. At the moment the tricuspid valve opens (beginning of diastole and beginning of y descent), the right atrium empties rapidly and with no resistance (causing a prominent y descent), although eventually the relaxing ventricle meets the limits of the rigid pericardial shell and pressures again rise.[30] This finding contrasts with that observed in tamponade, which impairs diastolic filling throughout diastole and thus eliminates the y descent.

B. Kussmaul's sign. Kussmaul's sign is the paradoxical increase in venous pressure during inspiration. This sign, present in 50% of patients with constriction, is discussed in Chapter 31.

C. Pericardial knock. The pericardial knock is a loud, high-frequency early diastolic sound heard between the apex and left lower sternal border. It is discussed in Chapter 37.

D. Other findings. Up to 90% of patients with constrictive pericarditis have systolic retraction of the apical impulse (see Chapter 33).[27,31]

According to traditional teachings, pulsus paradoxus is not a finding of constrictive pericarditis, yet the studies reviewed in Table 42-2 show that pulsus paradoxus is present in 17% to 43% of patients with constrictive pericarditis.[16,21,26,28] This seeming contradiction probably reflects different definitions for pulsus paradoxus. If pulsus paradoxus is defined as >10 mm Hg inspiratory fall in systolic blood pressure (i.e., the usual definition), 17% to 43% of patients in these studies had the finding[16,28]; if instead it is defined as >20 mm Hg inspiratory fall, no patient had the finding.[16] In contrast, the usual pulsus paradoxus in patients with tamponade is 20 to 50 mm Hg (see Table 42-1).[12]

Therefore, mild degrees of pulsus paradoxus (10 to 20 mm Hg) are commonly observed in patients with constrictive pericarditis, but larger degrees (>20 mm Hg) are not and suggest tamponade or another cause of the finding (see Chapter 13).

REFERENCES

1. Stokes W. *An introduction to the use of the stethoscope* (facsimile edition by the Classics of Cardiology Library), Edinburgh, 1825, Maclachlin and Stewart.
2. Harvey WP. Auscultatory findings in diseases of the pericardium, *Am J Cardiol* 7:15-20, 1961.

3. Spodick DH. Pericardial rub: prospective, multiple observer investigation of pericardial friction in 100 patients, *Am J Cardiol* 35:357-362, 1975.

4. Permanyer-Miralda G, Sagrista-Sauleda J, and Soler-Soler J. Primary acute pericardial disease: a prospective series of 231 consecutive patients, *Am J Cardiol* 56:623-630, 1985.

5. Posner MR, Cohen GI, and Skarin AT. Pericardial disease in patients with cancer: the differentiation of malignant from idiopathic and radiation-induced pericarditis, *Am J Med* 71:407-413, 1981.

6. Tofler GH and others. Pericarditis in acute myocardial infarction: characterization and clinical significance, *Am Heart J* 117:86-91, 1989.

7. Lichstein E, Liu HM, and Gupta P. Pericarditis complication acute myocardial infarction: incidence of complications and significance of electrocardiogram on admission, *Am Heart J* 87:246-252, 1974.

8. Wall TC and others. Usefulness of a pericardial friction rub after thrombolytic therapy during acute myocardial infarction in predicting amount of myocardial damage, *Am J Cardiol* 66:1418-1421, 1990.

9. Dubois C and others. Frequency and clinical significance of pericardial friction rubs in the acute phase of myocardial infarction, *Eur Heart J* 6:766-768, 1985.

10. Beck CS. Two cardiac compression triads, *JAMA* 104:714-716, 1935.

11. Fowler NO. Cardiac tamponade: a clinical or an echocardiographic diagnosis? *Circulation* 87:1738-1741, 1993.

12. Guberman BA and others. Cardiac tamponade in medical patients, *Circulation* 64:633-640, 1981.

13. Himelman RB and others. Inferior vena cava plethora with blunted respiratory response: a sensitive echocardiographic sign of cardiac tamponade, *J Am Coll Cardiol* 12:1470-1477, 1988.

14. Levine MJ and others. Implications of echocardiographically assisted diagnosis of pericardial tamponade in contemporary medical patients: detection before hemodynamic embarrassment, *J Am Coll Cardiol* 17:59-65, 1991.

15. Hancock EW. Cardiac tamponade, *Heart Dis Stroke* 3:155-158, 1994.

16. Lange RL and others. Diagnostic signs in compressive cardiac disorders: constrictive pericarditis, pericardial effusion, and tamponade, *Circulation* 33:763-777, 1966.

17. Reddy PS and others. Cardiac tamponade: hemodynamic observations in man, *Circulation* 58:265-272, 1978.

18. Brown J and others. Elevated arterial blood pressure in cardiac tamponade, *N Engl J Med* 327:463-466, 1992.

19. Markiewicz W, Borovik R, and Ecker S. Cardiac tamponade in medical patients: treatment and prognosis in the echocardiographic era, *Am Heart J* 111:1138-1142, 1986.

20. Curtiss EI and others. Pulsus paradoxus: definition and relation to the severity of cardiac tamponade, *Am Heart J* 115:391-398, 1988.

21. Paul O, Castleman B, and White PD. Chronic constrictive pericarditis: a study of 53 cases, *Am J Med Sci* 216:361-377, 1948.

22. Mounsey P. The early diastolic sound of constrictive pericarditis, *Br Heart J* 17:143-152, 1955.

23. Tyberg TI, Goodyer AVN, and Langou RA. Genesis of pericardial knock in constrictive pericarditis, *Am J Cardiol* 46:570-575, 1980.

24. Schiavone WA. The changing etiology of constrictive pericarditis in a large referral center, *Am J Cardiol* 58:373-375, 1986.

25. Evans W and Jackson F. Constrictive pericarditis, *Br Heart J* 14:53-69, 1952.

26. Wood P. Chronic constrictive pericarditis, *Am J Cardiol* 7:48-61, 1961.

27. El-Sherif A and El-Said G. Jugular, hepatic, and praecordial pulsations in constrictive pericarditis, *Br Heart J* 33:305-312, 1971.

28. Cameron J and others. The etiologic spectrum of constrictive pericarditis, *Am Heart J* 113:354-360, 1987.

29. Coralli RJ and Crawley IS. Hepatic pulsations in constrictive pericarditis, *Am J Cardiol* 58:370-373, 1986.

30. Shabetai R, Fowler NO, and Guntheroth WG. The hemodynamics of cardiac tamponade and constrictive pericarditis, *Am J Cardiol* 26:480-489, 1970.

31. Boicourt OW, Nagle RE, and Mounsey JPD. The clinical significance of systolic retraction of the apical impulse, *Br Heart J* 27:379-391, 1965.

CHAPTER 43

Congestive Heart Failure

I. INTRODUCTION. Heart failure is a clinical syndrome characterized by impaired ventricular performance, elevated diastolic filling pressures, and diminished exercise capacity. Patients with heart failure and ventricular disease may have a low ventricular ejection fraction ("systolic dysfunction") or normal ejection fraction ("diastolic dysfunction").

Clear descriptions of the signs of heart failure date to the Middle Ages.[1] In the seventeenth century, just after Harvey published his discovery of the circulation of blood, clinicians began to correlate the pathologic observation of large heart chambers and congested lungs with the clinical observations of dyspnea and edema.[2]

II. THE FINDINGS. Many of the findings of heart failure are discussed fully in other chapters of this text, including pulsus alternans and the dicrotic pulse (see Chapter 13), Cheyne-Stokes respirations (see Chapter 17), crackles (see Chapter 26), elevated neck veins (see Chapter 31), the abdominojugular test (see Chapter 31), displaced apical impulse (see Chapter 33), and third heart sound (see Chapter 36).

This chapter reviews one finding not discussed extensively elsewhere, the abnormal Valsalva response, and then presents the diagnostic accuracy of all findings of congestive heart failure.

III. THE VALSALVA RESPONSE

A. Introduction. The "Valsalva maneuver" consists of forced expiration against a closed glottis after a full inspiration.[3] The "Valsalva response" refers to the changes in blood pressure and pulse that occur during both the strain phase of the maneuver and the recovery period after the strain is released.

Valsalva introduced his maneuver in 1704 as a technique to expel pus from the middle ear.[3,4] The maneuver was forgotten, however, until 1859, when Weber showed he could use it to interrupt his arterial pulse at will (an experiment he stopped after he made himself faint and develop convulsions).[4] Beginning in the 1950s, many different investigators reported that the Valsalva response was distinctly abnormal in patients with congestive heart failure.[5-9]

B. Technique. To perform the maneuver, the patient should take a deep breath in and bear down, as if straining to have a bowel movement. The clinician measures the Valsalva response by using a blood pressure cuff, as described below. In clinical studies, the straining phase is standardized by having the patient's mouthpiece connected to a pressure transducer, which should demonstrate an increment of 30 to 40 mm Hg for at least 10 seconds.

The Valsalva maneuver is contraindicated in patients with recent eye or central nervous system surgery or hemorrhage. It is also unwise to perform the maneuver in patients with acute coronary ischemia, because it may induce arrhythmias, although in patients with chronic ischemic heart disease, the maneuver is safe and was once even used to terminate episodes of angina.[10]

C. The normal Valsalva response. The normal
Valsalva response is divided into 4 phases (Figure 43-1).[3] In phase 1, the arterial systolic blood
pressure rises temporarily because the increased
intrathoracic pressure is transmitted directly to
the aorta. In phase 2, blood pressure falls be-

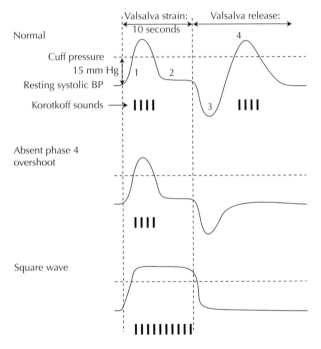

FIGURE 43-1 The Valsalva response. The *solid line* in each drawing
depicts changes in systolic blood pressure over time. The three types
of Valsalva responses are normal (*top*), absent phase 4 overshoot
(*middle*), and square wave (*bottom*). The clinician distinguishes these
responses by inflating the blood pressure cuff 15 mm Hg above the
patient's resting systolic blood pressure (horizontal dotted line) and
listening for Korotkoff sounds. Korotkoff sounds appear in phase
1 and 4 in the normal response, in phase 1 only in the absent phase
4 overshoot response, and in phases 1 and 2 only in the square wave
response. See text.

cause of reduced venous return with continuing straining. In phase 3, just after release of straining, pressure falls further because of temporary pooling of blood in the pulmonary veins. In phase 4, the arterial pressure overshoots to levels above the control values, primarily because of reflex sympathetic activity induced by previous hypotension. The changes in heart rate are exactly out of phase with the blood pressure: the heart rate increases during phases 2 and 3 and slows during phase 4.

The clinician identifies these 4 phases by inflating the blood pressure cuff on the patient's arm 15 mm Hg higher than the patient's resting systolic blood pressure and maintaining this cuff pressure during the straining phase and for 30 seconds afterwards, at the same time listening for Korotkoff sounds just as if measuring blood pressure. Korotkoff sounds appear whenever the patient's systolic pressure exceeds the cuff pressure. Therefore, during the normal Valsalva response, Korotkoff sounds appear during phase 1 and phase 4 but are absent during phases 2 and 3.

D. The abnormal Valsalva response (Figure 43-1). In patients with congestive heart failure, there are two abnormal Valsalva responses: **(1) absent phase 4 overshoot**, in which the arterial pressure fails to rise during phase 4 (Korotkoff sounds during phase 1 only), and **(2) square wave response**, in which the arterial pressure rises in parallel with intrathoracic pressure (Korotkoff sounds during phases 1 and 2 only).

In all three interpretable responses—normal, absent phase 4 overshoot, and square wave response—Korotkoff sounds appear during phase 1. If sounds do not appear during this phase, the intrathoracic pressure did not increase high enough during the maneuver, and the test is therefore *not* interpretable.

β-Blocker medications cause a false-positive response, primarily by eliminating the phase 4 overshoot.[11]

E. Pathogenesis of the abnormal Valsalva response. In patients with congestive heart failure, Korotkoff sounds fail to appear during phase 4 because the weakened heart cannot increase cardiac output in response to hypotension (there is a direct relationship between the degree of overshoot and patient's ejection fraction, $r = 0.72$).[11] Although the cause of the square wave response is still debated, it probably represents the combined effect of neurohormonal activation, peripheral venoconstriction, and increased central blood volume.[7,8,12] When central blood volume and central venous pressure are increased, the Valsalva maneuver may be unable to reduce venous return to the right heart and the congested lungs may have an ample supply of blood for the left heart, thus preventing phase 2 hypotension.[a]

IV. CLINICAL SIGNIFICANCE. Tables 43-1 and 43-2 present the diagnostic accuracy of physical signs for congestive heart failure. Table 43-1 refers to the diagnosis of elevated left heart filling pressures, and therefore applies to the diagnosis of systolic or diastolic dysfunction. The ability to accurately detect elevated left heart filling pressures is especially important in patients with dyspnea, because elevated pressures implicate the heart as the cause of the patient's symptoms. Table 43-2 refers to the diagnosis of depressed left ventricular ejection fraction and therefore applies only to the diagnosis of systolic dysfunction.

---

[a] The same pathophysiology probably explains the finding of reversed pulsus paradoxus in some patients with congestive heart failure receiving positive pressure ventilation (see Chapter 13).

TABLE 43-1 Congestive heart failure—elevated left heart filling pressures*

FINDING (REF)†	SENSITIVITY (%)	SPECIFICITY (%)	POSITIVE LR	NEGATIVE LR
Vital Signs				
Heart rate >100 beats/min at rest[13]	6	99	5.5	NS
Abnormal Valsalva response[14]	95	88	7.6	0.1
Lung Examination				
Crackles[11,13,15,16]	12-23	88-96	NS	NS
Heart Examination				
Elevated jugular venous pressure[11,13,16]	10-58	96-97	3.9	NS
Positive abdominojugular test[16-18]	55-84	83-98	8.0	0.3
Supine apical impulse lateral to MCL[15]	42	93	5.8	NS
S_3 gallop[11,13,15]	12-32	95-96	5.7	NS
S_4 gallop[11]	71	50	NS	NS
Other Findings				
Edema[11,13]	10	93-96	NS	NS

NS, Not significant; MCL, midclavicular line.

*Diagnostic standard: For elevated left heart filling pressures, pulmonary capillary wedge pressure >12 mm Hg[15] or >15 mm Hg,[14,16-18] or left ventricular end diastolic pressure >15 mm Hg.[11,13]

†Definition of findings: For abnormal Valsalva response, absent phase 4 overshoot or square wave response (see text); for positive abdominojugular test, sustained rise in jugular venous pressure during 10 to 15 seconds of midabdominal pressure (see text).

TABLE 43-2 Congestive heart failure—low ejection fraction*

Finding (ref)†	Sensitivity (%)	Specificity (%)	Positive LR	Negative LR
Vital Signs				
Abnormal Valsalva response[19,20]	69-88	90-91	7.6	0.3
Lung Examination				
Crackles[21,22]	10-24	90-98	NS	NS
Heart Examination				
Elevated neck veins[21]	7	98	NS	NS
Supine apical impulse lateral to MCL[21,22]	24-31	93-98	5.7	0.8
S_3 [21-23]	11-51	86-98	3.8	NS
Murmur of mitral regurgitation[22]	25	89	NS	NS
Other				
Hepatomegaly[21]	3	97	NS	NS
Edema[21]	8	98	NS	NS

NS, Not significant; MCL, midclavicular line.

*Diagnostic standards: For low ejection fraction, radionuclide left ventricular ejection fraction <0.50[19,20,22] or 0.53.[21]

†Definition of findings: For abnormal Valsalva response, absent phase 4 overshoot or square wave response (see text).

This information should only be used when evaluating patients similar to those enrolled in the studies cited in the Tables 43-1 and 43-2. These patients were all adults who presented to the clinician primarily for evaluation of chest pain or dyspnea. Most had no prior history of congestive heart failure, and many had an alternative explanation for dyspnea, such as lung disease.

A. **Detecting elevated left heart filling pressures.** In descending order of their positive LRs, the findings arguing most for the diagnosis of elevated filling pressures are a positive abdominojugular test (LR = 8.0; see Table 43-1), abnormal Valsalva response (i.e., either absent phase 4 overshoot or square wave response, LR = 7.6), displaced apical impulse (LR = 5.8), third heart sound (LR = 5.7), tachycardia (LR = 5.5), and elevated venous pressure (LR = 3.9). The absence of any of these findings (excepting the abnormal Valsalva response and positive abdominojugular test) provides the clinician no useful diagnostic information because many patients with heart failure lack these findings.

The presence of crackles, fourth heart sound, or edema does not indicate elevated left heart filling pressures in these patients. Crackles are unhelpful because they are infrequent in chronic heart failure and because many other disorders causing dyspnea also produce crackles. If the finding of crackles is instead just applied to patients with known cardiomyopathy (e.g., those awaiting cardiac transplantation), they become a more accurate sign of elevated filling pressure, detecting pulmonary capillary wedge pressures of 20 mm Hg or more with a sensitivity of 19% to 64%, specificity of 82% to 94%, and positive LR of 3.4. The finding is more accurate in this setting probably because other diagnoses causing crackles have already been excluded.[16,24,25]

B. **Detecting depressed left ventricular ejection fraction.** In comparison to the diagnosis of elevated left heart filling pressures, relatively few signs accurately indicate depressed ejection fraction (i.e., ejection fraction <50%): these are abnormal Valsalva response (either absent phase 4 overshoot or square wave response, LR = 7.6; see Table 43-2), a displaced apical impulse (LR = 5.7), and a third heart sound (LR = 3.8). The *absence* of any of these findings (excepting Valsalva response) is not particularly compelling because many patients with ejection fractions less than 50% lack these findings. However, the absence of the third heart sounds does argue against ejection fractions less than 30% (LR = 0.3; see Chapter 36).[22,23]

Some investigators believe that the abnormal Valsalva response is primarily a sign of elevated filling pressures, not low ejection fractions, citing data correlating the degree of Valsalva abnormality with left atrial pressure ($r = 0.77$, $p = .005$) but not ejection fraction.[14,26,27] This apparent contradiction may reflect varying prevalences of diastolic dysfunction in different investigators' practices. Assuming that the sign is primarily one of elevated filling pressures, it therefore also will be a good sign of depressed ejection fraction if most patients with heart failure in the clinician's practice have systolic dysfunction (Table 43-2),[19,20] but it will not predict ejection fraction if there is a mixture of patients with systolic and diastolic dysfunction.[14,26,27]

Several findings provide no useful diagnostic information when assessing the patient's ejection fraction: crackles, elevated neck veins, murmur of mitral regurgitation, hepatomegaly, or edema (all LRs not significant; see Table 43-2).

C. **Proportional pulse pressure.** In patients with known dilated cardiomyopathy and severe left ventricular dysfunction, a proportional pulse pressure (i.e., arterial pulse pressure divided by the systolic blood pressure) less than 0.25 detects a low cardiac index (of 2.2 L/min/m^2) with a sensitivity of 91%, specificity of 83%, positive LR of 5.4 and negative LR of 0.1.[25]

D. Prognosis in heart failure. In patients with clinically suspected ischemic heart disease, the physical signs of heart failure are independent predictors of mortality, adding prognostic information to that already provided by the patient's age, exercise capacity, and measured ejection fraction.[28,29] One-year cardiac mortality is higher for those with a displaced apical impulse (39% vs. 12% without the finding, $p = .005$) or the third heart sound (57% vs. 14% without the finding, $p = .002$).[15]

REFERENCES

1. Lutz JE. A XII century description of congestive heart failure, *Am J Cardiol* 61:494-495, 1988.
2. Nolan J. A historical review of heart failure, *Scot Med J* 38:53-57, 1993.
3. Nishimura RA and Tajik AJ. The Valsalva maneuver and response revisited, *Mayo Clin Proc* 61:211-217, 1986.
4. Dawson PM. An historical sketch of the Valsalva experiment, *Bull Hist Med* 14:295-320, 1943.
5. Ard RW and Twining RH. Evaluation of Valsalva test in bedside diagnosis of dyspnea, *Am J Med Sci* 234:403-412, 1957.
6. Burroughs RW and Bruce RA. Significance of abnormal phase II response to Valsalva maneuver in cardiac patients, *Circulation* 14:72-76, 1956.
7. Gorlin R, Knowled JH, and Storey CF. The Valsalva maneuver as a test of cardiac function, *Am J Med* 22:197-212, 1957.
8. Judson WE, Hatcher JD, and Wilkins RW. Blood pressure responses to the Valsalva maneuver in cardiac patients with and without congestive failure, *Circulation* 11:889-899, 1955.
9. Irvin CW. Valsalva maneuver as a diagnostic aid, *JAMA* 170:787-791, 1959.

10. Levine HJ, McIntryre KM, and Glovsky MM. Relief of angina pectoris by Valsalva maneuver, *N Engl J Med* 275:487-488, 1966.

11. Zema MJ and others. Left ventricular dysfunction: bedside Valsalva manoevre, *Br Heart J* 44:560-569, 1980.

12. Brunner-LaRocca H and others. Is blood pressure response to the Valsalva maneuver related to neurohormones, exercise capacity, and clinical findings in heart failure? *Chest* 116:861-867, 1999.

13. Harlan WR and others. Chronic congestive heart failure in coronary artery disease: clinical criteria, *Ann Intern Med* 86:133-138, 1977.

14. Schmidt DE and Shah PK. Accurate detection of elevated left ventricular filling pressure by a simplified bedside application of the Valsalva maneuver, *Am J Cardiol* 71:462-464, 1993.

15. Gadsboll N and others. Symptoms and signs of heart failure in patients with myocardial infarction: reproducibility and relationship to chest x-ray, radionuclide ventriculography and right heart catheterization, *Eur Heart J* 10:1017-1028, 1989.

16. Butman SM and others. Bedside cardiovascular examination in patients with severe chronic heart failure: importance of rest or inducible jugular venous distension, *J Am Coll Cardiol* 22:968-974, 1993.

17. Sochowski RA, Dubbin JD, and Naqvi SZ. Clinical and hemodynamic assessment of the hepatojugular reflux, *Am J Cardiol* 66:1002-1006, 1990.

18. Ewy GA. The abdominojugular test: technique and hemodynamic correlates, *Ann Intern Med* 109:456-460, 1988.

19. Zema MJ, Caccavano M, and Kligfield P. Detection of left ventricular dysfunction in ambulatory subjects with the bedside Valsalva maneuver, *Am J Med* 75:241-248, 1983.

20. Zema MJ, Masters AP, and Margouleff D. Dyspnea: the heart or the lungs? Differentiation at bedside by use of the simple Valsalva maneuver, *Chest* 85:59-64, 1984.

21. Gadsboll N and others. Interobserver agreement and accuracy of bedside estimation of right and left ventricular ejection fraction in acute myocardial infarction, *Am J Cardiol* 63:1301-1307, 1989.

22. Mattleman SJ and others. Reliability of bedside evaluation in determining left ventricular function: correlation with left ventricular ejection fraction determined by radionuclide ventriculography, *J Am Coll Cardiol* 1:417-420, 1983.

23. Patel R, Bushnell DL, and Sobotka PA. Implications of an audible third heart sound in evaluating cardiac function, *West J Med* 158:606-609, 1993.

24. Chakko S and others. Clinical, radiographic, and hemodynamic correlations in chronic congestive heart failure: conflicting results may lead to inappropriate care, *Am J Med* 90:353-359, 1991.

25. Stevenson LW and Perloff JK. The limited reliability of physical signs for estimating hemodynamics in chronic heart failure, *JAMA* 261:884-888, 1989.

26. McIntyre KM and others. A noninvasive method of predicting pulmonary-capillary wedge pressure, *N Engl J Med* 327:1715-1720, 1992.

27. Bernardi L, Saviolo R, and Spodick DH. Do hemodynamic responses to the Valsalva maneuver reflect myocardial dysfunction? *Chest* 95:986-991, 1989.

28. Marantz PR and others. Prognosis in ischemic heart disease. Can you tell as much at the bedside as in the nuclear laboratory? *Arch Intern Med* 152:2433-2437, 1992.

29. Likoff MJ, Chandler SL, and Kay HR. Clinical determinants of mortality in chronic congestive heart failure secondary to idiopathic dilated or to ischemic cardiomyopathy, *Am J Cardiol* 59:634-638, 1987.

PART NINE

Abdomen

CHAPTER 44

Inspection of the Abdomen

This chapter reviews two physical signs, ecchymosis of the abdominal wall and Sister Mary Joseph's nodule. Jaundice and dilated abdominal veins are discussed in Chapter 6, the signs of malnutrition in Chapter 10, and abnormal respiratory movements of the abdominal wall in Chapter 17.

ECCHYMOSIS OF THE ABDOMINAL WALL

I. THE FINDINGS. Ecchymosis of the abdominal wall is an important sign of retroperitoneal or intraperitoneal hemorrhage. Periumbilical ecchymosis is called "Cullen's sign," after the American pathologist and clinician who first described the finding in a patient with ectopic pregnancy in 1918.[a] Flank ecchymosis is often called "Grey Turner's sign" or "Turner's sign," after the British surgeon Gilbert Grey Turner who described the sign in a patient with hemorrhagic pancreatitis in 1920.[3] Nonetheless, Cullen's and Turner's signs are

---

[a] Cullen was well versed in the anatomy of the umbilicus, having just 2 years before his report published the book *Embryology, Anatomy, and Diseases of the Umbilicus, Together with the Urachus*, which contained 27 chapters on the umbilicus.[1,2]

rare, occurring in less than 3% of patients with pancreatitis[4] and less than 1% of patients with ruptured ectopic pregnancy.[5] Both signs have since been described in a wide variety of other disorders, including intrahepatic hemorrhage from tumor,[6,7] ischemic bowel,[8] splenic rupture,[9] rectus sheath hematoma,[10] perforated duodenal ulcer,[11] ruptured abdominal aortic aneurysm,[12] and after percutaneous liver biopsy.[13]

II. PATHOGENESIS. The discoloration of the skin is actually due to the collection of blood in the subcutaneous fascial planes, not the dispersion of red cells within lymphatics as has been sometimes surmised.[14] In patients with pancreatitis, computed tomography often reveals collections of fluid within the fascial planes behind the kidney, which at some point may reach the lateral border of the quadratus lumborum muscle, from where they may pass to the subcutaneous tissues of the lateral abdominal wall.[15] Presumably, the mechanism of Grey Turner's sign in other causes of retroperitoneal hemorrhage is the same. In most patients with Cullen's signs, blood travels to the periumbilical area through the falciform ligament, which connects to the retroperitoneum via the lesser omentum and transverse mesocolon (the falciform ligament and lesser omentum are the embryologic remnants of the ventral mesentery, into which the liver has grown).

In patients with ectopic pregnancy, however, the falciform ligament is probably not responsible for Cullen's sign because the ecchymosis of these patients is often located on the abdominal wall below the umbilicus, yet the falciform ligament attaches to the abdominal wall above the umbilicus. Some investigators have hypothesized that fascial planes connecting the broad ligament and the lower abdominal wall are responsible for Cullen's sign in ectopic pregnancy,[15] although this does not explain why the sign sometimes appears in patients with free rupture into the peritoneal cavity outside of the broad ligament.[5]

SISTER MARY JOSEPH'S NODULE

I. THE FINDING. Sister Mary Joseph's nodule is metastatic carcinoma of the umbilicus. It usually presents as a hard, dermal or subcutaneous nodule, and in about 20% of patients with the lesion, it represents the initial sign of malignancy.[16] Most patients have metastatic adenocarcinoma, usually from the stomach, large bowel, pancreas, or ovary.[16,17] It is an ominous sign, the average survival after discovery being only 10 to 11 months.[16,17]

The finding is named after Sister Mary Joseph, who, as first surgical assistant to William J. Mayo, noted the association between the umbilical nodule and intraabdominal malignancy (Sister Mary Joseph was born Julia Dempsey in 1856; before Vatican II in 1965, all Franciscan nuns took the name of Mary as a prefix to an additional name).[18,19] Dr. Mayo discussed the sign as early as 1928, calling it the "pants-button umbilicus,"[20] and it was not until Sir Hamilton Bailey's 1949 edition of *Physical Signs in Clinical Surgery* (10 years after Sister Mary Joseph's death) that the term "Sister Joseph's nodule" was used.[21]

A mimic of the Sister Mary Joseph nodule is an omphalith, which is the hardened concretion of keratin and sebum in the umbilicus from inadequate hygiene.[22] Careful examination of these patients, however, manages to extract the debris.

II. PATHOGENESIS. There are many potential avenues of spread to the umbilicus: vascular and lymphatic connections to the retroperitoneum, axilla, and inguinal regions, and embryologic remnants that connect the umbilicus to the bladder and retroperitoneum.[23] Nonetheless, the umbilicus and periumbilical tissues represent the thinnest part of the abdominal wall, and in one series of patients, direct spread from peritoneal tumor implants through the abdominal wall was the most common cause of the umbilical nodule.[16]

REFERENCES

1. Young RH. History of gynecological pathology. I. Dr. Thomas S. Cullen, *Int J Gynecol Pathol* 15:181-186, 1996.
2. Cullen TS. *Embryology, anatomy, and diseases of the umbilicus, together with the urachus,* Philadelphia, 1916, WB Saunders.
3. Turner GG. Local discoloration of the abdominal wall as a sign of acute pancreatitis, *Br J Surg* 7:394-395, 1920.
4. Dickson AP and Imrie CW. The incidence and prognosis of body wall ecchymosis in acute pancreatitis, *Surg Gynecol Obstet* 159:343-347, 1984.
5. Merrill JA. Cullen's sign: a historical review and report of histologic observations, *Obstet Gynecol* 12:317-324, 1958.
6. Mabin TA and Gelfand M. Cullen's signs, a feature in liver disease, *Br Med J* 1:493-494, 1974.
7. Marinella MA. Cullen's sign associated with metastatic thyroid cancer, *N Engl J Med* 340:149-150, 1999.
8. Kelley ML. Discolorations of flanks and abdominal wall, *Arch Intern Med* 108:132-135, 1961.
9. Chung MA, Oung C, and Szilagyi A. Cullen's sign: it doesn't always mean hemorrhagic pancreatitis, *Am J Gastroenterol* 87:1026-1028, 1992.
10. Guthrie CM and Stanfey HA. Rectus sheath haematoma presenting with Cullen's sign and Grey-Turner's sign, *Scot Med J* 41:54-55, 1996.
11. Evans DM. Cullen's sign in perforated duodenal ulcer, *Br Med J* 1:154, 1971.
12. Armour RH, Clifton MA, and Marsh CH. Balloon catheter control of a rupture abdominal aortic aneurysm in a patient with Cullen's sign, *Br J Surg* 65:350, 1978.
13. Capron JP and others. Cullen's sign after percutaneous liver biopsy, *Gastroenterology* 73:1185-1191, 1977.
14. Bem J and Bradley EL. Subcutaneous manifestations of severe acute pancreatitis, *Pancreas* 16:551-555, 1998.
15. Meyers MA, Feldberg MAM, and Oliphant M. Grey Turner's sign and Cullen's sign in acute pancreatitis, *Gastrointest Radiol* 14:31-37, 1989.

16. Powell FC and others. Sister Mary Joseph's nodule: a clinical and histologic study, *J Am Acad Dermatol* 10:610-615, 1984.

17. Dubreuil A and others. Umbilical metastasis or Sister Mary Joseph's nodule, *Int J Dermatol* 37:7-13, 1998.

18. Nelson CW. Historical profiles of Mayo: 100th anniversary of Sister Mary Joseph Dempsey, *Mayo Clin Proc* 67:512, 1992.

19. O'Neill TW and O'Brien AAJ. Sister (Mary) Joseph's nodule, *Ir Med J* 80:296, 1987.

20. Key JD, Shephard DAE, and Walters W. Sister Mary Joseph's nodule and its relationship to diagnosis of carcinoma of the umbilicus, *Minn Med* 59:561-566, 1976.

21. Bailey H. *Demonstrations of physical signs in clinical surgery,* ed 11, Baltimore, 1949 Williams & Wilkins, p. 426.

22. Amaro R and others. Pseudo Sister Mary Joseph's Nodule, *Am J Gastroenterol* 94:1949-1950, 1999.

23. Coll DM and others. Imaging appearances of Sister Mary Joseph's nodule, *Br J Radiol* 72:1230-1233, 1999.

Palpation and Percussion of the Abdomen

I. INTRODUCTORY COMMENTS ON TECHNIQUE.

Palpation of the abdomen may reveal abnormal tenderness, tumors, hernias, aneurysms, or organomegaly (i.e., of the liver, spleen, or gallbladder). To help the patient relax and to minimize pain during palpation, experienced clinicians all recommend that the clinician's hands should be warm, the technique soft and gentle, and the expected tender areas palpated last. Other maneuvers designed to help the patient relax include drawing up the patient's knees, encouraging deep breathing, or engaging the patient in conversation.

In the days before clinical imaging, palpation of a relaxed abdomen was so essential that patients with tense abdominal muscles were often reexamined after immersion in a hot bath or after anesthesia had been induced with ether or chloroform to determine whether an abnormality was present or not.[1]

II. LIVER

A. Liver span

1. The finding. The liver span is the distance in centimeters between the upper border of the liver in the right midclavicular line, as determined by percussion (i.e., where lung resonance changes to liver dullness), and the lower border, as determined by either percussion or palpation. Clinicians have been measuring the liver span ever since Piorry introduced topographic percussion in 1828.[2-4] After introduction of the x-ray, however, it became apparent that the estimated span often differed from the actual span, and most clinicians instead adopted the view that the percussed liver span was just an index of liver size, not a precise measurement.[5]

2. **Clinical significance.** The clinician's assessment of liver span almost always underestimates the actual value. Clinicians place the upper border too low (2 to 5 cm)[6,7] and lower border too high (>2 cm in about half of patients),[6,8] except in patients with chronic obstructive lung disease, in whom the error with the top border is less.[6] The liver span is the same whether the patient is percussed during quiet respirations or full held expiration.[9]

Nonetheless, most studies of liver span make two important points: (1) The estimated span correlates modestly with actual span, as determined by ultrasonography or scintigraphy ($r = 0.6$ to 0.7).[5,7,8,10] This correlation is much better in patients with diseased livers than with healthy livers.[7,10] (2) The percussed liver span is very dependent on the clinician's technique, and consequently, one clinician's "normal liver span" is not the same as another's. The heavier the clinician's percussion stroke, the smaller the measured span, and the greater the error in underestimating the actual liver size (see also Chapter 25).[6,9] This explains why published estimates of the "normal liver span" range from as low as 6 cm to as high as 15 cm[a,8,12-14] and why experienced clinicians in one study, each examining the same patient, differed in their estimate of the patient's span, *on average*, by 8 cm.[15]

Each clinician should therefore determine for himself or herself what the "normal liver span" is, using his or her own percussion technique on hundreds of healthy persons. This span then becomes the benchmark to indicate whether a patient's span is abnormally large or not.

B. Palpable liver edge

1. **The finding.** To palpate the liver edge, the clinician begins by gently palpating the patient's right *lower* quadrant. As the patient breathes in and out, the clinician moves the palpating hand upward 1 to 2 centimeters at a time, at each location searching for a liver edge that moves down during inspiration and strikes the clinician's fingers. Once the edge is located, the clinician should note its consistency (a cirrhotic liver is firmer than a healthy one)[10] and whether the edge has any irregularities or masses.[16]

   Anatomically, the normal liver extends on average 5 cm below the right costal margin at the midclavicular line.[7]

2. **Clinical significance.** If clinicians palpate what they believe is the patient's liver edge extending below the costal margin, they are virtually always correct (LR = 233.7; Table 45-1). Nonetheless, the distance between the liver edge and costal margin has little to do with the overall liver size, and the finding of a palpable liver edge is an unreliable sign of hepatomegaly (LR = only 1.7; see Table

---

[a] The normal upper limit for the cephalocaudad dimension of the liver on ultrasonography is 13 cm.[11]

TABLE 45-1 Palpation and percussion of liver and spleen*

Finding (ref)†	Sensitivity (%)	Specificity (%)	Positive LR	Negative LR
Liver				
Palpable Liver				
Detecting liver edge below costal margin[17]	48	100	233.7	0.5
Detecting enlarged liver[18-20]	50-71	56-77	1.7	0.5
Spleen				
Palpable Spleen				
Detecting enlarged spleen[18,19,21-25]	18-69	89-99	9.6	0.6
Splenic Percussion Signs				
Detecting enlarged spleen[22,23,26]				
Spleen percussion sign (Castell's)	25-81	46-94	1.9	0.7
Nixon method	25-65	68-95	NS	NS
Traube's space dullness	11-62	72-95	2.0	NS

NS, Not significant.

*Diagnostic standard: For enlarged liver, liver enlarged by scintigraphy[18,20] or postmortem weight of liver >2000 g[19]; for enlarged spleen, spleen enlarged by ultrasonography,[22,23] scintigraphy,[18,21,24,26] or postmortem weight >200 g[19] or >250 g.[25]

†Definition of findings: For splenic percussion signs, see text.

45-1). Moreover, about half of livers that extend below the costal margin are not palpable.[10,17] The *consistency* of the liver parenchyma probably determines in part whether a liver is palpable because in patients with cirrhosis, whose livers are smaller but firmer than normal, the liver's edge is palpable 95% of the time.[10]

C. Auscultatory percussion—"scratch test"

1. The finding.
Auscultatory percussion (see also Chapter 25) is frequently used to locate the lower border of the liver. According to traditional teachings, the moment the clinician's percussing digit crosses the border of the liver and begins to strike abdominal wall over the liver, the sound heard through the stethoscope becomes louder.

Nonetheless, the lack of consensus on the proper technique of locating the liver will quickly discourage the serious student of auscultatory percussion. Various experts recommend placing the stethoscope on the xiphoid,[6,27] near the umbilicus,[28] superior to[29] or at the costal margin,[30] at four separate positions over the liver,[31] or above the suspected center.[32] According to various authorities, the clinician should percuss with a finger and pleximeter,[32] a finger alone,[29] a bristle brush,[31] or a corrugated rod.[31] The direction of the stroke should be circular,[1] centripetal,[32] centrifugal,[31] left to right,[30] or always in a longitudinal axis and toward the liver.[6,29]

2. Clinical significance.
The evidence supporting auscultatory percussion of the liver is mixed and meager. Only one study supports the technique, showing that 78% of estimates of the lower border are within 2 cm of the actual border (by ultrasonography), compared with 44% for conventional percussion and palpation.[29] Another study

showed that palpation of the liver was more accurate than auscultatory percussion.[6] A third study showed that there was no correlation whatsoever between the distance of the liver edge below the costal margin, located by auscultatory percussion, and the actual distance (by ultrasonography) for any of 11 different examiners.[27]

D. Pulsatile liver. The finding of a pulsatile liver has been described in tricuspid regurgitation with high pulmonary pressures (30% to 91% of patients; see Chapter 41)[33-37] and constrictive pericarditis (55% of patients in one study).[38,39] In patients with the holosystolic murmur of tricuspid regurgitation, the finding of a pulsatile liver argues that the regurgitation is moderate to severe (LR = 3.9).[37]

III. THE SPLEEN

A. Palpable spleen

1. The finding. Experts recommend many different ways to palpate the spleen: some palpate from the patient's right side and others from the patient's left side (curling the fingers over the costal margin to "hook" the spleen edge); some position the patient supine, others position the patient supine with the patient's left fist under his or her left posterior chest, and still others position the patient in the right lateral decubitus position. One study comparing the three different positions found all to be equivalent,[23] and the approach the clinician uses probably depends most on personal preference.

2. Clinical significance

a. Detection of splenomegaly. Table 45-1 indicates that the finding of a palpable spleen argues strongly *for* splenomegaly (LR = 9.6; see Table 45-1). Although many enlarged spleens are not palpable (sensitivity is only 18% to 69%), virtually all massively enlarged spleens (i.e., weight >1 g or scintigraphic span >22 cm) are detectable by palpation.[25,40]

b. Etiology of splenomegaly. The common causes of splenomegaly are hepatic disease (i.e., portal hypertension), hematologic disorders (e.g., leukemias, lymphomas, myelofibrosis), infectious disease (e.g., HIV infection), and primary splenic disorders (e.g., splenic infarction or hematoma).[41,42] The presence of left upper quadrant tenderness and pain argues *for* a primary splenic disorder or hematologic disorder.[42] Associated lymphadenopathy practically excludes hepatic disease and points to one of the other disorders (LR = 0.04).[42] The finding of a palpable liver argues *for* hepatic disease (LR = 2.7), and the finding of massive splenomegaly (i.e., spleen extends to level of umbilicus) argues modestly for hematologic disease (LR = 2.1).[42]

B. Splenic percussion signs

1. The findings. There are three commonly used splenic percussion signs:

a. Spleen percussion sign. Castell described this sign in 1967,[13] finding it a useful way to measure splenic size in patients with infectious mononucleosis. The clinician percusses the lowest left intercostal space in the anterior axillary line (usually the eighth or ninth); if the percussion note in this location, usually resonant, becomes dull with a full inspiration, the test is positive. Since Castell's original description, other investigators have regarded any dullness at this location as a positive response (i.e., whether during inspiration or expiration).

b. Nixon's method. Nixon described this sign in 1954,[43] finding it accurate in his experience of 60 splenic aspiration biopsies. The patient is positioned in the right lateral decubitus position, and the clinician percusses from the lower level of pulmonary resonance in the posterior axillary line downwards obliquely to the lower midanterior costal margin. The test is positive if the border of dullness on this line lies more than 8 cm from the costal margin.

c. **Traube's space dullness.** Traube's space is the triangular space, normally tympanic, that is over the left lower anterior part of the chest. Its upper border is marked by the limits of cardiac dullness (usually the sixth rib), its lower border is the costal margin, and its lateral border is the anterior axillary line. Although Traube suggested that dullness in this space was a sign of pleural effusion,[44] Parrino in 1987 suggested that it could be a sign of splenic enlargement.[45]

2. **Clinical significance.** Positive percussion signs are much less convincing than palpation (positive LRs = 2.0 to insignificant; see Table 45-1). Traube's space dullness becomes even less accurate in overweight patients or those who have recently eaten.[46]

IV. GALLBLADDER: COURVOISIER'S SIGN

A. **The finding.** Courvoisier's sign is a *palpable nontender* gallbladder in a patient with *jaundice,* a finding that has been traditionally associated with malignant obstruction of the biliary system. Many textbooks call the sign "Courvoisier's law," as if the positive result were pathognomonic of malignancy, although the Swiss surgeon Courvoisier originally presented the finding in 1890 as only an interesting observation.[47] Writing in a monograph on biliary tract disorders, he stated that, among 187 patients with jaundice and common duct obstruction, a dilated gallbladder was found in only 20% of patients with stones, compared with 92% of patients having other disorders, mostly malignancy.[48,49]

B. Clinical significance. Summarizing the information about Courvoisier's sign is difficult because various authors define the sign differently. Some apply it to patients without jaundice (clearly not what Courvoisier intended)[50]; others define the positive sign as any palpable gallbladder, tender or nontender (some patients with cholecystitis have tender enlarged gallbladders)[51-53]; and still others expand the positive sign to include a dilated gallbladder discovered during surgery, clinical imaging, or even autopsy.[54]

Restricting analysis to those studies defining the positive sign as a palpable gallbladder in a jaundiced patient, Table 45-2 indicates that Courvoisier's sign is a compelling argument *for* extrahepatic obstruction of the biliary system (i.e., stones or malignancy, LR = 26.0) and *against* hepatocellular jaundice. Among patients with biliary obstruction, however, the sign argues only modestly for malignancy and against stones (LR = 2.6). Consequently, if there is a "law" to Courvoisier's sign, it is that the palpable gallbladder in a jaundiced patient indicates extrahepatic obstruction, not that the obstruction is caused by malignancy.

C. Pathogenesis. Courvoisier's original hypothesis—that the gallbladder of choledocholithiasis fails to dilate because its walls are fibrotic from chronic cholecystitis—is probably incorrect because experiments with gallbladders of jaundiced patients show that the wall stiffness of dilated and nondilated gallbladders is similar.[64] Instead, patients with dilated gallbladders have (1) much higher operative intraduc-

TABLE 45-2 Palpation of gallbladder and aorta*

Finding (ref)	Sensitivity (%)	Specificity (%)	Positive LR	Negative LR
Gallbladder				
Palpable Gallbladder				
Detecting obstructed bile ducts in patients with jaundice[55]	31	99	26.0	0.7
Detecting malignant obstruction in patients with obstructive jaundice[50,52,55,56]	26-55	83-90	2.6	0.7
Aorta				
Expansile Pulsating Epigastric Mass				
Detecting abdominal aortic aneurysm[57-63]	22-68	75-99	7.6	0.6

*Diagnostic standard: For *obstructive jaundice and malignant obstruction*, needle biopsy of liver, surgical exploration, or autopsy; for *abdominal aortic aneurysm*, ultrasonography revealing focal dilation of infrarenal aorta >3 cm in diameter,[59,61-63] >4 cm in diameter,[60] or >1.5 cm larger than proximal aorta.[57]

tal pressures and (2) longer duration of jaundice than those with normal-sized gallbladders.

The relationship between duration of jaundice and dilation of gallbladder explains why Courvoisier's original findings are different from the studies in Table 45-2. When analysis is restricted to just those patients with extrahepatic obstruction, the sensitivity of the dilated gallbladder in malignant obstruction today (25% to 55%) is lower than it was for Courvoisier (i.e., 92%) (although the specificity is similar, 80% to 90%). The reduced sensitivity may simply reflect the fact that patients with malignant obstruction today, compared with those from a century ago, are diagnosed sooner with clinical imaging, before pressures rise enough to enlarge the gallbladder greatly.

V. BLADDER VOLUME. For over a century clinicians have investigated percussing the suprapubic area to detect bladder volume, most studies revealing that the bladder volume must be about 400 to 600 ml before dullness reliably appears.[65] Although the extent of dullness above the symphysis pubis does correlate with bladder volume,[65,66] overall the sign is unreliable because the results vary tremendously among individual patients and because many patients have inexplicable dullness of the lower abdomen, even without bladder distention.[4,65]

VI. ASCITES
  A. The findings. In patients with ascites lying supine, peritoneal fluid gravitates to the flanks, and the air-filled intestines float up to occupy the periumbilical space. This distribution of fluid and air causes four characteristic signs of ascites: **(1) Bulging flanks. (2) Flank dullness.** Flank dullness is positive if there is a *horizontal* border between dullness in the flank area and resonance or tympany in the periumbilical

area. **(3) Shifting dullness.** Shifting dullness describes flank dullness whose position shifts as the patient changes position, usually by rolling on to one side. The sign is based on the principle that the air-filled loops of intestine, floating on peritoneal fluid, move to the uppermost position in the abdomen. In a patient with a positive response, the border between resonance and dullness shifts away from the side that is most dependent. To be positive, the shifting border should remain horizontal. **(4) Fluid wave.** To elicit the fluid wave, the clinician places one hand against the lateral wall of the abdomen and uses the other hand to tap firmly on the opposite lateral wall. In the positive response, the tap generates a wave that is transmitted through the abdomen and felt as a sudden shock by the other hand. Since a false-positive response may result from waves traveling through the subcutaneous tissue of the anterior abdominal wall, the clinician should always use the patient's hand or that of an assistant to apply firm pressure during the test against the anterior abdominal wall.

In addition to these four signs, most patients with ascites also have edema, from hypoalbuminemia and the weight of the peritoneal fluid compressing the veins to the legs.[67]

B. Pathogenesis. In experiments with cadavers performed a century ago, Müller showed that 1000 ml of fluid injected into the peritoneal space was undetectable by physical examination (i.e., flank or shifting dullness), 1500 ml resulted in some flank dullness, and 2000 ml was the smallest volume to cause shifting dullness.[65] The living abdominal wall is probably more elastic than the cadaver's, and it is likely that the careful clinician can detect smaller amounts of ascites in patients, but one small study of healthy volunteers still showed that injection of 500 to 1100 ml of fluid was necessary before shifting dullness appeared.[68] A significant cause of false-positive flank dullness or shifting dullness is accumulation of fluid within loops of the colon.[68,69] This condition, called "pseudoascites" in the days before clinical imaging,[69] typically occurred in patients with diarrheal illnesses.

C. **Clinical significance.** In patients with abdominal distention, the findings arguing the most *for* ascites are the positive fluid wave (LR = 5.0; Table 45-3) and presence of edema (LR = 3.8). The strongest arguments *against* the presence of ascites are the absence of edema (LR = 0.2) and the absence of flank dullness (LR = 0.3). Shifting dullness shifts the probability of ascites modestly upward when present (LR = 2.3) and modestly downward when absent (LR = 0.4). Findings having relatively little diagnostic value are positive flank dullness, positive bulging flanks, and negative fluid wave. The finding of a flat or everted umbilicus was also diagnostically unhelpful in one study.[71]

Auscultatory percussion also has been recommended to detect ascites,[73-75] although only the puddle sign (auscultatory percussion of the prone patient) has been formally tested,[70,71] proving to be diagnostically unhelpful.

VII. ABDOMINAL AORTIC ANEURYSM

A. **Introduction.** Abdominal aortic aneurysm is a focal ballooning of the infrarenal abdominal aorta, traditionally defined as a diameter greater than 3 to 4 cm. It is a disorder of elderly patients, affecting 1% to 2% of patients over the age of 50.[76,77] Abdominal aortic aneurysms tend to enlarge slowly, but some rupture catastrophically with an overall mortality of up to 90%.[78]

B. **The finding.** Because the normal aorta bifurcates at the level of the umbilicus, palpable aortic aneurysms usually are found in the

TABLE 45-3 Ascites*

Finding (ref)†	Sensitivity (%)	Specificity (%)	Positive LR	Negative LR
Inspection				
Bulging flanks[70-72]	73-93	44-70	1.9	0.4
Edema[71]	87	77	3.8	0.2
Palpation and Percussion				
Flank dullness[70,71]	80-94	29-69	NS	0.3
Shifting dullness[70-72]	60-87	56-90	2.3	0.4
Fluid wave[70-72]	50-80	82-92	5.0	0.5

NS, Not significant.

Diagnostic standard: For *ascites*, peritoneal fluid by ultrasonography

†*Definition of findings:* For *shifting dullness*, border between resonance and dullness "shifts" when patient rolls from supine to left lateral decubitus position or right lateral decubitus position; Cattau required a shift in both positions,[70] Simel in only 1 of 2 positions,[71] and Cummings used only the right lateral decubitus position at 45 degrees and required a shift >1 cm.[72]

epigastrium. The clinician should place one hand on each side of the aorta and measure its diameter, subtracting the estimated thickness of two layers of skin and subcutaneous tissue. Most studies do not specifically define the positive finding (instead stating simply the positive finding is "aortic aneurysm present by palpation"), although others define it as an estimated diameter greater than 3 cm using the previously described method.[58]

Importantly, an aortic aneurysm pushes the two hands *apart*, a finding called *expansile* pulsation.[79] Other prominent epigastric pulsations sometimes occur in patients with thin abdomens or in those with epigastric masses overlying the normal aorta, but unless these pulsations are expansile, they do not indicate an aneurysm.

C. Clinical significance. According to Table 45-2, the finding of a palpable epigastric pulsation suggestive of aneurysm argues strongly that one is present (LR = 7.6; see Table 45-1). In contrast, the absence of this finding is much less helpful (LR is only 0.6), simply because the sensitivity for the finding is as low as 22% (i.e., up to 78% of patients with aneurysms lack a prominent pulsation).

The two most important variables governing whether an aneurysm is palpable are (1) the size of the aneurysm and (2) the girth of the patient's abdomen. Aneurysms between 3 and 5 cm in diameter are the most difficult ones to detect, and if "aneurysm" is instead defined as a focal bulging greater than 5 cm in diameter—the diameter usually indicating surgical repair—the sensitivity of bedside examination increases to over 80% in almost all series.[58,77,80] Aneurysms are also more difficult to detect in patients with larger abdominal girths.[57,58,80,81] After restricting the analysis to just those patients with an abdominal girth less than 100 cm (measured at the umbilicus)[57,58] or to patients in whom the clinician can palpate the aorta,[58,81,82] the sensitivity of the examination exceeds 88% in all studies. These results indicate that the negative examination argues strongly against an aneurysm greater than 5 cm in diameter, especially if the patient has a girth less than 100 cm or has a palpable aorta.

The most common cause for a false-positive examination is an abnormally tortuous aorta.[83,84] Rare causes are a horseshoe kidney, intraabdominal tumor, or paraaortic adenopathy.[83,84]

REFERENCES

1. Cabot RC. *Physical diagnosis,* New York, 1926, William Wood & Co.
2. Risse GB. Pierre A. Piorry (1794-1879): the French "master of percussion," *Chest* 60:484-488, 1971.
3. Sakula A. Pierre Adolphe Piorry (1794-1879): pioneer of percussion and pleximetry, *Thorax* 34:575-581, 1979.
4. McGee S. Percussion and physical diagnosis: separating myth from science, *Disease-a-Month* 41:643-692, 1995.
5. Zelman S and Pickard CM. Roentgen and autopsy evaluation of percussion of the liver and spleen, *Gastroenterology* 29:1037-1045, 1955.
6. Sullivan S, Krasner N, and Williams R. The clinical estimation of liver size: a comparison of techniques and an analysis of the source of error, *Br Med J* 2:1042-1043, 1976.
7. Peternel WW, Schaefer JW, and Schiff L. Clinical evaluation of liver size and hepatic scintiscan, *Am J Dig Dis* 11:346-350, 1966.
8. Sapira JD and Williamson DL. How big is the normal liver? *Arch Intern Med* 139:971-973, 1979.
9. Castell DO and others. Estimation of liver size by percussion in normal individuals, *Ann Intern Med* 70:1183-1189, 1969.
10. Zoli M and others. Physical examination of the liver: is it still worth it? *Am J Gastroenterol* 90:1428-1432, 1995.
11. Niederau C and others. Sonographic measurements of the normal liver, spleen, pancreas, and portal vein, *Radiology* 149:537-540, 1983.

12. Goodman JL. The enlarged liver in diabetes mellitus: its determination by percussion, *Am J Digest Dis* 18:181-185, 1950.

13. Castell DO. The spleen percussion sign: a useful diagnostic technique, *Ann Intern Med* 67:1265-1267, 1967.

14. Naftalis J and Leevy CM. Clinical estimation of liver size, *Am J Dig Dis* 8:236-243, 1963.

15. Blendis LM and others. Observer variation in the clinical and radiological assessment of hepatosplenomegaly, *Br Med J* 1:727-730, 1970.

16. Fenster F and Klatskin G. Manifestations of metastatic tumors of the liver: a study of eighty-one patients subjected to needle biopsy, *Am J Med* 31:238-248, 1961.

17. Ariel IM and Briceno M. The disparity of the size of the liver as determined by physical examination and by hepatic gamma scanning in 504 patients, *Med Ped Oncol* 2:69-73, 1976.

18. Halpern S and others. Correlation of liver and spleen size: determinations by nuclear medicine studies and physical examination, *Arch Intern Med* 134:123-124, 1974.

19. Riemenschneider PA and Whalen JP. The relative accuracy of estimation of enlargement of the liver and spleen by radiologic and clinical methods, *Am J Roentgen Rad Ther Nuc Med* 94:462-468, 1965.

20. Rosenfield AT, Laufer I, and Schneider PB. The significance of a palpable liver: a correlation of clinical and radioisotope studies, *Am J Roent Rad Ther Nuc Med* 122: 313-317, 1974.

21. Westin J and others. Spleen size in polycythemia: a clinical and scintigraphic study, *Acta Med Scand* 191:263-271, 1972.

22. Tamayo SG and others. Examiner dependence on physical diagnostic tests for the detection of splenomegaly: a prospective study with multiple observers, *J Gen Intern Med* 8:69-75, 1993.

23. Barkun AN and others. The bedside assessment of splenic enlargement, *Am J Med* 91:512-518, 1991.

24. Holzbach RT and others. Evaluation of spleen size by radioactive scanning, *J Lab Clin Med* 60:902-913, 1962.

25. Ingeberg S, Stockel M, and Sorensen PJ. Prediction of spleen size by routine radioisotope scintigraphy, *Acta Haemat* 69:243-248, 1983.

26. Sullivan S and Williams R. Reliability of clinical techniques for detecting splenic enlargement, *Br Med J* 2:1043-1044, 1976.

27. Tucker WN and others. The scratch test is unreliable for detecting the liver edge, *J Clin Gastroenterol* 25:410-414, 1997.
28. Kukowka A. Auskultatorische Methode zur bestimmung der Lebergroesse—ein einfaches, probates Schnellverfahren, *Z Allgemeinmedizin* 48:1645-1646, 1972.
29. Fuller GN, Hargreaves MR, and King DM. Scratch test in clinical examination of liver, *Lancet* 1:181, 1988.
30. Rinzler SH. Re-emphasis of the auscultatory method for ascertaining the size of the liver, *NY State J Med* 50:300, 1950.
31. Sehrwald. Ueber die Brauchbarkeit des Phonoendoskopes, *Dtsch Arch Klin Med* 79:450-467, 1904.
32. Camman GP and Clark A. A new mode of ascertaining the dimensions, form, and condition of internal organs by percussion, *N Y J Med Surg* 3:62-96, 1840.
33. Terry RB. Coupled hepatic pulsations in tricuspid incompetence (a new physical sign), *Am Heart J* 57:158-159, 1959.
34. Salazar E and Levine HD. Rheumatic tricuspid regurgitation: the clinical spectrum, *Am J Med* 33:111-129, 1962.
35. Lingamneni R and others. Tricuspid regurgitation: clinical and angiographic assessment, *Cath Cardiovasc Diag* 5:7-17, 1979.
36. Müller O and Shillingford J. Tricuspid incompetence, *Br Heart J* 16:195-207, 1954.
37. Cha SD and Gooch AS. Diagnosis of tricuspid regurgitation, *Arch Intern Med* 143:1763-1768, 1983.
38. El-Sherif A and El-Said G. Jugular, hepatic, and praecordial pulsations in constrictive pericarditis, *Br Heart J* 33:305-312, 1971.
39. Coralli RJ and Crawley IS. Hepatic pulsations in constrictive pericarditis, *Am J Cardiol* 58:370-373, 1986.
40. Arkles LB, Gill GD, and Molan MP. A palpable spleen is not necessarily enlarged or pathological, *Med J Austral* 145:15-17, 1986.
41. Lipp WF, Eckstein EH, and Aaron AH. The clinical significance of the palpable spleen, *Gastroenterology* 3:287-291, 1944.
42. O'Reilly RA. Splenomegaly at a United States county hospital: diagnostic evaluation of 170 patients, *Am J Med Sci* 312:160-165, 1996.
43. Nixon RK. The detection of splenomegaly by percussion, *N Engl J Med* 250:166-167, 1954.
44. Verghese A, Krish G, and Karnad A. Ludwig Traube: the man and his space, *Arch Intern Med* 152:701-703, 1992.

45. Parrino TA. The art and science of percussion, *Hosp Pract* 99:25-36, 1987.

46. Barkun AN and others. Splenic enlargement and Traube's space: how useful is percussion? *Am J Med* 87:562-566, 1989.

47. Ludwig Courvoisier (1843-1918): Courvoisier's sign, *JAMA* 204:165, 1968.

48. Verghese A, Dison C, and Berk SL. Courvoisier's "Law"— A eponym in evolution, *Am J Gastroenterol* 82:248-250, 1987.

49. Delpre G and Kadish U. Courvoisier's gallbladder: "Render unto Caesar that which is Caesar's," *Dig Dis Sci* 32:446, 1987.

50. Viteri AL. Courvoisier's law and evaluation of the jaundiced patient, *Tex Med* 76:60-61, 1980.

51. Gunn A and Keddie N. Some clinical observations on patients with gallstones, *Lancet* 2:239-241, 1972.

52. Chen JJ and others. Gallbladder volume in patients with common hepatic duct dilatation: an evaluation of Courvoisier's sign using ultrasonography, *Scand J Gastroenterol* 29:284-288, 1994.

53. Fournier AM and Michel J. Courvoisier's sign revisited: two patients with palpable gallbladder, *South Med J* 85:548-550, 1992.

54. Mikal S and Campbell AJA. Carcinoma of the pancreas: diagnostic and operative criteria based on one hundred consecutive autopsies, *Surgery* 28:963-969, 1950.

55. Shenker S, Balint J, and Schiff L. Differential diagnosis of jaundice: report of a prospective study of 61 proved cases, *Am J Dig Dis* 7:449-463, 1962.

56. Zollinger R and Kevorkian AY. Surgical aspects of obstructive jaundice, *N Engl J Med* 221:486-488, 1939.

57. Lederle FA, Walker JM, and Reinke DB. Selective screening for abdominal aortic aneurysms with physical examination and ultrasound, *Arch Intern Med* 148:1753-1756, 1988.

58. Fink HA and others. The accuracy of physical examination to detect abdominal aortic aneurysm, *Arch Intern Med* 160:833-836, 2000.

59. Twomey A and others. Unrecognized aneurysmal disease in male hypertensive patients, *Inter Angiol* 5:269-273, 1986.

60. Collin J and others. Oxford screening programme for abdominal aortic aneurysm in men aged 65 to 74 years, *Lancet* 2:613-615, 1988.

61. Allen PIM and others. Population screening for aortic aneurysms, *Lancet* 2:736, 1987.

62. Al Zahrani HA and others. Screening for abdominal aortic aneurysm in the Jeddah area, western Saudi Arabia, *Cardiovasc Surg* 4:87-92, 1996.

63. Andersson AP and others. Screening for abdominal aortic aneurysm in 295 outpatients with intermittent claudication, *Vasc Surg* 25:516-520, 1991.

64. Chung RS. Pathogenesis of the "Courvoisier gallbladder," *Dig Dis Sci* 28:33-38, 1983.

65. Müller F. Einige Beobachtungen aus dem Percussionscurs, *Berl Klin Wochenschr*, 32:278-280, 1895.

66. Guarino JR. Auscultatory percussion of the urinary bladder, *Arch Intern Med* 145:1823-1825, 1985.

67. Hussey HH and Jeghers H. Practical considerations of venous pressure, *N Engl J Med* 237:776-782; 812-818, 1947.

68. Moses WR. Shifting dullness in the abdomen, *South Med J* 39:985-987, 1946.

69. Sahli H. *A treatise on diagnostic methods of examination*, Philadelphia, 1911, WB Saunders.

70. Cattau EL and others. The accuracy of the physical examination in the diagnosis of suspected ascites, *JAMA* 247: 1164-1166, 1982.

71. Simel DL, Halvorsen RA, and Feussner JR. Quantitating bedside diagnosis: Clinical evaluation of ascites *J Gen Intern Med* 3:423-428, 1988.

72. Cummings S and others. The predictive value of physical examination for ascites, *West J Med* 142:633-636, 1985.

73. Guarino JR. Auscultatory percussion to detect ascites, *N Engl J Med* 315:1555-1556, 1986.

74. McLean ACJ. Diagnosis of ascites by auscultatory percussion and hand-held ultrasound unit, *Lancet* 2:1526-1527, 1987.

75. Lawson JD and Weissbein AS. The puddle sign—an aid in the diagnosis of minimal ascites, *N Engl J Med* 260:652-654, 1959.

76. Lederle FA and others. Prevalence and associations of abdominal aortic aneurysm detected through screening, *Ann Intern Med* 126:441-449, 1997.

77. Lederle FA and Simel DL. Does this patient have abdominal aortic aneurysm? *JAMA* 281:77-82, 1999.

78. Ernst CB. Abdominal aortic aneurysm, *N Engl J Med* 328:1167-1172, 1993.

79. Osler W. Aneurysm of the abdominal aorta, *Lancet* 2:1089-1096, 1905.

80. Chervu A and others. Role of physical examination in detection of abdominal aortic aneurysms, *Surgery* 117:454-457, 1995.

81. Arnell TD and others. Abdominal aortic aneurysm screening in elderly males with atherosclerosis: the value of the physical exam, *Am Surg* 62:861-864, 1996.

82. Cabellon S and others. Incidence of abdominal aortic aneurysms in patients with atheromatous arterial disease, *Am J Surg* 146:575-576, 1983.

83. Nusbaum JW, Freimanis AK, and Thomford NR. Echography in the diagnosis of abdominal aortic aneurysm, *Arch Surg* 102:385-388, 1971.

84. Robicsek F and others. The value of angiography in the diagnosis of unruptured aneurysms of the abdominal aorta, *Ann Thor Surg* 11:538-550, 1971.

CHAPTER 46

Abdominal Pain and Tenderness

ACUTE ABDOMINAL PAIN

I. INTRODUCTION. Among patients presenting with acute abdominal pain and tenderness (i.e., pain lasting <7 days), the most common diagnoses are nonspecific abdominal pain (43% of patients), acute appendicitis (4% to 20%), acute cholecystitis (3% to 9%), small bowel obstruction (4%), and ureterolithiasis (4%).[1-4] The term "acute abdomen" usually refers to those conditions causing abrupt abdominal pain and tenderness and requiring urgent diagnosis and surgical intervention, such as appendicitis, bowel obstruction, and perforated intraabdominal organs.

Today, diagnosis of the acute abdomen combines bedside evaluation, laboratory testing, and clinical imaging. Because modern imaging tools are imperfect, however—in one study, for example, ultrasonography detected appendicitis with a sensitivity of only 49% and specificity of only 88%[5]—the fundamental diagnostic tool in patients with the acute abdomen remains careful analysis of the patient's symptoms and signs.[6]

II. THE FINDINGS. The two most common causes of the acute abdomen are (1) peritonitis, from inflammation (appendicitis, cholecystitis) or perforation of a viscus (appendix, peptic ulcer of stomach or duodenum, diverticulum) and (2) bowel obstruction. Both peritonitis and obstruction cause abdominal tenderness. Additional findings are discussed below.

A. Peritonitis. The additional findings of peritonitis are guarding and rigidity, rebound tenderness, a positive cough test, and a *negative* abdominal wall tenderness test.

  1. Guarding and rigidity. Guarding refers to *voluntary contraction* of the abdominal wall musculature, usually the result of fear, anxiety, or the laying on of cold hands.[7] Rigidity refers to *involuntary contraction* of the abdominal musculature in response to peritoneal inflammation, a reflex the patient cannot control.[7] Experienced surgeons distinguish guarding from rigidity in two ways. First, they attempt to distract the patient during examination, often by engaging the patient in conversation or using the stethoscope to gently palpate the abdomen.[8,9] Second, they examine the patient repeatedly over time. Guarding, but not rigidity, diminishes as the patient is distracted and fluctuates in intensity over time, sometimes even disappearing.

      The first clinician to clearly describe rigidity was the Roman physician Celsus, writing in 30 A.D.[10]

  2. Rebound tenderness. To elicit rebound tenderness, the clinician maintains pressure over an area of tenderness and then withdraws the hand abruptly. If the patient winces with pain upon withdrawal of the hand, the test is positive. Many expert surgeons discourage using the rebound tenderness test, regarding it "unnecessary,"[7,11] "cruel,"[6] or a "popular and somewhat unkind way of emphasizing what is already obvious."[12]

Rebound tenderness was originally described by J. Moritz Blumberg (1873-1955), a German surgeon and gynecologist, who believed that pain in the lower abdomen after abrupt withdrawal of the hand from the *left* lower abdominal quadrant was a sign of appendicitis (i.e., Blumberg's sign).[13]

3. **Cough test.** In patients with peritonitis, sudden movements that jar the abdomen, like coughing, cause pain. The cough test is positive if the patient, in response to a cough, shows signs of pain, such as flinching, grimacing, or moving hands toward the abdomen.[14]

4. **Abdominal wall tenderness test.** In 1926 Carnett[15] introduced the abdominal wall tenderness test as a way to diagnose lesions in the abdominal wall that cause abdominal pain and tenderness and sometimes mimic peritonitis. In this test, the clinician locates the area of maximal tenderness by gentle palpation and then applies enough pressure to elicit moderate tenderness. The patient is then asked to fold the arms on the chest and lift the head and shoulders, as if performing a partial sit-up. If this maneuver causes increased tenderness at the site of palpation, the test is positive,[16] which traditionally argues against peritonitis because tense abdominal wall muscles should protect the peritoneum from the clinician's hands.

One well-recognized cause of acute abdominal wall tenderness is diabetic neuropathy (i.e., "thoracoabdominal neuropathy" involving nerve roots T7 to T11; lesions of T1-T6 cause chest pain).[17-22] In addition to a positive abdominal wall tenderness test, characteristic signs of this disorder are cutaneous hypersensitivity, often of contiguous dermatomes, and weakness of the abdominal muscles, causing ipsilateral bulging of the abdominal wall that sometimes resembles a hernia.[18,19,21]

B. Appendicitis

1. **McBurney's point tenderness.** In a paper read before the New York Surgical Society in 1889 that cited the advantages of early operation in appendicitis, Charles McBurney stated that all patients with appendicitis have maximal pain and tenderness "determined by the pressure of the finger (at a point) very exactly between an inch and a half and two inches from the anterior superior spinous process of the ilium on a straight line drawn from that process to the umbilicus."[23,24]

2. **Rovsing's sign.** Rovsing's sign (Neils T. Rovsing, 1862-1927, Danish surgeon) is positive when pressure over the patient's *left* lower quadrant causes pain in the right lower quadrant.[7] This sign is sometimes called indirect tenderness.

3. **Rectal tenderness.** In patients with appendicitis whose inflammation is confined to the pelvis, rectal examination may reveal tenderness, especially on the right side, and some patients with perforation may have a rectal mass (i.e., pelvic abscess).

4. **Psoas sign.** The inflamed appendix may lie against the right psoas muscle, causing the patient to shorten that muscle by drawing up the right knee. To elicit the psoas sign, the patient lies on the left side and the clinician hyperextends the right hip. Painful hip extension is the positive response.[7,11]

5. **Obturator sign.** The obturator sign is based on the same principle as the psoas sign, that stretching a pelvic muscle irritated by an inflamed appendix causes pain. To stretch the right obturator internus muscle and elicit the sign, the clinician flexes the

patient's right hip and knee and then internally rotates the right hip.[7,11]

C. Cholecystitis and Murphy's sign. Patients with acute cholecystitis present with continuous epigastric or right upper quadrant pain, nausea, and vomiting. The traditional physical signs are fever, right upper quadrant tenderness, and a positive Murphy's sign. In 1903, the American surgeon Charles Murphy stated that the hypersensitive gallbladder of cholecystitis prevents the patient from taking in a "full, deep inspiration when the clinician's fingers are hooked up beneath the right costal arch below the hepatic margin. The diaphragm forces the liver down until the sensitive gallbladder reaches the examining fingers, when the inspiration suddenly ceases as though it had been shut off."[25]

Most clinicians elicit Murphy's sign by palpating the right upper quadrant of the supine patient. In his original description, Murphy proposed other methods, such as the "deep grip palpation" technique, in which the clinician examines the seated patient from behind and curls the finger tips of his or her right hand under the right costal margin, and the "hammer stroke percussion" technique, in which the clinician strikes a finger pointed into the right upper quadrant with the ulnar aspect of the other hand.[25]

D. Small bowel obstruction. Patients with small bowel obstruction present with abdominal pain and vomiting. The traditional physical signs are abdominal distention and tenderness, visible peristalsis, and abnormal bowel sounds (initially, high-pitched tickling sounds followed by diminished or absent bowel sounds).[7,11] Signs of peritonitis (e.g., rigidity, rebound) may appear if portions of the bowel become ischemic.

III. CLINICAL SIGNIFICANCE. Tables 46-1 through 46-4 present the physical findings of the acute

Text continued on p. 624

TABLE 46-1 Acute abdominal pain, signs detecting peritonitis*

Finding (ref)†	Sensitivity (%)	Specificity (%)	Positive LR	Negative LR
Abdominal Examination				
Guarding[2,26-32]	13-69	56-97	2.6	0.6
Rigidity[2,30-32]	6-31	96-100	5.1	NS
Rebound tenderness[2,26-36]	40-95	20-89	2.1	0.5
Abnormal bowel sounds[2,32]	25-61	44-95	NS	0.8
Rectal Examination				
Rectal tenderness[2,5,29,30,32-34]	20-53	41-96	NS	NS
Other Tests				
Positive abdominal wall tenderness test[16,37]	1-5	32-72	0.1	NS
Positive cough test[14,26]	77-82	50-79	2.4	0.3

NS, Not significant.

*Diagnostic standard: For peritonitis, surgical exploration and follow-up of patients not operated on; causes of peritonitis included appendicitis (most common), cholecystitis, and perforated ulcer. One study also included patients with pancreatitis.[32]

†Definition of findings: For abnormal bowel sounds, absent, diminished, or hyperactive; for abdominal wall tenderness test, see text; for positive cough test, the patient is asked to cough, and during the cough shows signs of pain or clearly reduces the intensity of the cough to avoid pain.[26]

TABLE 46-2 Acute right lower quadrant tenderness, signs detecting appendicitis*

Finding (ref)†	Sensitivity (%)	Specificity (%)	Positive LR	Negative LR
Vital Signs				
Fever[26,34]	70-74	50-70	1.8	0.5
Abdominal Examination				
Severe right lower quadrant tenderness[26,27]	87-99	8-65	NS	0.2
McBurney's point tenderness[26,27,38]	50-94	75-86	3.4	0.4
Rovsing's sign[5,27,28,31]	22-68	58-96	2.5	0.7
Rectal Examination				
Rectal tenderness[5,29,30,33,34]	38-53	41-62	NS	NS
Other Signs				
Psoas sign[28,29]	13-15	91-97	NS	NS
Obturator sign[29]	8	94	NS	NS

NS, Not significant.

Diagnostic standard: For appendicitis, surgical findings, histology, and follow-up of patients not operated on.

†*Definition of findings:* For fever, temperature >37.3° C[34] or not defined[26]; for *positive cough test,* see Table 46-1.

TABLE 46-3 Acute right upper quadrant tenderness, signs detecting cholecystitis*

Finding (ref)	Sensitivity (%)	Specificity (%)	Positive LR	Negative LR
Murphy's sign[39,40]	48-97	48-79	2.0	NS
Back tenderness[41]	27	36	0.4	2.0
Right upper quadrant mass[41,42]	14-23	70-83	NS	NS

NS, Not significant.

*Diagnostic standard: For cholecystitis, positive hepatobiliary scintiscan[40] or surgical findings and histology.[39,41,42]

TABLE 46-4 Acute abdominal pain, signs detecting bowel obstruction*

Finding (ref)†	Sensitivity (%)	Specificity (%)	Positive LR	Negative LR
Inspection of Abdomen				
Visible peristalsis[3]	6	100	18.8	NS
Distended abdomen[1,3,32]	58-67	89-96	9.6	0.4
Palpation of Abdomen				
Guarding[1,2,32]	20-63	47-78	NS	NS
Rigidity[1-3,32]	6-18	75-99	NS	NS
Rebound tenderness[1,2,32]	22-40	52-82	NS	NS
Auscultation of Abdomen				
Hyperactive bowel sounds[3,32]	40-42	89-94	5.0	0.6
Abnormal bowel sounds[1-3,32]	63-93	43-88	3.2	0.4
Rectal Examination				
Rectal tenderness[1,2,32]	4-26	72-94	NS	NS

NS, Not significant.

**Diagnostic standard:* For *small bowel obstruction,* surgical findings, abdominal radiographs, and clinical follow-up.

†*Definition of findings:* For *abnormal bowel sounds,* hyperactive, absent, or diminished bowel sounds.

abdomen. Tables 46-1 and 46-4 apply to all patients with acute abdominal pain and tenderness and address how well physical signs identify peritonitis (Table 46-1) and small bowel obstruction (Table 46-4) (these studies included almost 4000 patients). Tables 46-2 and 46-3 refer to only a subset of patients with abdominal pain: Table 46-2 applies to patients *hospitalized* with right lower quadrant tenderness and suspected appendicitis, and Table 46-3 applies to patients *hospitalized* with right upper quadrant pain and suspected cholecystitis.

A. Peritonitis (see Table 46-1). The primary cause of peritonitis in the studies of Table 46-1 was appendicitis, although some patients had perforated ulcers, perforated diverticuli, or cholecystitis. According to these studies, the most compelling findings arguing *for* peritonitis are rigidity (LR = 5.1), guarding (LR = 2.6), and a positive cough test (LR = 2.4). The findings arguing the most *against* peritonitis are a *positive* abdominal wall tenderness test (LR = 0.1) and a *negative* cough test (LR = 0.3). The presence or absence of rebound tenderness (positive LR = 2.1, negative LR = 0.5) shifts probability relatively little, confirming the long-held opinion of expert surgeons that rebound tenderness adds little to what clinicians already know from gentle palpation.

Findings that do not help diagnose peritonitis are the character of the bowel sounds and the presence or absence of rectal tenderness.

B. Appendicitis. The finding of right lower quadrant tenderness in a patient with acute abdominal pain discriminates well between those with and without appendicitis (sensitivity 94%, specificity 87%, positive LR = 7.3, negative LR = 0.1).[43]

1. Individual findings (see Table 46-2). Just as rigidity and guarding argue for peritonitis in patients with acute abdominal pain (see Table 46-1), these findings also argue for appendicitis in patients with right lower quadrant pain (the positive LR for rigidity is 4.0; for guarding, 2.2).[26-31] Other findings that argue *for* appendicitis are McBurney's point tenderness (LR = 3.4) and a positive Rovsing's sign (LR = 2.5). The absence of severe right lower quadrant tenderness (LR = 0.2), the absence of McBurney's point tenderness (LR = 0.4), and the negative cough test argue *against* appendicitis (LR = 0.4).[26] Again, rebound tenderness is one of the least discriminating of signs (positive LR = 2.0, negative LR = 0.5).[a]

Findings having little or no diagnostic value in diagnosing appendicitis are rectal tenderness (whether the tenderness is generalized or confined to the right rectum), the psoas sign, and the obturator sign. Nonetheless, a rectal examination should still be performed to detect the rare patient (2% or less) with a pelvic abscess and rectal mass.[30,32]

2. **Combination of findings.** Many scoring systems have been developed to improve diagnostic accuracy and reduce the negative appendectomy rate in patients with acute right lower quadrant tenderness.[5,27,28,34,43-49] Most of these scoring systems, however, are suboptimal because they are based on either simple conversion of individual LRs to "diagnostic weights," without first performing tests of independence,[5,28,34,44,45,47] or on arbitrary diagnostic weights based on traditional teachings.[46] The few studies available that looked at the independence of

---

[a]The figures for rigidity, guarding, rebound tenderness, and cough test do not appear in Table 46-2, because they are similar to those already shown in Table 46-1.

findings investigated relatively few physical signs.[27,43,49]

C. Cholecystitis (Table 46-3). In patients with right upper quadrant pain and suspected cholecystitis, a positive Murphy's sign argues modestly *for* cholecystitis (LR = 2.0). The presence of back tenderness argues somewhat *against* cholecystitis (LR = 0.4), probably because it is more commonly found in alternative diagnoses such as renal disease or pancreatitis.[41] The presence or absence of a right upper quadrant mass is unhelpful, probably because a palpable tender gallbladder is uncommon in cholecystitis (sensitivity less than 25%) and because the sensation of a right upper quadrant mass may occur in other diagnoses, such as liver disease or localized rigidity of the abdominal wall from other disorders.

There is also a "sonographic Murphy's sign," elicited during ultrasonography of the right upper quadrant, which is simply the finding of maximal tenderness over the gallbladder. Studies of this sign in patients with right upper quadrant pain reveal much better diagnostic accuracy than conventional palpation: sensitivity = 63%, specificity = 94%, positive LR = 9.9, and negative LR = 0.4.[50] The superior accuracy of this sign, which also relies on palpation of the abdominal wall, suggests that the poorer accuracy of conventional palpation is due to the difficulty precisely locating the position of the gallbladder.

Murphy's sign may be even less accurate in elderly patients, because up to 25% of patients over 60 years of age with cholecystitis lack any abdominal tenderness whatsoever.[51] Although most of these patients have abdominal pain, some have altered mental status and lack pain as well.

D. Small bowel obstruction (see Table 46-4). In patients with acute abdominal pain, the findings of visible peristalsis (LR = 18.8), abdominal distention (LR = 9.6), and hyperactive bowel sounds (LR = 5.0) all argue *for* bowel obstruction (although visible peristalsis is a rare finding, occurring in only 6% of patients). Diminished or absent bowel sounds also occur in obstruction, being found in 1 of 4 patients.[3,32]

The findings arguing somewhat *against* obstruction are normal bowel sounds (i.e., not hyperactive, absent, or diminished) and the absence of a distended abdomen (both LRs = 0.4). Nonetheless, 30% to 40% of patients with obstruction lack abdominal distention, especially early in the course or if the obstruction is high in the intestines. The findings of peritoneal irritation—rigidity and rebound tenderness—argue neither for nor against the diagnosis of obstruction.

E. Renal colic. In one study of 1333 patients presenting with acute abdominal pain, two findings were accurate signs of ureterolithiasis (as diagnosed by imaging or follow-up): loin tenderness (sensitivity 15%, specificity 99%, positive LR = 27.7, negative LR = 0.9) and renal tenderness (sensitivity 86%, specificity 76%, positive LR = 3.6, negative LR = 0.2). As compelling as these findings are, they are less important than the finding of microscopic hematuria, which has a sensitivity of 75%, specificity of 99%, positive LR of 73.1, and negative LR of 0.3.[52]

CHRONIC ABDOMINAL PAIN

There is relatively little information on the accuracy of examination in diagnosing chronic abdominal pain. What is available, however, suggests that the finding of abdominal tenderness is common in many nonorganic disorders and has little diagnostic value. In patients with suspected biliary colic, right upper quadrant tenderness does not distinguish patients with cholelithiasis

TABLE 46-5 Chronic upper abdominal pain*

Finding (ref)	Sensitivity (%)	Specificity (%)	Positive LR	Negative LR
Right upper quadrant tenderness, detecting cholelithiasis[53]	53	51	NS	NS
Lower abdominal tenderness, detecting cholelithiasis[53]	21	57	0.5	1.4
Epigastric tenderness, detecting positive upper endoscopy[54]	63	31	NS	NS

NS, Not significant.

*Diagnostic standard: For cholelithiasis, ultrasonography or oral cholecystogram[53]; for positive upper endoscopy, findings on upper gastrointestinal endoscopy, most of which were peptic ulcers.

from those without, although lower abdominal tenderness argues modestly against cholelithiasis (LR = 0.5; Table 46-5). In patients with dyspepsia, epigastric tenderness does not help predict whether upper endoscopy will reveal an ulcer, some other abnormality, or normal findings.

Even if the finding of tenderness has little value, abdominal examination is still important in these patients, to detect masses, organomegaly, and signs of a surgical abdomen (see above).

REFERENCES

1. Eskelinen M, Ikonen J, and Lipponen P. Contributions of history-taking, physical examination, and computer assistance to diagnosis of acute small-bowel obstruction: a prospective study of 1333 patients with acute abdominal pain, *Scand J Gastroenterol* 29:715-721, 1994.

2. Brewer RJ and others. Abdominal pain: an analysis of 1000 consecutive cases in a university hospital emergency room, *Am J Surg* 131:219-223, 1976.

3. Böhner H and others. Simple data from history and physical examination help to exclude bowel obstruction and to avoid radiographic studies in patients with acute abdominal pain, *Eur J Surg* 164:777-784, 1998.

4. Ohmann C, Yang Q, and Franke C. Diagnostic scores for acute appendicitis, *Eur J Surg* 161:273-281, 1995.

5. Jahn H and others. Comparison of clinical judgment and diagnostic ultrasonography in the diagnosis of acute appendicitis: experience with a score-aided diagnosis, *Eur J Surg* 163:433-443, 1997.

6. Silen W. Pitfalls to avoid when evaluating severe abdominal pain, *J Crit Ill* 7:685-689, 1992.

7. Clain A. *Hamilton Bailey's demonstrations of physical signs in clinical surgery,* Bristol, 1986, Wright.

8. Meyerowitz BR. Abdominal palpation by stethoscope, *Arch Surg* 111:831, 1976.

9. Mellinkoff SM. "Stethoscope sign," *N Engl J Med* 271:630, 1964.

10. Celsus. *De Medicina* (English translation of Latin edition written between A.D. 25 and 35, printed in 1478), Cambridge, 1953, Harvard University Press.

11. Cope Z. *The early diagnosis of the acute abdomen,* London, 1972, Oxford University Press.

12. Lawrie R. Acute peritonitis, *Practitioner* 192:759-765, 1964.

13. Bailey H. *Demonstrations of physical signs in clinical surgery,* ed 11, Baltimore, 1949, Williams & Wilkins.

14. Bennett DH, Tambeur LJMT, and Campbell WB. Use of coughing test to diagnose peritonitis, *Br Med J* 308:1336, 1994.

15. Carnett JB. Intercostal neuralgia as a cause of abdominal pain and tenderness, *Surg Gynecol Obstet* 42:625-632, 1926.

16. Gray DWR and others. Is abdominal wall tenderness a useful sign in the diagnosis of non-specific abdominal pain? *Ann Roy Coll Surg Eng* 70:233-234, 1988.

17. Hershfield NB. The abdominal wall: a frequently overlooked source of abdominal pain, *J Clin Gastroenterol* 14: 199-202, 1992.

18. Chaudhuri KR and others. Unilateral abdominal muscle herniation with pain: a distinctive variant of diabetic radiculopathy, *Diab Med* 14:803-807, 1997.

19. Stewart JD. Diabetic truncal neuropathy: topography of the sensory deficit, *Ann Neurol* 25:233-238, 1989.

20. Sun SF and Streib EW. Diabetic thoracoabdominal neuropathy: clinical and electrodiagnostic features, *Ann Neurol* 9:75-79, 1981.

21. Parry GJ and Floberg J. Diabetic truncal neuropathy presenting as abdominal hernia, *Neurology* 39:1488-1490, 1989.

22. Kikta DG, Breuer AC, and Wilbourn AJ. Thoracic root pain in diabetes: the spectrum of clinical and electromyographic findings, *Ann Neurol* 11:80-85, 1982.

23. McBurney C. Experience with early operative interference in cases of disease of the vermiform appendix (reprinted in Classic articles in colonic and rectal surgery), *Dis Colon Rect* 26:291-303, 1998.

24. Cope Z. *A history of the acute abdomen,* London, 1965, Oxford University Press.

25. Aldea PA, Meehan JP, and Sternbach G. The acute abdomen and Murphy's signs, *J Emerg Med* 4:57-63, 1986.

26. Golledge J and others. Assessment of peritonism in appendicitis, *Ann R Coll Surg Engl* 78:11-14, 1996.

27. Andersson RE and others. Diagnostic value of disease history, clinical presentation, and inflammatory parameters of appendicitis, *World J Surg* 23:133-140, 1999.

28. Izbicki JR and others. Accurate diagnosis of acute appendicitis: a retrospective and prospective analysis of 686 patients, *Eur J Surg* 158:227-231, 1992.

29. Berry J and Malt RA. Appendicitis near its centenary, *Ann Surg* 200:567-575, 1984.

30. Dixon JM and others. Rectal examination in patients with pain in the right lower quadrant of the abdomen, *Br Med J* 302:386-388, 1991.

31. Alshehri MY and others. Value of rebound tenderness in acute appendicitis, *East Afr Med J* 72:504-507, 1995.

32. Staniland JR, Ditchburn J, and De Dombal FT. Clinical presentation of acute abdomen: study of 600 patients, *Br Med J* 3:393-398, 1972.

33. Nauta RJ and Magnant C. Observation versus operation for abdominal pain in the right lower quadrant: Roles of the clinical examination and the leukocyte count, *Am J Surg* 151:746-748, 1986.

34. Alvarado A. A practical score for the early diagnosis of acute appendicitis, *Ann Emerg Med* 15:557-564, 1986.

35. Liddington MI and Thomson WHF. Rebound tenderness test, *Br J Surg* 78:795-796, 1991.

36. Prout WG. The significance of rebound tenderness in the acute abdomen, *Br J Surg* 57:508-510, 1970.

37. Thomson H and Francis DMA. Abdominal-wall tenderness: a useful sign in the acute abdomen, *Lancet* 2:1053-1054, 1977.

38. Lane R and Grabham J. A useful sign for the diagnosis of peritoneal irritation in the right iliac fossa, *Ann R Coll Surg Eng* 79:128-129, 1997.

39. Adedeji OA and McAdam WAF. Murphy's sign, acute cholecystitis and elderly people, *J Roy Coll Surg Eng* 41:88-89, 1996.

40. Singer AJ and others. Correlation among clinical, laboratory, and hepatobiliary scanning findings in patients with suspected acute cholecystitis, *Ann Emerg Med* 28:267-272, 1996.

41. Halasz NA. Counterfeit cholecystitis: a common diagnostic dilemma, *Am J Surg* 130:189-193, 1975.

42. Schofield PF, Hulton NR, and Baildam AD. Is it acute cholecystitis? *Ann Roy Coll Surg Eng* 68:14-16, 1986.

43. Eskelinen M, Ikonen J, and Lipponen P. The value of history-taking, physical examination, and computer assistance in the diagnosis of acute appendicitis in patients more than 50 years old, *Scand J Gastroenterol* 30:349-355, 1995.

44. Arnbjörnsson E. Scoring system for computer-aided diagnosis of acute appendicitis: the value of prospective versus retrospective studies, *Ann Chir Gynaecol* 74:159-166, 1985.

45. Teicher I and others. Scoring system to aid in diagnoses of appendicitis, *Ann Surg* 198:753-759, 1982.

46. Christian F and Christian GP. A simple scoring system to reduce the negative appendicectomy rate, *Ann Roy Coll Surg Eng* 74:281-285, 1992.

47. Fenyo G. Routine use of a scoring system for decision-making in suspected acute appendicitis in adults, *Acta Chir Scand* 153:545-551, 1987.

48. Van Way CW and others. A feasibility study of computer aided diagnosis in appendicitis, *Surg Gynecol Obstet* 155: 685-688, 1982.

49. Ohmann C, Franke C, and Yang Q. Clinical benefit of a diagnostic score for appendicitis: results of a prospective interventional study, *Arch Surg* 134:993-996, 1999.

50. Ralls PW and others. Prospective evaluation of the sonographic Murphy sign in suspected acute cholecystitis, *J Clin Ultrasound* 10:113-115, 1982.

51. Morrow DJ, Thompson J, and Wilson SE. Acute cholecystitis in the elderly: a surgical emergency, *Arch Surg* 113: 1149-1152, 1978.

52. Eskelinen M, Ikonen J, and Lipponen P. Usefulness of history-taking, physical examination and diagnostic scoring in acute renal colic, *Eur Urol* 34:467-473, 1998.

53. Diehl AK, Sugarek NJ, and Todd KH. Clinical evaluation for gallstone disease: usefulness of symptoms and signs in diagnosis, *Am J Med* 89:29-33, 1990.

54. Priebe WM, DaCosta LR, and Beck IT. Is epigastric tenderness a sign of peptic ulcer disease? *Gastroenterology* 82:16-19, 1982.

CHAPTER 47

Auscultation of the Abdomen

ABDOMINAL BRUITS

I. THE FINDING. Abdominal bruits are murmurs heard during auscultation of the abdomen. Like any murmur generated outside the four heart chambers, abdominal bruits may extend beyond the confines of the first and second heart sounds from systole into diastole (i.e., they may be "continuous"; see Chapter 38). Most bruits are detected in the epigastrium or upper abdominal quadrants.

II. CLINICAL SIGNIFICANCE

A. Bruits in healthy persons. Bruits occur in 4% to 20% of healthy persons in most large series.[1-5] Abdominal bruits are more common in those younger than 40 years of age than in older persons.[1,4-6]

Characteristically, the abdominal bruit of a healthy individual is systolic, medium to low pitched, and audible between the xiphoid process and umbilicus.[1] Only rarely does it spread to the patient's sides, in contrast to abnormal bruits, which are often loudest away from the epigastrium (see below). Arteriograms reveal that the most common source for the normal abdominal bruit is the patient's celiac artery.[6]

B. Renovascular hypertension. In patients with renal artery stenosis and renovascular hypertension, an abdominal bruit may be heard in the epigastrium, although the sound sometimes radiates to one side.[1] In one study of patients referred because of severe hypertension that was difficult to control—a setting suggesting renovascular hypertension—the finding of a *systolic/diastolic* abdominal bruit was virtually diagnostic for renovascular hypertension (LR = 38.9; Table 47-1). In contrast, the finding in similar patients of *any* abdominal bruit (i.e., one not necessarily extending into diastole) was less compelling (LR = 4.8), probably because they also occur in persons without renovascular hypertension (see above).

The abdominal bruit of renovascular hypertension, however, does not always originate in the renal artery. In one study of patients undergoing surgery for renal artery stenosis, intraoperative auscultation localized the bruit to the renal arteries as the sole source only about half the time.[1] In the remaining patients, other vessels alone or with the renal artery generated the sound. Possibly, bruits in these patients are general markers of vascular disease, just as the finding of a carotid bruit has been associated with disease in other distant vascular beds, such as the coronary vasculature.[9]

C. Other disorders. Harsh, epigastric, or right upper quadrant bruits (systolic and continuous) have been repeatedly described in patients with hepatic malignancies[10,11] and hepatic cirrhosis.[10,12] In these patients, the sound may represent extrinsic compression of vessels by tumor or regenerating nodules, the hypervascular tumor, or portosystemic collateral vessels. Left upper quadrant bruits occur in patients with carcinoma of the body of the pancreas (8 of 21 patients in one study).[13] Other rare causes of abdominal bruits are renal artery aneu-

TABLE 47-1 Auscultation of abdomen*

Finding (Ref)	Sensitivity (%)	Specificity (%)	Positive LR	Negative LR
Abdominal Bruit—Any				
Detecting renovascular hypertension[2,3]	27-38	89-96	4.8	0.7
Detecting abdominal aortic aneurysm[7]	11	95	NS	NS
Abdominal Bruit—Systolic/Diastolic				
Detecting renovascular hypertension[8]	39	99	38.9	0.6

NS, Not significant.

*Diagnostic standard: For renovascular hypertension, >50% stenosis on renal arteriogram alone[2,3] or combined with renal vein renin ratio >1.5[8]; for abdominal aortic aneurysm, see Table 45-2 in Chapter 45.

rysms,[14] aortocaval fistulae,[15] ischemic bowel disease,[16] and celiac compression syndrome.[17] Although an abdominal bruit is traditionally associated with abdominal aortic aneurysm, the finding had no diagnostic value in one study (Table 47-1).[7]

HEPATIC RUB

In the absence of recent liver biopsy, the finding of a hepatic friction rub has been repeatedly associated with intrahepatic malignancy, either hepatoma or metastatic disease.[11,18] In one study of tumors metastatic to the liver, 10% of patients had a hepatic friction rub.[19]

BOWEL SOUNDS

I. THE FINDING. Most clinicians have great difficulty making any sense out of a patient's bowel sounds, for two reasons: (1) Normal bowel sounds, from moment to moment, vary greatly in pitch, intensity, and frequency. One healthy person may have no bowel sounds for up to 4 minutes, but when examined later may have more than 30 discrete sounds per minute.[20] The activity of normal bowel sounds may cycle with peak-to-peak periods as long as 50 to 60 minutes,[21] meaning that any analysis based on even several minutes of bedside auscultation is a very incomplete sample. (2) Bowel sounds generated at one point of the intestinal tract radiate widely over the entire abdominal wall.[20,22] The sounds heard in the right lower quadrant, for example, may actually originate in the stomach. This dissemination of bowel sounds makes the practice of listening to them in all four quadrants fundamentally unsound because, as an example, the left lower quadrant may be quieter than the left upper quadrant not because the descending colon is making less noise than the stomach, but instead because the entire abdomen has become quieter, at least for the moment the clinician is listening to the lower quadrant.

Most bowel sounds are generated in the stomach, followed by the large intestine and then the small bowel.[23] The overall frequency of bowel sounds increases after a meal.[24] The actual cause of bowel sounds is still debated; experiments with exteriorized loops of bowel in dogs show many intestinal contractions to be silent, although sound often occurs when contractions propel contents through a bowel segment that is not relaxed.[20]

II. CLINICAL SIGNIFICANCE. Analysis of the bowel sounds has modest value in diagnosing small bowel obstruction. After experimental complete bowel obstruction in animals, bowel sounds are hyperactive for about 30 minutes before becoming diminished or absent.[21] In patients with small bowel obstruction, clinical observation shows that about 40% have hyperactive bowel sounds and about 25% have diminished or absent bowel sounds.[25,26] Consequently, since most patients with small bowel obstruction have abnormal bowel sounds, the finding of *normal* bowel sounds in a patient with acute abdominal pain argues somewhat *against* the diagnosis of bowel obstruction (LR = 0.4, see Table 46-4 in Chapter 46).

A traditional finding of peritonitis is diminished or absent bowel sounds, although studies of patients with acute abdominal pain show this finding to be unreliable (see Chapter 46).

REFERENCES

1. Julius S and Stewart BH. Diagnostic significance of abdominal murmurs, *N Engl J Med* 276:1175-1178, 1967.
2. Krijnen P and others. A clinical prediction rule for renal artery stenosis, *Ann Intern Med* 129:705-711, 1998.
3. Carmichael DJS and others. Detection and investigation of renal artery stenosis, *Lancet* 1:667-670, 1986.
4. McSherry JA. The prevalence of epigastric bruit, *J Roy Coll Gen Pract* 29:170-172, 1979.

5. Rivin AU. Abdominal vascular sounds, *JAMA* 221:688-690, 1972.

6. McLoughlin MJ, Colapinto RF, and Hobbs BB. Abdominal bruits: clinical and angiographic correlation, *JAMA* 232: 1238-1242, 1975.

7. Lederle FA, Walker JM, and Reinke DB. Selective screening for abdominal aortic aneurysms with physical examination and ultrasound, *Arch Intern Med* 148:1753-1756, 1988.

8. Grim CE and others. Sensitivity and specificity of screening tests for renal vascular hypertension, *Ann Intern Med* 91:617-622, 1979.

9. Heymann A and others. Risk of stroke in asymptomatic persons with cervical arterial bruits: a population study in Evans County, Georgia, *N Engl J Med* 302:838-841, 1980.

10. Clain D, Wartnaby K, and Sherlock S. Abdominal arterial murmurs in liver disease, *Lancet* 2:516-519, 1966.

11. Sherman HI and Hardison JE. The importance of a coexistent hepatic rub and bruit: a clue to the diagnosis of cancer of the liver, *JAMA* 241:1495, 1979.

12. McFadzean AJS and Gray J. Hepatic venous hum in cirrhosis of liver, *Lancet* 2:1128-1130, 1953.

13. Serebro H. A diagnostic sign of carcinoma of the body of the pancreas, *Lancet* 1:85-86, 1965.

14. Okamoto M and others. Renal artery aneurysm: the significance of abdominal bruit and use of color Doppler, *Intern Med* 31:1217-1219, 1992.

15. Potyk DK and Guthrie CR. Spontaneous aortocaval fistula, *Ann Emerg Med* 25:424-427, 1995.

16. Sarr MG, Dickson Er, and Newcomer AD. Diastolic bruit in chronic intestinal ischemia: recognition by abdominal phonoangiography, *Dig Dis Sci* 25:761-762, 1980.

17. Gutnik LM. Celiac artery compression syndrome, *Am J Med* 76:334-336, 1984.

18. Fred HL and Brown GR. The hepatic friction rub, *N Engl J Med* 266:554-555, 1962.

19. Fenster F and Klatskin G. Manifestations of metastatic tumors of the liver: a study of eighty-one patients subjected to needle biopsy, *Am J Med* 31:238-248, 1961.

20. Milton GW. Normal bowel sounds, *Med J Aust* 2:490-493, 1958.

21. Mynors JM. The bowel sounds, *S Afr J Surg* 7:87-91, 1969.

22. Watson WC and Knox EC. Phonoenterography: the recording and analysis of bowel sounds, *Gut* 8:88-94, 1967.

23. Politzer JP and others. The genesis of bowel sounds: influence of viscus and gastrointestinal content, *Gastroenterology* 71:282-285, 1976.
24. Vasseur C and others. Postprandial bowel sounds, *IEEE Trans Biomed Eng* 22:443-448, 1975.
25. Bohner H and others. Simple data from history and physical examination help to exclude bowel obstruction and to avoid radiographic studies in patients with acute abdominal pain, *Eur J Surg* 164:777-784, 1998.
26. Staniland JR, Ditchburn J, and De Dombal FT. Clinical presentation of acute abdomen: study of 600 patients, *Br Med J* 3:393-398, 1972.

PART TEN

Extremities

CHAPTER 48

Peripheral Vascular Disease

I. **INTRODUCTION.** Chronic arterial disease usually affects three distinct segments in the lower limbs: (1) the aortoiliac (especially the infrarenal abdominal aorta and common iliac arteries), (2) the femoropopliteal (especially the superficial femoral artery in the adductor canal), and (3) the peroneotibial (below the knee).[1] Disease in each segment produces distinct patterns of claudication (Table 48-1). Most patients have aortoiliac disease, femoropopliteal disease, or both.[2] Disease below the knee is uncommon, except in diabetics and patients with thromboangiitis obliterans.

The diagnostic standard for chronic lower-extremity ischemia is the ankle-to-arm systolic pressure index (AAI), which is obtained by measuring the highest systolic blood pressure at the ankle (dorsalis pedis and posterior tibial arteries) with a hand-held Doppler flowmeter and dividing it by the blood pressure in the brachial artery. Values below 0.97 are abnormal (i.e., the lower 2.5% of measurements from large numbers of young, nonsmoking, asymptomatic persons).[3-5] Most patients with claudication have AAIs between 0.5 and 0.8 and disease in only a single segment; those with limb-threatening ischemia (i.e., rest pain,

643

TABLE 48-1 Diagnosis of peripheral arterial disease: traditional approach

Anatomic Segment	Location of Claudication	Pulse Examination		
		Femoral*	Popliteal	Pedal
Aortoiliac	Buttock, thigh, calf†	Absent	Absent	Absent
Femoropopliteal*	Calf	Present	Absent	Absent
Peroneotibial	None or foot‡	Present	Present	Absent

Adapted from reference 1.

*"Femoro" of "femoropopliteal" indicates the superficial femoral artery; of "femoral pulse," the common femoral artery.

†May cause erectile dysfunction if internal iliac arteries are involved.

‡Disease in this segment usually causes no claudication in patients with diabetes but causes foot pain in those with thromboangiitis obliterans (Buerger's disease).

gangrene) have AAIs less than 0.5 and disease in at least 2 segments.[4,5]

II. THE FINDINGS

A. Appearance of the foot.
In contrast to earlier writers on peripheral vascular disease who emphasized the physical sign of gangrene, the American surgeon Leo Buerger wrote in his 1924 book *The Circulatory Disturbances of the Extremities* that there were various "prodromal" signs of vascular disease, including toe and foot ulcers, poor capillary refill, impaired nail growth, atrophic skin, foot pallor with elevation, and foot rubor in the lowered position.[6] Clinicians have since regarded these findings as characteristic of chronic lower limb ischemia, although some of them—especially poor capillary refill and dependent rubor—were controversial even in Buerger's time.[7,8]

B. Pulses.
In studies of large numbers of healthy individuals, the dorsalis pedis pulse is not palpable 3% to 14% of the time and the posterior tibial pulse is not palpable 0% to 10% of the time.[9-14] Even so, when one of these arteries is congenitally small or absent, the other enlarges to make up the difference, explaining why only 0% to 2% of healthy individuals are missing both pedal pulses.[9,10,13]

The absence of both pedal pulses is common to disease of each of the three vascular segments and thus represents the best screening test for peripheral vascular disease (see Table 48-1).

C. Bruits.
A traditional finding of stenosis of a peripheral vessel is a limb bruit, either iliac (above the inguinal crease), femoral (in the thigh), or popliteal. Complete occlusion of a vessel should make the bruit disappear.

D. Ancillary tests
1. Venous filling time.
In patients with peripheral vascular disease, the veins of the feet fill abnormally slowly once they are

emptied. After positioning the patient supine and identifying a prominent vein on the top of the foot, the clinician empties this vein by elevating the patient's leg to 45 degrees above the table surface for 1 minute. The patient then sits up and dangles the foot over the edge of the examining table, and the clinician records how long in seconds it takes for the vein to rise above the level of the skin surface. Times greater than 20 seconds are abnormal.[15]

2. **Capillary refill time.** To perform this test, the clinician applies firm pressure to the plantar skin of the distal great toe for 5 seconds and then times how long it takes for the normal skin color to return after releasing the pressure. In the great toe, times greater than 5 seconds are regarded abnormal.[15]

3. **Buerger's test.** In the Buerger test, the clinician observes the color of the patient's leg when it is elevated and then when it is lowered. Abnormal pallor with elevation and a deep rubor in the lowered position are features of vascular disease.[1,6] In Buerger's version of the test, the clinician elevated the leg to produce pallor and then simply recorded the angle at which the reddish hue returned as the limb was lowered (his "angle of circulatory sufficiency").[6] In the only investigated version of this test (see below), the clinician elevated the leg 90 degrees from the table surface for 2 minutes and then dangled it perpendicular to the table edge for another 2 minutes. The positive response was abnormal pallor with elevation and the appearance of a dusky red flush spreading proximally from the toes in the dependent position.[20]

III. CLINICAL SIGNIFICANCE
A. Diagnosis of peripheral vascular disease.
Table 48-2 shows that the most compelling

TABLE 48-2 Peripheral vascular disease*

Finding (ref)†	Sensitivity (%)	Specificity (%)	Positive LR	Negative LR
Inspection				
Wounds or sores on foot[16]	2	100	7.0	NS
Foot color abnormally pale, red, or blue[16]	35	87	2.8	0.7
Atrophic skin[15]	50	70	1.7	NS
Absent lower limb hair[15]	48	71	1.7	NS
Palpation				
Foot asymmetrically cooler[16]	10	98	6.1	0.9
Absent femoral pulse[16]	7	99	6.1	NS
Absent posterior tibial and dorsalis pedis pulses[16,17]	63-72	92-99	14.9	0.3
Auscultation				
Limb bruit present[16,18,19]	20-50	95-99	7.3	0.7
Ancillary Tests				
Capillary refill time ≥5 seconds[15]	28	85	1.9	NS
Venous filling time >20 seconds[15]	22	94	3.6	NS

NS, Not significant.

*Diagnostic standard: For peripheral vascular disease, ankle-arm index <0.8 to 0.97 except for the study by Boyko[15] (i.e., atrophic skin, absent lower limb hair, capillary refill time, and venous filling time), which recruited diabetic patients exclusively and defined disease as AAI <0.5.

†Definition of findings: For limb bruit present, femoral artery bruit[16,19] or iliac, femoral, or popliteal bruit.[18]

physical signs arguing *for* the presence of peripheral vascular disease in the symptomatic leg (i.e., AAI <0.9) are the absence of both pedal pulses (likelihood ratio [LR] = 14.9), the presence of any limb bruit (LR = 7.3), the presence of wounds or sores on the foot (LR = 7.0), the absence of the femoral pulse (LR = 6.1), and the presence of asymmetric coolness of the foot (LR = 6.1). In another study,[15] the presence of a cool foot was not diagnostically helpful, although this study defined the abnormal finding as a foot cooler than the ipsilateral calf, which is actually a normal finding (i.e., in healthy individuals, the skin surface temperature diminishes toward the feet because of reduced cutaneous blood flow to conserve body heat).[1]

The only finding arguing *against* peripheral vascular disease is the presence of one or both pedal pulses (LR = 0.3), although studies show that up to 1 in 3 patients with disease have this finding. In these patients, however, the pulses often disappear during exercise (e.g., running in place, walking, toe-stands, or ankle flexion repeatedly against resistance), just as normal resting coronary blood flow in a patient with coronary artery disease may become abnormal after exercise.[21-23]

Findings that are unhelpful diagnostically are atrophic skin, hairless lower limbs,[24] and a prolonged capillary refill time. Writing soon after Buerger introduced the capillary refill time as a test of peripheral vascular disease (his "expression test"), Lewis[8] and Pickering[7] also showed it was an unreliable sign because prompt refill could occur from the veins of a limb rendered completely ischemic experimentally.[a]

---

[a] In adults, the capillary refill time is still looking for a disease. It has been proven unhelpful not only in peripheral vascular disease, but also in the assessment of blood loss and hypovolemia (see Chapter 9).

B. Distribution of peripheral vascular disease.

One study showed that vascular surgeons using traditional methods accurately localized the distribution of disease in 96% of 102 symptomatic patients, although the study omitted information about the relative value of specific findings.[25] Of the few studies available, one confirms the traditional teaching (Table 48-1) that the finding of an absent or severely diminished femoral pulse in a symptomatic limb argues strongly *for* aortoiliac disease (sensitivity 39%, specificity 99%, positive LR = 31.0, negative LR = 0.6).[26] Also, in symptomatic limbs with a preserved popliteal pulse (i.e., a finding arguing against *occlusion* of the aortoiliac or femoropopliteal segments), the presence of a limb bruit argues *for* the presence of stenoses on angiography, a finding of therapeutic importance because these patients may be candidates for angioplasty (sensitivity 80%, specificity 75%, positive LR = 3.2, negative LR = 0.3).[27] Finally, patients who have a positive Buerger test have more extensive disease than those who are test negative, including more rest pain (60% vs. 8%) and gangrene (23% vs. 0%) and lower AAIs (mean ± SD, 0.37 ± 0.29 vs. 0.62 ± 0.23).[20]

REFERENCES

1. McGee SR and Boyko EJ. Physical examination and chronic lower-extremity ischemia: a critical review, *Arch Intern Med* 158:1357-1364, 1998.
2. Mannick JA. Evaluation of chronic lower-extremity ischemia, *N Engl J Med* 309:841-843, 1983.
3. Hiatt WR, Hoag S, and Hamman RF. Effect of diagnostic criteria on the prevalence of peripheral arterial disease: the San Luis Valley diabetes study, *Circulation* 91:1472-1479, 1995.
4. Carter SA. Indirect systolic pressures and pulse waves in arterial occlusive disease of the lower extremities, *Circulation* 37:624-637, 1968.

5. Ouriel K and others. A critical evaluation of stress testing in the diagnosis of peripheral vascular disease, *Surgery* 91:686-693, 1982.

6. Buerger L. *The circulatory disturbances of the extremities: including gangrene, vasomotor and trophic changes,* Philadelphia, 1924, WB Saunders.

7. Pickering GW. On the clinical recognition of structural disease of the peripheral vessels, *Br Med J* 2:1106-1110, 1933.

8. Lewis T. *Vascular disorders of the limbs,* New York, 1936, Macmillan.

9. Barnhorst DA and Barner HB. Prevalence of congenitally absent pedal pulses, *N Engl J Med* 278:264-265, 1968.

10. Morrison H. A study of the dorsalis pedis and posterior tibial pulses in one thousand individuals without symptoms of circulatory affections of the extremities, *N Engl J Med* 208:438-440, 1933.

11. Nuzzaci G and others. A study of the semeiological reliability of dorsalis pedis artery and posterior tibial artery in the diagnosis of lower limb arterial occlusive disease, *Angiology* 35:767-772, 1984.

12. Robertson GSM, Ristic CD, and Bullen BR. The incidence of congenitally absent foot pulses, *Ann Roy Coll Surg Eng* 72:99-100, 1990.

13. Silverman JJ. The incidence of palpable dorsalis pedis and posterior tibial pulsations in soldiers: an analysis of over 1000 infantry soldiers, *Am Heart J* 32:82-87, 1946.

14. Stephens GL. Palpable dorsalis pedis and posterior tibial pulses: incidence in young men, *Arch Surg* 84:662-664, 1962.

15. Boyko EJ and others. Diagnostic utility of the history and physical examination for peripheral vascular disease among patients with diabetes mellitus, *J Clin Epidemiol* 50:659-668, 1997.

16. Stoffers HEJH and others. Diagnostic value of signs and symptoms associated with peripheral arterial occlusive disease seen in general practice: a multivariable approach, *Med Decis Making* 17:61-70, 1997.

17. Christensen JH and others. Clinical relevance of pedal pulse palpation in patients suspected of peripheral arterial insufficiency, *J Intern Med* 226:95-99, 1989.

18. Carter SA. Arterial auscultation in peripheral vascular disease, *JAMA* 246:1682-1686, 1981.

19. Criqui MH and others. The sensitivity, specificity, and predictive value of traditional clinical evaluation of peripheral arterial disease: results from noninvasive testing in a defined population, *Circulation* 71:516-522, 1985.
20. Insall RL, Davies RJ, and Prout WG. Significance of Buerger's test in the assessment of lower limb ischaemia, *J Roy Soc Med* 82:729-731, 1989.
21. Barner HB and others. Intermittent claudication with pedal pulses, *JAMA* 204:100-104, 1968.
22. Carter SA. Response of ankle systolic pressure to leg exercise in mild or questionable arterial disease, *N Engl J Med* 287:578-582, 1972.
23. DeWeese JA. Pedal pulses disappearing with exercise: a test for intermittent claudication. *N Engl J Med* 262:1214-1217, 1960.
24. Parfrey N and others. Hairless lower limbs and occlusive arterial disease, *Lancet* 1:276, 1976.
25. Baker WH and others. Diagnosis of peripheral occlusive disease: comparison of clinical evaluation and noninvasive laboratory, *Arch Surg* 113:1308-1310, 1978.
26. Johnston KW, Demorais D, and Colapinto RF. Difficulty in assessing the severity of aorto-iliac disease by clinical and arteriographic methods, *Angiology* 32:609-614, 1981.
27. Nicholson ML and others. Predictive value of bruits and Doppler pressure measurements in detecting lower limb arterial stenosis, *Eur J Vasc Surg* 7:59-62, 1993.

CHAPTER 49

The Diabetic Foot

I. **INTRODUCTION.** The term "diabetic foot" refers to complications in a foot rendered hypesthetic from diabetic polyneuropathy. These complications include ulceration, Charcot arthropathy, and infection. Each year, 2.5% of diabetics develop a foot ulcer,[1] and the diabetic foot is the leading cause of hospitalization among diabetics and the overall leading cause of amputation in the United States.[2,3]

II. **THE FINDINGS**
   A. **Foot ulceration.** Over 75% of diabetic ulcers develop on the toes or on the plantar surface of the metatarsal heads.[4,5] Most of the remaining ulcers appear over the heel, plantar midfoot, or previous amputation sites. "Ulcer area" refers to the product of the maximum ulcer width and maximum ulcer length.
   B. **Diabetic neuropathy and Semmes-Weinstein monofilaments.** Although neuropathy, ischemia, and infection all contribute to ulceration, the most important is neuropathy.[3,6] Conventional examination often fails to detect diabetic polyneuropathy, however, and about half of patients with diabetic ulceration lack complaints of numbness or pain[7] and can still detect the touch of a cotton wisp or pinprick.[4,8] Consequently, most diabetologists use a simple and more sensitive bedside tool, the Semmes-

Weinstein monofilament, to identify which patients have sufficient neuropathy placing them at risk for ulceration.

According to traditional teachings, a foot that is able to sense the 5.07 monofilament[a] is protected from ulceration, whereas one that fails to perceive the 5.07 monofilament is predisposed to ulceration. To use the monofilament, the patient should be lying supine with eyes closed, and the monofilament should be applied perpendicular to the skin with enough force to buckle it for approximately 1 second.[10] The patient responds "yes" each time he senses the monofilament, as the clinician randomly tests each site on the foot multiple times.[11] In clinical studies, anywhere from 1 to 10 different sites on the foot are tested,[12] but each study defines the abnormal result as inability to consistently sense the monofilament at *any* site. Testing the plantar surface of the first and fifth metatarsal heads may be the most efficient and overall accurate bedside maneuver.[12]

Monofilaments were first developed by von Frey in 1898 who glued thorns to hairs of various stiffnesses and calibrated them with a chemical balance ("von Frey hairs").[9] Nylon monofilaments were introduced in 1960 by Josephine Semmes and Sidney Weinstein, who used filaments of 20 different diameters (from 0.06 to 1.14 mm) to study sensation in patients with penetrating brain injuries.[13,14] Although the 5.07 monofilament is firmly entrenched as the standard for testing diabetic feet, this is based on an older study of patients

---

[a]The nominal value of a monofilament represents the common logarithm of 10 times the force in milligrams required to bow it (e.g., the 5.07 monofilament will buckle with 11.8 g of pressure, $\log_{10} (10 \times 11,800) = 5.07$).[9] Therefore, monofilaments with higher numbers are stiffer and more easily perceived than those with lower numbers.

with neuropathic foot ulcers from diabetes or leprosy, which used just 3 of the 20 monofilaments available.[10] The monofilaments studied were the 4.17 monofilament, which was selected because virtually all normal persons are able to sense it, and the stiffer 5.07 and 6.10 monofilaments. In the study, none of the patients with ulcers could sense the 4.17 or 5.07 monofilaments, although some could sense the 6.10 monofilament. These findings led the investigators to conclude that the ability to sense the 5.07 monofilament was protective (i.e., 6.10 was not protective and 4.17 was normal sensation). It is also possible, however, that a better indicator of protective sensation is one of the other 7 monofilaments between 6.10 and 4.17 not used in the study, and in support of this hypothesis, one study has suggested that the 4.21 monofilament may be a better discriminatory threshold.[4]

C. **Charcot joint.** Charcot joint (neuroarthropathy) refers to accelerated degenerative changes and ultimate joint destruction that follows repetitive trauma to insensitive, neuropathic joints. Although historically the most common causes were syphilis (affecting the larger joints of the lower extremity) and syringomyelia (affecting the larger joints of the upper extremity), the most common cause today is diabetes. In diabetic patients, Charcot joint characteristically affects the foot, including ankle, tarsometatarsal, and metatarsophalangeal joints.[15,16]

Most patients present with a limp, difficulty putting on shoes, or soft tissue swelling suggesting fracture, acute arthritis, or sprain.[16] The characteristic physical findings are anesthetic or hypesthetic feet (100% of patients), bony deformities (69% of patients), and soft tissue swelling (17% of patients). Many patients also have ulceration and abnormal callus formation. The most common bony deformities are abnormal projections on the plantar arch ("rocker sole") or other unusual prominence of the dorsal or medial arches of the midfoot or the metatarsophalangeal (MTP) joint. Soft tissue swelling typically appears at the ankle and midfoot, sometimes with marked rubor and warmth that mimics arthritis.

Jean-Martin Charcot described Charcot neuroarthropathy in 1868 in patients with tabes dorsalis,[17] although he credited the American Mitchell (1831) with the original description.[18]

D. Osteomyelitis. In diabetic patients with foot ulceration and underlying radiographic abnormalities of the bone, it is very difficult to distinguish Charcot foot from osteomyelitis. One proposed test is the "probe test," in which the clinician gently probes the ulcer base with a sterile, blunt, 14.0 cm 5 Fr stainless steel eye probe. The test is positive, suggesting osteomyelitis, if the clinician detects a rock-hard, often gritty structure at the ulcer base without any intervening soft tissue.[5]

III. CLINICAL SIGNIFICANCE

A. The Semmes-Weinstein monofilament. According to the information presented in Table 49-1, the *inability* to feel the 5.07 monofilament is a modest predictor of ulceration during a 3- to 4-year follow-up (LR = 2.9; Table 49-1). Another study has demonstrated that the *presence* of 5.07-monofilament sensation argues *against* subsequent amputation during 3 to 4 years follow-up (LR = 0.3).[22] Monofilament sensation predicts complications better than other quantitative measures of sensation, including the 128 Hz tuning fork[23] and graded vibratory or thermal stimuli.[4,24]

B. Osteomyelitis. In diabetic patients with foot ulceration, three findings argue *for* underlying osteomyelitis (defined by bone biopsy): the finding of an ulcer depth greater than 3 mm or

TABLE 49-1 The diabetic foot*

Finding (ref)†	Sensitivity (%)	Specificity (%)	Positive LR	Negative LR
Predictors of Subsequent Foot Ulceration				
Unable to sense the 5.07 monofilament[19,20]	66-68	61-86	2.9	0.5
Predictors of Osteomyelitis, in Patients with Foot Ulcers				
Positive probe test[5]	66	85	4.3	0.4
Ulcer area >2 cm^2 [21]	56	92	7.2	0.5
Ulcer deeper than 3 mm or bone exposed[21]	82	77	3.6	0.2
Accompanying erythema, swelling, purulence[21]	36	77	NS	NS

NS, Not significant.

*Diagnostic standard: For foot ulceration, the appearance of an ulcer during 3- to 4-year follow-up interval; for osteomyelitis, biopsy of the bone.

†Definition of findings: For positive probe test and ulcer area, see text.

bone exposed (LR = 3.6), a positive probe test (LR = 4.3), and an ulcer area >2 cm^2 (LR = 7.2). The findings of erythema, swelling, or purulence are unhelpful in diagnosing osteomyelitis.[21]

REFERENCES

1. Moss SE, Klein R, and Klein BEK. The prevalence and incidence of lower extremity amputation in a diabetic population, *Arch Intern Med* 152:610-616, 1992.

2. Lipsky BA. Osteomyelitis of the foot in diabetic patients, *Clin Infect Dis* 25:1318-1326, 1997.

3. Shaw JE and Boulton AJ. The pathogenesis of diabetic foot problems: an overview, *Diabetes* 46(suppl)2:S58-S61, 1997.

4. Sosenko JM and others. Comparison of quantitative sensory-threshold measures for their association with foot ulceration in diabetic patients, *Diab Care* 13:1057-1061, 1990.

5. Grayson ML and others. Probing to bone in infected pedal ulcers: a clinical sign of underlying osteomyelitis in diabetic patients, *JAMA* 273:721-723, 1995.

6. Caputo GM and others. Assessment and management of foot disease in patients with diabetes, *N Engl J Med* 331:854-860, 1994.

7. Kumar S and others. The prevalence of foot ulceration and its correlates in type 2 diabetic patients: a population-based study, *Diabetic Med* 11:480-484, 1994.

8. Valk GC and others. Clinical examination versus neurophysiological examination in the diagnosis of diabetic polyneuropathy, *Diab Med* 9:716-721, 1992.

9. Levin S, Pearsall G, and Ruderman RJ. Von Frey's method of measuring pressure sensibility in the hand: an engineering analysis of the Weinstein-Semmes pressure aesthesiometer, *J Hand Surg (Amer)* 3:211-216, 1978.

10. Birke JA and Sims DS. Plantar sensory threshold in the ulcerative foot, *Lepr Rev* 57:261-267, 1986.

11. Mueller MJ. Identifying patients with diabetes mellitus who are at risk for lower-extremity complications: use of Semmes-Weinstein monofilaments, *Phys Ther* 76:68-71, 1996.

12. McGill M and others. Possible sources of discrepancies in the use of the Semmes-Weinstein monofilament. Impact on prevalence of insensate foot and workload requirements, *Diabetes Care* 22:598-602, 1999.

13. Semmes J and others. *Somatosensory changes after penetrating brain wounds in man,* Cambridge, 1960, Harvard University Press.

14. Weinstein S and Sersen EA. Tactual sensitivity as a function of handedness and laterality, *J Compar Physiolog Psychol* 54:665-669, 1961.

15. Gupta R. A short history of neuropathic arthropathy, *Clin Orthop* 296:43-49, 1993.

16. Sinha S, Munichoodappa CS, and Kozak GP. Neuroarthropathy (Charcot joints) in diabetes mellitus (clinical study of 101 cases), *Medicine (Baltimore)* 51:191-210, 1972.

17. Charcot JM. The classic: on arthropathies of cerebral or spinal origin, *Clin Orthop Relat Res* 296:4-7, 1993.

18. Kelly M. John Kearsley Mitchell (1793-1858) and the neurogenic theory of arthritis, *J History Med* 20:151-156, 1965.

19. Boyko EJ and others. A prospective study of risk factors for diabetic foot ulcer. The Seattle Diabetic Foot study, *Diabetes Care* 22:1036-1042, 1999.

20. Rith-Najarian SJ, Stolusky T, and Gohdes DM. Identifying diabetic patients at high risk for lower-extremity amputation in a primary health care setting. A prospective evaluation of simple screening criteria, *Diabetes Care* 15:1386-1389, 1992.

21. Newman LG and others. Unsuspected osteomyelitis in diabetic foot ulcers: diagnosis and monitoring by leukocyte scanning with indium In 111 oxyquinoline, *JAMA* 266:1246-1251, 1991.

22. Adler AI and others. Lower-extremity amputation in diabetes. The independent effects of peripheral vascular disease, sensory neuropathy, and foot ulcers, *Diabetes Care* 22:1029-1035, 1999.

23. McNeely MJ and others. The independent contributions of diabetic neuropathy and vasculopathy in foot ulceration, *Diabetes Care* 18:216-219, 1995.

24. Litzelman DK, Marriott DJ, and Vinicor F. Independent physiological predictors of foot lesions in patients with NIDDM, *Diabetes Care* 20:1273-1278, 1997.

CHAPTER 50

Edema and Deep Vein Thrombosis

EDEMA

I. INTRODUCTION. Edema of a limb may occur because of increased venous pressure (venous insufficiency, congestive heart failure), increased vascular permeability (e.g., inflammation), decreased oncotic pressure (e.g., hypoalbuminemia), lymphatic obstruction (i.e., lymphedema), and deposition of additional tissue (e.g., lipedema). The most common causes of bilateral edema are congestive heart failure, chronic venous insufficiency, pulmonary hypertension without left heart failure, and drug-induced edema (e.g., nifedipine, nonsteroidal antiinflammatory medications).[1,2] The most common causes of unilateral swelling of the leg are deep vein thrombosis, Baker's cyst, and cellulitis (see below).[3-5]

II. THE FINDINGS. The pitting characteristics of edema reflect the viscosity of the edema fluid, which in turn depends largely on its protein concentration.[6-9] Edema fluid with low protein levels (e.g., hypoalbuminemia, congestive heart failure) pits easily and recovers relatively quickly compared with edema fluid that has higher protein levels (lymphedema, inflammatory edema).[7,8] A clue to "low protein edema" (i.e., edema associated with a serum albumin level <3.5 g/dl) is edema that pits easily with just 1 to 2 seconds of thumb pressure over the tibia, and then, after removal of the thumb, begins to recover within 2 to 3 seconds.[9]

Lymphedema is painless, firm edema that characteristically causes squaring of the toes and a dorsal hump on the foot. In contrast to venous edema, lymphedema varies little during the day and ulceration is uncommon unless there is secondary infection. Even though lymphedema has high protein levels, clinical experience shows it does pit early in its course although it eventually becomes nonpitting, hard, and "woody" as a secondary fibrous reaction ensues.[6]

Lipedema consists of bilateral deposition of excess subcutaneous fatty tissue in the legs that does not pit with pressure and whose most characteristic feature is sparing of the feet.[10] Lipedema occurs exclusively in obese women.

III. CLINICAL SIGNIFICANCE

A. Pitting edema. In patients with bilateral pitting edema of the legs, the most important diagnostic finding is the patient's venous pressure, estimated from examination of the neck veins. If the neck veins are abnormally distended, cardiac disease or pulmonary hypertension is at least partly responsible for the patient's edema; if they are normal, another cause is responsible, such as liver disease, nephrosis, chronic venous insufficiency, or one of the medications the patient is taking. Clinicians' estimates of venous pressure are accurate, with studies showing that the finding of elevated neck veins predicts an abnormally increased central venous pressure (i.e., >8 cm H_2O) with a positive LR of 9.0 (see Chapter 31).

In contrast, the finding of pitting edema by itself and without knowledge of the patient's venous pressure is an unreliable sign of cardiac disease. For example, in a study of patients undergoing cardiac catheterization because of chest pain or dyspnea, the finding of edema (without knowledge of venous pressure) lacked any significant relationship with the patient's left heart pressures (see Chapter 43).[11,12]

B. Lymphedema. Lymphedema is classified as "primary" (i.e., congenital abnormality of the lymphatic systems) or "secondary" (damage to the lymphatics from previous radiation or surgery, malignant obstruction, or recurrent episodes of cellulitis). Primary lymphedema begins before the age of 40 years, may be bilateral (50% of cases), and affects women 10 times more often than men.[13] Secondary lymphedema from infection, radiation, or surgery affects men and women of all ages, is usually unilateral, and is preceded by the characteristic history. Malignant obstruction affects patients older than 40 years and is almost always unilateral (>95% of cases).[13] The most common cause of malignant lymphedema in the leg of men is metastatic prostate carcinoma; in women, it is lymphoma.[13] Lymphedema of the arm is almost always due to breast cancer, either the tumor itself, or combined treatment with surgery and radiation.[14]

DEEP VEIN THROMBOSIS

I. INTRODUCTION. Deep vein thrombosis is conventionally divided into *proximal* thrombosis (popliteal vein and above) and *distal* thrombosis (calf veins). Several studies have shown that only proximal thrombi are associated with clinically significant pulmonary emboli, and thus only these thrombi require treatment with anticoagulation.[15]

In patients with acutely painful and swollen calves, accurate diagnosis is essential, not only because untreated proximal thrombi may cause fatal pulmonary emboli, but also because inappropriate administration of anticoagulation to persons without proximal thrombi risks unnecessarily life-threatening hemorrhage.

II. THE FINDINGS

A. Inspection and palpation.

The most important signs of vein thrombosis are tenderness and swelling. Calf asymmetry >1.5 cm is abnormal, indicating significant edema of the larger limb or atrophy of the smaller one.[16]

Other traditional signs associated with deep vein thrombosis are a palpable cord, dilated superficial veins, Homan's sign, skin erythema, and altered skin temperature (both coolness and warmth have been proposed by different authorities). The basis for these signs, however, seems dubious. Since large muscles and dense fascial tissues encompass the deep veins of the legs, concealing them from the examiner's eyes and hands, it is difficult to conceive how a clinician could ever palpate the cord of a thrombosed deep vein. The increased collateral flow around an obstruction could make the superficial veins more conspicuous, but skin surface temperature and color reflect blood flow and vessel size of the minute vessels *of the dermis*,[17] which should not necessarily be different after venous obstruction.

B. Homans' sign.

In his extensive writings about venous thrombosis, the American surgeon John Homans contrasted two forms of the disease: bland thrombosis of the calf veins, which caused few symptoms other than mild swelling and pain, and iliofemoral thrombophlebitis ("phlegmasia alba dolens"), which caused generalized leg edema and cyanosis.[18-20] Homans believed that most pulmonary emboli originated in the bland calf thrombi, and that once diagnosed, the disorder should be treated by femoral vein ligation to prevent pulmonary emboli (anticoagulation was not yet being used). In 1941, Homans proposed that the "dorsiflexion sign"—"discomfort behind the knee on forced dorsiflexion of the foot"—was a sign of these difficult-to-diagnose calf thrombi.[19] Although contemporaries called the sign "Homans' sign,"[21] Homans never did and instead later credited another clinician for making the original description.[22]

Surgeons soon learned that there were many examples of a false-positive Homans' sign (i.e., positive dorsiflexion sign but no clot found at surgery),[21,23] and in 1944, Homans redefined the positive response, stating that "discomfort need have no part in the reaction." Eventually, Homans became unenthusiastic about the sign[24,25] and has been quoted as saying "if you wanted to name a sign after me, why didn't you pick a good one?"[26]

C. Pseudothrombophlebitis. In a large series of patients presenting with suspected deep vein thrombosis, only 1 out of every 4 or 5 patients actually has the diagnosis.[27-31] An important mimic of deep vein thrombosis (i.e., "pseudothrombophlebitis") is Baker's cyst, which is a distended gastrocnemius-semimembranosus bursa that has dissected or ruptured into the calf or is compressing the popliteal vein.[32,33] A telltale sign of this disorder (and any other cause of calf hematoma) is crescent-shaped ecchymosis near either malleolus.[34,35]

III. CLINICAL SIGNIFICANCE

A. Individual findings. Table 50-1 presents the diagnostic accuracy of physical signs for deep vein thrombosis, as applied to thousands of patients with acute calf pain, swelling, or both. Although some studies recruited outpatients[27,37] and others both inpatients and outpatients,[29,30,39] the accuracy of individual signs is the same whether or not inpatients are included in the analysis. In some studies, "deep vein thrombosis" refers only to proximal thrombosis

TABLE 50-1 Deep vein thrombosis*

Finding (ref)†	Sensitivity (%)	Specificity (%)	Positive LR	Negative LR
Inspection				
Any calf or ankle swelling[24,25,30,36-38]	41-90	8-74	NS	0.7
Asymmetric calf swelling, ≥2 cm difference[29]	61	71	2.1	0.6
Thigh swelling[30]	50	80	2.5	0.6
Superficial venous dilation[25,39]	29-33	82-85	1.9	NS
Erythema[36,37,39]	16-48	61-87	NS	NS
Superficial thrombophlebitis[38]	5	95	NS	NS
Palpation				
Tenderness[24,25,36-39]	42-85	10-65	NS	NS
Asymmetric skin coolness[25]	42	63	NS	NS
Asymmetric skin warmth[36,39]	29-71	51-77	1.4	NS
Palpable cord[30,39]	15-30	73-85	NS	NS
Other Tests				
Homans' sign[24,25,30,36-39]	10-54	39-89	NS	NS

NS, Not significant.

*Diagnostic standard: For deep venous thrombosis, positive contrast venography[24,25,30,36-39] or compression ultrasonography.[29]

†Definition of findings: All findings refer to the symptomatic leg.

(popliteal vein or higher),[30,36,37] whereas others included patients with proximal vein or isolated calf vein thrombosis (but in these studies, only 15% to 29% had isolated calf thrombosis).[29,38,39]

According to these studies, only the findings of thigh swelling (LR = 2.5), asymmetric calf swelling ($\geq$2 cm difference, LR = 2.1), superficial vein dilation (LR = 1.9), and asymmetric skin warmth (LR = 1.4) argue significantly *for* thrombosis, although the discriminatory value of all of these signs is slight. The presence or absence of erythema, tenderness, skin coolness, palpable cord, and Homans' sign have no diagnostic value. As expected, the finding of superficial thrombophlebitis (i.e., visibly inflamed and tender subcutaneous veins) has no relationship to pathology in the deep veins. No finding argues convincingly *against* the diagnosis of thrombosis (no LR <0.5).

These same studies show that the presence of certain risk factors assists diagnosis. For example, the knowledge of active cancer in a patient with calf swelling detects deep vein thrombosis with a sensitivity of 20% to 39%, specificity of 90% to 92%, and positive LR of 3.2.[27,29,30] Similarly, the finding "recent immobilization" has a sensitivity of 24% to 41%, specificity of 82% to 90%, and positive LR of 2.3.[27,30]

B. Combined findings. Given the meager accuracy of individual findings, Wells and others developed a simple scoring scheme (Table 50-2) that combines findings, stratifying patients into groups of "low," "moderate," or "high" probability for deep vein thrombosis.[27] The findings in his model were all proven to be independent predictors in an earlier analysis.[28,40] According to two studies applying this scheme to over 850 outpatients, a low pretest probability (0 or fewer points) argues convincingly against deep vein thrombosis (LR = 0.2; Table 50-3), and a high pretest probability (3 or more points) argues

TABLE 50-2 Wells scoring scheme for pretest probability of deep-vein thrombosis[27]*

Clinical Feature	Points
Risk Factors	
Active cancer	1
Paralysis, paresis, or recent plaster immobilization of the lower extremities	1
Recently bedridden >3 days or major surgery within 4 wk	1
Signs	
Localized tenderness along the distribution of the deep venous system	1
Entire leg swollen	1
Asymmetric calf swelling (>3 cm difference, 10 cm below tibial tuberosity)	1
Asymmetric pitting edema	1
Collateral superficial veins (nonvaricose)	1
Alternative Diagnosis	
Alternative diagnosis as likely or more likely than deep venous thrombosis	−2

*Interpretation of score: High probability if 3 points or more, moderate probability if 1 or 2 points, and low probability if 0 points or less.

strongly *for* the diagnosis (LR = 13.2). The finding of a moderate pretest probability is diagnostically unhelpful.

Because the hazards of misdiagnosis are great, however, clinicians should still use compression ultrasonography when diagnosing deep vein thrombosis and reserve Wells' scheme for deciding whether additional tests are necessary. For example, in patients with low clinical probability and negative compression ultrasonography, the clinician can safely avoid serial ultrasonography (a common practice after a single negative ultrasound, to detect proximal propagation of clot missed on the first ultrasound). Also, in patients with high clinical probability but negative ultrasonography, the

TABLE 50-3 Wells scoring scheme for deep vein thrombosis*

Pretest Probability[27,31]†	Sensitivity (%)	Specificity (%)	Positive LR
Low pretest probability	7-11	36-43	0.2
Moderate pretest probability	33-34	—	NS
High pretest probability	56-60	94-96	13.2

NS, Not significant.

Diagnostic standard: For deep vein thrombosis, compression ultrasonography,[27,31] sometimes with contrast venography.[27]

†*Definition of findings: For pretest probability, see Table 50-2.*

probability of deep vein thrombosis is so high that further testing may be necessary (e.g., venography).[27]

This diagnostic scheme should not be applied to inpatients or to any patients with prior deep vein thrombosis or suspected pulmonary embolism because these patients were excluded from the studies in Table 50-3.

REFERENCES

1. Ciocon JO, Galindo-Ciocon D, and Galindo DJ. Raised leg exercises for leg edema in the elderly, *Angiology* 46:19-25, 1995.
2. Blankfield RP and others. Etiology and diagnosis of bilateral leg edema in primary care, *Am J Med* 105:192-197, 1998.
3. Belch JJF and others. Combined phlebography and arthrography in patients with painful swollen calf, *Br Med J* 282:949, 1981.
4. Hall S and others. The painful swollen calf: a comparative evaluation of four investigative techniques, *Med J Austr* 144:356-358, 1986.
5. Simpson FG and others. Prospective study of thrombophlebitis and "pseudothrombophlebitis," *Lancet* 1:331-333, 1980.
6. Bates DO, Levick JR, and Mortimer PS. Quantification of rate and depth of pitting in human edema using an electronic tonometer, *Lymphology* 27:159-172, 1994.
7. Berlyne GM and others. Oedema protein concentrations for differentiation of cellulitis and deep vein thrombosis, *Lancet* 2:728-729, 1989.
8. Crockett DJ. The protein levels of oedema fluids, *Lancet* 2:1179-1182, 1956.
9. Henry JA and Altmann P. Assessment of hypoproteinaemic oedema: a simple physical sign, *Br Med J* 1:890-891, 1978.
10. Allen EV and Hines EA. Lipedema of the legs: a syndrome characterized by fat legs and orthostatic edema, *Proc Staff Mayo Clin* 15:184-187, 1940.
11. Harlan WR and others. Chronic congestive heart failure in coronary artery disease: clinical criteria, *Ann Intern Med* 86:133-138, 1977.

12. Zema MJ and others. Left ventricular dysfunction: bedside Valsalva manoevre, *Br Heart J* 44:560-569, 1980.

13. Smith RD, Spittell JA, and Schirger A. Secondary lymphedema of the leg: its characteristics and diagnostic implications, *JAMA* 185:80-82, 1963.

14. Browse NL. Lymphoedema of the arm, *Br Med J* 295:3-4, 1987.

15. Huisman MV and others. Serial impedance plethysmography for suspected deep venous thrombosis in outpatients: the Amsterdam general practitioner study, *N Engl J Med* 314:823-828, 1986.

16. Stein PD and others. Asymmetry of calves in the assessment of patients with suspected acute pulmonary embolism, *Chest* 107:936-939, 1995.

17. Lewis T. *The blood vessels of the human skin and their responses,* London, 1927, Shaw & Sons.

18. Homans J. Thrombosis of the deep veins of the lower leg, causing pulmonary embolism, *N Engl J Med* 211:993-997, 1934.

19. Homans J. Exploration and division of the femoral and iliac veins in the treatment of thrombophlebitis of the leg, *N Engl J Med* 224:179-186, 1941.

20. Homans J. Thrombosis as a complication of venography, *JAMA* 119:136, 1942.

21. Moses WR. The early diagnosis of phlebothrombosis, *N Engl J Med* 234:288-291, 1946.

22. Homans J. Venous thrombosis and pulmonary embolism, *N Engl J Med* 236:196-201, 1947.

23. Allen AW, Linton RR, and Donaldson GA. Thrombosis and embolism: review of 202 patients treated by femoral vein interruption, *Ann Surg* 118:728-740, 1943.

24. Cranley JJ, Canos AJ, Sull WJ. The diagnosis of deep venous thrombosis: fallibility of clinical signs, *Arch Surg* 111:34-36, 1976.

25. Haeger K. Problems of acute deep venous thrombosis: I. The interpretation of signs and symptoms, *Angiology* 20:219-223, 1969.

26. Barker WF. To the memory of John Homans, M.D., 1877-1954, *Maj Probl Clin Surg* 4:v-vii, 1966.

27. Wells PS and others. Value of assessment of pretest probability of deep-vein thrombosis in clinical management, *Lancet* 350:1795-1798, 1997.

28. Wells PS and others. Accuracy of clinical assessment of deep-vein thrombosis, *Lancet* 345:1326-1330, 1995.

29. Criado E and Burnham CB. Predictive value of clinical criteria for the diagnosis of deep vein thrombosis, *Surgery* 122:578-583, 1997.

30. Landefeld CS, McGuire E, and Cohen AM. Clinical findings associated with acute proximal deep vein thrombosis: a basis for quantifying clinical judgment, *Am J Med* 88:382-388, 1990.

31. Miron MJ, Perrier A, and Bounameaux H. Clinical assessment of suspected deep vein thrombosis: comparison between a score and empirical assessment, *J Intern Med* 247:249-254, 2000.

32. Katz RS and others. The pseudothrombophlebitis syndrome, *Medicine* 56:151-164, 1977.

33. Wigley RD. Popliteal cysts: variations on a theme by Baker, *Semin Arthritis Rheum* 12:1-10, 1982.

34. Tibbutt DA and Gunning AJ. Calf haematoma: a new sign in differential diagnosis from deep vein thrombosis, *Br Med J* 4:204, 1974.

35. Kraag G and others. The hemorrhagic crescent sign of acute synovial rupture, *Ann Intern Med* 85:477-478, 1976.

36. Vaccaro P and others. Shortcomings of physical examination and impedance plethysmography in the diagnosis of lower extremity deep venous thrombosis, *Angiology* 38: 232-235, 1981.

37. O'Donnell TF and others. Diagnosis of deep venous thrombosis in the outpatient by venography, *Surg Gynecol Obstet* 150:69-74, 1980.

38. Molloy W and others. Clinical findings in the diagnosis of proximal deep vein thrombosis, *Ir Med J* 75:119-120, 1982.

39. Kahn SR and others. Clinical prediction of deep vein thrombosis in patients with leg symptoms, *Thromb Haemost* 81:353-357, 1999.

40. Wells PS and others. A simple clinical model for the diagnosis of deep-vein thrombosis combined with impedance plethysmography: potential for an improvement in the diagnostic process, *J Intern Med* 243:15-23, 1998.

PART ELEVEN

Neurologic Examination

CHAPTER 51

Visual Field Testing

I. **INTRODUCTION.** Abnormalities of peripheral vision are called "visual field defects." These defects, many of which can be detected at the bedside, provide important clues to the diagnosis of lesions throughout the visual pathways—retina, optic nerve, optic chiasm, optic tracts, optic radiations (parietal and temporal lobes), and occipital cortex (Figure 51-1).

II. **DEFINITION.** The term **hemianopia** describes visual defects that occupy about one half of an eye's visual space. **Quadrantanopia** describes defects confined mostly to about one fourth of an eye's visual space. **Homonymous** describes defects that affect the same side of the vertical meridian (i.e., right or left side) of both eyes. For example, a right homonymous hemianopia affects the right visual space of both eyes (i.e., the temporal field of the right eye and the nasal field of the left eye). "Homonymous" implies the defect does not cross the vertical meridian.

III. **THE ANATOMY OF THE VISUAL PATHWAYS.** The key anatomic points in Figure 51-1 are (1) Images from the visual fields are inverted throughout the retina and all neural pathways. Images from the temporal visual field fall on the nasal retina, and those from the nasal field on the temporal retina.

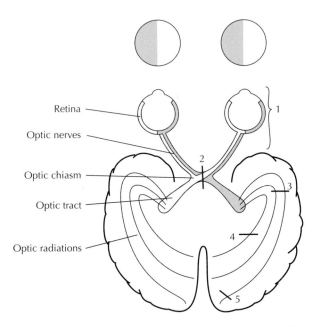

FIGURE 51-1 Anatomy of the visual pathways. The anatomy of the visual pathways appears at the top of the figure, the light gray shading indicating how visual information from the left visual space eventually courses to the right brain. Visual field defects are on the facing page. Anterior defects (labeled "1," from disease of the optic nerve or retina) characteristically affect one eye and cause defects (the *black shading*) that may cross the vertical meridian (i.e., the vertical meridian is the vertical line bisecting each visual field). Chiasmal defects (labeled "2") and postchiasmal defects (labeled "3" for a lesion in the anterior temporal lobe, "4" for the parietal lobe, and "5" for the occipital cortex) characteristically affect both eyes and respect the vertical meridian.

Images from the superior visual fields are transmitted throughout the inferior visual pathways (inferior retina, inferior optic nerve and chiasm, and temporal lobe), and those from the inferior visual fields throughout the superior visual pathways (superior retina, superior optic nerve and chiasm,

ANTERIOR LESIONS:

CHIASMAL LESIONS:

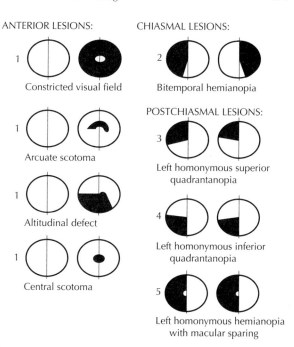

POSTCHIASMAL LESIONS:

1 Constricted visual field

1 Arcuate scotoma

1 Altitudinal defect

1 Central scotoma

2 Bitemporal hemianopia

3 Left homonymous superior quadrantanopia

4 Left homonymous inferior quadrantanopia

5 Left homonymous hemianopia with macular sparing

FIGURE 51-1, cont'd For legend see opposite page.

parietal lobe). (2) The nasal retinal fibers cross in the chiasms; therefore, disease of the optic chiasm causes defects in both temporal visual fields ("bitemporal hemianopia"). (3) The visual pathways posterior to the optic chiasm contain information from the same visual space of each eye: lesions in the right postchiasmal pathways cause defects in the left visual space of each eye (i.e., temporal field of left eye and nasal field of right eye), and those of the left postchiasmal pathways cause defects in the right visual space. Such defects, respecting the vertical meridian in each eye, are called "homonymous." (4) The visual pathways in the occipital cortex that contain information from the macula (point of fixation) are distant from those connected to the more peripheral fields.[1] Therefore, lesions of the occipital cortex may cause either homonymous defects sparing the macula or visual defects confined just to central vision.

IV. **TECHNIQUE.** There are two traditional ways to test visual fields at the bedside: static confrontational testing and kinetic confrontational testing. In both techniques, the patient sits about 70 to 100 cm from the clinician and fixes on the clinician's own eye. Only one eye of the patient is tested at a time; the other is occluded with a card or the patient's hand.

A. **Static technique.** Using this technique, the clinician presents objects at a fixed point in the visual field, usually about 20 to 30 degrees from fixation. Typically, the clinician presents his hands to two visual quadrants simultaneously and asks the patient to count the number of fingers shown or indicate which index finger is wiggling.[2] Testing two quadrants simultaneously has the advantage of detecting some parietal lobe lesions, which may allow patients to see an object in the contralateral field if it appears alone, but not if another object is presented simultaneously to the healthy visual field.[3]

Throughout the examination, the clinician focuses on whether a defect respects the vertical or horizontal meridians of the visual field (see below). Defects crossing the vertical meridian are due to anterior disease (see below), whereas those respecting the vertical meridian are due to chiasmal disease (if the defect is bitemporal) or postchiasmal disease (if it is homonymous).

B. **Kinetic technique.** In this technique, the clinician tests one quadrant at a time by slowly moving an object (e.g., wiggling finger) from an extreme peripheral field toward fixation, the patient then indicating the moment he sees the object.

V. THE FINDINGS. Visual field defects are classified as "prechiasmal" (from disease in retina or optic nerves, often called "anterior defects"), "chiasmal," and "postchiasmal" (optic tracts, optic radiations, and occipital cortex).

A. Anterior or prechiasmal defects. The characteristic features follow:

   1. **One eye is affected (unless the retinal or optic nerve disorder is bilateral).**

   2. **Visual acuity is poor.** Most patients have diminished acuity or, if acuity is normal, other signs of anterior disease, such as an afferent pupillary defect (see Chapter 19), red color desaturation, abnormal retina examination, or an abnormal optic disc (drusen, cupping, or atrophy).

   3. **The defects may cross the vertical meridian.** This occurs because retinal nerve fibers from the temporal retina arch across the vertical meridian to reach the optic disc and nerve (which lie on the nasal side of the retina). Damage to these fibers thus may cause a defect that crosses the vertical meridian. Small nerve fiber defects may cause an "arcuate defect" (see Figure 51-1), larger ones an "altitudinal defect" (having a sharp horizontal border in the nasal field). Damage to fibers from the macula may cause "central scotomas" and, to those preferentially affecting the most peripheral vision, "constricted visual fields."[4]

B. Chiasmal defects. These defects are bitemporal hemianopias (see Figure 51-1).

C. Postchiasmal defects. The characteristics of these defects are the following:

   1. **Both eyes are affected, causing homonymous hemianopias or quadrantanopias.**

   2. **Visual acuity is normal.** This is true in greater than 90% of cases. If visual acuity is abnormal, it is because of bilateral disease and thus the acuity in both eyes is the same.[5]

3. **Pupil and retinal examination are normal.** One important exception is the occasional finding of papilledema, caused by brain tumors affecting the optic radiations.

VI. CLINICAL SIGNIFICANCE

A. **Etiology.** Most anterior defects are caused by severe glaucoma, retinal emboli, and optic neuritis. Chiasmal defects are often due to a pituitary tumor just below the optic chiasm. Over 95% of postchiasmal defects are due to lesions of the temporal, parietal, and occipital lobes. Lesions of the optic tracts are rare.[5]

Although parietal and temporal lobe disease may cause inferior and superior quadrantanopias, respectively (see Figure 51-1), lesions in these areas more often cause dense hemianopias or hemianopias that are denser inferiorly or superiorly, respectively.[5,6]

B. **Diagnostic accuracy.** Table 51-1 summarizes the diagnostic accuracy of the confrontational technique for diagnosing visual field defects. The only study comparing static and kinetic techniques found the two methods were equivalent, although this study excluded patients with hemispheral disease.[9]

Table 51-1 reveals that, if the clinician finds a defect by confrontation, one is likely present by perimetry (LRs = 4.2 to 6.8). The absence of a defect, on the other hand, is less helpful, especially in patients with suspected anterior defects or those with chiasmal disease.

C. **Differential diagnosis of postchiasmal defects.** Homonymous hemianopias may be either an isolated finding or associated with other neurologic findings. The most common cause of an *isolated* homonymous hemianopia is an ischemic infarct of the occipital cortex.[10,11] In patients with associated hemiparesis, aphasia, or asymmetric optokinetic nystagmus, the most common diagnosis is parietal lobe

TABLE 51-1 Visual field defects*

Finding (ref)	Sensitivity (%)	Specificity (%)	Positive LR	Negative LR
Confrontation Technique, Detecting the Following Visual Field Defects[7-9]				
Anterior defects (retina and optic nerve)	11-58	93-98	4.2	0.7
Patchy defects	6			
Constriction of visual fields	58			
Arcuate defects	20-51			
Altitudinal defects	88			
Posterior defects (optic chiasm to occipital cortex)	43-86	86-95	6.8	0.4
Bitemporal hemianopia	45			
Homonymous hemianopia	80			
Patients with Homonymous Hemianopias, Detecting Parietal Lobe Disease				
Asymmetric optokinetic nystagmus[5]	93	84	5.7	0.1
Associated hemiparesis or aphasia[10]	90	95	18.3	0.1

Diagnostic standard: For visual field defects, conventional perimetry.

disease.[5,10,12,13] Optokinetic nystagmus is a normal horizontal nystagmus that occurs when patients look at a vertically striped tape moving in front of them. The clinician moves the tape first to one side and then the other, comparing the amplitude of horizontal nystagmus produced, which should be equal in each direction. Parietal lobe lesions reduce or eliminate optokinetic nystagmus when the tape is moved toward the side with the lesion. (Barany first made this observation in 1921.)

In patients with homonymous defects, the presence of asymmetric optokinetic nystagmus, associated aphasia or hemiparesis, argues strongly *for* a parietal lobe lesion (LR = 5.7 for optokinetic nystagmus and 18.3 for hemiparesis or aphasia), whereas the absence of these findings argues against it (both LRs = 0.1) and makes an occipital or temporal lobe lesion most likely.

D. Improving detection of visual field defects.
Confrontation fails to detect some defects because they are too small, lack a sharp linear border (e.g., patchy defects of anterior disease), or are too peripheral (e.g., constricted visual fields; confrontation only tests the most central 20 to 30 degrees of visual space). To increase sensitivity of bedside examination, some experts have proposed the following techniques, each of which supplement routine confrontational testing:

1. Perform confrontational testing with red-colored squares or lights instead of fingers. In areas of early defects, patients may describe that the red light appears orange, pale yellow, or white.[14] In one study, this method detected chiasmal defects with an overall sensitivity of 79%.[9]

2. Repeat confrontational testing from 4 meters away. Routine confrontational testing is performed from 1 meter away; increasing the distance to 4 meters may improve sensitivity for subtle arcuate scotomata (glaucoma or optic nerve disease) or macular sparing (some occipital cortex lesions).[15]

3. **Examine the patient's perceptions of the clinician's face, positioned about 30 cm away.** The clinician tests one eye at a time and asks whether any areas of the clinician's face are missing or distorted.[7,16]

REFERENCES

1. Trauzettel-Klosinski S and Reinhard J. The vertical field border in hemianopia and its significance for fixation and reading, *Invest Ophthalmol Vis Sci* 39:2177-2186, 1998.

2. Welsh RC. Finger counting in the four quadrants as a method of visual field gross screening, *Arch Ophthalmol* 66:678-679, 1961.

3. Bender MB and Furlow LT. Phenomenon of visual extinction in homonymous fields and psychologic principles involved, *Arch Neurol Psych* 53:29-45, 1945.

4. Kitazawa Y and Yamamoto T. Glaucomatous visual field defects: their characteristics and how to detect them, *Clin Neurosci* 4:279-283, 1997.

5. Smith JL. Homonymous hemianopia: a review of one hundred cases, *Am J Ophthalmol* 54:616-623, 1962.

6. McFadzean RM and Hadley DM. Homonymous quadrantanopia respecting the horizontal meridian: a feature of striate and extrastriate cortical disease, *Neurology* 49:1741-1746, 1997.

7. Johnson LN and Baloh FG. The accuracy of confrontation visual field test in comparison with automated perimetry, *J Natl Med Assoc* 83:895-898, 1991.

8. Shahinfar S, Johnson LN, and Madsen RW. Confrontation visual field loss as a function of decibel sensitivity loss on automated static perimetry: implications on the accuracy of confrontation visual field testing, *Ophthalmology* 102: 872-877, 1995.

9. Trobe JD and others. Confrontation visual field techniques in the detection of anterior visual pathway lesions, *Ann Neurol* 10:28-34, 1981.

10. Jacobsen DM. The localizing value of a quadrantanopia, *Arch Neurol* 54:401-404, 1997.

11. Trobe JD, Lorber ML, and Schlezinger NS. Isolated homonymous hemianopia, *Arch Ophthalmol* 89:377-381, 1973.

12. Smith JL and Cogan DG. Optokinetic nystagmus: a test for parietal lobe lesions (a study of 31 anatomically verified cases), *Am J Ophthalmol* 48:187-193, 1959.

13. Baloh RW, Yee RD, and Honrubia V. Optokinetic nystagmus and parietal lobe lesions, *Ann Neurol* 7:269-276, 1980.

14. Frisen L. A versatile color confrontation test for the central visual field: a comparison with quantitative perimetry, *Arch Ophthalmol* 89:3-9, 1973.

15. Kodsi SR and Younge BR. The four-meter confrontation visual field test, *J Clin Neuroophthalmology* 13:40-43, 1993.

16. Reader AL and Harper DG. Confrontation visual-field testing, *JAMA* 236:250, 1976.

CHAPTER 52

Nerves of the Eye Muscles (III, IV, and VI): Approach to Diplopia

DIPLOPIA

I. INTRODUCTION. Patients with lesions of cranial nerves 3, 4, and 6 have paralysis of one or more ocular muscles, which prevents the eyes from aligning properly and causes double vision, or diplopia. The most common mistake in analyzing diplopia, however, is to prematurely conclude that the patient must have neuropathy of one of these three nerves. Because less than half of the patients with diplopia actually have a cranial neuropathy, this chapter first emphasizes the general approach to *all* causes of diplopia.

II. DEFINITIONS. Diplopia may be **monocular** or **binocular**. Monocular diplopia persists after occluding one eye. Binocular diplopia depends on the visual axes of each eye being out of alignment and therefore disappears when one eye is occluded.

Several other terms are used to describe the findings of patients with *binocular diplopia*. **Heterotropia** is a general term for the finding of visual axes that are not parallel (synonyms are "squint" or "strabismus"). **Esotropia** means that one eye is converging or is deviated toward the nose (e.g., a

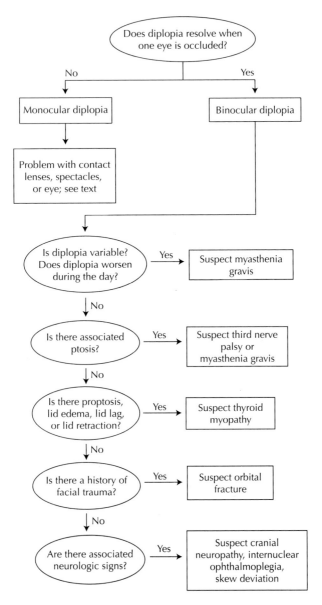

FIGURE 52-1 For legend see opposite page.

FIGURE 52-1 General approach to diplopia. The clinician should first distinguish monocular from binocular diplopia and, in patients with binocular diplopia, address the 5 questions on the right side of the figure. Only then should the clinician identify which muscle is weak, although this is unnecessary if the clinician already suspects myasthenia (from fatigability) or full third nerve palsy (from weakness of the medial rectus, superior rectus, inferior rectus, and inferior oblique muscles, with or without a dilated pupil).

Uncommon causes of diplopia and associated *ptosis*, not presented in the figure, are botulism, the Fisher variant of Guillain-Barré syndrome, and aberrant regeneration of the third nerve.[1,2] Uncommon causes of diplopia and associated *orbital findings* (e.g., proptosis) are carotid-cavernous fistula (which causes an orbital bruit),[3] orbital tumor, and pseudotumor.

---

left esotropia means that the left eye is deviated toward the nose). **Exotropia** means that one eye is diverging or is deviated toward the temple (e.g., a right exotropia means that the right eye is deviated out). **Hypertropia** means that one eye is deviated upwards (e.g., a left hypertropia means that the left eye is elevated with respect to the right eye). Diplopia may be **horizontal**, with the two images side by side, or **vertical**, with one image higher than the other (the term "vertical diplopia" also encompasses diplopia with images separated both vertically and horizontally).

III. TECHNIQUE

A. General approach. Figure 52-1 outlines the general approach to diplopia. The most important initial question is whether the diplopia is monocular or binocular, which can easily be addressed by covering one of the patient's eyes. Overall, 25% of all diplopia is monocular and 75% is binocular.[4]

In patients with binocular diplopia, the clinician can avoid misdiagnosing cranial neuropathy by first addressing the five questions listed in Figure 52-1. Only after asking these questions should the clinician attempt to identify which eye muscle is weak.

B. Identifying the weak muscle. When examining the eye muscles, the clinician holds up his index finger or penlight and asks the patient to track it toward each of the six cardinal directions of gaze (i.e., left, left and up, left and down, right, right and up, right and down). These directions parallel the principle action of the six eye muscles, as described in Figure 52-2.

There are two steps in identifying which eye muscle is weak. Step 1 reduces the number of possible weak eye muscles from 12 to 2. Step 2 then identifies which of these two muscles is causing the diplopia.

1. Step 1: The worst diplopia (and heterotropia) occurs when the patient looks in the direction of the weak muscle. The clinician asks the patient which of the six cardinal directions most aggravates the diplopia. According to this rule, the weak muscle is then one of the two muscles that are responsible for this movement, one of which moves the right eye and the other the left eye. For example, diplopia that is worse on far right lateral gaze indicates weakness of the right lateral rectus or the left medial

FIGURE 52-2 Principle actions of ocular muscles. There are 12 ocular muscles, 6 in each eye. The actions of the medial rectus (MR) and lateral rectus (LR) are simple right and left lateral movements. Although the actions of the 4 vertical eye muscles—the superior rectus (SR), inferior rectus (IR), superior oblique (SO), and inferior oblique (IO)—are more complex, there is one direction of gaze, indicated in the figure, in which weakness is most apparent.

rectus. Diplopia that is worse when the patient looks to the left and down indicates a problem of the left inferior rectus or the right superior oblique.[a]

2. **Step 2 identifies which of the two identified muscles is weak.** There are three techniques:

   a. **Inspection of the eyes.** In patients with diplopia on far right lateral gaze, the weak muscle is the right lateral rectus if there is an esotropia, but the left medial rectus is weak if there is an exotropia. In patients with diplopia that is worse when looking up and to the right, the weak muscle is the right superior rectus if there is a left hypertropia but the left inferior oblique if there is a right hypertropia.

   Often, however, the heterotropia is not obvious, either because the visual axes are only out of line by a degree or two (too small to see) or because the patient can compensate and temporarily pull the visual axes back into line. In these patients, the following techniques are helpful:

   b. **The affected eye is the one with the most peripheral image.** By placing a red glass over one eye (usually the right eye), the patient is less likely to fuse the images, and, when looking at a penlight in the direction of maximal diplopia, sees two images, one red and one white. The most peripheral image belongs to the weak eye.

   For example, in a patient whose maximal diplopia is to the left and down (and

---

[a] Because the actions of the four vertical muscles are sometimes difficult to recall, a mnemonic by Maddox (1907) may be helpful: the affected muscle is "either the same-named rectus muscle or the most crossed-named oblique muscle." For example, if diplopia is worse when the patient looks to the *left* in a *superior* direction, the affected muscles are either the *left superior* rectus or *right inferior* oblique.

who has the red glass over the right eye), the weak muscle is the right superior oblique if the red image is most peripheral, but the left inferior rectus is weak if the white image is most peripheral.

c. **The cover/uncover test.** To perform this test the clinician covers one eye while the patient looks in the direction of maximal diplopia. Covering one eye prevents fusion of the images, and any heterotropia that exists will return, although it is now obscured by occlusion of the eye. The clinician then observes which way that eye moves to pick up the image after it is uncovered. If it moves out, there was an esotropia; if it moves in, there was a exotropia, and if it moves down, that eye had a hypertropia.

IV. CLINICAL SIGNIFICANCE

A. **Monocular diplopia.** Almost all patients with monocular diplopia have "extraocular" or "ocular" causes.[4-7] Common extraocular causes are the patient's spectacles (e.g., reflections off one or both surfaces of the lenses) or contact lenses (e.g., air bubble in the pupillary area, abnormal curves, or uneven thicknesses). This diplopia resolves after removal of the lenses and, in patients with spectacles, varies as the spectacles are moved in and out or up and down. Common "ocular" causes include problems in the lens (e.g., fluid clefts, early cataracts), cornea (e.g., astigmatism, keratitis), and eyelids (e.g., chalazion, prolonged reading which may allow drooping lids to temporarily deform the cornea). The diplopia of these patients resolves when patients look through a pinhole or when a card is held over half of the pupillary aperture (the diplopia resolves because it depends on irregularities of the optic media acting as tiny prisms that divert some rays off the fovea; the pinhole or card blocks these wayward rays and thus eliminates the problem).

Rare patients with monocular diplopia have a cerebral disease.[8,9] Despite traditional teachings, hysteria is a rare cause of monocular diplopia.

B. Binocular diplopia

1. **Etiology.** Among patients with binocular diplopia, common final diagnoses are cranial neuropathy (3, 4, or 6; 40% of patients), eye muscle disease (thyroid ophthalmopathy, myasthenia gravis; 15% of patients), trauma (14%), supranuclear causes (internuclear ophthalmoplegia, skew deviation, 7%), other causes (12%), and unknown (12%).[4]

2. **Weak muscles and their clinical significance.** Incomplete palsies of the third cranial nerve are rare (in one study of 579 patients with third nerve palsies, less than 1% were partial).[10,11] Therefore, if only one or two of the third nerve muscles (i.e., superior rectus, inferior rectus, medial rectus, and inferior oblique) are weak, the diagnosis is almost certainly *not* a partial third nerve palsy but instead one of the diagnoses listed below.

   a. **Weak superior rectus muscle.** The clinician should consider **myasthenia gravis**. Sixty-five percent of patients with myasthenia gravis present with ocular symptoms, usually diplopia and ptosis.[12] Symptoms often have a fluctuating course, worsen at the end of the day, or even alternate between the eyes. The most common muscles affected are the superior rectus and medial rectus, whose weakness clinicians can often bring out by having the patient sustain an upward or far lateral gaze for 30 seconds or more.[13,14]

In myasthenia gravis, the pupils are always normal.

b. Weak inferior rectus muscle. The clinician should consider thyroid myopathy and orbital floor fracture.

(1) *Thyroid myopathy.* Patients may have associated proptosis, lid lag, lid retraction, chemosis, and hyperemia at the insertions of the recti muscles (see Chapter 22). These findings are sometimes subtle, and because many patients are also clinically euthyroid, the only finding of thyroid myopathy may be heterotropia. The cause of diplopia is mechanical restriction of the eye muscles, which ophthalmologists confirm using the "forced duction test" (i.e., after anesthetization of the conjunctiva, the ophthalmologist grasps the conjunctiva with toothed forceps and attempts to passively rotate the eye, detecting abnormal resistance in patients with thyroid myopathy).[10,15]

(2) *Orbital fracture.* Diplopia is a complication of 58% of blowout fractures of the orbit and 20% of all midfacial fractures.[16] The heterotropia occurs because of swelling or entrapment of one of the eye muscles, most often the inferior rectus. In addition to the history of previous trauma, some patients have an additional clue, hypesthesia of the ipsilateral infraorbital area, which results from accompanying injury to the infraorbital branch of the trigeminal nerve. Diplopia may first become a problem for the patient days after the injury, when the swelling has had time to partially resolve.[10]

c. **Weak medial rectus.** The clinician should consider internuclear ophthalmoplegia and myasthenia gravis.

(1) ***Internuclear ophthalmoplegia ("INO").***[17,18] Lesions in the medial longitudinal fasciculus (the periaqueductal pathway in the brain stem that links the nuclei of cranial nerves 3, 4, and 6 and coordinates conjugate eye movements) cause internuclear ophthalmoplegia, whose features are (1) Incomplete adduction of one eye on lateral gaze (i.e., the "weak" medial rectus) and (2) jerk nystagmus of the contralateral abducting eye. Many patients also have vertical nystagmus on upward gaze. The finding is named according to the side with weak adduction. For example, in efforts to look to the far right, if the patient's left eye is unable to completely adduct and the right eye develops a jerk nystagmus, the patient has a left internuclear ophthalmoplegia (and a lesion in the left medial longitudinal fasciculus).

Ninety-seven percent of patients with *bilateral* INOs have multiple sclerosis whereas *unilateral* INO has many causes, although the most common one is vertebral-basilar cerebrovascular disease.[18]

(2) ***Myasthenia gravis*** (see Section 2a above) sometimes causes medial rectus weakness. In contrast to the finding in patients with internuclear ophthalmoplegia, there is no jerk nystagmus of the abducting eye.

d. **Weak lateral rectus.** Weakness of this muscle almost always indicates damage to the **sixth cranial nerve** (see below), although mimics include myasthenia gravis and thyroid myopathy.[19]

   e. Weak superior oblique indicates damage to the **fourth cranial nerve** (see below).

   f. Weak inferior oblique usually indicates **Brown's syndrome.**[20,21] These patients appear to have a weak inferior oblique muscle, but the problem actually is in the superior oblique muscle and tendon, which are unable to move freely through their pulley (i.e., the trochlea). In some patients, Brown's syndrome is congenital. Acquired Brown's syndrome is a complication of orbital inflammation, surgery, and metastases.

  3. Skew deviation. Skew deviation has the following diagnostic features: (1) there is an acquired hypertropia, (2) there is associated cerebellar or brain stem disease, and (3) no other cause is apparent. The disease is usually ipsilateral to the lower eye, but the finding has no other localizing value. Skew deviation mimics weakness of the inferior rectus 40% of the time, of the inferior oblique 25% of the time, superior rectus 17% of the time, and superior oblique 17% of the time (although the head tilt test, described below, is negative).[10,22]

DISORDERS OF CRANIAL NERVES 3, 4, AND 6

I. INTRODUCTION. Table 52-1 reviews the causes of *isolated* palsies of these three cranial nerves, based on analysis of over 3500 patients reported in the literature.[23-31] Major causes are ischemic infarcts (all three nerves), intracranial aneurysms (especially the third nerve), head trauma (especially the fourth nerve), and tumors (especially when more than one of these nerves are affected). At least one fourth of isolated cranial neuropathies affecting

TABLE 52-1 Etiology of isolated palsies of cranial nerves 3, 4, and 6

	Oculomotor Nerve	Trochlear Nerve	Abducens Nerve	Mixed*
Proportion (%)†	31	10	45	14
Etiology (%)				
Head trauma	13	34	11	18
Neoplasm	11	5	19	29
Ischemic	25	22	17	7
Aneurysm	17	1	3	11
Other	13	9	22	19
Idiopathic	21	29	28	16

Based on references 23 to 31.

*"Mixed" means combinations of cranial nerves 3, 4, or 6.

†"Proportion" is ratio of palsies affecting this cranial nerve to total number of palsies affecting cranial nerves 3, 4, or 6.

these nerves remain idiopathic, even in our modern era of clinical imaging.[31]

II. RULES FOR DIAGNOSING ISCHEMIC INFARCTS.

One of the most common causes of *isolated* palsies of cranial nerves 3, 4, or 6 is ischemic infarction, a diagnosis made at the bedside based on the following criteria: (1) the palsy is isolated (i.e., no other neurologic or ophthalmologic findings), (2) the onset is abrupt, (3) the patient has risk factors for cerebrovascular disease (i.e., is older than 50 years, has hypertension or diabetes), (4) no other cause is apparent, and (5) the palsy is self-limited (i.e., it resolves over several months). Seventy-five percent of ischemic mononeuropathies resolve within 4 months; persistence beyond this should prompt evaluation for other causes.

III. OCULOMOTOR NERVE (CRANIAL NERVE 3)

A. The finding. Complete weakness causes downward and outward deviation of the affected eye and ptosis. The pupil may or may not be dilated, depending on the etiology of the patient's neuropathy.

B. Clinical significance

1. Pupil-sparing rule.[32,33] The most common causes of *isolated* third nerve paralysis are posterior communicating artery aneurysm (which must be managed aggressively) and ischemic infarction of the third nerve (which is managed conservatively). In over 95% of aneurysmal palsies, the pupil reacts sluggishly to light or is fixed and dilated, but in 73% of ischemic palsies, the pupil is spared.[25,26,28,34-37] These observations have led to the "pupil-sparing rule," which states that patients who have third nerve palsies that spare the pupil do not have aneurysms and can be safely managed expectantly.

Before applying this rule, however, there are three important caveats: (1) The rule applies only to patients with *complete* paralysis of the ocular muscles of the third nerve and *complete* sparing of the pupil. Up to 4% of patients with aneurysms do have sparing of the pupil although the third nerve muscles are only partially paralyzed[26,28,35,37-42]; (2) The rule should be applied very cautiously to patients aged 20 to 50 years, an age group in which ischemic infarcts are uncommon, and (3) The rule only applies to patients with isolated third nerve palsies. Any other neurologic or ophthalmologic finding (e.g., hemiparesis, proptosis, other cranial neuropathy) disqualifies the rule.

2. **Clinical syndromes.** Associated findings distinguish the different causes of third nerve palsy.[43]

   a. **Ipsilateral brain stem.** Damage to the third nerve fascicle as it exits the ipsilateral brain stem causes accompanying ipsilateral cerebellar signs (Nothnagel's syndrome, involving the superior cerebellar peduncle), contralateral hemitremor (Benedikt's syndrome, involving the red nucleus), or contralateral hemiparesis (Weber's syndrome, involving the cerebral peduncle).

   b. **Damage to the nerve in the subarachnoid space.** Important causes include uncal herniation (i.e., patient is comatose) and internal carotid-posterior communicating artery aneurysm (i.e., the third nerve palsy is isolated).

   c. **Ipsilateral cavernous sinus or orbit.** Lesions of the cavernous sinus or orbit cause simultaneous injury to cranial nerves 3, 4, and 6 (which causes total ophthalmoplegia), to the sympathetic nerves of the iris (contributing to a pupil that is small and unreactive), and to the ophthalmic distribution of the trigeminal nerve (causing hypesthesia of upper third of face). Orbital disease also causes early, prominent proptosis.

d. Ischemic infarcts. Ischemic infarction causes an isolated third nerve palsy (see "rules for diagnosing ischemic infarcts" in Section II above and "pupil sparing rule" in Section III-B-1 above).

IV. TROCHLEAR NERVE (CRANIAL NERVE 4)

A. The finding. Paralysis of cranial nerve 4 causes vertical diplopia and hypertropia of the affected eye. The hypertropia may not be evident on examination, however, and often the clinician will have to tilt the patient's head toward the affected side to bring out the finding. Tilting the head aggravates the diplopia because it requires the ipsilateral eye to intort, which calls upon simultaneous contraction of the superior oblique and superior rectus muscles. These two muscles work together, and the tendency of the superior oblique to depress the eye is normally balanced by that of the superior rectus to elevate the eye. If the superior oblique is weak, however, attempts to intort the eye (e.g., during tilting of the head) instead bring about unopposed action of the superior rectus, which elevates the eye and aggravates the vertical diplopia and hypertropia.

B. Clinical significance

1. Head position. In studies of patients with isolated fourth nerve palsies, 45% actually habitually tilt their head away from the side of the lesion (to minimize any need for intorsion in the affected eye).[30,44,45] This habitual head tilting is often apparent in old photographs of patients with chronic fourth nerve palsies. As expected, when the head is tilted toward the affected side, the diplopia and hypertropia worsen in 96% of patients.[30,45]

2. **Clinical syndromes.** The trochlear nerve has the longest intracranial course of any cranial nerve, in part explaining why trauma is the most common explanation for isolated lesions. Associated findings distinguish the different clinical syndromes.

a. **Contralateral midbrain.** Associated findings are contralateral Horner's syndrome, contralateral dysmetria, and contralateral internuclear ophthalmoplegia. In all of these syndromes, the associated findings are contralateral because the trochlear nerves cross on their way to the eyes (i.e., the fourth cranial nerve innervating the right eye originates in the left brain stem).[46,47]

b. **Ipsilateral cavernous sinus or orbit.** These lesions cause combinations of findings discussed in Section III-B-2-c above.

c. **Ischemic infarcts** (see Section II above). Ischemic infarction cause an isolated fourth nerve palsy (see "rules for diagnosing ischemic infarcts" in Section II above).

V. ABDUCENS NERVE (CRANIAL NERVE 6).

A. **The finding.** Paralysis of the sixth cranial nerve causes esotropia and an inability to fully abduct the affected eye.

B. **Clinical significance.** The various clinical syndromes are distinguished by their associated findings.

1. **Ipsilateral pons.** Associated findings are contralateral hemiparesis (Raymond's syndrome), ipsilateral seventh nerve palsy and contralateral hemiparesis (Millard-Gubler syndrome), or ipsilateral Horner's syndrome, ipsilateral horizontal gaze palsy, and ipsilateral involvement of cranial nerves 5, 7, and 8 (Foville's syndrome).

2. **Damage to the nerve in the subarach-noid space** often causes an isolated sixth nerve palsy. Examples are meningitis, recent lumbar puncture (with subsequent leak of cerebrospinal fluid that leads to stretching of the nerve),[48] and pseudotumor cerebri (also from stretching of the nerve, brought on by elevated intracranial pressure; these patients may have associated papilledema).

3. **At the petrous apex.** Examples are complicated otitis media (Gradenigo's syndrome: associated ipsilateral decreased hearing, facial pain from involvement of the fifth cranial nerve, and ipsilateral seventh nerve palsy), petrous bone fracture (associated hemotympanum and Battle's sign), and nasopharyngeal carcinoma.[49]

4. **Ipsilateral cavernous sinus or orbit.** These lesions cause combinations of findings discussed in Section III-B-2-c above.

5. **Ischemic infarcts.** Ischemic infarction causes an isolated sixth nerve palsy (see "rules for diagnosing ischemic infarcts" in Section II above).

REFERENCES

1. Forster RK, Schatz NJ, and Smith JL. A subtle eyelid sign in aberrant regeneration of the third nerve, *Am J Ophthalmol* 67:696-698, 1969.

2. Fisher M. An unusual variant of acute idiopathic polyneuritis (syndrome of ophthalmoplegia, ataxia, and areflexia), *N Engl J Med* 255:57-65, 1956.

3. Henderson JW and Schneider RC. The ocular findings in carotid-cavernous fistula in a series of 17 cases, *Am J Ophthalmol* 48:585-597, 1959.

4. Morris RJ. Double vision as a presenting symptom in an ophthalmic casualty department, *Eye* 5:124-129, 1991.

5. Coffeen P and Guyton DL. Monocular diplopia accompanying ordinary refractive errors, *Am J Ophthalmol* 105:451-459, 1988.

6. Amos JF. Diagnosis and management of monocular diplopia, *J Am Optometric Assoc* 53:101-115, 1982.
7. Records RE. Monocular diplopia, *Surv Ophthalmol* 24:303-306, 1980.
8. Bender MB. Polyopia and monocular diplopia of cerebral origin, *Arch Neurol Psych* 54:323-328, 1945.
9. Meadows JC. Observations on a case of monocular diplopia of cerebral origin, *J Neurol Sci* 18:249-253, 1973.
10. Keane JR. Vertical diplopia, *Semin Neurol* 6:147-154, 1986.
11. Trobe JD. Isolated third nerve palsies, *Semin Neurol* 6:135-141, 1986.
12. Oosterhuis HJGH. The ocular signs and symptoms of myasthenia gravis, *Doc Ophthalmol* 52:363-378, 1982.
13. Osher RH. Myasthenic "oculomotor" palsy, *Arch Ophthalmol* 11:31-34, 1979.
14. Glaser JS. Myasthenic pseudo-internuclear ophthalmoplegia, *Arch Ophthalmol* 75:363-366, 1966.
15. Appen RE, Wendelborn D, and Nolten WE. Diplopia in autoimmune thyroid disease, *Arch Intern Med* 142:898-901, 1982.
16. Al-Qurainy IA and others. Diplopia following midfacial fractures, *Br J Oral Maxillofac Surg* 29:302-307, 1991.
17. Cogan DG. Internuclear ophthalmoplegia, *Arch Ophthalmol* 84:583-589, 1970.
18. Smith JL and Cogan DG. Internuclear ophthalmoplegia: a review of 58 cases, *Arch Ophthalmol* 61:687-694, 1959.
19. Galetta SL and Smith JL. Chronic isolated sixth nerve palsies, *Arch Neurol* 46:79-82, 1989.
20. Wilson ME, Eustis HS, and Parks MM. Brown's syndrome, *Surv Ophthalmol* 34:153-172, 1989.
21. Brown HW. True and simulated superior oblique tendon sheath syndromes, *Doc Ophthalmol* 34:123-136, 1973.
22. Keane JR. Ocular skew deviation: analysis of 100 cases, *Arch Neurol* 32:185-190, 1975.
23. Tiffin PAC and others. Acquired palsy of the oculomotor, trochlear and abducens nerves, *Eye* 10:377-384, 1996.
24. Rush JA and Younge BR. Paralysis of cranial nerves III, IV, and VI, *Arch Ophthalmol* 99:76-79, 1981.
25. Rucker CW. Paralysis of the third, fourth and sixth cranial nerves, *Am J Ophthalmol* 46:787-794, 1958.
26. Rucker CW. The causes of paralysis of the third, fourth and sixth cranial nerves, *Am J Ophthalmol* 61:1293-1298, 1966.
27. Berlit P. Isolated and combined pareses of cranial nerves III, IV, and VI: a retrospective study of 412 patients, *J Neurol Sci* 103:10-15, 1991.

28. Green WR, Hackett ER, and Schlezinger NS. Neuro-ophthalmologic evaluation of oculomotor nerve paralysis, *Arch Ophthalmol* 72:154-167, 1964.

29. Burger LJ, Kalvin NH, and Smith JL. Acquired lesions of the fourth cranial nerve, *Brain* 93:567-574, 1970.

30. Khawam E, Scott AB, and Jamplosky A. Acquired superior oblique palsy, *Arch Ophthalmol* 77:761-768, 1967.

31. Richards BW, Jones FR, and Younge BR. Causes and prognosis in 4278 cases of paralysis of the oculomotor, trochlear, and abducens cranial nerves, *Am J Ophthalmol* 113:489-496, 1992.

32. Trobe JD. Third nerve palsy and the pupil, *Arch Ophthalmol* 106:601-602, 1988.

33. Trobe JD. Isolated pupil-sparing third nerve palsy, *Ophthalmology* 92:58-61, 1985.

34. Zorrilla E and Kozak GP. Ophthalmoplegia in diabetes mellitus, *Ann Intern Med* 67:968-976, 1967.

35. Capo H, Warren F, and Kupersmith MJ. Evolution of oculomotor nerve palsies, *J Clin Neuro-ophthalmol* 12:12-15, 1992.

36. Hopf HC and Gutmann L. Diabetic 3rd nerve palsy: evidence for a mesencephalic lesion, *Neurology* 40:1041-1045, 1990.

37. Cogan DG and Mount HTJ. Intracranial aneurysms causing ophthalmoplegia, *Arch Ophthalmol* 70:757-771, 1963.

38. Fujiwara S and others. Oculomotor nerve palsy in patients with cerebral aneurysms, *Neurosurg Rev* 12:123-132, 1989.

39. Kissel JT and others. Pupil-sparing oculomotor palsies with internal carotid-posterior communicating artery aneurysms, *Ann Neurol* 13:149-154, 1983.

40. Raja IA. Aneurysm-induced third nerve palsy, *J Neurosurg* 36:548-551, 1972.

41. Keane JR. Aneurysms and third nerve palsies, *Ann Neurol* 14:696-697, 1983.

42. Botterell EH, Lloyd LA, and Hoffman HJ. Oculomotor palsy due to supraclinoid internal carotid artery berry aneurysm, *Am J Ophthalmol* 54:609-616, 1962.

43. Brazis PW. Localization of lesions of the oculomotor nerve: recent concepts, *Mayo Clin Proc* 66:1029-1035, 1991.

44. Urist MJ. Head tilt in vertical muscle paresis, *Am J Ophthalmol* 69:440-442, 1970.

45. Younge BR and Sutula F. Analysis of trochlear nerve palsies: diagnosis, etiology, and treatment, *Mayo Clin Proc* 52:11-18, 1977.

46. Brazis PW. Palsies of the trochlear nerve: diagnosis and localization—recent concepts, *Mayo Clin Proc* 68:501-509, 1993.

47. Guy J and others. Contralateral trochlear nerve paresis and ipsilateral Horner's syndrome, *Am J Ophthalmol* 107: 73-76, 1989.

48. Bryce-Smith R, Macintosh RR. Sixth-nerve palsy after lumbar puncture and spinal analgesia, *Br Med J* 1:275-276, 1951.

49. Smith JL and Wheliss JA. Ocular manifestations of nasopharyngeal tumors, *Trans Am Acad Ophthalmol Otol* 66:659-664, 1962.

CHAPTER 53

Miscellaneous Cranial Nerves

Table 53-1 reviews the physical examination of the 12 cranial nerves. Cranial nerves 1, 5, 7, and 9 through 12 are discussed in this chapter. Cranial nerve 2 is discussed in Chapters 19 and 51; cranial nerve 8, in Chapter 21; and cranial nerves 3, 4, and 6, in Chapter 52.

OLFACTORY NERVE (I)

I. TECHNIQUE. The usual test for the sense of smell is placing a nonirritative substance, such as wintergreen or cloves, under one nostril at a time. Pungent substances like ammonia should not be used because they stimulate trigeminal nerve endings (i.e., cranial nerve 5).

II. CLINICAL SIGNIFICANCE

A. Anosmia. Anosmia is the complete absence of smell. The most common causes are upper respiratory infection and sinus disease (which obstructs the nasal passages) and previous head trauma (which damages the olfactory fibers).[1] Less common causes are Kallman's syndrome (hypogonadotropic hypogonadism) and sphenoid ridge masses (e.g., meningioma causing the ipsilateral anosmia, ipsilateral optic atrophy,

TABLE 53-1 The 12 cranial nerves

CRANIAL NERVE	MOTOR EXAMINATION	SENSORY EXAMINATION	REFLEX EXAMINATION
Olfactory nerve (I)		Detection of nonirritating odors	
Optic nerve (II)		Visual acuity Retinal examination	Afferent pupillary defect ("swinging flashlight test")
Nerves of the eye muscles: Oculomotor nerve (III) Trochlear nerve (IV) Abducens nerve (VI)	Extraocular movements (III, IV, and VI) Lid elevation (III only)		Pupillary constriction (III only)
Trigeminal nerve (V)	Masseter muscle Lateral pterygoid muscle	Pain, temperature, and touch sensation of the ipsilateral face	Corneal reflex (afferent limb) Jaw jerk (afferent and efferent limb) Glabellar reflex (afferent limb)

Continued

TABLE 53-1 The 12 cranial nerves—cont'd

CRANIAL NERVE	MOTOR EXAMINATION	SENSORY EXAMINATION	REFLEX EXAMINATION
Facial nerve (VII)	All facial movements except lid elevation	Taste sensation to anterior 2/3 of the tongue	Corneal reflex (efferent limb) Glabellar reflex (efferent limb)
Vestibulocochlear nerve (VIII)		Tests of hearing (cochlear component)	Vestibuloocular reflex (vestibular component)
Glossopharyngeal nerve (IX)	Ipsilateral palate elevation (with X)	Sensation posterior pharynx Taste sensation to posterior 2/3 of the tongue	Gag reflex (afferent limb and, with X, efferent limb)
Vagus nerve (X)	Ipsilateral palate elevation (with IX)		Gag reflex (efferent limb with IX)
Spinal accessory nerve (XI)	Trapezius muscle Sternocleidomastoid muscle		
Hypoglossal nerve (XII)	Genioglossus muscle		

and contralateral papilledema of the Foster-Kennedy syndrome).[1,2]

B. Olfactory dysfunction. Patients with olfactory dysfunction are able to detect odors but frequently misidentify them. Olfactory dysfunction is common in patients with Parkinson's disease[3,4] or after frontal or temporal lobectomies.[5]

TRIGEMINAL NERVE (V)

I. INTRODUCTION. The trigeminal sensory and motor nuclei are located in the pons, although the sensory nucleus extends through the medulla into the cervical spinal cord. The sensory branches of the trigeminal nerve innervate the upper face (V_1, ophthalmic division), midface (V_2, maxillary division), and lower face (V_3, mandibular division). The motor fibers to masseter and lateral pterygoid muscles travel with the mandibular division (V_3).

II. THE FINDING

A. Motor weakness. Lesions of the motor component of the trigeminal nerve affect the masseter muscle (causing difficulty clenching that side of the jaw, sometimes with atrophy that flattens the contour of the cheek) and lateral pterygoid muscle (causing difficulty deviating the jaw to the opposite side; at rest the jaw may deviate toward the weak side).

B. Sensory loss. Lesions of the sensory component cause diminished pain, temperature, and touch sensation in any or all of the three divisions on one side of the face. Sensation to most of the external ear (excluding the tragus) and the angle of the jaw is preserved in trigeminal lesions because these areas are supplied by cervical sensory roots (see Figure 55-1 in Chapter 55).

C. Corneal reflex. Unilateral gentle stimulation of the cornea normally causes bilateral blinking.

The afferent limb of this reflex is the ipsilateral trigeminal nerve (only V_1 and V_2) and the efferent limb is both facial nerves (i.e., both eyes blink after stimulation of one cornea).

III. CLINICAL SIGNIFICANCE

A. Motor weakness. *Unilateral* weakness of the trigeminal muscles indicates disease of the proximal mandibular division (e.g., skull metastases) or a lesion in the ipsilateral pons (patients with pontine lesions have other associated neurologic findings, such as abnormalities of cranial nerves 6 or 7, or contralateral hemiparesis). Unilateral weakness of the trigeminal muscles does not occur with cerebral hemispheric lesions because each trigeminal nucleus receives bilateral cortical innervation.[6] *Bilateral* weakness, however, may occur in bilateral cerebral hemispheric disease and cause great difficulty chewing (see Pseudobulbar Palsy below).

B. Sensory loss. Sensory loss of the face may be part of a broader neurologic syndrome affecting sensation of the whole body and other neurologic functions (lesions of the cerebral hemisphere, thalamus, or brain stem) or may be isolated to the face (lesions of the peripheral nerve and its branches).

1. Sensory loss of face and body. In thalamic and cerebral hemispheric lesions, sensation of the face and body is abnormal on the *same* side, contralateral to the lesion. There is often associated hemiparesis, aphasia, or both.[7-9] In brain stem lesions, the sensory abnormalities of the face and body are on *opposite* sides: sensation is diminished on the ipsilateral face but *contralateral* body (see Figure 55-2 and Table 55-2 in Chapter 55).[10-14] Pontine lesions affect intraoral more than facial sensation, whereas medullary lesions affect facial more than intraoral sensation.[15]

2. **Sensory loss isolated to the face.** Sensory loss isolated to the face is part of syndromes affecting the apex of the temporal bone (see Chapter 52, cranial nerve 6), the cavernous sinus syndrome (V_1 division only, see Chapter 52), and "numb chin syndrome." The numb chin syndrome, which describes the loss of sensation on the lower lip and chin, has an ominous prognosis in cancer patients and suggests the presence of metastatic disease to the ipsilateral mandible, base of skull, or leptomeninges.[16] These patients sometimes have abnormalities of other cranial nerves.

C. **Abnormal corneal reflex.** The two limbs of the corneal reflex are cranial nerves 5 and 7. According to traditional teachings, unilateral trigeminal nerve dysfunction (i.e., in the ipsilateral brain stem, V_1, or V_2 divisions) prevents both eyes from blinking after stimulation of the ipsilateral cornea, whereas unilateral facial nerve dysfunction prevents the ipsilateral eye from blinking when its cornea is stimulated, although the contralateral eye blinks normally. The absent corneal reflex is felt to be particularly important in patients with unilateral sensorineural hearing loss, in whom it raises the possibility of cerebellopontine angle tumors, such as acoustic neuroma.

Nonetheless, the clinical utility of the asymmetric corneal reflex is limited. The reflex is inexplicably absent unilaterally in 8% of healthy elderly patients,[17] and the sensitivity of the absent reflex for acoustic neuroma is only 33%, the finding usually indicating the tumor has already grown to a large size (>2 cm in diameter).[18]

D. **Herpes zoster infection and the nasociliary branch of the trigeminal nerve ("Hutchinson's sign").** About half of patients with *Herpes zoster* infection of the ophthalmic division of the trigeminal nerve ("herpes zoster ophthalmicus") develop vision-threatening complications such as uveitis and keratitis within 1 to 4 weeks of the onset of the rash (mean onset = 1.8 weeks).[19] In 1865, Hutchinson noted that the tip of the nose, cornea, and iris all share the same branch of the trigeminal nerve (the nasociliary nerve) and that if a patient with Herpes zoster ophthalmicus developed vesicles on the tip of the nose (i.e., "Hutchinson's sign"), there was an increased risk of ocular complications.[20] The clinical utility of this sign, however, is limited: its accuracy is only modest (sensitivity 57%, specificity 82%, positive LR = 3.2, negative LR = 0.5),[19] and today all patients with herpes zoster ophthalmicus, whether or not the tip of the nose or the eye is involved, should receive antiviral medications.[21]

FACIAL NERVE

I. THE FINDING. Lesions of the facial nerve may cause facial asymmetry (diminished ipsilateral nasolabial fold and widened ipsilateral palpebral fissure) and weakness of most ipsilateral facial muscles (muscles used during speaking, blinking, raising eyebrows, smiling, wrinkling the forehead, closing the eyes, showing teeth, and retracting the chin). There may be abnormalities of ipsilateral tearing (lacrimal gland), hearing (stapedius muscle), taste (anterior 2/3 of the tongue), and the corneal and glabellar reflexes.

Facial nerve lesions do not cause ptosis, because the lid muscles are not innervated by the facial nerve but rather by sympathetic nerves and cranial nerve 3.

II. CLINICAL SIGNIFICANCE

A. Central vs. peripheral facial weakness. Unilateral facial weakness may be "central" (i.e., in upper motor neurons, from lesions in the contralateral motor cortex or descending pyramidal tracts) or "peripheral" (i.e., in lower motor neurons, from lesions in the peripheral nerve or facial nucleus in the ipsilateral pons).[a] These lesions are distinguished by the following two features:

1. **Distribution of weakness.** Peripheral lesions affect both upper and lower facial muscles, whereas central lesions affect predominately the lower facial muscles. Wrinkling of the forehead is relatively spared in central lesions because the facial nuclei innervating these muscles receive bilateral cortical innervation.

2. **Movements affected.** Peripheral lesions paralyze all facial movements on the side affected, whereas central lesions affect voluntary movements but spare emotional ones. The patient with central weakness (e.g., cerebral hemispheric stroke) may be unable to wrinkle one corner of the mouth volitionally yet can move it normally during laughter or crying. This occurs because emotional input to the facial nuclei does not come from the motor cortex.[b22,23]

B. **Peripheral nerve lesions**

1. **Etiology.** The causes of isolated peripheral facial palsies are idiopathic (50% to 87%), surgical or accidental trauma (5% to 22%), herpes zoster infections (Ramsey Hunt syndrome, 7% to 13%), tumors (e.g., cholesteatoma, parotid tumors, 1% to 6%), and miscellaneous disorders (8% to 11%). (These figures originate in specialty referral centers and may overrepresent unusual etiologies).[24-29] "Bell's palsy" refers to the

---

[a] Chapter 54 defines "upper" and "lower" motor neurons.
[b] The opposite clinical finding, emotional paralysis without volitional paralysis, occurs with lesions of the thalamus or frontal lobe.[22,23]

idiopathic disorders, although evidence is mounting that it represents response to viral infection.[30]

2. **Associated findings.** In patients with Bell's palsy, associated findings are diminished taste (52%), hyperacusis (8% to 30%), increased tearing (19% to 34%), and decreased tearing (2% to 17%).[25-28,31-33] Increased tear production occurs because the weak orbicularis oculi muscle cannot contain and direct the tears down the nasolacrimal duct; decreased tearing reflects diminished lacrimal gland function. Although 23% of patients also have sensory complaints, the finding of hypesthesia of the face (i.e., cranial nerve 5) is variable: some investigators, arguing that Bell's palsy is part of a multiple cranial neuropathy, have found hypesthesia in as many as 48% of patients,[27,31] while other investigators have never found associated hypesthesia of the face.[25]

3. **Topographic diagnosis.** The branches of the facial nerve diverge from the main trunk in predictable order: they are, proximally to distally, branches to the lacrimal gland, stapedius muscle, tongue (taste), and facial muscles.[27] Therefore, tests of tearing (Schirmer's tear test), stapedius function (stapedius reflex during audiometry), and taste should pinpoint the location of the lesion, although this is only accurate when the nerve is completely severed. In patients with patchy lesions (Bell's palsy or partial injuries), topographic diagnosis is often nonsensical (e.g., tearing reduced but taste and stapedius function preserved) and has minimal clinical value.[27,31,34]

4. **Complications of Bell's palsy.**[26,28,32,33] Three complications occur after recovery from Bell's palsy:

   a. **Associated movements** ("synkinesis," 55% to 94% of patients). These are unexpected movements that probably result from aberrant regeneration. Examples are narrowing of the palpebral fissure when the patient smiles or motion of the corner of the mouth when the patient closes the eyes tightly.

b. Contracture (3% to 36%). Despite the name, this is increased muscle tone, not a fibrotic scar, which often restores facial symmetry even though some weakness persists.

c. Crocodile tears (2% to 6%), from aberrant regeneration of salivary gland fibers to the lacrimal gland. When affected patients eat, tears form and run down the cheek or collect in the nose.

GLOSSOPHARYNGEAL (IX) AND VAGUS (X) NERVES

I. FINDING. These nerves are considered together because their function is difficult to separate at the bedside and because clinical disorders usually affect both nerves simultaneously. There are three abnormal findings: **(1) Absent pharyngeal sensation,** which is usually tested with a cotton applicator stick touching the posterior oropharynx. **(2) Diminished velar movement.** The posterior edge of the soft palate is called the "velum" and its elevation, "velar movement." The soft palate should elevate as the patient vocalizes a prolonged "ah." **(3) Gag reflex.** During stimulation of the posterior tongue, pharynx, or soft palate, there is reflex elevation of the tongue and soft palate and constriction of the pharyngeal muscles. The gag reflex is labeled abnormal when it is diminished, absent, hyperactive, or asymmetric.

II. CLINICAL SIGNIFICANCE. Abnormalities of these nerves may occur because of *bilateral* cerebral hemispheric disease or because of disease in the *ipsilateral* medulla or peripheral nerves (i.e., cranial nerves 9 and 10). *Unilateral* cerebral hemispheric disease does not ordinarily cause palatal weakness because each nucleus of these nerves receives bilateral corticobulbar innervation.

A. Bilateral cerebral hemispheric lesions: Pseudobulbar palsy. Bilateral lesions above the level of the pons that disrupt the descending pyramidal tracts innervating brain stem motor nuclei may cause significant paralysis of the palate and pharynx, along with paralysis of the tongue, face, and muscles of chewing. This syndrome, "pseudobulbar palsy," affects about 4% of patients with cerebrovascular disease, who mostly have lacunar infarcts in both internal capsules.[35,36] The main clinical features are dysarthria, dysphagia, and paralysis of voluntary movements of the face.[37,38] Other findings are hyperactive jaw jerk (70% of patients), absent gag reflex (70%), and hyperactive emotional reflexes that cause spasmodic and often inappropriate crying and laughing (24%).[35,36,39-41] The animated facial movements that appear while the patient laughs or cries uncontrollably contrast markedly with the lack of voluntary facial movement and the patient's inability to mimic gestures.

The term "pseudobulbar," coined by Lepine in 1877,[36] is used because the lesion is supranuclear, to distinguish this syndrome from similar motor paralysis that may occur after damage to the brain stem nuclei themselves (i.e., "bulbar" paralysis).[36,37] The term is a misnomer, however, because "bulbar" refers to the medulla and two motor nuclei prominently affected in pseudobulbar palsy—those of the facial muscles (VII) and of chewing (V)—reside in the pons.

B. Bedside predictors of risk of aspiration after stroke. In patients who have suffered bilateral strokes, significant dysfunction of cranial nerves 9 and 10 makes the airway vulnerable to aspiration during swallowing. Table 53-2 presents the accuracy of several bedside signs as predictors of aspiration in patients with strokes. The presence of normal pharyngeal sensation (LR = 0.03) and a normal water swallow test (LR = 0.2) argue significantly *against* the risk for aspiration (see footnote to Table 53-2 for definitions of findings). An *abnormal* water swallow test, however, argues *for* risk of aspiration (LR = 5.6). The accuracy of other findings, including the abnormal gag reflex, dysphonia, drowsiness, and abnormal cough, are only modest (Table 53-2). Findings with no predictive value are bilateral cranial nerve findings,[42] abnormal sensation of face and tongue,[42] dysarthria,[45,48] and abnormal chest radiograph.[42]

The poor predictive value of the absent gag reflex is not surprising because the pharyngeal muscles involved in this reflex are not necessarily the same ones activated during normal swallowing to protect the airway. Moreover, the gag reflex is often absent in normal individuals, especially elderly patients.[49,50] Pharyngeal sensation, on the other hand, is rarely absent in normal individuals.[49]

C. **Lesions of ipsilateral brain stem or peripheral nerve.** The lateral medullary syndrome causes ipsilateral absence of pharyngeal sensation and reduced velar elevation, associated with Horner's syndrome and other sensory and cerebellar signs (see Table 55-2 in Chapter 55). The jugular foramen syndrome (e.g., basilar skull fracture or glomus jugulare tumors) simultaneously disrupts cranial nerves 9, 10, and 11, causing ipsilateral paralysis of the palate, vocal cords (hoarseness), and trapezius and sternocleidomastoid muscles.

SPINAL ACCESSORY NERVE (XI)

I. **FINDING.** The primary findings are a weakness or atrophy, or both, of the sternocleidomastoid muscle (which turns the head to the opposite side) and

TABLE 53-2 Aspiration after stroke*

Finding (ref)†	Sensitivity (%)	Specificity (%)	Positive LR	Negative LR
Voice and Cough				
Abnormal voluntary cough[42-46]	48-89	36-94	1.9	0.5
Dysphonia[42-46]	60-97	9-68	NS	0.4
Neurologic Examination				
Drowsiness[47]	76	65	2.2	0.4
Absent pharyngeal sensation[47]	98	60	2.4	0.03
Abnormal gag reflex[42-46,48]	60-87	45-82	1.8	0.5
Other Tests				
Water swallow test[47]	80	86	5.6	0.2

NS, Not significant.

*Diagnostic standard: For aspiration, barium material entering the airway below the larynx during videofluoroscopy.

†Definition of findings: For abnormal voluntary cough, the patient is asked to cough as hard as possible and the resulting cough is absent, weak, breathy, or sluggish; for dysphonia, the patient is asked to sing a prolonged "ah" and the voice is breathy, hoarse, wet, harsh, or strained; for absent pharyngeal sensation, the patient cannot sense an applicator stick applied to the posterior oropharynx, on one or both sides; for abnormal gag reflex, the gag reflex is diminished, absent, hyperactive, or asymmetric; for water swallow test, drinking 50 ml of water in 5 ml aliquots causes coughing, choking, or alteration of the voice.

trapezius muscle (which elevates the ipsilateral shoulder).

II. **CLINICAL SIGNIFICANCE.** Unilateral weakness of these muscles may represent disease of the cerebral hemispheres, brain stem, spinal cord, or peripheral nerve. Atrophy indicates that the lesion is in the nucleus (i.e., brain stem or high cervical spinal cord) or peripheral nerve (i.e., the lesion is *not* in the cerebral hemispheres).

A. **Cerebral hemisphere.** Lesions of the cerebral hemispheres affect the trapezius and sternocleidomastoid muscles differently: lesions in one cerebral hemisphere weaken the *contralateral* trapezius but the *ipsilateral* sternocleidomastoid muscle.[c][51] Therefore, in a hemispheric stroke, the patient may demonstrate weakness turning the head toward the hemiparetic side.[52] In a focal seizure, the head often deviates toward the seizing limbs.

B. **Brain stem or high cervical spinal cord.** Lesions of the accessory nucleus, located in the medulla and high cervical spinal cord (e.g., syringomyelia), may cause atrophy and weakness of the *ipsilateral* trapezius and sternocleidomastoid muscle.

C. **Peripheral nerve.** Injuries to the peripheral nerve, which occur from trauma to the posterior triangle of the neck (e.g., surgical excision of lymph nodes, blunt trauma), may paralyze the *ipsilateral* trapezius or sternocleidomastoid muscles, although the sternocleidomastoid muscle is often spared because its branches diverge

---

[c] Descending corticobulbar fibers to the sternocleidomastoid muscle are believed to cross twice to innervate the ipsilateral side. This innervation makes teleological sense because the sternocleidmastoid muscle turns the head to the opposite side, and the cerebral hemisphere is interested in turning the head to same side whose visual fields, eye movements, and motor function it controls.[51]

early from the main trunk of the nerve.[53] The jugular foramen syndrome, discussed above under the glossopharyngeal nerve, also affects cranial nerve 11 along with cranial nerves 9 and 10.

HYPOGLOSSAL NERVE

I. FINDING. During protrusion of the tongue, each genioglossus muscle acts to push the tongue out and toward the opposite side. Normally these laterally directed forces balance each other, and the tongue remains in the midline. With unilateral hypoglossal weakness, however, the intact genioglossus muscle acts to deviate the tongue toward the opposite, or weak, side.

II. CLINICAL SIGNIFICANCE. Weakness of the genioglossus may represent disease in the cerebral hemisphere, brain stem, or peripheral nerve. Atrophy or fasciculations of the tongue indicate the lesion is either in the hypoglossal nucleus (brain stem) or hypoglossal nerve (i.e., *not* cerebral hemispheres).

A. Cerebral hemisphere. Lesions of the cerebral hemisphere may cause weakness of the contralateral genioglossus. Therefore, the tongue deviates toward the side of the weak arm and leg.

B. Brain stem. The medial medullary syndrome causes ipsilateral hypoglossal paralysis, contralateral hemiparesis, and contralateral loss of proprioceptive and vibratory sensation (preserving pain and temperature sensation). Therefore, the tongue deviates away from the side of the weak arm and leg.

C. Peripheral nerve. The most common causes of lesions of the hypoglossal nerve are metastatic cancer (to base of skull, subarachnoid space, or neck) and trauma (e.g., gunshot wounds to the neck, radical neck surgery, carotid endarterectomy).[54]

Hypoglossal palsy in association with other cranial nerve findings occurs with both brain stem and peripheral nerve disorders, and therefore has little localizing value.[54]

REFERENCES

1. Deems DA and others. Smell and taste disorders: a study of 750 patients from the University of Pennsylvania smell and taste center, *Arch Otolaryngol Head Neck Surg* 117:519-528, 1991.
2. Shiffman SS. Taste and smell in disease, *N Engl J Med* 308:1275-1279; 1337-1343, 1983.
3. Doty RL, Deems DA, and Stellar S. Olfactory dysfunction in parkinsonism: a general deficit unrelated to neurologic signs, disease stage, or disease duration, *Neurology* 38:1237-1244, 1988.
4. Hawkes CH, Shephard BC, and Daniel SE. Olfactory dysfunction in Parkinson's disease, *J Neurol Neurosurg Psych* 62:436-446, 1997.
5. Zatorre RJ and Jones-Gotman M. Human olfactory discrimination after unilateral frontal or temporal lobectomy, *Brain* 114:71-84, 1991.
6. Cruccu G, Fornarelli M, and Manfredi M. Impairment of masticatory function in hemiplegia, *Neurology* 38:301-306, 1988.
7. Barraquer-Bordas L and others. Thalamic hemorrhage. A study of 23 patients with diagnosis by computed tomography, *Stroke* 12:524-527, 1981.
8. Kim JS. Pure sensory stroke: clinical-radiological correlates of 21 cases, *Stroke* 23:983-987, 1992.
9. Walshe TM, Davis KR, and Fisher CM. Thalamic hemorrhage: a computed tomographic-clinical correlation, *Neurology* 27:217-222, 1977.
10. Kim JS and others. Spectrum of lateral medullary syndrome: correlation between clinical findings and magnetic resonance imaging in 33 subjects, *Stroke* 25:1405-1410, 1994.
11. Norrving B and Cronqvist S. Lateral medullary infarction: prognosis in an unselected series, *Neurology* 41:244-248, 1991.

12. Peterman AF and Siekert RG. The lateral medullary (Wallenberg) syndrome: clinical features and prognosis, *Med Clin North Am* 44:887-895, 1960.

13. Sacco RL and others. Wallenberg's lateral medullary syndrome: clinical-magnetic resonance imaging correlations, *Arch Neurol* 50:609-614, 1993.

14. Fisher CM, Karnes WE, and Kubik CS. Lateral medullary infarction: the pattern of vascular occlusion, *J Neuropathol Exp Neurol* 20:323-379, 1961.

15. Graham SH, Sharp FR, and Dillon W. Intraoral sensation in patients with brainstem lesions: role of the rostral spinal trigeminal nuclei in pons, *Neurology* 38:1529-1533, 1988.

16. Lossos A and Siegal T. Numb chin syndrome in cancer patients: etiology, response to treatment, and prognostic significance, *Neurology* 42:1181-1184, 1992.

17. Rai GS and Elias-Jones A. The corneal reflex in elderly patients, *J Am Geriatr Soc* 27:317-318, 1979.

18. Harner SG and Laws ER. Clinical findings in patients with acoustic neuroma, *Mayo Clin Proc* 58:721-728, 1983.

19. Harding SP, Lipton JR, and Wells JCD. Natural history of herpes zoster ophthalmicus: predictors of postherpetic neuralgia and ocular involvement, *Br J Ophthalmol* 71:353-358, 1987.

20. Tomkinson A, Doblin DG, and Brown MJKM. Huchinson's sign and its importance in rhinology, *Rhinology* 33:180-182, 1995.

21. Pavan-Langston D. Herpes zoster ophthalmicus, *Neurology* 45 (suppl 8):S50-S51, 1995.

22. Hopf HC, Mueller-Forell W, and Hopf NJ. Localization of emotional and volitional facial paresis, *Neurology* 42:1918-1923, 1992.

23. Ross RT and Mathiesen R. Volitional and emotional supra-nuclear facial weakness, *N Engl J Med* 338:1515, 1998.

24. Mountain RE and others. The Edinburgh facial palsy clinic: a review of three years' activity, *J Roy Coll Surg Edinb* 39:275-279, 1994.

25. Hauser WA and others. Incidence and prognosis of Bell's palsy in the population of Rochester, Minnesota, *Mayo Clin Proc* 46:258-264, 1971.

26. Devriese PP and others. Incidence, prognosis and recovery of Bell's palsy: a survey of about 1000 patients (1974-1983), *Clin Otolaryngol* 15:15-27, 1990.

27. Adour KK. Diagnosis and management of facial paralysis, *N Engl J Med* 307:348-351, 1982.

28. Park HW and Watkins AL. Facial paralysis: analysis of 500 cases, *Arch Phys Med* 30:749-762, 1949.

29. May M and Klein SR. Differential diagnosis of facial nerve palsy, *Otolaryngol Clin North Am* 24:613-645, 1991.

30. Murakami S and others. Bell palsy and Herpes simplex virus: identification of viral DNA in endoneurial fluid and muscle, *Ann Intern Med* 124:27-30, 1996.

31. Adour KK and others. The true nature of Bell's palsy: analysis of 1000 consecutive patients, *Laryngoscope* 88:787-801, 1978.

32. Katusic SK and others. Incidence, clinical features, and prognosis in Bell's palsy, Rochester, Minnesota, 1968-1982, *Ann Neurol* 20:622-627, 1986.

33. Taverner D. Bell's palsy: a clinical and electromyographic study, *Brain* 78:209-228, 1955.

34. Tonning FM. The reliability of level-diagnostic examinations in acute, peripheral facial palsy, *Acta Otolaryngol* 84:414-415, 1977.

35. Loeb C and others. Pseudobulbar palsy: a clinical computed tomography study, *Eur Neurol* 30:42-46, 1990.

36. Besson G and others. Acute pseudobulbar or suprabulbar palsy, *Arch Neurol* 48:501-507, 1991.

37. Flora GC. Pseudobulbar palsy, *Minn Med* 53:569-572, 1970.

38. Langworthy OR and Hesser FH. Syndrome of pseudobulbar palsy: an anatomic and physiologic analysis, *Arch Intern Med* 65:106-121, 1940.

39. Black DW. Pathological laughter, *J Nerv Ment Dis* 170:67-71, 1982.

40. Asfora WT and others. Is the syndrome of pathological laughing and crying a manifestation of pseudobulbar palsy? *J Neurol Neurosurg Psych* 52:523-525, 1989.

41. Lieberman A and Benson F. Control of emotional expression in pseudobulbar palsy: a personal experience, *Arch Neurol* 34:717-719, 1977.

42. Horner J and others. Aspiration following stroke: clinical correlates and outcome, *Neurology* 38:1359-1362, 1988.

43. Horner J, Massey EW, and Brazer SR. Aspiration in bilateral stroke patients, *Neurology* 40:1686-1688, 1990.

44. Horner J, Brazer ST, and Massey EW. Aspiration in bilateral stroke patients: a validation study, *Neurology* 43:430-433, 1993.

45. Daniels SK and others. Aspiration in patients with acute stroke, *Arch Phys Med Rehabil* 79:14-19, 1998.

46. Stanners AJ, Chapman AN, and Bamford JM. Clinical predictors of aspiration soon after stroke, *Age Ageing* 22(suppl 2):P17-P18, 1993.

47. Kidd K and others. Aspiration in acute stroke: a clinical study with videofluoroscopy, *Q J Med* 86:825-829, 1993.

48. Horner J and others. Dysphagia following brain-stem stroke: clinical correlates and outcome, *Arch Neurol* 48:1170-1173, 1991.

49. Davies AE and others. Pharyngeal sensation and gag reflex in healthy subjects, *Lancet* 345:487-488, 1995.

50. Leder SB. Gag reflex and dysphagia, *Head Neck* 18:138-140, 1996.

51. Manon-Espaillart R and Ruff RL. Dissociated weakness of sternocleidomastoid and trapezius muscles with lesions in the CNS, *Neurology* 38:796-797, 1988.

52. Mastaglia FL, Knezevic W, and Thompson PD. Weakness of head turning in hemiplegia, *J Neurol Neurosurg Psych* 49:195-197, 1986.

53. Berry H, MacDonald EA, and Mrazek AC. Accessory nerve palsy: a review of 23 cases, *Can J Neurol Sci* 18:337-341, 1991.

54. Keane JR. Twelfth-nerve palsy, *Arch Neurol* 53:561-566, 1996.

CHAPTER 54

Examination of the Motor System: Approach to Weakness

THE MOTOR EXAMINATION

Examination of the muscles includes inspection (for atrophy, hypertrophy, fasciculations), percussion (for myotonia), full flexion and extension of the elbows and knees (to detect abnormal tone and nonneurologic restrictions to movement, such as contractures or joint disease), and tests of muscle strength.

I. MUSCLE STRENGTH

A. Definitions. **Paralysis** refers to loss of power of any degree, from mild weakness to complete loss. The suffixes **-plegia** and **-paresis** also indicate paralysis (e.g., "hemiplegia"), although "-paresis" is usually used to indicate incomplete paralysis. **Tetraparesis** indicates weakness of all four limbs (specialists in spinal cord disorders prefer this term over "quadriparesis"); **paraparesis**, weakness of both legs; **hemiparesis**, weakness of an arm and leg on one side of the body; and **monoparesis**, weakness of just one arm or leg.

B. The findings

1. Technique. The clinician tests single muscles at a time by asking the patient to contract the muscle strongly while the clinician tries to resist any movement. Unilateral weakness is recognized by comparing the muscle to its companion on the opposite side; bilateral weakness, by comparing the strength to some standard recalled from clinical experience. The clinician grades the muscle's strength according to a 6-point system (0 through 5), as described below.

In patients with weakness, the clinician should systematically test all the muscles from head to foot, paying particular attention to which muscles are weak, whether the proximal and distal muscles of a limb differ in strength, and whether the weakness of a monoparetic limb involves only muscles from a single spinal segment or peripheral nerve (see Chapter 57). An excellent, inexpensive handbook describes the proper technique for testing all of the important muscles of the arms and legs.[1]

Testing muscles by resisting their action, however, tends to overlook significant weakness of the muscles of the hip, powerful muscles that can easily overcome the physician's resistance even when significant weakness is present.[2] A better way to test these muscles is to have the patient rise up from a chair and sit down 10 times. Patients with normal strength who are 50 years old or younger accomplish this in less than 20 seconds; those older than 50 years of age accomplish it in less than 25 seconds.[3] If patients require more time than this, proximal weakness of the legs is present unless an alternative explanation is present, such as joint or bone disease.

2. **Grading muscle strength.** Muscle strength is graded using a conventional scale developed by the British Medical Research Council (MRC) during World War II (Table 54-1).[1]

TABLE 54-1 Grading muscle strength

Grade	Finding
0	No contraction
1	Flicker or trace of contraction
2	Active movement with gravity eliminated
3	Active movement against gravity
4	Active movement against gravity and resistance
5	Normal power

From reference 1.

This scale, which is used universally, has one drawback: it assigns a disproportionate amount of a muscle's power to grade 4 strength. For example, the biceps muscle uses just 2% of its full power to overcome gravity (i.e., grade 3 strength), meaning almost 98% of the remaining range of power is grade 4.[4] Because of this drawback, many neurologists subdivide grade 4 into 3 more grades: "4 minus" (i.e., moves barely against resistance), "4," and "4 plus" (i.e., almost full power).

3. **Special tests for cerebral lesions.** In patients with cerebral lesions, measures of muscle power alone often underestimate the size of the lesion and the patient's functional disability. The following tests have been developed as more sensitive tests of motor function in these patients.

   a. **Upper limb drift.** The patient stretches out both arms directly in front of him or her and closes his or her eyes. In patients with hemispheric lesions, the contralateral arm drifts downward and pronates.

   b. **Forearm rolling test.**[5] The patient bends each elbow and places both forearms parallel to each other. He or she then rotates the forearms about each other in a rapid rolling motion for 5 to 10 seconds in each direction. In the abnormal response, seen in patients with hemispheric lesions, the forearm contralateral to the lesion is held still while the other arm "orbits" around it.

    c. Rapid finger tapping. The patient taps rapidly the tip of his index finger against the interphalangeal joint of the thumb. In patients with hemispheric lesions, the speed of finger tapping is asymmetric, the contralateral hand being slower.

C. Clinical significance. See "approach to weakness" below.

II. ATROPHY AND HYPERTROPHY
A. Atrophy
    1. Definition. Atrophy describes muscles that are emaciated or wasted.

    2. Technique. Atrophy is detected during inspection of the muscle. Examples are (1) a thenar eminence appearing abnormally flat when viewed from the side (e.g., cervical radiculopathy or carpal tunnel syndrome), (2) the anterior neck missing shadows because of atrophic sternocleidomastoid muscles (e.g., syringomyelia), or (3) metacarpal bones appearing unusually prominent on the back of the hand, from atrophic intrinsic muscles (e.g., polyneuropathy).

      Significant asymmetry of the circumference of the arms or legs indicates atrophy of the smaller side (or edema of the other side). In normal persons, the difference in calf circumference between the right and left sides is less than 1 cm in 90% and less than 1.5 cm in 100% (measured 10 cm below the tibial tuberosity).[6] Measurements of thigh circumference correlate well with the muscle's cross-sectional area as measured by computed tomography ($r = 0.694$, $p < .01$).[7]

3. **Clinical significance.** Atrophy is a feature of lower motor neuron disease[a] and muscle disuse (especially from adjacent joint disease or trauma).[8-10] In patients with sciatica, the finding of ipsilateral calf wasting (i.e., maximum circumference at least 1 cm less than contralateral side) accurately indicates lumbosacral nerve compression from disc herniation (LR = 5.2; see Chapter 57).

B. **Hypertrophy.** Hypertrophy describes abnormal enlargement of a muscle. Bilateral calf hypertrophy is a typical feature of some muscular dystrophies, although it also is found in a wide variety of other neuromuscular diseases.[11]

III. FASCICULATIONS

A. **Definition.** Fasciculations are involuntary rapid muscle twitches that are too weak to move a limb but are easily felt by patients and seen by clinicians. Most healthy people experience fasciculations at some time, especially in the muscles around their eyelids.

B. **Clinical significance.** Isolated fasciculations without other neurologic findings are benign.[12,13] When accompanied by weakness or atrophy, however, fasciculations indicate lower motor neuron disease, usually of the anterior horn cell or proximal peripheral nerve. Tongue fasciculations occur in up to one third of patients with amyotrophic lateral sclerosis (see Approach to Weakness below).[14]

---

[a] In the evaluation of weakness, a fundamental distinction is the separation of upper motor neuron lesions (i.e., located in the cerebral cortex, brain stem, or descending motor pathways of the spinal cord) from lower motor neuron lesions (i.e., located in the peripheral nerves and anterior horn cells of the spinal cord). See Figure 54-1 and Approach to Weakness at the end of this chapter.

IV. MUSCLE TONE. Muscle tone refers to involuntary muscle tension that clinicians perceive when repeatedly flexing and extending one of the patient's limbs. Assessing muscle tone assumes that the patient is relaxed and that any limitation is not due to bone or joint abnormalities. Muscle tone may be increased (e.g., spasticity, rigidity, or paratonia) or diminished (flaccidity).

A. Increased muscle tone

  1. Spasticity

   a. Definition. Spasticity is increased muscle tone that develops in patients with upper motor neuron lesions.[15-18] The increased muscle tone of spasticity has three characteristic features: **(1) Velocity-dependence.** The amount of muscle tone depends on the velocity of movement. There is more resistance with rapid movements and less resistance with slow ones. **(2) Flexor and extensor tone differ.** The tone in the flexors and extensors of a limb is not balanced, which commonly causes characteristic resting postures of that limb (see below). **(3) Associated weakness.** The muscle with spasticity is also weak. In addition, muscles shortened by spasticity eventually develop fixed contractures, unless the spasticity is treated.

   b. Characteristic postures. In spasticity, an imbalance in flexor and extensor tone, commonly causes abnormal postures of the resting limb. In hemiplegia, for example, there is excess tone in the *flexors* of the arms and *extensors* of the legs, which causes the arm and hand to be fixed against the chest, flexed and internally rotated, and the leg to extend with the foot pointed.[19] In contrast, some patients with complete spinal cord lesions have excess tone in the *flexors* of the legs, which causes the legs to flex up onto the abdomen ("paraplegia-in-flexion").[b20]

c. **Clasp-knife phenomenon.** Up to half of patients with spasticity have the "clasp-knife phenomenon," which is usually observed in the extensors of the knee, less often in the elbow flexors.[17,19] To elicit this phenomenon, the clinician extends the patient's knee using a constant velocity, but as the patient's knee nears full extension, the muscle tone of the quadriceps muscles increases dramatically and completes the movement, just as the blade of a pocket knife opens under the influence of its spring.[21] The clasp-knife phenomenon occurs because muscle tone is dependent on the muscle's length, the tone diminishing with stretching and increasing with shortening.

d. **Relationship of spasticity to weakness.** Although spasticity is a sign of upper motor neuron disease, its severity correlates poorly with the degree of weakness or hyperreflexia.[22,23] Patients with slowly developing cerebral hemisphere lesions usually develop spasticity and weakness in concert.[24] Patients with strokes or spinal cord injury, in contrast,

---

[b] These hemiplegic and paraplegic postures recall the neurologic development of normal infants. Paraplegia-in-flexion resembles the initial posture of babies, their legs flexed against their chest. The infant eventually is able to extend the leg and stand (resembling extensor tone of hemiplegia), after descending pathways from the brain stem mature enough to overcome the spinal reflexes responsible for the flexed position. The infant eventually walks after cerebral connections mature enough to provide fine motor control. Damage to the cerebral hemispheres (e.g., stroke) disrupts this fine motor control and uncovers the extensor posture; damage to the spinal cord (e.g., severe multiple sclerosis or complete spinal cord transection) removes all supraspinal input, uncovering the original flexed posture of the legs.[16]

develop immediate weakness and flaccidity, spasticity appearing only days to weeks later.[19] Some elderly patients with large strokes have persistent "flaccid hemiplegia," in which the paralyzed muscles never develop increased muscle tone despite being hyperreflexic.[24]

2. Rigidity

a. Definition. Rigidity is increased muscle tension that has three characteristic features: **(1) No velocity-dependence.** The resistance to movement is the same with slow and rapid movements. **(2) Flexor and extensor tone are the same. (3) No associated weakness**. Patients with rigidity lack the clasp-knife phenomenon.[16] "Cogwheel rigidity" refers to rigidity that gives way intermittently as if the patient's limb were the lever pulling over a ratchet.

b. Distinguishing spasticity from rigidity. Most clinicians distinguish spasticity from rigidity by repeatedly extending and flexing the patient's limbs and observing the characteristics noted above. In the 1950s, Wartenberg introduced a simple bedside test to assess motor tone and to distinguish spasticity from rigidity.[c,25,26] In this test, the patient is seated on the edge of the examining table, which is open underneath to allow the legs to swing unobstructed back and forth. The clinician lifts both feet to extend the knees, instructs the patient to relax, and then releases the legs. The normal lower limb swings back and forth six or seven

---

[c] Robert Wartenberg, who wrote many popular neurology textbooks in the 1950s, was an ardent opponent of eponyms and called his test the "test for pendulousness of the legs."

times, smoothly and regularly in a perfect sagittal plane. In patients with spasticity, the limbs drop with normal velocity, but their movements are jerky and fall out of the sagittal plane, the great toe tracing zigzags or ellipses. In patients with rigidity, the swinging time and velocity are significantly reduced, resulting in a total of only one or two swings. Others have confirmed Wartenberg's findings.[25,27-31]

c. **Clinical significance—Parkinson's disease.** Rigidity is a common finding of extrapyramidal disease, the most common example of which is Parkinson's disease. The diagnosis of Parkinson's disease is still a bedside diagnosis that traditionally requires the presence of 2 of the following 3 signs: (1) rigidity, (2) bradykinesia, and (3) tremor (the classic "pill-rolling" tremor is about 4 to 6 Hz). Some experts require that bradykinesia be present to prevent misdiagnosis of Parkinson's disease in elderly patients with essential tremor and other causes of cogwheeling.[32] Of the many ways to assess bradykinesia, one is the blink rate: Normal persons blink about 24 ±15 times per minute, whereas patients with Parkinson's disease blink more slowly, about 12 ±10 times per minute. Severely symptomatic patients blink only 5 to 6 times per minute.[33,34]

Nonetheless, when these conventional diagnostic criteria (i.e., 2 of 3 classic signs) are compared with the postmortem pathologic diagnosis of Parkinson's disease, there is a false-positive rate of about 25%.[35] Bedside findings that improve diagnostic accuracy are presented in Table 54-2.[35] Among patients who have 2 of the 3 classic signs, the strongest additional

TABLE 54-2 Parkinson's disease*

FINDING[35]†	SENSITIVITY (%)	SPECIFICITY (%)	POSITIVE LR	NEGATIVE LR
All three traditional findings present	64	71	2.2	0.5
Asymmetric onset and no atypical features	75	75	3.0	0.3
Asymmetric onset, no atypical features, and no alternative diagnosis	68	83	4.1	0.4

*Diagnostic standard: For Parkinson's disease, postmortem examination of brain revealing depletion of nigral pigmented neurons with Lewy bodies in some of remaining nerve cells.

†Definition of findings: For traditional findings, characteristic tremor, rigidity, or bradykinesia; for atypical features and alternative diagnosis, see text. These LRs apply only to patients who have 2 of the 3 traditional findings.

bedside argument *for* Parkinson's disease (LR = 4.1; Table 54-2) is the combination of (1) asymmetric onset, (2) *no* atypical features (i.e., atypical features are early marked autonomic disturbance, early severe dementia, upper motor neuron findings, or gaze palsies), and (3) *no* alternative diagnosis (i.e., alternative diagnoses are use of neuroleptic medication, history of multiple previous cerebrovascular accidents, history of encephalitis at time of onset of symptoms).

3. Paratonia

a. Definition. Paratonia is excess muscle tension that is *not present at rest* but develops when the patient's limb *contacts* another object, as if such contact makes the patient unable to relax. There are two forms: oppositional paratonia **("gegenhalten")** and facilitatory paratonia **("mitgehen")**. In patients with oppositional paratonia, the clinician feels a stiffening of the limb with every applied movement, but unlike rigidity the stiffening depends entirely on contact and its force is proportional and opposite to the examiner's. Patients with facilitatory paratonia, in contrast, actively aid movements guided by the examiner.

b. Technique. One simple test of facilitatory paratonia is to take the arm of the seated patient and bend the elbow back and forth three times, from full flexion to 90 degrees extension. The clinician then releases the arm at the patient's lap and scores any further movement, 0 being no movement, 4 full flexion or more, and 1 to 3 intermediate movements.[36]

c. Clinical significance. Both oppositional and facilitatory paratonia are associated with extensive frontal lobe disease and often appear in dementing illnesses.[36-40] Among patients with dementia, the severity of oppositional or facilitatory paratonia (including the score for the paratonia test described in Section b above) correlates inversely with the Folstein mini-mental status score ($r = -0.5$ to -0.7, $p < .05$).[36]

B. Decreased muscle tone: hypotonia ("flaccidity")

1. **Definition.** Hypotonia refers to reduced or absent muscle tension.

2. **Technique.** There are many ways to detect the flaccid muscle: the limb feels like a "rag doll," the muscles feel soft and flabby, the outstretched arm when tapped demonstrates wider than normal excursions, or the knee jerks are abnormally pendular. The original definition of abnormally pendular knee jerks—more than three back-and-forth swings of the patient's leg during testing of the knee jerk—has to be revised because many normal individuals have this finding.[30]

3. **Clinical significance.** Hypotonia is a feature of lower motor neuron disease and cerebellar disease.

4. **Pathogenesis.** There is some evidence that "normal" muscle tone actually consists of tiny muscle contractions that assist the clinician in moving the extremity (even though the patient is trying to relax).[41] Clinicians perceive reduced muscle tension in hypotonic limbs because these contractions are absent.

V. MUSCLE PERCUSSION.

Striking the muscle with a reflex hammer may elicit 2 abnormal findings, percussion myotonia and myoedema.

A. Percussion myotonia

1. **The finding.** Percussion myotonia is a prolonged muscle contraction that lasts several

seconds and causes a sustained dimple to appear on the skin. Percussion myotonia of the thenar eminence may actually draw the thumb into sustained opposition with the fingers.

2. **Clinical significance.** Percussion myotonia is a feature of some myotonic syndromes, such as myotonia congenita and myotonic dystrophy.[42]

B. Myoedema

1. **The finding.** Myoedema is a focal mounding of muscle lasting seconds at the point of percussion. Unlike myotonia, myoedema causes a lump instead of a dimple, and the lump may be oriented crosswise or diagonal to the direction of muscle fibers.

   Graves and Stokes originally described myoedema in 1830.

2. **Clinical significance.** Myoedema is a normal physiologic response and does not indicate disease.[43] Its historical association with undernourished patients simply reflects the ease with which the response appears when there is no intervening subcutaneous fat.[43-45]

APPROACH TO WEAKNESS

I. CAUSE OF WEAKNESS. Neuromuscular weakness has four principal causes: (1) upper motor neuron disease ("pyramidal tract disease" or "central weakness"), (2) lower motor neuron disease ("denervation disease" or "peripheral weakness"), (3) neuromuscular junction disorders, and (4) muscle disease. Each disorder is associated with distinct physical signs (Table 54-3), neuroanatomy (Figure 54-1), and etiologies (Table 54-4).

Most patients with weakness have disorders of the upper and lower motor neuron lesions. Clinicians should consider muscle disease in any patient with *symmetric* weakness of the *proximal* muscles of the arms and legs (sometimes associated with

TABLE 54-3 Differential diagnosis of weakness*

| Location of Lesion | Motor Examination: | | Sensory Changes | Muscle Stretch Reflexes | Other Findings |
	Muscle Tone	Atrophy or Fasciculations?			
Upper motor neuron	Spasticity	No	Sometimes	Increased	Babinski sign
Lower motor neuron	Hypotonia	Yes	Usually†	Decreased/absent	
Neuromuscular junction	Normal or hypotonia	No	No	Normal/decreased	Ptosis, diplopia
Muscle	Normal	No‡	No	Normal/decreased	Myotonia

*These characteristics are *specific* but not *sensitive*, and thus are helpful when *present*, not when absent. See Section III-A.

†Sensory findings are in distribution of spinal segment, plexus, or peripheral nerve. See Chapter 57.

‡Atrophy may be a late finding.

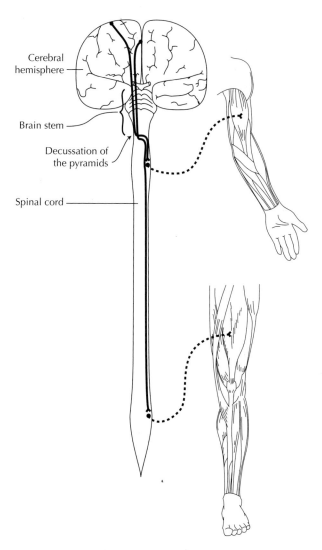

Cerebral hemisphere

Brain stem

Decussation of the pyramids

Spinal cord

FIGURE 54-1 For legend see p. 736.

FIGURE 54-1 Anatomy of upper motor and lower motor neurons.
The figure illustrates the entire pathway of nerves responsible for
movement, from cerebral cortex to muscle. *Upper motor neurons*
(*solid line*) extend from the cerebral cortex through the brain stem to
the spinal cord. *Lower motor neurons* (*dotted line*) originate in the
spinal cord and travel to muscles within peripheral nerves. Because
the upper motor neurons cross to the contralateral side at the border
between the brain stem and spinal cord ("decussation of the pyramids"), weakness of the upper motor neuron type may result from
lesions in the *ipsilateral* spinal cord, *contralateral* brain stem, or
contralateral cerebral hemisphere disease. Lesions of the spinal cord,
where both upper and lower motor neurons reside, may cause weakness of both types: of the *lower motor neuron* type *at* the level of the
lesion and of the *upper motor neuron* type in muscles whose peripheral nerves originate *below* the level of the lesion.

**TABLE 54-4 Common etiologies of neuromuscular
weakness**

LOCATION OF LESION	COMMON ETIOLOGY
Upper motor neuron	Cerebrovascular disease
	Multiple sclerosis
	Brain tumor
Lower motor neuron	Polyneuropathy (diabetes, alcoholism)
	Entrapment neuropathy
	Trauma
Neuromuscular junction	Myasthenia gravis
Muscle	Drug-induced myopathy
	Thyroid disease
	Polymyositis

---

muscle pain, dysphagia, and weakness of the neck
muscles). Disorders of the neuromuscular junction
should be considered in patients whose weakness
varies during the day or who have *ptosis* or *diplopia*.
Associated abnormalities sensation, tone, or reflexes of the weak limb exclude muscle or neuromuscular junction disease and argue for upper or
lower motor neuron lesions.

II. THE FINDINGS

A. Upper vs. lower motor neuron lesions.

Both upper motor neuron weakness and lower motor neuron weakness tend to affect *distal* muscles in either a symmetric or asymmetric pattern.[46-48] The bedside findings that distinguish these two disorders are other neurologic findings in the weak limb, certain localizing signs of upper motor neuron disease, the Babinski sign, and the type of weakness produced.

1. **Associated findings in the weak limb (see Table 54-3).** Spasticity and hyperreflexia indicate central weakness; hypotonia, atrophy, fasciculations, and absent muscle stretch reflexes indicate peripheral weakness. In patients with central weakness, sensory abnormalities vary from the isolated loss of cortical sensations in the distal limb to dense loss of all sensation throughout the limb; if sensory abnormalities occur in peripheral weakness, they follow the distribution of spinal segments or peripheral nerves (see Chapter 55).

2. **Localizing signs of upper motor neuron weakness.** The upper motor neuron pathway extends from the cerebral cortex down through the spinal cord (Figure 54-1), traveling in tight quarters with central neurons innervating other structures. Consequently, in addition to producing central weakness, lesions along this pathway cause characteristic additional physical signs (Table 54-5) that confirm the weakness is of the central type and pinpoint its location.

3. **Babinski sign.** The Babinski sign (Chapter 56) indicates central weakness. In the positive response, the great toe moves upward after a scratching stimulus to the sole of the patient's foot.

4. **Distribution of weakness**

   a. **Limbs affected.** The findings of monoparesis, paraparesis, and tetraparesis are,

TABLE 54-5 Localizing signs in upper motor neuron weakness

Anatomic Location	Associated Finding
Cerebral hemisphere	Seizures
	Hemianopia
	Aphasia (right hemiparesis)
	Inattention to left body, apraxia (left hemiparesis)
	Cortical sensory loss*
	Hyperactive jaw jerk
Brain stem	Crossed motor findings†
	Contralateral third nerve palsy (midbrain)
	Contralateral sixth nerve palsy (pons)
	Sensory loss on contralateral face*
Spinal cord	Sensory level*
	Pain and temperature sensory loss on contralateral arm and leg*
	No sensory or motor findings in face
	Additional lower motor neuron findings (atrophy, fasciculations)

*Chapter 55 describes the different sensory syndromes.

†Crossed motor findings refers to unilateral cranial nerve palsy opposite the side of weakness.

by themselves, unhelpful because they are features of both central and peripheral weakness. Only hemiparesis is specific, indicating a central lesion.

b. Movement vs. muscle. Central lesions paralyze *movements*; peripheral lesions paralyze *muscles*. This occurs because neurons from a single area of the cerebral cortex connect to many different spinal cord segments and muscles to accomplish a particular movement. A single muscle has many movements and thus receives information from many different upper segments, all of which converge on the single peripheral nerve traveling to the muscle. A lesion in that nerve, therefore, obliterates a muscle's entire repertoire of movement; a lesion in an upper segment eliminates only one of many possible movements.[26]

One example of this is the contrast between peripheral facial weakness (Bell's palsy), which paralyzes all ipsilateral facial movements, and central facial weakness (e.g., strokes), which paralyzes voluntary movements but spares emotional ones (e.g., during laughing or crying).[49] Another example is the contrast between the peripheral paraparesis of Guillain-Barré syndrome, which paralyzes all leg movements, and the central paraparesis of spinal cord injury, which eliminates volitional movements of the legs but allows the powerful flexor spasms induced by a mild scratching of the patient's foot.[20]

B. The diagnostic process

1. **Upper motor neuron weakness.** In patients with upper motor neuron weakness, associated neurologic findings indicate the *level* of the lesion (see Table 54-5); the distribution of weakness indicates the *side* of the lesion. For example, bilateral weakness (paraparesis or tetraparesis) indicates *bilateral* lesions (in the thoracic cord or higher if paraparesis, and in the cervical cord or higher if tetraparesis). Monoparesis or hemiparesis indicates a *unilateral* lesion, either in the *contralateral* cerebral hemisphere or brain stem or the *ipsilateral* spinal cord.[d]

---

[d] It is the contralateral cerebral hemisphere and brain stem because the descending central motor pathways originate in the contralateral hemisphere, but it is the ipsilateral spinal cord because these pathways cross just below the brain stem (Figure 54-1).

Table 54-6 illustrates this diagnostic process in the analysis of central weakness. In
the first column is the distribution of central
weakness for hypothetical patients, which
narrows the diagnostic possibilities to a
smaller region of the central motor pathway
(second column). The associated findings
(third column) identify the level of the lesion
within that region, thus pinpointing the lesion's location (fourth column).

2. **Lower motor neuron weakness.** In patients with monoparesis of the lower motor
   neuron type, the clinician should determine
   whether the muscles affected are supplied by
   a single spinal segment (radiculopathy), peripheral nerve (peripheral neuropathy) or
   combination of the two (plexopathy). Further evaluation of these patients is discussed
   in Chapter 57.

   In lower motor neuron weakness, the lesion is always *ipsilateral* to the side of the
   weakness.

3. **Combined upper and lower motor neuron weakness.** Combined upper and lower
   motor neuron findings indicate disease in
   the spinal cord, the only anatomic location where both segments reside. Common
   causes are myelopathy and amyotrophic lateral sclerosis.

   a. **Myelopathy.** Myelopathy is a term de-
      scribing a spinal cord lesion confined to
      a discrete level (e.g., trauma, tumor, disc
      disease). The lesion causes motor, sen-
      sory, and reflex abnormalities *at* the level
      of the lesion and *below* it. The weakness is
      of the peripheral type *at* the level of the
      lesion (from damage to anterior horn
      cells and spinal roots),[e] and of the central

---

[e] Exceptions to this are lesions at the foramen magnum and C3-C4
level, which sometimes produce atrophy in the hands.[50]

TABLE 54-6 Diagnostic approach to upper motor neuron weakness

STEP ONE:		STEP TWO:	
DISTRIBUTION OF WEAKNESS	DIAGNOSTIC POSSIBILITIES	ADDITIONAL FINDING	LOCATION OF LESION
Left monoparesis	Right cerebral hemisphere Right brain stem Left spinal cord	New seizures	Right cerebral hemisphere
Right hemiparesis	Left cerebral hemisphere Left brain stem Right spinal cord	Aphasia	Left cerebral hemisphere
		Right homonymous hemianopia	Left cerebral hemisphere
		Left sixth nerve palsy	Left brain stem
		Loss of sensation left arm and leg; face spared	Right spinal cord
Paraparesis	Bilateral lesion of thoracic cord or above	Sensory level at midchest; normal arm strength and reflexes; spine tenderness between scapulae	Bilateral lesion, thoracic cord
Tetraparesis	Bilateral lesion of cervical cord or above	Hyperactive jaw jerk; dementia	Bilateral lesion, cerebral hemispheres
		Sensory level upper chest; absent biceps reflexes but hyperactive triceps reflexes	Bilateral lesion, cervical cord

type *below* the level of the lesion (from damage to the descending upper motor neuron paths).

Identifying the level of the lesion requires knowledge of which spinal segments innervate which muscle. Table 54-7 presents the standardized segmental innervation used internationally by spinal cord specialists (Chapter 57 discusses the derivation of this table). For example, in a patient with a lesion involving the C7 segment of the spinal cord, there is peripheral weakness in the C7 muscles (i.e., atrophy and weakness of the elbow extensors) but central weakness of all the muscles below this level (hyperreflexia and increased tone of the hands, legs, and feet, and a positive Babinski sign). The

TABLE 54-7 Segmental innervation of muscles*

Spinal Level	Muscles
Arm	
C5	Elbow flexors (biceps, brachialis)
C6	Wrist extensors (extensor carpi radialis longus and brevis)
C7	Elbow extensors (triceps)
C8	Finger flexors (flexor digitorum profundus of middle finger)
T1	Small finger abductors (abductor digiti minimi)
Leg	
L2	Hip flexors (iliopsoas)
L3	Knee extensors (quadriceps)
L4	Ankle dorsiflexors (tibialis anterior)
L5	Long toe extensors (extensor hallucis longus)
S1	Ankle plantar flexors (gastrocnemius, soleus)

*Most muscles are innervated by nerves from more than one spinal root. This table, based on reference 51, simplifies this innervation to standardize the description of spinal cord injury. A more thorough description of segmental innervation of muscle appears in Tables 57-1 and 57-5 of Chapter 57.

muscles from segments above C7, the biceps and wrist extensors, are normal.[f]

b. Amyotrophic lateral sclerosis. Amyotrophic lateral sclerosis is a degenerative disorder of descending motor tracts and motor nuclei of the spinal cord. The disorder causes both lower motor neuron findings (atrophy, fasciculations) and upper motor neuron findings (hyperreflexia). About half of patients have a Babinski response.[14] The disease may start in the arms (44%), legs (37%), or bulbar muscles (causing tongue fasciculations, change in voice, and difficulty swallowing, 19%).[14] There are no sensory findings.

Amyotrophic lateral sclerosis and cervical myelopathy are commonly confused at the bedside, even by experienced neurologists.[52] In patients with both upper and lower motor neuron signs, findings that argue in favor of amyotrophic lateral sclerosis are (1) prominent fasciculations, (2) absence of sensory findings, and (3) signs of lower motor neuron degeneration affecting more than one level of the spinal cord simultaneously.[g53,54]

III. CLINICAL SIGNIFICANCE. The clinical significance of the motor examination cannot be tested in the conventional manner of this book because bedside criteria alone are sufficient to diagnose many causes of weakness (e.g., cerebrovascular

---

[f] By convention, the neurologic level in spinal cord injury refers to the most caudal level with *normal* function, rather than the first level with abnormal function.[51] The motor level for this hypothetical patient is C6.

[g] The four spinal cord levels are bulbar (jaw, face, tongue, larynx), cervical (neck, arm, hand, diaphragm), thoracic (back, abdomen), and lumbosacral (back, abdomen, leg, and foot).

disease, amyotrophic lateral sclerosis, and peripheral nerve injuries are routinely diagnosed by bedside criteria).

Nonetheless, investigations of these signs do allow a few additional points.

A. Clinical syndromes are often incomplete.
Most studies show that the full lower motor or upper motor neuron syndromes, as depicted in Table 54-3, are often incomplete. In upper motor neuron weakness, up to 25% of patients lack exaggerated reflexes[47,55] and the absence of spasticity is common, especially in acute lesions (see above). Similarly, in many examples of lower motor weakness, the nerve affected does not even innervate a clinical reflex (e.g., L5 radiculopathy, median or ulnar neuropathy), and therefore, the reflexes of the limbs are normal. Therefore, in the evaluation of weak patients, the *absence* of spasticity or hyperreflexia does *not* argue against the presence of upper motor neuron disease, nor does the *absence* of hypotonicity of hyporeflexia argue against the presence of lower motor neuron disease.

On the other hand, the *presence* of abnormal reflexes is very helpful: In one study of patients with weakness, 87% had abnormal reflexes, and in every case, areflexia correctly predicted lower motor neuron disease and hyperreflexia correctly predicted upper motor neuron disease.[47]

The fact that syndromes are often incomplete emphasizes the importance of the complete neurologic examination. For example, in a patient with weakness of the fingertips, in whom the absence of sensory or reflex changes prevents classifying the weakness as peripheral or central using the criteria of Table 54-3, the discovery of any additional neurologic finding from Table 54-5 indicates the lesion is central, and pinpoints its location precisely.

B. Proximal weakness indicates muscle disease. If "proximal weakness" is defined as strength of a limb's proximal muscles being one MRC grade less than the distal muscles, proximal weakness is seen in 92% of patients with muscle disease.[47] This means that the *absence* of proximal weakness is a strong argument against muscle disease.

C. For cerebral hemispheric lesions, the special tests are very sensitive. Table 54-8 presents the diagnostic accuracy of various physical signs for detecting unilateral cerebral hemispheric lesions, as detected by computed tomography. According to this table, the traditional findings of a contralateral cerebral lesion—hemiparesis, Babinski response, hemianopia, hemisensory disturbance—are indeed very compelling (LRs = 11.0 to 36.3). A more important point is that arm rolling test, upper limb drift, and finger tapping test are slightly more sensitive than hemiparesis (although it is an insignificant difference), and that all four of these findings are much more sensitive than the Babinski response, hemianopia, or hemisensory disturbance (p <.0001). This means that the *normal* arm rolling test, *absence* of upper limb drift, *normal* finger tapping test and *normal* *strength* argue much more convincingly *against* the presence of a contralateral cerebral lesion (LRs = 0.1 to 0.3) than does the *absent* Babinski response, *normal* visual fields, or *normal* sensory examination (LRs = 0.6 to 0.7).

The LRs on Table 54-8 are spectacular compared with many of those in the general medicine section of this book, simply because, in the field of neurology, the clinical signs still largely define the clinical problem. A cerebral lesion on imaging is "significant" (and therefore is called "disease") because it causes hemiparesis or some other neurologic sign. In contrast, we cannot say this about many signs from general

TABLE 54-8 Unilateral cerebral hemispheric disease*

Finding (ref)†	Sensitivity (%)	Specificity (%)	Positive LR	Negative LR
Arm rolling test	87	98	36.3	0.1
Upper limb drift	79	98	33.0	0.2
Finger tapping test	79	93	11.0	0.2
Facial weakness	77	98	32.3	0.2
Hemiparesis	75	98	31.7	0.3
Wrist extensor weakness	69	98	29.0	0.3
Babinski response	45	98	19.0	0.6
Hemianopia	30	98	NS	0.7
Hemisensory disturbance	29	98	NS	0.7

NS, Not significant.

*Diagnostic standard: For unilateral cerebral hemispheric disease, computed tomography; from reference 5.

†Definition of findings: For arm rolling test, upper limb drift, and finger tapping test, see text.

medicine (e.g., aortic stenosis is not significant because it causes a heart murmur, but instead because it overloads the left ventricle and causes cardiac symptoms and death).

D. Diagnosis of peripheral nerve disorders. Chapter 57 discusses the clinical significance of muscle weakness and its localizing value to the diagnosis of peripheral nerve disorders.

REFERENCES

1. Medical Research Council. *Aids to the examination of the peripheral nervous system,* London, 1986, Bailliere Tindall.
2. Beasley WC. Quantitative muscle testing: principles and applications to research and clinical services, *Arch Phys Med Rehab* 42:398-425, 1961.
3. Csuka M and McCarty DJ. Simple method for measurement of lower extremity muscle strength, *Am J Med* 78:77-81, 1985.
4. van der Ploeg RJO, Oosterhuis HJGH, and Reuvekamp J. Measuring muscle strength, *J Neurol* 231:200-203, 1984.
5. Sawyer RN and others. Asymmetry of forearm rolling as a sign of unilateral cerebral dysfunction, *Neurology* 43:1596-1598, 1993.
6. Stein PD and others. Asymmetry of calves in the assessment of patients with suspected acute pulmonary embolism, *Chest* 107:936-939, 1995.
7. Lorentzon R and others. Thigh musculature in relation to chronic anterior cruciate ligament tear: muscle size, morphology, and mechanical output before reconstruction, *Am J Sport Med* 17:423-429, 1989.
8. Stokes M and Young A. The contribution of reflex inhibition to arthrogenous muscle weakness, *Clin Sci* 67:7-14, 1984.
9. Ross M and Worrell TW. Thigh and calf girth following knee injury and surgery, *J Occup Sport Phys Ther* 27:9-15, 1998.
10. Helliwell PS and Jackson S. Relationship between weakness and muscle wasting in rheumatoid arthritis, *Ann Rheum Dis* 53:726-728, 1994.
11. Reimers CD and others. Calf enlargement in neuromuscular diseases: a quantitative ultrasound study in 350 patients and review of the literature, *J Neurol Sci* 143:46-56, 1996.

12. Blexrud MD, Windebank AJ, and Daube JR. Long-term follow-up of 121 patients with benign fasciculations, *Ann Neurol* 34:622-625, 1993.

13. Reed DM and Kurland LT. Muscle fasciculations in a healthy population, *Arch Neurol* 9:363-367, 1963.

14. Li TM, Alberman E, and Swash M. Clinical features and associations of 560 cases of motor neuron disease, *J Neurol Neurosurg Psych* 53:1043-1045, 1990.

15. Young RR. Spasticity: a review, *Neurology* 44:S12-S20, 1994.

16. Lance JW. The control of muscle tone, reflexes, and movement: Robert Wartenberg lecture, *Neurology* 30:1303-1313, 1980.

17. Burke D, Gillies JD, and Lance JW. The quadriceps stretch reflex in human spasticity, *J Neurol Neurosurg Psych* 33:216-223, 1970.

18. Burke D, Gillies JD, and Lance JW. Hamstrings stretch reflex in human spasticity, *J Neurol Neurosurg Psych* 34:231-235, 1971.

19. Twitchell TE. The restoration of motor function following hemiplegia in man, *Brain* 74:443-480, 1951.

20. Marshall J. Observations on reflex changes in the lower limbs in spastic paraplegia in man, *Brain* 77:290-304, 1954.

21. Gowers WR. *A manual of diseases of the nervous system* (1981 facsimile by Classics of Medicine Library), Philadelphia, 1888, P. Blakiston, Son & Co.

22. Fellows SJ, Ross HF, and Thilmann AF. The limitations of the tendon jerk as a marker of pathological stretch reflex activity in human spasticity, *J Neurol Neurosurg Psych* 56:531-537, 1993.

23. Dohrmann GJ and Norwack WJ. Relationship between various clinical signs in lesions of the descending motor system, *Dis Nerv Sys* 35:375-377, 1974.

24. Landau WM. Spasticity: the fable of a neurological demon and the emperor's new therapy, *Arch Neurol* 31:217-219, 1974.

25. Wartenberg R. Pendulousness of the legs as a diagnostic test, *Neurology* 1:18-24, 1951.

26. Wartenberg R. *Diagnostic tests in neurology: a selection for office use*, Chicago, 1953, Year Book Publishers, Inc.

27. Brown RA and others. Observations on the applicability of the Wartenberg pendulum test to healthy, elderly subjects, *J Neurol Neurosurg Psych* 51:1171-1177, 1988.

28. Bajd T and Vodovnik L. Pendulum testing of spasticity, *J Biomed Eng* 6:9-16, 1984.

29. Boczko M and Mumenthaler M. Modified pendulousness test to assess tonus of thigh muscles in spasticity, *Neurology* 8:846-851, 1958.

30. Pickett JB and Tatum EJ. Pendular knee reflexes: a reliable sign of hypotonia? *Lancet* 2:236-237, 1984.

31. Brown RA and others. Does the Wartenberg pendulum test differentiate quantitatively between spasticity and rigidity? A study in elderly stroke and Parkinson's patients, *J Neurol Neurosurg Psych* 51:1178-1186, 1988.

32. Hughes AJ and others. Accuracy of clinical diagnosis of idiopathic Parkinson's disease: a clinico-pathological study of 100 cases, *J Neurol Neurosurg Psych* 55:181-184, 1992.

33. Karson CN and others. Blink rates and disorders of movement, *Neurology* 34:677-678, 1984.

34. Bentivoglio AR and others. Analysis of blink rate patterns in normal subjects, *Mov Dis* 12:1028-1034, 1997.

35. Hughes AJ and others. What features improve the accuracy of clinical diagnosis in Parkinson's disease: a clinico-pathologic study, *Neurology* 42:1142-1146, 1992.

36. Beversdorf DQ and Heilman KM. Facilitory paratonic and frontal lobe functioning, *Neurology* 51:968-971, 1998.

37. Tyrrell P and Rossor M. The association of gegenhalten in the upper limbs with dyspraxia, *J Neurol Neurosurg Psych* 51:995-997, 1988.

38. O'Keefe ST and others. Gait disturbance in Alzheimer's disease: a clinical study, *Age Ageing* 25:313-316, 1996.

39. Denny-Brown D. The nature of apraxia, *J Nerv Ment Dis* 126:9-32, 1958.

40. Chatterjee A. Feeling frontal dysfunction: facilitory paratonia and the regulation of motor behavior, *Neurology* 51:937-939, 1998.

41. van der Meche FGA, van Gijn J. Hypotonia: an erroneous clinical concept? *Brain* 109:1169-1178, 1986.

42. Barchi RL. Myotonia, *Neurol Clin* 6:473-484, 1988.

43. Hornung K and Nix WA. Myoedema: a clinical and electrophysiological evaluation, *Eur Neurol* 32:130-133, 1992.

44. Conn RD and Smith RH. Malnutrition, myoedema, and Muehrcke's lines, *Arch Intern Med* 116:875-878, 1965.

45. Jones MP and Parkes WE. Myoedema, *Clin Sci* 14:97-100, 1955.

46. Adams RW, Gandevia SC, and Skuse NF. The distribution of muscle weakness in upper motoneuron lesions affecting the lower limb, *Brain* 113:1459-1476, 1990.

47. Thijs RD and others. Distribution of muscle weakness of central and peripheral origin, *J Neurol Neurosurg Psych* 65:794-796, 1998.

48. Colebatch JG and Gandevia SC. The distribution of muscular weakness in upper motor neuron lesions affecting the arm, *Brain* 112:749-763, 1989.

49. Ross RT and Mathiesen R. Volitional and emotional supranuclear facial weakness, *N Engl J Med* 338:1515, 1998.

50. Sonstein WJ and others. False localizing signs in upper cervical spinal cord compression, *Neurosurg* 38:445-449, 1996.

51. Maynard FM and others. International standards for neurological and functional classification of spinal cord injury, *Spinal Cord* 35:266-274, 1997.

52. Davenport RJ and others. Avoiding false positive diagnoses of motor neuron disease: lessons from the Scottish Motor Neuron Disease Register, *J Neurol Neurosurg Psych* 60:147-151, 1996.

53. World Federation of Neurology Research Group on Neuromuscular Diseases. El Escorial World Federation of Neurology criteria for the diagnosis of amyotrophic lateral sclerosis, *J Neurol Sci* 124(suppl):96-107, 1994.

54. Li TM and others. Differential diagnosis of motoneurone disease from other neurological conditions, *Lancet* 2:731-733, 1986.

55. van Gijn J. The Babinski sign and the pyramidal syndrome, *J Neurol Neurosurg Psych* 41:865-873, 1978.

Examination of the Sensory System

SIMPLE SENSATIONS

I. DEFINITIONS. There are four simple sensations: pain, temperature, touch, and vibration. These sensations are all called "simple" because their perception does not require a healthy contralateral cerebral cortex. Excepting the sense of vibration, the simple sensations have distinct sensory organs in the skin and, excepting touch, their pathways in the spinal cord are well defined.

Hypesthesia refers to a diminished ability to perceive a simple sensation; **anesthesia** refers to the complete inability to perceive a simple sensation. Although both "hypesthesia" and "anesthesia" originally referred only to the sensation of touch, many clinicians use the terms when reporting any of the simple sensations. **Hypalgesia** means there is a decreased sensitivity to painful stimuli; **analgesia**, a complete insensitivity. **Hyperpathia, hyperesthesia**, and **allodynia** all refer to an increased sensitivity to sensory stimuli, often with unpleasant qualities, although some experts restrict "hyperpathia" to increased sensitivity from *painful* stimuli and allodynia to discomfort from *tactile* stimuli.

II. TECHNIQUE. Which sensory tests to include in the physical examination depends on the clinical

751

setting. For screening examinations in patients with no sensory complaints, testing only for touch on all four extremities usually suffices. For sensory complaints confined to one limb, testing for touch and pain sensation is usually performed, although testing for pain sensation has a better chance of detecting subtle radiculopathies and peripheral nerve disorders (see "Dermatomes" below).[1,2] For screening diabetic feet and limbs at risk for neuropathic ulcers and arthropathy, clinicians should use Semmes-Weinstein monofilaments (see Chapter 49). Finally, for any patients with sensory complaints involving large portions of a limb or the trunk, testing for all simple sensations is necessary to uncover "sensory dissociation" (i.e., perception of one modality but not another), which is an important clue to spinal cord disease (see Sensory Syndromes later in this chapter).

During sensory testing, the patient's perceptions are compared either with a known standard of normal sensation (e.g., Semmes-Weinstein monofilaments for tactile sensation and tuning fork tests for vibratory sensation), to the contralateral companion part of the patient's body, or to the clinician's own sense of what is normal, as gathered from previous experience.

A. Touch. The sensation of touch is usually tested qualitatively by stimulating the patient's skin lightly with a cotton wisp, piece of tissue paper, or the clinician's finger, or quantitatively by using Semmes-Weinstein monofilaments (see Chapter 49).

B. Pain and temperature. The usual techniques for testing pain sensation are a safety pin bent at right angles or the sharp edge of a broken wooden applicator stick, both of which must be discarded after use to prevent the transmission of infection.[3] It is no longer permissible to use the built-in pin of many reflex hammers or the traditional tailor's pinwheel, because of the risk of transmitting infection.

The traditional test for temperature sensation uses tubes of warm and cold water, although testing the patient's ability to distinguish the cold stem of the tuning fork from the warmer index finger is much simpler.[4]

C. Vibration. Vibratory sensation is tested with a tuning fork (usually 128 Hz, less often 256 Hz). There is no compelling reason for using one tuning fork over the other, except that standards have been developed for the 128 Hz fork. Humans are most sensitive to vibration frequencies of 200 to 300 Hz and have difficulty consistently detecting frequencies below 100 Hz.[5,6] Traditionally, the tuning fork is applied against bony prominences, although this is based on the mistaken belief that bones contain the "vibration receptors"; vibratory sensation is just as good, or even better, over soft tissues without underlying bone (the clinician can easily demonstrate this by testing sensation on the abdominal wall).[7]

When a 128 Hz tuning fork is struck from a distance of 20 cm against the heel of the clinician's palm, a healthy 40 year-old person should perceive vibrations for at least 11 seconds when the stem of the fork is held against the lateral malleolus, and for at least 15 seconds when it is held against the ulnar styloid.[8] These values decrease 2 seconds for every decade of age greater than 40 years.

One disadvantage to vibratory testing is that the vibrating impulse is conducted away from the tuning fork, thus preventing precise definition of sensory boundaries in patients with peripheral nerve injuries.[7]

Rumpf introduced the tuning fork to bedside neurology in 1889.[9]

III. CLINICAL SIGNIFICANCE
A. Touch, pain, and temperature sensation.
Abnormalities of the simple sensations define

all important clinical sensory syndromes: peripheral nerve injury, radiculopathy, spinal cord syndromes, lateral medullary infarction, and thalamic and cerebral hemispheric syndromes (see Sensory Syndromes). No diagnostic test has proved superior to bedside examination. In patients with neuropathy, the clinician's bedside assessment of hypesthesia is a more specific predictor of fiber loss on nerve biopsy than automated touch-pressure esthesiometers.[10] In some ways, physical examination is even superior to nerve conduction testing, which evaluates only the larger myelinated peripheral nerve fibers, not the smaller unmyelinated fibers, which carry pain and temperature sensations and from which many uncomfortable sensory syndromes originate.[11]

Diabetic feet insensate to the 5.07 monofilament have increased risk of subsequent foot ulceration and amputation[12-14] (see Chapter 49).

B. **Vibratory sensation.** Vibratory sensation is often diminished in peripheral neuropathy and spinal cord disease but spared in disease confined to the cerebral cortex.[7] Although it is a highly developed sensation—Helen Keller could interpret speech by feeling the vibrations of the speaker's larynx, lips, and nose—it lacks distinct sense organs and its neuroanatomic pathways remain obscure.[7,15] Traditionally, it is associated with proprioception because impulses from both sensations ascend in the posterior columns of the spinal cord, but there are many clinical examples of dissociation of vibratory and proprioceptive loss, both in peripheral neuropathy and cord disease (see "proprioception").[7,16]

C. **Hyperpathia and allodynia are nonspecific findings.** Hyperpathia and allodynia occur in many different painful conditions, including peripheral neuropathy, brain stem infarction, and thalamic stroke, and by themselves have no localizing value.[17,18]

PROPRIOCEPTION

I. DEFINITION. Proprioception allows individuals to detect joint motion and limb position when their eyes are closed.[19] Like most of the simple sensations, proprioception has distinct sense organs and ascending pathways in the spinal cord. Unlike simple sensations, however, full perception requires a healthy contralateral cerebral cortex; in this way, it resembles cortical sensations (see Cortical Sensations).[20,21]

Sir Charles Bell originally called proprioception the "sixth sense." In 1906, Sherrington introduced the term "proprioception" to describe this sensation.[19,22]

II. TECHNIQUE. The conventional test of proprioception is to lightly hold the sides of the patient's finger or toe and bend it slowly up and down. The patient is asked to indicate any sensation of movement and the movement's direction. Because normal persons perceive motion much more easily than direction, a normal person may accurately indicate the presence of motion all of the time but indicate the wrong direction up to 10% of the time.[23] Normal individuals can detect 1 to 2 degrees of movement in most joints, the hips being the most sensitive.[23,24]

Another test of proprioception tests the ability to direct a limb to a given point, again with eyes closed: in one version, the clinician positions the patient's outstretched index finger on the clinician's own index finger. The patient then drops the arm to the side and attempts to find the previous position. Normal individuals consistently come within 5 cm of the target.[22]

Patients with severe proprioceptive loss depend on vision for balance and thus become very unstable when they close their eyes or walk in darkness. This dependence on vision forms the basis for another test of proprioceptive loss, "Romberg's sign," which is discussed fully in Chapter 5.

III. CLINICAL SIGNIFICANCE. Proprioceptive loss is common in peripheral neuropathy (e.g., diabetes mellitus), spinal cord disease (e.g., multiple sclerosis, B_{12} deficiency, tabes dorsalis), and severe hemispheral disease. In unilateral disease of the spinal cord (e.g., the Brown-Séquard syndrome), proprioception is lost on the side of weakness, opposite the side with the pain and temperature loss (see Sensory Syndromes below). In patients with strokes, proprioceptive loss indicates extensive damage and correlates with a poorer functional recovery and higher mortality.[25]

According to traditional teachings, a disproportionate loss of vibration sensation and proprioception (compared with pain and temperature sensation) occurs in diseases of the dorsal columns of the spinal cord (e.g., tabes dorsalis, multiple sclerosis, B_{12} deficiency) and some peripheral neuropathies (e.g., diabetic polyneuropathy). Although this teaching is true, most patients with these disorders also have abnormalities of pain and temperature sensation as well.[7,26]

CORTICAL SENSATIONS

I. DEFINITION. Cortical sensations are those sensations requiring higher integration and processing for them to be perceived properly. Consequently, perception of cortical sensations requires a healthy contralateral cerebral cortex. They may become abnormal in cerebral hemispheric disease, *even though* the simple sensations are preserved.

II. TECHNIQUE. Testing for cortical sensations has three requirements: (1) the patient's eyes are closed; (2) the patient lacks dementia; and (3) most of the simple sensations, especially touch, are preserved. If the simple sensations are profoundly altered, as in severe peripheral neuropathy, no sensory information will reach the cerebral hemisphere and tests for cortical sensation become uninterpretable.

A. **Two-point discrimination.** Two-point discrimination is the ability to distinguish two compass points simultaneously applied to the skin. The normal minimal distance is 3 cm for the hand or foot and 0.6 cm for the fingertips.[16,20,27,28]

B. **Tactile recognition ("stereognosis").** Tactile recognition is the ability to recognize common objects like a key, paper clip, coin, tweezers, or rubber ball placed in the hand. Normal individuals can name >90% of objects within 5 seconds or less.[29,30]

C. **Graphesthesia.** Graphesthesia is the ability to identify letters or numbers traced on the hand or foot. Normal individuals can easily recognize symbols 1 cm in height on the fingertips and 6 cm tall elsewhere.[20]

D. **Localization.** Localization is the ability to accurately point to a spot on the body just touched by the clinician.

E. **Bilateral simultaneous tactile stimulation.** This tests the patient's ability to recognize that both sides of the body are being touched simultaneously. The term "tactile extinction" refers to the patient's consistent failure to detect the stimulus on one side of the body.[31]

F. **Appreciation of weights.** Appreciation of weights is the ability to perceive differences in weight between two objects, placed sequentially in the patient's hand. This test was used more often several decades ago than it is now.[32]

III. **CLINICAL SIGNIFICANCE.** Lesions of the posterior parietal lobe may preserve the simple sensations but eliminate proprioception and cortical sensations, the loss typically confined to just the contralateral distal parts of the limbs, sparing the face and trunk.[21,32-34]

It is important to note that cortical disease also may eliminate any or all of the simple sensations, especially if the lesion involves the anterior parietal lobe (postcentral gyrus) or deeper white matter.[7,21,32,35] These lesions often cause a dense sensory loss on the opposite side of the body, involving the trunk, limbs, and face, sometimes referred to as the "pseudothalamic syndrome" because of its resemblance to the sensory loss of thalamic disease (see Sensory Syndromes below).[21]

DERMATOMES

I. DEFINITION. Dermatomes define the area of skin innervated by a single nerve root or spinal segment. They are primarily used to determine whether the sensory loss on a limb corresponds to a single spinal segment, implying the lesion is of that nerve root (i.e., radiculopathy), and to assign the neurologic "level" to a spinal cord lesion.

II. DERIVATION OF THE DERMATOMAL MAPS. The original human dermatomal maps emerged from Sherrington's experiments with monkeys and Head's observations of patients with *Herpes zoster* infection.[2,36] These maps have been subsequently revised, based on several types of evidence collected over the last century, including neurosurgical observations (by Cushing, Foester, and Keegan), experiments injecting novocaine next to the roots of medical student volunteers, and electrical stimulation of the skin while recording potentials at the nerve roots.[1,2,36-38] Differences among dermatomal maps, which are minor and primarily deal with how far proximally some limb dermatomes extend, probably reflect biologic variation and differences in experimental method (i.e., sensory loss from a herniated disc or novocaine injection is not necessarily the same as that from root resection).

III. TECHNIQUE. The dermatomal map in Figure 55-1 is the international standard used for classifying patients with spinal cord injury (see also Table

FIGURE 55-1 Dermatomes. This is the dermatome map recommended by the American Spinal Injury Association.[39] Note that the C2 dermatome includes the angle of the jaw and most of the ear. The precise boundaries of the S1 and S2 dermatomes are the most controversial.[37]

55-1).[39] Two principles apply when evaluating the dermatomal pattern of sensory loss: (1) Contiguous dermatomes overlap, which means that damage to one nerve root may cause either no anesthesia or a sensory loss confined to a small area. These small areas, which are referred to as "signature zones," define the sensory level in patients with spinal cord

TABLE 55-1 Dermatomes and their signature zones

Spinal Level	Signature Zone
Cervical	
C3	Supraclavicular fossa
C4	Top of acromioclavicular joint
C5	Lateral side of antecubital fossa
C6	Thumb
C7	Middle finger
C8	Little finger
Thoracic (selected levels)	
T1	Medial (ulnar) side of the antecubital fossa
T2	Apex of axilla
T4	Fourth intercostal space (nipple line)
T10	Tenth intercostal space (umbilicus)
T12	Inguinal ligament at midpoint
Lumbar	
L1	Half the distance between T12 and L2
L2	Mid-anterior thigh
L3	Medial femoral condyle
L4	Medial malleolus
L5	Dorsum of the foot at the third metatarsal phalangeal joint
Sacral	
S1	Lateral heel
S2	Popliteal fossa in the mid-line
S3	Ischial tuberosity
S4-5	Perianal level

Based on reference 39 and original work cited in text.

disease[a]; (2) Tactile dermatomes are larger than pain dermatomes. This suggests that, when only one or two segments are affected, testing for pain sensibility is a more sensitive method of examination than testing for abnormal touch.[1,2]

---

[a] In sensory testing, as in motor testing, the neurologic "level" refers to the most caudal level with *normal* function, rather than the first level with abnormal function. For example, a patient with sensation in the nipple line, but none below it, has a "T4 sensory level."

IV. CLINICAL SIGNIFICANCE

A. **The sensory level in spinal cord disease.**

The patient's sensory level is often several segments *below* the actual level of the lesion in the spinal cord (e.g., the patient with a T8 sensory level may have a lesion in the T3 segment of the spinal cord).[b40-42] There are two explanations for this phenomenon: one is that the organization of the ascending spinothalamic pathway (carrying pain and temperature sensation) makes the more lateral fibers carrying lower body sensations more vulnerable to external injury. Another is that the actual spinal lesion causes injury by compromising the cord's blood supply, thereby causing injury at a distant segment.[40,41]

When the sensory and motor levels disagree, the motor level is a more reliable indicator of level of injury and future disability for the patient.[44] In some patients with spinal cord disease, the best indicator of the level of disease is the location of their pain or vertebral tenderness.[42]

B. **Dermatomal loss in radiculopathy.** The

clinical significance of dermatomal sensory loss in disorders of the nerve roots is discussed in Chapter 57.

SENSORY SYNDROMES

I. TECHNIQUE. Figure 55-2 depicts the sensory loss

of the important sensory syndromes. Sensory loss confined to a *portion* of a limb suggests injury to a peripheral nerve, plexus, or spinal root, subjects discussed in Chapter 57. When sensory loss involves *most of a limb* or the *trunk*, a systematic

---

[b] During the first successful operation to remove a spinal tumor, in 1887, the surgeon's initial incision, which had been based on the patient's sensory level at T5, had to be revised upward twice before the tumor was found at the T2 level.[43]

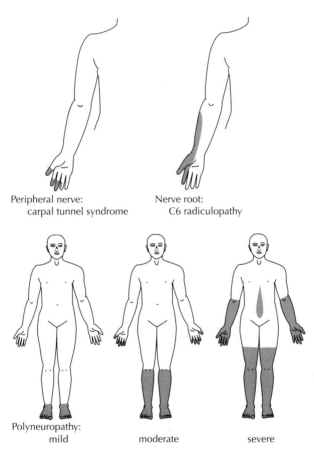

Peripheral nerve:
    carpal tunnel syndrome

Nerve root:
    C6 radiculopathy

Polyneuropathy:
    mild   moderate   severe

FIGURE 55-2 Sensory syndromes. In these figures, the gray shading indicates hypalgesia (loss of pain temperature sensation) and the arrows indicate limbs with significant accompanying weakness. In the Brown-Séquard syndrome (hemisection of the cord, *top row, right*), there is often diminished tactile sensation on the side of weakness and opposite the side with hypalgesia.

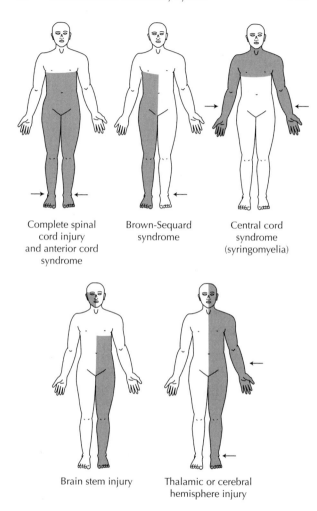

Complete spinal
cord injury
and anterior cord
syndrome

Brown-Sequard
syndrome

Central cord
syndrome
(syringomyelia)

Brain stem injury

Thalamic or cerebral
hemisphere injury

FIGURE 55-2, cont'd For legend see opposite page.

approach using the following questions defines the syndrome.

A. **Does the sensory loss involve both sides of the body?** Involvement of *both* sides indicates polyneuropathy or spinal cord disease. Involvement of *one* side indicates contralateral disease of the brain stem, thalamus, or cerebral cortex. In patients with pure hemisection of the spinal cord (i.e., Brown-Séquard syndrome), there is sensory loss on both sides of the body, although pain and temperature sensation is lost on the side *opposite to* the lesion and tactile sensation is lost on the side *of* the lesion.

B. **Is there a sensory level?** A sensory level is a distinct border on the trunk, below which sensory testing is abnormal and above which it is normal. A sensory level indicates spinal cord disease, although the finding sometimes also occurs in lateral medullary infarction.[17,45,46]

C. **Is there sensory dissociation?** Sensory dissociation is a disproportionate loss of one or more simple sensations with preservation of others. Loss of pain and temperature sensation with preservation of touch and vibration sensation is a feature of some *incomplete* spinal cord syndromes (e.g., syringomyelia, spinal stroke, and Brown-Séquard syndrome).

D. **Is there sensory loss on the face?** Sensory loss on the face indicates disease above the spinal cord, in the brain stem, thalamus, or cerebral hemispheres. In brain stem disease (e.g., lateral medullary syndrome), the sensory loss on the patient's face is *opposite* the side of sensory loss on the body; in disease of the thalamus or cerebral hemisphere, the sensory loss on the face and body are on the *same* side.

E. **Are there associated neurologic signs?** Most disorders causing the sensory syndromes depicted in Figure 55-2 also cause significant weakness (indicated by the arrows in Figure

55-2), a major exception being the lateral medullary syndrome.

The presence of an associated **Horner's syndrome** (see Chapter 19 for definition) indicates disease of the ipsilateral brain stem or cervical spinal cord.[47]

II. DEFINITION OF THE SENSORY SYNDROMES.

Peripheral nerve and spinal root disorders are discussed in Chapter 57.

A. Polyneuropathy. Polyneuropathy is a bilateral "stocking-glove" sensory loss that spares the face (the sensory loss resembles the pattern of a stocking or glove because polyneuropathy affects all nerves of the same length equally). Because the sensory loss of polyneuropathy affects the longest nerves first, hypesthesia initially appears in the feet; later in the fingertips; and, only after extensive involvement of the arms and legs, the anterior trunk.[48] Atrophy of the small muscles of the feet and hands and absent ankle reflexes are common. Distal weakness may occur, but because the nerves to the foot dorsiflexors are longer than those to plantar flexors, patients with polyneuropathy have more trouble walking on their heels than on their toes (the opposite finding, trouble walking on toes but not on heels, suggests an alternative diagnosis).[49]

B. Spinal cord syndromes

1. Complete spinal cord lesion. A complete spinal cord lesion causes a sensory level with loss of all simple sensations below that level, weakness (tetraparesis or paraparesis), and urinary retention.

2. Incomplete spinal cord lesions

a. Anterior cord syndrome. Spinal stroke, which may follow prolonged hypotension or trauma to the aorta, resembles the complete spinal cord lesion, except there is a disproportionate loss of pain and temperature sensation and relative sparing of touch and vibration, owing to the more vulnerable blood supply of the ventral cord.[50]

b. Brown-Séquard syndrome describes injury to one-half of the cord, causing *contralateral* loss of pain and temperature sensation but *ipsilateral* paralysis and diminished touch sensation.[47] Unilateral disease of the cervicothoracic region may involve the ascending sympathetic fibers and cause an ipsilateral Horner's syndrome.[47]

The pure Brown-Séquard syndrome is rare. Instead, most patients with unilateral disease of the spinal cord present with bilateral weakness and sensory loss, although the weakness is greatest on the side of the lesion and the hypalgesia is greatest opposite the lesion.[47]

c. Central cord syndrome. In syringomyelia, the sensory loss typically involves one or both arms. Seventy-five percent of patients have atrophy and weakness of one or both hands or sternocleidomastoid muscles.[51,52]

C. Lateral medullary infarct ("Wallenberg's syndrome") is a dramatic syndrome presenting with dizziness and causing sensory loss on opposite sides of face and body but no weakness (the lesion is ipsilateral to the facial analgesia). Common associated signs are diminished corneal reflex, ipsilateral limb ataxia, nystagmus, ipsilateral Horner's syndrome, gait ataxia, and ipsilateral palate weakness (see Table 55-2).[45,53-57]

D. Thalamic disease. A lesion in the thalamus may cause loss of all simple sensations on the opposite side of the body, associated with hemiparesis, vertical gaze abnormalities, miosis, and aphasia.[35,58,59]

TABLE 55-2 Lateral medullary syndrome (Wallenberg's syndrome)

Physical Finding	Frequency (%)*
Cranial Nerves	
Diminished corneal reflex (V and VII)	91
Ipsilateral Horner's syndrome†	71-95
Ipsilateral face analgesia (V)	58-86
Nystagmus	57-100
Ipsilateral palate weakness (IX, X)	52-86
Ipsilateral facial weakness (VII)	36
Sensory	
Contralateral body analgesia	91
Coordination	
Ipsilateral limb ataxia	95
Gait ataxia	88

Data obtained from 160 patients from references 53 to 57.

*Results are overall mean frequency or, if statistically heterogeneous, the range of values.

†Strictly speaking, Horner's syndrome does not involve cranial nerves, although it is discovered during examination of the pupils and eyelids.

E. Cerebral hemispheric disease. Cerebral hemispheral disease may cause a dense sensory loss and hemiparesis identical to thalamic disease ("pseudothalamic syndrome"),[21] or the selective loss of cortical sensations in the distal parts of the extremities (see Cortical Sensations above).

REFERENCES

1. Inouye Y and Buchthal F. Segmental sensory innervation determined by potentials recorded from cervical spinal nerves, *Brain* 100:731-748, 1977.
2. Foester O. The dermatomes in man, *Brain* 56 part 1:1-39, 1933.
3. Finelli PF. Reflex hammer with built-in pin, *Neurology* 41:344, 1991.

4. DeMyer W. Pointers and pitfalls in the neurologic examination, *Semin Neurol* 18:161-168, 1998.

5. Loefvenberg J and Johansson RS. Regional differences and interindividual variability in sensitivity to vibration in the glabrous skin of the human hand, *Brain Res* 301:65-72, 1984.

6. Plumb CS and Meigs JW. Human vibration perception, *Arch Gen Psych* 4:611-614, 1961.

7. Fox JC and Klemperer WW. Vibratory sensibility: a quantitative study of its thresholds in nervous disorders, *Arch Neurol Psych* 48:612-645, 1942.

8. De Michele G and others. Influence of age, gender, height and education on vibration sense: a study by tuning fork in 192 normal subjects, *J Neurol Sci* 105:155-158, 1991.

9. Pearce JMS. Early days of the tuning fork, *J Neurol Neurosurg Psych* 65:728-733, 1998.

10. Dyck PJ and others. Clinical vs. quantitative evaluation of cutaneous sensation, *Arch Neurol* 33:651-655, 1976.

11. Gilliat RW and Sears TA. Sensory nerve action potentials in patients with peripheral nerve lesions, *J Neurol Neurosurg Psych* 21:109-118, 1958.

12. Rith-Najarian SJ, Stolusky T, and Gohdes DM. Identifying diabetic patients at high risk for lower-extremity amputation in a primary health care setting. A prospective evaluation of simple screening criteria, *Diabetes Care* 15:1386-1389, 1992.

13. Boyko EJ and others. A prospective study of risk factors for diabetic foot ulcer. The Seattle Diabetic Foot study, *Diabetes Care* 22:1036-1042, 1999.

14. Adler AI and others. Lower-extremity amputation in diabetes: the independent effects of peripheral vascular disease, sensory neuropathy, and foot ulcers, *Diabetes Care* 22:1029-1035, 1999.

15. Calne DB and Pallis CA. Vibratory sense: a critical review, *Brain* 89:723-746, 1966.

16. Renfrew S and Cavanagh D. The discrimination between pinching and pressing of the skin: the basis of a clinical test, *Brain* 77:305-313, 1954.

17. Soffin G, Feldman M, and Bender MB. Alterations of sensory levels in vascular lesions of lateral medulla, *Arch Neurol* 18:178-190, 1968.

18. Archer AG and others. The natural history of acute painful neuropathy in diabetes mellitus, *J Neurol Neurosurg Psych* 46:491-499, 1983.

19. McCloskey DI. Kinesthetic sensibility, *Physiol Rev* 58:763-820, 1978.

20. Bender MB, Stacy C, and Cohen J. Agraphesthesia: a disorder of directional cutaneous kinesthesia or a disorientation in cutaneous space, *J Neurol Sci* 53:531-555, 1982.

21. Bassetti C, Bogousslavsky J, and Regli F. Sensory syndromes in parietal stroke, *Neurology* 43:1942-1949, 1993.

22. Cohen LA. Analysis of position sense in human shoulders, *J Neurophysiol* 21:550-568, 1957.

23. Laidlaw RW and Hamilton MA. A study of thresholds in apperception of passive movement among normal control subjects, *Bull Neurol Inst NY* 6:268-273, 1937.

24. Laidlaw RW and Hamilton MA. The quantitative measurement of apperception of passive movement, *Bull Neurol Inst NY* 6:145-153, 1937.

25. Smith DL, Akhtar AJ, and Garraway WM. Proprioception and spatial neglect after stroke, *Age Ageing* 12:63-69, 1983.

26. Harati Y. Diabetic peripheral neuropathies, *Ann Intern Med* 107:546-559, 1987.

27. Gellman H and others. Carpal tunnel syndrome: an evaluation of the provocative diagnostic tests, *J Bone Joint Surg* 68A:735-737, 1986.

28. Buch-Jaeger N and Foucher G. Correlation of clinical signs with nerve conduction tests in the diagnosis of carpal tunnel syndrome, *J Hand Surg (Br)* 19B:720-724, 1994.

29. Dannenbaum RM and Jones LA. The assessment and treatment of patients who have sensory loss following cortical lesions, *J Hand Ther* 6:130-138, 1993.

30. Corkin S, Milner B, and Rasmussen T. Somatosensory thresholds: contrasting effects of postcentral-gyrus and posterior parietal-lobe excisions, *Arch Neurol* 23:41-58, 1970.

31. Schwartz AS and others. The asymmetric lateralization of tactile extinction in patients with unilateral cerebral dysfunction, *Brain* 102:669-684, 1979.

32. Holmes G. Disorders of sensation produced by cortical lesions, *Brain* 50:413-427, 1927.

33. Pause M and others. Sensorimotor disturbances in patients with lesions of the parietal cortex, *Brain* 112:1599-1625, 1989.

34. Derouesne C and others. Pure sensory stroke caused by a small cortical infarct in the middle cerebral artery territory, *Stroke* 15:660-662, 1984.

35. Kim JS. Pure sensory stroke: clinical-radiological correlates of 21 cases, *Stroke* 23:983-987, 1992.

36. Wolf JK. *Segmental neurology: a guide to the examination and interpretation of sensory and motor function,* Baltimore, 1981, University Park Press.

37. Keegan JJ and Garrett FD. The segmental distribution of the cutaneous nerves in the limbs of man, *Anat Rec* 102:409-437, 1948.

38. Young JH. The revision of the dermatomes, *Aust N Z J Surg* 18:171-186, 1949.

39. Maynard FM and others. International standards for neurological and functional classification of spinal cord injury, *Spinal Cord* 35:266-274, 1997.

40. Sonstein WJ and others. False localizing signs in upper cervical spinal cord compression, *Neurosurg* 38:445-449, 1996.

41. Jamieson DRS, Teasdale E, and Willison HJ. False localising signs in the spinal cord, *Br Med J* 312:243-244, 1996.

42. Barron KD and others. Experiences with metastatic neoplasms involving the spinal cord, *Neurology* 38:91-106, 1988.

43. Spillane JD. *The doctrine of the nerves: chapters in the history of neurology,* Oxford, 1981, Oxford University Press.

44. Marino RJ and others. Superiority of motor level over single neurological level in categorizing tetraplegia, *Paraplegia* 33:510-513, 1995.

45. Matsumoto S and others. A sensory level on the trunk in lower lateral brainstem lesions, *Neurology* 38:1515-1519, 1988.

46. Currier RD, Giles CL, and DeJong RN. Some comments on Wallenberg's lateral medullary syndrome, *Neurology* 11: 778-791, 1961.

47. Koehler PJ and Endtz LJ. The Brown-Sequard syndrome: true or false? *Arch Neurol* 43:921-924, 1986.

48. Waxman SG and Sabin TD. Diabetic truncal polyneuropathy, *Arch Neurol* 38:46-47, 1981.

49. Bourque PR and Dyck PJ. Selective calf weakness suggests intraspinal pathology, not peripheral neuropathy, *Arch Neurol* 47:79-80, 1990.

50. Silver JR and Buxton PH. Spinal stroke, *Brain* 97:539-550, 1974.

51. McIlroy WJ and Richardson JC. Syringomyelia: a clinical review of 75 cases, *Can Med Assoc J* 93:731-734, 1965.

52. Tashiro K and others. Syringomyelic syndrome: clinical features in 31 cases confirmed by CT myelography or magnetic resonance imaging, *J Neurol* 235:26-30, 1987.

53. Kim JS and others. Spectrum of lateral medullary syndrome: correlation between clinical findings and magnetic resonance imaging in 33 subjects, *Stroke* 25:1405-1410, 1994.

54. Norrving B and Cronqvist S. Lateral medullary infarction: prognosis in an unselected series, *Neurology* 41:244-248, 1991.

55. Peterman AF and Siekert RG. The lateral medullary (Wallenberg) syndrome: clinical features and prognosis, *Med Clin North Am* 44:887-895, 1960.

56. Sacco RL and others. Wallenberg's lateral medullary syndrome: clinical-magnetic resonance imaging correlations, *Arch Neurol* 50:609-614, 1993.

57. Fisher CM, Karnes WE, and Kubik CS. Lateral medullary infarction: the pattern of vascular occlusion, *J Neuropathol Exp Neurol* 20:323-379, 1961.

58. Barraquer-Bordas L and others. Thalamic hemorrhage. A study of 23 patients with diagnosis by computed tomography, *Stroke* 12:524-527, 1981.

59. Walshe TM, Davis KR, and Fisher CM. Thalamic hemorrhage: a computed tomographic-clinical correlation, *Neurology* 27:217-222, 1977.

CHAPTER 56

Examination of the Reflexes

Reflexes are involuntary contractions of muscles, induced by specific stimuli. In the neurologic examination, there are three types of reflexes: (1) muscle-stretch reflexes ("deep tendon" or "myotatic" reflexes), (2) cutaneous reflexes, and (3) primitive reflexes (or "release" reflexes). This chapter also discusses the Babinski response, which is an abnormal cutaneous reflex of the foot that appears in upper motor neuron disease.

REFLEX HAMMERS

I. TYPES OF REFLEX HAMMERS. Early in the history of reflex testing,[a] clinicians used various implements to elicit reflexes: The great British neurologist Gowers used the ulnar aspect of his hand or his rigid stethoscope. Other clinicians were less selective, using paper weights, laboratory stands, or even table lamps.[1-3] In the late 1800s and early 1900s, many different reflex hammers were produced, some of which remain popular today.

A. Taylor hammer (developed in 1888 by J.M. Taylor, personal assistant to S. Weir Mitchell at

---

[a] Reflex testing became common after Erb and Westphal simultaneously discovered the value of muscle stretch reflexes in 1875.

the Philadelphia Orthopedic Hospital and Infirmary for Nervous Disease). This hammer has a tomahawk-shaped soft rubber hammer with a broad edge for percussing most tendons and a rounded point for reaching the biceps tendon or percussing muscles directly. The original handle ended in an open loop; the pointed end was added about 1920 for use in eliciting cutaneous reflexes.[3]

B. **Queen Square hammer** (developed by a Miss Wintle, a head nurse at the National Hospital for Nervous Diseases at Queen's Square, London, who for years made hammers from ring pessaries, solid brass wheels, and bamboo rods to sell to resident medical officers). This hammer has a rubber-lined disc attached to the end of a long rod, like a wheel on an axle.[1]

C. **Babinski hammer** (or "Babinski/Rabiner" hammer). This hammer has a handle that can be removed and attached either perpendicular or parallel to the disc-shaped head. Babinski's name probably reflects marketing more that innovation.[3]

D. **Troemner hammer.** This hammer, the only one of the four that actually resembles a hammer, was made popular in this country by the Mayo Clinic, where the neurologist Woltman introduced it in 1927.[4]

II. **CLINICAL SIGNIFICANCE.** No study has demonstrated any hammer to be superior to another, and selection depends more on personal preference and tradition. The Taylor is popular in America, the Queen Square in England, and the Troemner in continental Europe.[5] Some models (e.g., Babinski hammer) have built-in pins, designed for testing pain sensation and cutaneous reflexes. Because these pins could transmit infections, however, they should not be used.[6]

MUSCLE STRETCH REFLEXES

I. DEFINITION. Muscle stretch reflexes are involuntary contractions of muscles induced by a brisk stretch of the muscle. Muscle stretch reflexes are usually named after the muscle being tested (Table 56-1), the one notable exception being the Achilles or ankle jerk. Although these reflexes are often called "deep tendon reflexes," this name is a misnomer because tendons have little to do with the response, other than being responsible for mechanically transmitting the sudden stretch from the reflex hammer to the muscle spindle. In addition, some muscles with stretch reflexes have no tendons (e.g., "jaw jerk" of the masseter muscle).

Most healthy persons have the muscle stretch reflexes listed in Table 56-1.

II. TECHNIQUE

A. Method. The usual stimulus is a sharp tap with the reflex hammer on the muscle's tendon, near where the tendon inserts distally on bone. The Achilles reflex also is elicited sometimes by the plantar strike method, in which the reflex hammer strikes the clinician's hand, which is resting on the ball of the foot. In clinical studies of the Achilles reflex, both the plantar strike and tendon strike methods are equivalent.[18,19]

B. Grading reflex amplitude. The most important observation during reflex examination is the reflex's amplitude. Unlike examination of

TABLE 56-1 Common muscle stretch reflexes

Name of Reflex	Peripheral Nerve	Spinal Level
Brachioradialis	Radial	C5-C6
Biceps	Musculocutaneous	C5-C6
Triceps	Radial	C7-C8
Quadriceps (patellar)	Femoral	L2-L4
Achilles (ankle)	Tibial	S1

Based on references 7 to 17.

motor strength, examination of reflexes lacks a single universally accepted grading system. Proposed schemes range from S. Weir Mitchell's original 4 grades[3] to the Mayo Clinic's 9 grades.[20] A 5-point grading system (i.e., grades 0 through 4), reproduced in Table 56-2, is recommended by the National Institute of Neurological Disorders and Stroke.[21]

C. Reinforcement: the Jendrassik maneuver.
According to the NINDS scale (see Table 56-2), grade 1 reflexes include reflexes brought out only during reinforcement, and grade 0 reflexes are those that are absent despite reinforcement. The most common method of reinforcing reflexes is the Jendrassik maneuver. In 1885, Erno Jendrassik reported that having the patient "hook together the flexed fingers of his right and left hands and pull them apart as strongly as possible" while the clinician taps on the tendon enhances the reflexes of normal patients.[1] Reflex enhancement with this maneuver persists as long as the patient is pulling apart the arms, up to 10 seconds in some studies.[22,23] In one study of normal elderly patients, the absent ankle jerk was made to appear 70% of the time using reinforcing maneuvers.[24]

TABLE 56-2 NINDS muscle stretch reflex scale

Grade	Finding
0	Reflex absent
1	Reflex small, less than normal; includes a trace response or a response brought out only with reinforcement
2	Reflex in lower half of normal range
3	Reflex in upper half of normal range
4	Reflex enhanced, more than normal; includes clonus if present, which optionally can be noted in an added verbal description of the reflex

NINDS, National Institute of Neurological Disorders and Stroke, from reference 21.

III. CLINICAL SIGNIFICANCE

A. **Amplitude of reflex.** The amplitude of muscle stretch reflexes depends on the integrity of the lower and upper motor neurons innervating the reflex (see Figure 54-1 in Chapter 54 for definition of lower and upper motor neurons). (1) The lower motor neurons of a reflex are its peripheral nerve (second column in Table 56-1) and its spinal segment (third column in Table 56-1): disease at either of these locations *reduces* or *abolishes* the relevant reflex. (2) The upper motor neurons are the descending corticospinal pathways innervating the reflex: disease anywhere along this pathway (e.g., cerebral hemisphere, brain stem) *exaggerates* the reflex. (3) Disease of the *spinal cord*, where both upper and lower motor neurons reside, abolishes the reflex *at* the level of the lesion (lower motor neuron response) and exaggerates all reflexes from spinal levels *below* the level of the lesion (upper motor neuron response).

Nonetheless, absent or exaggerated reflexes, by themselves, do not signify neurologic disease.[25-27] For example, 6% to 50% of elderly persons without neurologic disease lack the ankle jerk bilaterally, despite the Jendrassik maneuver,[24,28] and a small percentage of normal individuals have generalized hyperreflexia.[25-27,29] Instead, the absent or exaggerated reflex is significant only when it is associated with one of the following clinical settings:

1. **The absent reflex is associated with other findings of lower motor neuron disease (weakness, atrophy, fasciculations).**

2. **The exaggerated reflex is associated with other findings of upper motor neuron disease (i.e., weakness, spasticity, Babinski sign).**

3. **The reflex amplitude is asymmetric**, which suggests either lower motor neuron

disease of the side with the diminished reflex or upper motor neuron disease of the side with exaggerated reflex.

4. The reflex is unusually brisk compared with reflexes from a higher spinal level, which raises the possibility of spinal cord disease at some level of the spinal cord between the segments with diminished reflexes and those with exaggerated ones.

B. Localizing value of diminished reflexes. In patients with nerve complaints of the arm or leg suggesting disorders of the cervical or lumbosacral nerve roots, the diminished reflex has important localizing value that indicates a lesion of the reflex's respective spinal root (see Table 56-1). A diminished biceps or brachioradialis reflex indicates C6 radiculopathy (LR = 14.2),[15] a diminished triceps reflex indicates C7 or C8 radiculopathy (LR = 28.3),[15] and diminished quadriceps reflex indicates L3 or L4 radiculopathy (LR = 6.9).[b30] Although the unilaterally diminished ankle jerk is a common finding in patients with L5 or S1 radiculopathy (45% of patients), the finding does not reliably distinguish lesions of the S1 root (the traditional spinal segment of the gastrocnemius-soleus muscles) from the L5 root (see also Chapter 57).[30,31]

C. Additional findings in the hyperreflexic patient. The physical finding of hyperreflexia has generated more eponyms in physical diagnosis than any other physical finding,[c] even though the basic pathophysiology for all exaggerated reflexes is the same (i.e., loss of cortico-

---

[b] A diminished biceps or brachioradialis reflex argues for a C6 lesion because C5 radiculopathies are rare.[15] L3 and L4 radiculopathies are also rare.[30]

[c] *Dorland's Medical Dictionary* lists 115 neurologic reflexes, 46 having eponyms.[32]

spinal inhibition) and the reflexes differ only by which muscle is stretched and which method the clinician uses to stretch the muscle. Of the many findings that have been described in hyperreflexic patients, commonly recognized ones are finger flexion reflexes, jaw jerks, clonus, and "irradiating" reflexes.

1. **Finger flexion reflexes** (introduced by Hoffman about 1900). In a positive response, sudden stretching of the finger flexors causes the finger flexors to involuntarily contract (the finger flexion reflex, therefore, is no different from any other muscle stretch reflex). There are many ways to elicit this finding, each with its own eponym (e.g., Hoffman's sign, Finger Rossolimo sign, Troemner's sign, von Bechterew's reflex). One of these methods is described in Figure 56-1. Like other exaggerated reflexes, finger flexion reflexes by themselves have little diagnostic value (i.e., they are detectable in 3% of healthy college students),[29] and to be significant, they must accompany one of the settings described in Section A above.

2. **Jaw jerk** (originally described by Lewis in 1882).[33] In a positive response, sudden stretching of the masseter muscle causes reflex contraction, moving the jaw briskly upward. With the patient's jaw slightly open, the clinician can elicit the reflex by tapping with a reflex hammer directly on the chin or on a tongue blade resting on the lower teeth or tongue. An exaggerated jaw jerk, sometimes appearing with clonus (see below), implies bilateral disease above the level of the pons (e.g., pseudobulbar palsy).[25] In patients with spastic tetraparesis, for example, an exaggerated jaw jerk excludes cervical cord disease and points to pyramidal tract disease above the pons.

FIGURE 56-1 Finger flexion reflex. After positioning the patient's hand in the supinated position with fingers slightly flexed, the clinician places his own index and middle fingers across the tips of the patient's fingers and taps them with the reflex hammer. Reflex contraction of the patient's finger flexor muscles is a positive response.

3. Clonus. Clonus is a self-sustained, oscillating stretch reflex induced when the clinician briskly stretches a hyperreflexic muscle and then continues to apply stretching force to that muscle. Each time the muscle relaxes from the previous reflex contraction, the applied stretching force renews the reflex, setting up a rhythmic series of muscle contractions that continue as long as the tension is applied. These rhythmic oscillations ("clonus") are most easily elicited in the foot (usually with oscillations of 5 to 8 Hz), by briskly dorsiflexing the patient's ankle. Clonus also may be elicited in the quadriceps, finger flexors, jaw, and other muscles.

As expected mathematically, the frequency of clonus varies inversely with the length of the reflex path ($r = -0.80$, $p<.001$). Clonus of the wrist has a higher frequency than that of the ankle, simply because the nerves to the forearm are shorter than those to the calf.[34]

4. **"Irradiation" of reflexes.** In some hyperreflexic patients, the blow of the reflex hammer is conducted mechanically through bone and tissues, where it may stretch hyperexcitable muscles at distant sites, thus producing additional, unexpected movements (e.g., "crossed adductor reflex").[26,35] Also, if this distant irradiation of a reflex is combined with paralysis of the reflex of interest, paradoxical movements or "inverted" reflexes may appear.

   a. **Crossed adductor reflex.** Tapping on the medial femoral condyle, patella, or patellar tendon causes the contralateral adductor muscle to contract, moving the contralateral knee medially.[36]

   b. **Inverted supinator reflex** (the "supinator reflex" is the brachioradialis reflex). Introduced by Babinski in 1910, this sign indicates spinal cord disease at the C5-C6 level.[26,37,38] In a positive response, tapping on the brachioradialis muscle causes no flexion at the elbow but instead flexion of the fingers. The lesion at C5-C6 eliminates the brachioradialis reflex (lower motor neuron) but exaggerates all reflexes below that level (upper motor neuron), including the finger flexion reflexes (C8), which are stimulated by mechanical conduction of the blow on the brachioradialis.

   c. **Inverted knee jerk.**[39] The inverted knee jerk indicates spinal cord disease at the L2-L4 level. In the positive response, attempts to elicit the knee jerk instead cause paradoxical knee flexion. Its two components are denervation of L2-L4 (thus paralyzing the quadriceps jerk) and conduction of the blow to the muscle spindles of the hamstrings (innervated by the L5-S1 level and made hyperexcitable by the same lesion).

CUTANEOUS REFLEXES ("SUPERFICIAL" REFLEXES)

I. **DEFINITION.** Cutaneous reflexes are involuntary muscle contractions that follow stimulation of the skin surface by scratching, stroking, or pinching.

II. **SUPERFICIAL ABDOMINAL REFLEX (T6 TO T11)**

A. **Technique.** In the superficial abdominal reflexes, stroking the skin of the abdomen causes the underlying abdominal wall muscle to contract, sometimes pulling the umbilicus toward the stimulus. The clinician usually tests one abdominal quadrant at a time using a side-to-side motion with a wooden applicator stick or the pointed end of the reflex hammer handle. The abdominal reflexes appear just as often whether the direction is medial-to-lateral or lateral-to-medial.[40]

B. **Clinical significance.** According to traditional teachings, superficial abdominal reflexes disappear with both upper and lower motor neuron disease. Their clinical value is slight, however, because they are also absent in about 20% of normal individuals, more so in the elderly.[40,41] Moreover, the observation of asymmetric reflexes or ones preserved only in the upper quadrants, patterns traditionally associated with neurologic disease, also are common findings in healthy persons.[40-42]

III. BULBOCAVERNOSUS REFLEX (S2 TO S4)

A. Technique. After positioning the patient in the lithotomy position, sudden manual compression of the glans penis or clitoris causes reflex contraction of the bulbocavernosus muscle and external anal sphincter. The reflex is detected either by palpating the skin behind the scrotum (bulbocavernosus muscle) or, more commonly, placing the index finger in the anal canal (external anal sphincter). Other effective stimuli are percussing the suprapubic area[43] or pulling the retention balloon of an indwelling Foley catheter against the bladder neck.[44]

B. Clinical significance. The bulbocavernosus reflex is one of the few ways to test the conus medullaris (distal end of the spinal cord) and the S2-S4 pelvic nerves (the only other bedside test of this region is testing sensation in the perineal, or "saddle" area).[44-46] Therefore, this reflex is particularly important in patients with urinary retention, which may be caused by disease of the pelvic nerves or cauda equina. In one study of consecutive patients referred for urodynamic studies,[44] most of whom had difficulty with urination, an *absent* reflex predicted disease in the S2-S4 segments only modestly in women (LR = 2.7) but much better in men (LR = 13.0). The modest accuracy of the sign in women may reflect damage to the pudendal nerve from prior childbirth or pelvic surgery.[44] In this study, the *presence* of a bulbocavernosus reflex was unhelpful: although the positive response is expected in patients with urinary retention from common disorders like prostate hypertrophy, it also is commonly found in incomplete lesions of the sacral nerves.

In spinal cord injury above the S2-S4 level (i.e., upper motor neuron lesion in the nerves innervating the S2-S4 segment), the bulbocavernosus reflex also disappears, but only temporarily for a period of 1 to 6 weeks.[44]

BABINSKI RESPONSE

I. DEFINITION. The Babinski response is an abnormal cutaneous reflex found in upper motor neuron disease affecting the muscles of the foot. In these patients, scratching the sole of the patient's foot causes an upward movement of the great toe, instead of the normal downward movement (Figure 56-2). Much revered and much researched, this reflex was originally described by Babinski in 1896.[47] It goes by various names, including "Babinski response," "Babinski sign," "Babinski reflex," "upgoing toe," and "extensor response."

In some patients with bilateral corticospinal tract disease, scratching the foot may even cause the contralateral great toe to move upward, a response termed "crossed dorsiflexion" or "crossed extensor" response.[47]

II. PATHOGENESIS. In response to painful stimuli applied to the lower limbs, most mammals rapidly withdraw that limb by flexing the hips and knees and dorsiflexing the feet and toes. This primitive reflex, the "flexion response," also occurs in human infants until the age of 1 or 2 years, after which the developing pyramidal tracts cause two important changes: (1) the flexion response becomes less brisk, and (2) the toes no longer move upward, but instead move downward because of the interval development of a normal plantar cutaneous re-

FIGURE 56-2 Babinski response. Drawing of the normal plantar cutaneous reflex (*left*) and the Babinski response (*right*), adapted from photographs taken by Babinski himself in 1900.[47]

flex.[48] If pyramidal tract disease develops later in the person's life, the normal plantar cutaneous reflex disappears, and instead, painful stimulation of the foot causes the great toe to again move upward.

The use of the term "extensor response" to describe the Babinski response is unfortunate and confusing: even though anatomists have always named the upward movement "extension" (e.g., great toe "extensor" muscle), physiologists have named the same upward movement "flexion" (e.g., the primitive "flexion response" discussed above).

III. TECHNIQUE

A. Eliciting the response. Of the many ways to elicit this reflex, a slow (i.e., 5 to 6 second) hockey-stick stroke beginning the lateral plantar surface is best, using a wooden applicator stick, key, or pointed handle of the reflex hammer (Figure 56-2). This method is superior to other methods, including scratching the lateral sole, scratching below the lateral malleolus (Chaddock method), rubbing the anterior shin (Oppenheim method) or—the least effective stimulus—squeezing the calf (Gordon method).[49]

B. Interpreting the response. Helpful guidelines in assessing an equivocal toe response, based on careful electrodiagnostic studies and patient follow-up, are as follows: (1) The pathologic upgoing toe results from contraction of the extensor hallucis longus muscle, whose tendon is conspicuous under the skin on top of the great toe.[50,51] Movement of the toe per se is not critical and may be prevented by joint disease. Moreover, the toe may seem to be upgoing—without contraction of the extensor hallucis longus muscle—when the ankle dorsiflexes or when the toe returns from an initial downward movement. (2) Over 90% of the time, the foot with the pathologic upgoing toe is weak or has difficulty with fine motor movements. An excellent test of fine motor movement is rapid foot tapping against the examiner's hand: normal persons accomplish 20 to 40 taps per 10 seconds. (3) The pathologic upgoing toe coincides with a flexion response in the whole limb, which may be slight but is evident in the ipsilateral tensor fascia lata and hamstrings. (4) The pathologic upgoing toe is reproducible.[48,52,53]

As Babinski himself pointed out, fanning of the toes is a normal phenomenon and not part of the pathologic response.[47,48]

IV. CLINICAL SIGNIFICANCE

A. Associated conditions. The Babinski response is found in both destructive lesions of the pyramidal tracts (see Chapter 54) and in many metabolic disorders affecting these tracts, most of which are associated with altered mental status, such as seizures, meningitis, drug overdose, renal, and hepatic failure.[47]

B. False-negative response. Patients may have pyramidal tract disease yet lack the upgoing toe (i.e., false-negative response) because they have (1) spinal shock,[50] (2) a peroneal palsy denervating the muscles that dorsiflex the great toe (a common problem in bedridden patients due to pressure against the head of the fibula),[50] or (3) pyramidal tract disease sparing the muscles of the foot (e.g., upper motor neuron weakness is confined to the arm of that side).[54]

PRIMITIVE REFLEXES

I. DEFINITION. Primitive reflexes (or "release" reflexes) are a hodgepodge of reflexes that are normally present in infants but disappear during normal development of the central nervous system, only to reappear sometimes later in life when neurologic disease or aging removes (or "releases") the inhibiting influences of the central nervous system.[55] Among many primitive reflexes, the more common ones are the palmomental reflex, glabellar reflex, grasp reflex, snout reflex, and suck reflex.

II. TECHNIQUE

A. Palmomental reflex.
In this reflex, a key or other blunt object is used to apply an unpleasant stimulus to the patient's thenar eminence, stroking it briskly in a proximal to distal direction. A positive response is a brief contraction of the ipsilateral mentalis muscle, causing the ipsilateral lower lip to protrude, rise, or wrinkle.

The wrinkle response at the corner of the mouth is probably the beginnings of a wince that would develop with more painful stimuli.[56] Theoretically, the stimulus could be applied anywhere on the skin of the patient's body, and in fact, descriptions of similar response after stimulation of the patient's arm, chest, trunk, sole of the foot, and tongue have all appeared.[56] The most sensitive area, however, is the thenar eminence.[57]

Marinesco and Radovici discovered the palmomental reflex in 1920.[56]

B. Glabellar reflex.
The stimulus for the glabellar reflex is light taps with the finger or soft rubber reflex hammer, about two times per second, over the patient's glabella. Although most normal persons respond to this by blinking bilaterally, the blinking stops after the first few taps in normal individuals. Persistent blinking is a positive response, although there is no consensus whether habituation should be indefinite or just beyond a certain number of blinks (e.g., >4 successive blinks).

The glabellar reflex is sometimes called the "blink reflex" or "Myerson's reflex," although the original description was by Overend in 1896.[58]

C. Grasp reflex.
In the grasp reflex, the clinician places his index and middle fingers over the

thenar aspect of the patient's wrist and exerts pressure on the skin while withdrawing the fingers between the patient's thumb and index finger. In a positive response, the patient grasps the clinician's fingers, and the grasp progressively increases as the clinician attempts to withdraw.

III. CLINICAL SIGNIFICANCE

A. General comments. Primitive reflexes are common findings in frontal lobe disease,[59] Parkinson's disease,[60,61] dementias,[62-66] and advanced HIV infection.[67] Other than the grasp reflex (see below), the precise neuroanatomic cause of these reflexes is unknown.

B. Palmomental reflex. The palmomental reflex is bilateral 75% of the time and unilateral 25% of the time. The side of the reflex does not correlate with the side of the lesion.[68] In patients with Parkinson's disease, the palmomental reflex correlates with the degree of akinesia, and the reflex often disappears with the onset of levodopa-induced dyskinesias.[60]

C. Glabellar reflex. The afferent limb of the glabellar reflex is the trigeminal nerve, and the efferent limb is the facial nerve. Lesions of either nerve may interrupt the reflex (although in facial nerve palsy, the blinking continues on the sound side). This reflex is also a common finding in Parkinson's disease, and in these patients, the positive response may reverse after administration of levodopa.[61]

D. Grasp reflex. A positive grasp reflex is common in frontal lobe disease and, if both arms can be tested (i.e., no paralysis), the grasp reflex when present is usually bilateral.[59] In patients with dementia, the sign correlates with more severe cognitive and functional impairment and greater loss of pyramidal cells in the frontal lobe.[62,63,66] Among patients admitted to a neurologic ward, a positive grasp reflex (defined as no habituation with three successive strokes) predicted discrete lesions in the frontal lobe or deep nuclei and subcortical white matter with a sensitivity of 13%, specificity 99%, and positive LR of 20.2.[59]

E. **Primitive reflexes and normal aging.** The palmomental and glabellar reflexes, but not the grasp reflex, also are described to occur in normal persons, although the reported frequencies from different studies vary widely.[64,65,67,69] The reported frequency for the palmomental sign in normal persons varies from 3% to 70%; that for the glabellar sign, from 3 to 33%.[60,65,67,69-72] A few of these "normal" persons with primitive reflexes undoubtedly have subclinical disease, as indicated by lesions in the basal ganglia or subcortical white matter on MRI imaging.[70] Others, however, have no evidence of neurologic disease, although importantly, their findings differ from the pathologic response in two important ways: (1) the primitive reflex of patients without neurologic lesions is weak and fatigable, disappearing after the first few repetitive stimuli spaced evenly apart,[55] and (2) the primitive reflex of patients without neurologic lesions is an isolated finding. For example, less than 1% of normal persons have a positive palmomental reflex, if it is defined as persistence beyond 5 or more strokes of the thenar eminence.[57,60] And, even if the definition of a positive response includes fatigable primitive reflexes, less than 12% of normal persons have two primitive reflexes, and less than 2% have three or more primitive reflexes.[67,69,71,72]

REFERENCES

1. Schiller F. The reflex hammer: In memoriam Robert Wartenberg (1887-1956), *Med Hist* 11:75-85, 1967.

2. Tyler KL and McHenry LC. Fragments of neurological history: the knee jerk and other tendon reflexes, *Neurology* 33:609-610, 1983.

3. Lanska DJ. The history of reflex hammers, *Neurology* 39: 1542-1549, 1989.

4. Rooke ED. The Tromner hammer: a historical postscript, *Proc Mayo Clin* 35:355-356, 1960.

5. Pryse-Phillips W. *Companion to clinical neurology,* Boston, 1995, Little, Brown & Co.

6. Finelli PF. Reflex hammer with built-in pin, *Neurology* 41:344, 1991.

7. Nieuwenhuys R. Bolk's studies of segmental anatomy, *Acta Morphol Neerl Scand* 13:7-33, 1975.

8. Wolf JK. *Segmental neurology: a guide to the examination and interpretation of sensory and motor function,* Baltimore, 1981, University Park Press.

9. Brendler SJ. The human cervical myotomes: functional anatomy studied at operation, *J Neurosurg* 28:105-111, 1968.

10. Levin KH, Maggiano HJ, and Wilbourn AJ. Cervical radiculopathies: comparison of surgical and EMG localization of single-root lesions, *Neurology* 46:1022-1025, 1996.

11. Liguori R, Krarup C, and Trojaborg W. Determination of the segmental sensory and motor innervation of lumbosacral spinal nerves, *Brain* 115:915-934, 1992.

12. Thage O. The myotomes L2-S2 in man, *Acta Neurol Scand* 41(suppl 13):241-243, 1965.

13. Wilbourn AJ and Aminoff MJ. AAEM minimonograph 32: the electrodiagnostic examination in patients with radiculopathies, *Musc Nerv* 21:1612-1631, 1998.

14. Young JH. The revision of the dermatomes, *Aust N Z J Surg* 18:171-186, 1949.

15. Yoss RE and others. Significance of symptoms and signs in localization of involved root in cervical disk protrusion, *Neurology* 7:673-683, 1957.

16. Makin GJV, Brown WF, and Ebers GC. C7 radiculopathy: importance of scapular winging in clinical diagnosis, *J Neurol Neurosurg Psych* 49:640-644, 1986.

17. Medical Research Council. *Aids to the examination of the peripheral nervous system,* London, 1986, Bailliere Tindall.

18. Schwartz RS and others. A comparison of two methods of eliciting the ankle jerk, *Aust N Z J Med* 20:116-119, 1990.

19. O'Keeffe STO and others. A comparison of two techniques for ankle jerk assessment in elderly subjects, *Lancet* 344: 1619-1620, 1994.

20. Wiebers DO and others, editors. Members of the Mayo Clinic Department of Neurology. *Mayo Clinic examinations in neurology,* ed 7, St Louis, 1998, Mosby.

21. Hallett M. NINDS myotatic reflex scale, *Neurology* 43:2723, 1993.

22. Gassel MM and Diamantopoulos E. The Jendrassik Maneuver: I. The pattern of reinforcement of monosynaptic reflexes in normal subjects and patients with spasticity or rigidity, *Neurology* 14:555-560, 1964.

23. Kawamura T and Watanabe S. Timing as a prominent factor of the Jandrassik manoeuvre on the H reflex, *J Neurol Neurosurg Psych* 38:508-516, 1975.

24. Impallomeni M and others. The elderly and their ankle jerks, *Lancet* 1:670-672, 1984.

25. Wartenberg R. Studies in reflexes: history, physiology, synthesis and nomenclature I, *Arch Neurol Psych* 51:113-133, 1944.

26. Wartenberg R. Studies in reflexes: history, physiology, synthesis and nomenclature II, *Arch Neurol Psych* 52:341-358, 1944.

27. Wartenberg R. Studies in reflexes: history, physiology, synthesis and nomenclature III, *Arch Neurol Psych* 52:359-382, 1944.

28. Bowditch MG, Sanderson P, and Livesey JP. The significance of an absent ankle reflex, *J Bone Joint Surg (Br)* 78B:276-279, 1996.

29. Echols DH. The Hoffman sign: its incidence in university students, *J Nerv Ment Dis* 84:427-431, 1936.

30. Kortelainen P and others. Symptoms and signs of sciatica and their relation to the localization of the lumbar disc herniation, *Spine* 10:88-92, 1985.

31. Kerr RSC, Cadoux-Hudson TA, and Adams CBT. The value of accurate clinical assessment in the surgical management of the lumbar disc protrusion, *J Neurol Neurosurg Psych* 51:169-173, 1988.

32. Friel JP. *Dorland's illustrated medical dictionary,* ed 25, Philadelphia, 1974, WB Saunders.

33. Lanska DJ. Morris James Lewis (1852-1928) and the description of the jaw jerk, *J Child Neurol* 6:235-236, 1991.

34. Iansek R. The effects of reflex path length on clonus frequency in spastic muscles, *J Neurol Neurosurg Psych* 47:1122-1124, 1984.

35. Lance JW and DeGail P. Spread of phasic muscle reflexes in normal and spastic subjects, *J Neurol Neurosurg Psych* 28:328-334, 1965.

36. Teasdall RD and van den Ende H. The crossed adductor reflex in humans: an EMG study, *Can J Neurol Sci* 8:81-85, 1981.

37. Estanol BV and Marin OSM. Mechanism of the inverted supinator reflex: a clinical and neurophysiological study. *J Neurol Neurosurg Psych* 39:905-908, 1976.

38. Lance JW. Mechanism of the inverted supinator reflex, *J Neurol Neurosurg Psych* 40:207, 1977.

39. Boyle RS and others. Inverted knee jerk: a neglected localising sign in spinal cord disease, *J Neurol Neurosurg Psych* 42:1005-1007, 1979.

40. Babu K and others. Statistical approach to a neurological problem, *J Indian Med Assoc* 62:344-347, 358-359, 1974.

41. Madonick MJ. Statistical control studies in neurology: 8. The cutaneous abdominal reflex, *Neurology* 7:459-465, 1957.

42. Yngve D. Abdominal reflexes, *J Pediatr Ortho* 17:105-108, 1997.

43. Hargrove GK and Bors E. The suprapubic abdominal reflex: a useful method to assess the function of the sacral reflex arcs, *J Urol* 107:243-244, 1972.

44. Blaivas JG, Zayed AAH, and Labib KB. The bulbocavernosus reflex in urology: a prospective study of 299 patients, *J Urol* 126:197-199, 1981.

45. Bors E and Blinn KA. Bulbocavernosus reflex, *J Urol* 82:128-130, 1959.

46. Lapides J and Bobbitt JM. Diagnostic value of bulbocavernous reflex, *JAMA* 162:971-972, 1956.

47. Van Gijn J. *The Babinski sign: a centenary,* Utrecht, 1996, Universiteit Utrecht.

48. Van Gijn J. The Babinski reflex, *Postgrad Med J* 71:645-648, 1995.

49. Dohrman GJ and Nowace WJ. The upgoing great toe: optimal method of elicitation, *Lancet* 1:339-341, 1973.

50. Landau WM and Clare MH. The plantar reflex in man, with special reference to some conditions where the extensor response is unexpectedly absent, *Brain* 82:321-355, 1959.

51. Van Gijn J. Babinski response: stimulus and effector, *J Neurol Neurosurg Psych* 38:180-186, 1975.

52. Van Gijn J. The Babinski sign and the pyramidal syndrome, *J Neurol Neurosurg Psych* 41:865-873, 1978.

53. Van Gijn J. Equivocal plantar responses: a clinical and electromyographic study, *J Neurol Neurosurg Psych* 39:275-282, 1976.

54. Fulton JF and Keller AD. *The sign of Babinski: a study of the evolution of cortical dominance in primates,* Springfield, 1932, Charles C Thomas.

55. Vreeling FW and others. Primitive reflexes in healthy, adult volunteers and neurological patients: methodological issues, *J Neurol* 240:495-504, 1993.

56. Reis DJ and Sweden S. The palmomental reflex, *Arch Neurol* 4:486-498, 1961.

57. Marti-Vilalta JL and Graus F. The palmomental reflex: clinical study of 300 cases, *Eur Neurol* 23:12-16, 1984.

58. Fine EJ, Sentz L, and Soria E. The history of the blink reflex, *Neurology* 42:450-454, 1992.

59. De Renzi E and Barbieri C. The incidence of the grasp reflex following hemispheric lesion and its relation to frontal damage, *Brain* 115:293-313, 1992.

60. De Noordhout AM and Delwaide PJ. The palmomental reflex in Parkinson's disease: comparisons with normal subjects and clinical relevance, *Arch Neurol* 45:425-427, 1988.

61. Klawans HL and Goodwin JA. Reversal of the glabellar reflex in Parkinsonism, *J Neurol Neurosurg Psych* 32:423-427, 1969.

62. Forstl H and others. Neurologic signs in Alzheimer's disease: results of a prospective clinical and neuropathologic study, *Arch Neurol* 49:1038-1042, 1992.

63. Molloy DW and others. Clinical significance of primitive reflexes in Alzheimer's disease, *J Am Geriatr Soc* 39:1160-1163, 1991.

64. Vreeling FW and others. Primitive reflexes in Alzheimer's disease and vascular dementia, *J Geriatr Psych Neurol* 8:111-117, 1995.

65. Hogan DB and Ebly EM. Primitive reflexes and dementia: results from the Canadian study of health and aging, *Age Ageing* 24:375-381, 1995.

66. Burns A, Jacoby R, and Levy R. Neurological signs in Alzheimer's disease, *Age Ageing* 20:45-51, 1991.

67. Tremont-Lukats IW, Teixeira GM, and Hernandez DE. Primitive reflexes in a case-control study of patients with advanced human immunodeficiency virus type 1, *J Neurol* 246:540-543, 1999.

68. Whittle IR and Miller JD. Clinical usefulness of the palmomental reflex, *Med J Aust* 146:137-139, 1987.

69. Brown DL, Smith TL, and Knepper LE. Evaluation of five primitive reflexes in 240 young adults, *Neurology* 51:322, 1998.

70. Kobayashi S and others. Primitive reflexes and MRI findings, cerebral blood flow in normal elderly, *Gerontology* 36:199-205, 1990.
71. Isakov E and others. The diagnostic value of three common primitive reflexes, *Eur Neurol* 23:17-21, 1984.
72. Jacobs L and Gossman MD. Three primitive reflexes in normal adults, *Neurology* 30:184-188, 1980.

CHAPTER 57

Disorders of the Nerve Roots, Plexi, and Peripheral Nerves

I. **INTRODUCTION.** Nerve roots destined to innervate the limbs exit through vertebral foramina and intermingle in plexi (i.e., the brachial and lumbosacral plexi) before emerging as peripheral nerves that extend to the fingers and toes. Lesions anywhere along this pathway—from spinal nerve roots to the final peripheral nerve branch—produce combinations of pain, *lower* motor neuron weakness, and sensory loss.

A lesion in the nerve root is called **radiculopathy**; one in the plexus, **plexopathy**, and; one in the peripheral nerve, **peripheral neuropathy.** This chapter emphasizes how to distinguish these lesions in patients with nerve complaints of the arms or legs. Because the neuroanatomy of these lesions is complex, accurate diagnosis requires systematic examination of all the limb's muscles, sensation, and reflexes.

II. **THE ARM**

    A. **Introduction.** In patients presenting with upper extremity nerve complaints, the most common neurologic diagnosis is carpal tunnel syndrome, followed by polyneuropathy, ulnar neuropathy, and cervical radiculopathy.[1,2] Other focal neuropathies and plexopathies are less common. Most cervical radiculopathies affect the C7 root (70% of cases) or C6 root (20% to 25% of cases).[3,4]

B. Neurologic findings

1. Motor. Most muscles of the arm are innervated by nerves from more than one spinal segment. Table 57-1 presents the relationship between the different peripheral nerves (grouped in rows) and their corresponding spinal roots (in columns). The spinal levels listed in Table 57-1 are based on several lines of evidence, including Bolk's detailed dissection of a single human subject,[5,6] electrodiagnostic studies,[7,8] and bedside observations of patients with documented spinal root lesions.[4,9]

a. Radiculopathy. Even though most muscles receive innervation from more than one spinal nerve root, injury to one root is usually sufficient to cause significant loss of power. The motor examination of radiculopathy has two characteristics: (1) Weakness affects two or more muscles from the same spinal segment but different peripheral nerves (i.e., all of the weak muscles are in the same *column* in Table 57-1). For example, a C6 radiculopathy may simultaneously weaken elbow flexion (biceps muscle, musculocutaneous nerve) and wrist extension (radial and ulnar wrist extensors, radial nerve).[4] (2) Weakness may involve muscles innervated by "proximal nerves," which are listed in the top rows of Table 57-1. Proximal nerves originate from the nerve roots but then promptly innervate muscles of the shoulder, thus moving away from the course of the peripheral nerves of the arm. Therefore, if a muscle inner-

TABLE 57-1 Innervation of muscles of the arm*

SPINAL SEGMENTS	C5	C6	C7	C8	T1
Proximal Nerves					
Rhomboids (dorsal scapular nerve)	■				
Supraspinatus (suprascapular nerve)	■				
Infraspinatus (suprascapular nerve)	■				
Deltoid (axillary nerve)	■	▨			
Serratus anterior (long thoracic nerve)	▨	▨	■		
Musculocutaneous Nerve					
Biceps	■	■			
Radial Nerve					
Triceps		▨	■	▨	
Brachioradialis	■	▨			
Extensor carpi radialis longus	▨	■	▨		
Extensors carpi ulnaris			■	▨	
Finger extensors			■	■	
Median Nerve					
Pronator teres		■	■		
Flexor carpi radialis		▨	■		
Flexor digitorum superficialis			▨	■	▨
Abductor pollicis brevis				■	■
Ulnar Nerve					
Flexor carpi ulnaris			▨	■	
Hypothenar muscles				■	▨
Interossei				■	▨

*Table 57-1 indicates those spinal levels that usually (black shade) and sometimes (grey shade) contribute to the corresponding muscle; based on references 3 to 11.

vated by one of these nerves is weak in a patient with nerve complaints of the arm or hand, the lesion must be a proximal one near the nerve roots. A common example is the finding of scapular winging (i.e., weak serratus anterior muscle, long thoracic nerve) in a patient with arm pain and triceps weakness. Involvement of the serratus anterior points to the C7 root and away from the radial nerve or brachial plexus.[10]

b. Brachial plexopathy. Lesions of the brachial plexus cause simultaneous weakness of muscles from two or more adjacent spinal segments (i.e., adjacent *columns* in Table 57-1) and from two or more peripheral nerves. Brachial plexus lesions usually affect either the upper plexus (C5-C6) as a group, causing weakness of the shoulder and upper arm but sparing all muscles of the hand, or the lower plexus (C7-T1) as a group, affecting all muscles of the hand but sparing those of the shoulder and upper arm.

c. Peripheral nerve disorders. These lesions weaken two or more muscles from a *single* peripheral nerve (which may have different spinal segments) and spare muscles from other nerves. For example, a complete radial nerve injury weakens the brachioradialis muscle (C5-C6),[a] elbow extension (triceps, C7), wrist extension (wrist extensors, C6-C7), and finger extension (finger extensors, C8).

In Table 57-1, the muscles belonging to each peripheral nerve are listed in the order that their branches diverge from the main trunk. Therefore, a proximal lesion of the radial nerve in the axilla would cause the findings described in the previous paragraph, but a lesion of the radial nerve at the elbow, after the branch to the extensor carpi radialis longus, spares the triceps and brachioradialis but weakens

---

[a] Testing elbow flexion with the forearm midway between supination and pronation reveals brachioradialis weakness.[11]

FIGURE 57-1 "Claw hand" of ulnar nerve palsy. All metacarpopha-
langeal joints are extended because of paralysis of all interossei and
unopposed action of finger extensors (radial nerve). The hyperextension is less prominent in the index and middle fingers because the
lumbricals of these digits, innervated by the median nerve, act to flex
the joint. Tethering from the flexor tendons causes all interphalangeal
joints to flex.

more distal muscles (i.e., wrist and finger
extensors).

Some peripheral nerve lesions can be
recognized at a glance, such as the wrist
drop of radial neuropathy and the "claw
hand" appearance of ulnar neuropathy
(Figure 57-1). A callus over the hypothenar eminence in a patient with ulnar
muscle weakness suggests damage to the
deep branch of the ulnar nerve, caused by
chronic pressure on the heel of the hand
from bicycling or using a walker.[12,13]

2. **Sensory findings.** Radiculopathy causes
sensory loss in a dermatomal pattern (see
Table 55-1 and Figure 55-1 in Chapter 55).
Brachial plexus lesions cause sensory loss
from adjacent dermatomes. Peripheral nerve
lesions cause the sensory loss described in
Table 57-2 (in Table 57-2, the branches are

TABLE 57-2 Sensory branches of peripheral nerves of the arm

Nerve	Sensory branches
Musculocutaneous nerve	Radial aspect forearm
Radial nerve	Dorsal arm and forearm
	Radial aspect dorsal hand
Median nerve	Radial palm
	First three digits and radial aspect ring finger
Ulnar nerve	Ulnar aspect of hand and digits

listed in proximal to distal order; therefore, a proximal radial nerve lesion affects sensation of the posterior arm, forearm, *and* hand; one at the elbow affects only the dorsal hand).

One pure sensory syndrome of the arm is "cheiralgia paresthetica," from injury to the superficial branch of the radial nerve, usually because of too tight a wrist band or hand cuffs. Sensory findings are confined to the radial aspect of the dorsal hand.[14]

3. **Reflexes.** The three muscle stretch reflexes of the arm are the biceps (musculocutaneous nerve, C5-C6), brachioradialis (radial nerve, C5-C6), and triceps (radial nerve, C7-C8).[b] Therefore, the finding of abnormal reflexes *excludes* both median and ulnar neuropathies and instead *argues for* radiculopathy or plexopathy. Radial nerve lesions usually spare the brachioradialis and triceps reflex because the branches to these muscles diverge from the main trunk proximally in the axilla, and most injuries to this nerve occur at a more

---

[b] Even though weakness of the triceps may follow lesions in the C6 or C7 roots (C7 is most common; see Table 57-1), the absent triceps jerk usually results from C7 or C8 lesions.[4]

distal point (e.g., humeral fracture or "Saturday night palsy.")

4. **Provocative tests.** One traditional test for cervical radiculopathy, "Spurling's sign" or "the neck compression test," should *not* be performed. In this test, the clinician turns and tilts the patient's head and neck toward the painful side and then adds a compressive force to the top of the head.[15] Aggravation of pain is a positive response. The sensitivity of the sign in documented cervical disc disease is only 9% to 16%[16,17]; its specificity has never been tested; and in patients with rheumatoid arthritis, cervical malformations, or metastatic disease, the test risks serious injury to the spine.

"Tinel's" and "Phalen's" signs, used traditionally to diagnose carpal tunnel syndrome, are discussed below.

C. **Additional diagnostic clues**

1. **The clavicle.** The brachial plexus lies just behind the clavicle. Therefore, additional physical findings in the supraclavicular space, such as mass, adenopathy, hemorrhage, or other evidence of trauma, suggest injury to the brachial plexus. Trauma *above* the clavicle injures roots; that *below* the clavicle injures peripheral nerves.

2. **Horner's syndrome** (see Chapter 19). An associated Horner's syndrome (i.e., ipsilateral small pupil and ptosis) indicates radiculopathy (C8-T1) or a lesion of the lower brachial plexus.

D. **Clinical significance**

1. **Radiculopathy.** Table 57-3 presents the diagnostic accuracy of the motor, sensory, and reflex examination in cervical radiculopathy, illustrating the accuracy of findings in predicting the level of the lesion. With respect to the motor examination, each of the indicator muscles discussed in Chapter 54 (i.e., elbow

TABLE 57-3 Localizing cervical radiculopathy*

Finding[4]	Sensitivity (%)	Specificity (%)	Positive LR	Negative LR
Motor Examination				
Weak elbow flexion, detecting C5 radiculopathy	83	84	5.3	NS
Weak wrist extension, detecting C6 radiculopathy	37	84	2.3	NS
Weak elbow extension, detecting C7 radiculopathy	65	84	4.0	0.4
Weak finger flexion, detecting C8 radiculopathy	50	87	3.8	NS
Sensory Examination				
Sensory loss affecting thumb, detecting C6 radiculopathy	32	96	8.5	NS
Sensory loss affecting middle finger, detecting C7 radiculopathy	5	98	NS	NS
Sensory loss affecting little finger, detecting C8 radiculopathy	23	99	41.4	NS
Reflex Examination				
Diminished biceps or brachioradialis reflex, detecting C6 radiculopathy	53	96	14.2	0.5
Diminished triceps reflex, detecting C7 or C8 radiculopathy	64	98	28.3	0.4

NS, Not significant.

Diagnostic standard: For level of radiculopathy; surgical findings.

flexion for C5, wrist extension for C6, elbow extension for C7, and finger flexion for C8) accurately predicts the level involved (LRs = 2.3 to 5.3). The weaker a muscle is, the more significant is its localizing value.[4] The presence of normal triceps strength argues *against* a lesion at C7 (LR = 0.4). Sensory loss on the thumb argues for C6 radiculopathy (LR = 8.5) and sensory loss on the little finger argues for C8 radiculopathy (LR = 41.4). Because fewer than 1 in 3 patients with cervical radiculopathy have sensory loss, however, the finding of normal sensation is never a compelling argument against cervical radiculopathy. A diminished biceps or brachioradialis reflex accurately points to the C6 level (LR = 14.2) and a diminished triceps reflex accurately indicates the C7 or C8 level (LR = 28.3).

Importantly, the LRs in Table 57-3 apply only to patients with cervical radiculopathy. Patients with carpal tunnel syndrome also may develop hypesthesia of the thumb and those with ulnar neuropathy may develop hypesthesia of the little finger, although in these patients, the arm reflexes and arm and wrist strength are normal.

2. **Plexopathy in cancer patients.** If brachial plexopathy develops in a patient with cancer who has received radiation near the shoulder, the question arises whether the plexopathy is due to metastatic disease or radiation injury. Findings arguing for *metastatic* involvement are motor and sensory findings confined to C7-T1 (LR = 30.9) and Horner's syndrome (LR = 4.1). Findings arguing for *radiation* injury are motor and sensory findings confined to C5-C6 (LR = 8.8) and lymphedema of the ipsilateral arm (LR = 4.9).[18]

3. **Peripheral nerve injury: diagnosis of carpal tunnel syndrome.** Table 57-4 summarizes the diagnostic accuracy of findings for the most common peripheral neuropathy of the arm, carpal tunnel syndrome. According to Table 57-4, two findings argue *for* carpal tunnel syndrome: a "classic" or "probable" hand diagram (LR = 2.4)[c] and diminished pain sensation in the distribution of the median nerve (LR = 3.1). The most compelling finding arguing *against* carpal tunnel syndrome is an "unlikely" hand diagram (LR = 0.2). Several traditional tests, such as Tinel's and Phalen's sign (defined in Table 57-4), do not help distinguish carpal tunnel syndrome from the electrodiagnosis of other common disorders causing hand dysesthesias (such as polyneuropathy, ulnar neuropathy, or radiculopathy).[1,28]

III. THE LEG

A. **Introduction.** Among patients presenting with lower extremity nerve complaints, the most common neurologic diagnosis is by far lumbosacral radiculopathy, which almost always affects the L5 or S1 roots (each are affected with about the same frequency).[3,30-34]

B. **Neurologic findings**
   1. **Motor.** Table 57-5 presents the innervation of the muscles of the leg, showing the rela-

---

[c] The Katz hand diagram is a self-administered diagram of the hand that depicts the patient's symptoms: the "classic" pattern depicts symptoms affecting at least 2 of digits 1, 2, or 3 but sparing the palm and dorsum of the hand; the "probable" pattern is similar to the classic pattern, although palm symptoms are allowed; the "unlikely" pattern depicts symptoms not involving digits 1, 2, or 3.[19] Palm symptoms are not part of the "classic" pattern because the palmar cutaneous branch of the median nerve does not travel through the carpal tunnel.[29]

TABLE 57-4 Diagnosing carpal tunnel syndrome*

FINDING (REF)†	SENSITIVITY (%)	SPECIFICITY (%)	POSITIVE LR	NEGATIVE LR
Hand Diagram				
"Classic" or "probable"[19]	64	73	2.4	0.5
"Unlikely"[19]	4	—	0.2	—
Motor Examination				
Weak thumb abduction[20,21]	63-66	62-66	1.8	0.5
Thenar atrophy[20,22,23]	4-28	82-99	NS	NS
Sensory Examination (median distribution)				
Hypalgesia[21,22]	15-51	85-93	3.1	NS
Abnormal 2-point discrimination[20,23,24]	6-32	64-99	NS	NS
Abnormal vibration sensation[20,24]	20-61	71-81	NS	NS
Other Tests				
Tinel's sign[20-25]	23-60	64-87	NS	NS
Phalen's sign[20-27]	10-91	33-86	1.3	0.7

NS, Not significant.

*Diagnostic standard: For *carpal tunnel syndrome,* abnormal motor or sensory conduction within the carpal tunnel, measured by nerve conduction testing.

†Definition of findings: For *hand diagram,* see text; for all *sensory findings,* perception diminished in index finger compared with ipsilateral little finger (*2-point discrimination* used compass points separated by 4 to 6 mm, *vibratory sensation* used 126 or 256 Hz tuning fork); for *Tinel's sign,* paresthesias in distribution of median nerve when clinician taps on the distal wrist crease over the median nerve; and for *Phalen's sign,* paresthesias in the distribution of the median nerve when the patient flexes both wrists 90 degrees for 60 seconds.[28]

TABLE 57-5 Innervation of the muscles of the leg*

Spinal Segments	L2	L3	L4	L5	S1	S2
Proximal Nerves						
Gluteus medius (gluteal nerves; internal rotation and abduction of hip)			■	■	▨	
Gluteus maximus (gluteal nerves; extension of hip)				■	■	▨
Femoral Nerve						
Iliopsoas	■	▨				
Quadriceps	▨	■	■			
Obturator nerve						
Thigh adductors	■	■	▨			
Sciatic Nerve Trunk†						
Hamstrings (knee flexion)				■	■	
Peroneal Nerve†						
Tibialis anterior (dorsiflexion of ankle)			■	■		
Extensors of toes				■	▨	
Peroneus longus (eversion of ankle)				■	■	
Tibial Nerve†						
Tibialis posterior (inversion of ankle)			■	■		
Gastrocnemius				▨	■	▨
Flexor digitorum (curl toes)					■	■

*Table 57-5 indicates those spinal levels that usually (black shade) and sometimes (grey shade) contribute to the corresponding muscle; based on references 3, 5, 6, 9, 11, 35, and 36.

†The sciatic nerve trunk divides above the knee into the peroneal and tibial nerves. Therefore, lesions of the sciatic nerve trunk affect muscles of all three branches (see text).

tionship between different spinal roots (in columns) and the different peripheral nerves (grouped in rows).

a. Radiculopathy. Like radiculopathy of the arm, radiculopathy of the leg has two characteristics: (1) Weakness affects 2 or more muscles from the same spinal segment but different peripheral nerves (i.e., all muscles innervated by same *column* in Table 57-5). For example, an L5 radiculopathy may affect both the dorsiflexors of the foot and toes (peroneal nerve) and inversion of the foot (tibial nerve). (2) Weakness may involve "proximal nerves" to the glutei muscles (which cause characteristic abnormalities of the gait; see Chapter 5).

b. **Lumbosacral plexopathy.** Unlike brachial plexus lesions, lumbosacral plexopathies tend to affect the entire leg (L2-S1) simultaneously, and discrete upper and lower plexus syndromes are rare.[37,38]

c. **Peripheral nerve disorders.** Peripheral nerve lesions weaken 2 or more muscles from a *single* peripheral nerve (which may belong to different spinal segments) and spare muscles from other nerves. For example, over 85% of patients with foot drop due to peroneal nerve injury have weak ankle dorsiflexion (L4-L5) and eversion (L5-S1) but preservation of inversion (i.e., foot inversion has the same spinal segments but a different nerve, the tibial nerve).[39]

The sciatic trunk divides into the peroneal and tibial nerves just above the knee. Therefore, lesions of the sciatic trunk may affect any of the muscles listed under "sciatic trunk," "peroneal nerve," and "tibial nerve" in Table 57-5. Most patients with sciatic neuropathy have greater peroneal involvement (75% of patients) or equal involvement of the peroneal and tibial divisions (20% of patients) A sciatic neuropathy with greater involvement of the tibial nerve muscles is uncommon.[40]

The finding of weakness predominantly of the proximal leg muscles argues against sciatic, peroneal, or tibial neuropathy because all of these nerves innervate muscles below the knee. Therefore, proximal weakness suggests femoral or obturator neuropathy; lumbosacral plexopathy or radiculopathy; or, if sensory findings are absent, muscle disease.

2. **Sensory findings.** Radiculopathy causes sensory loss in a dermatomal pattern (see Table 55-1 and Figure 55-1 in Chapter 55), peripheral nerve lesions cause the sensory loss described in Table 57-6, and lumbosacral plexopathies tend to affect the entire leg.

A pure sensory syndrome is "meralgia paresthetica," which consists of hypesthesia of the anterior and lateral thigh, usually caused by mechanical compression of the lateral femoral cutaneous nerve (e.g., obesity, pregnancy, or carpenter's belts).[41]

3. **Reflexes.** The two muscle stretch reflexes of the leg are the quadriceps reflex (femoral nerve, L2-L4) and Achilles reflex (tibial nerve, S1). The peroneal nerve does not contribute to the Achilles reflex. Consequently, in patients with foot drop, the finding of an

TABLE 57-6 Sensory branches of peripheral nerves of the leg

NERVE	SENSORY BRANCHES
Femoral nerve	Anterior thigh
	Medial calf
Obturator nerve	Medial thigh
Sciatic nerve trunk*	Posterior thigh
Peroneal nerve*	Lateral calf and dorsal foot
Tibial nerve*	Sole of foot

*The sciatic nerve trunk divides above the knee into the peroneal and tibial nerves. Therefore, lesions of the sciatic nerve trunk affect sensation from all three branches.

asymmetrically diminished or absent ankle jerk argues *against* peroneal palsy and *for* sciatic neuropathy (87% have abnormal ankle jerk)[40] or lumbosacral radiculopathy (45% have abnormal ankle jerk).[9,30,34]

4. **Provocative tests.** The "straight-leg raising" test is a traditional maneuver used to diagnose lumbosacral radiculopathy, which is usually caused by disc herniation. In the maneuver, the clinician lifts the extended leg of the supine patient, flexing the leg at the hip. In a positive response, the patient develops pain down the ipsilateral leg (if pain develops just in the hip or back, the test is considered negative). The "crossed straight-leg raising" maneuver consists of pain in the affected leg when the clinician lifts the contralateral healthy limb. The pathogenesis of the sign is believed to be stretching of the sciatic nerve and its nerve roots.[42]

A positive straight-leg raising test is sometimes called "Lasègue's sign," after the French clinician Charles Lasègue (1816 to 1883), although Lasègue never published a description of the sign. His student Forst described the maneuver in his 1881 doctoral thesis, crediting Lasègue. An earlier description of the sign was published by Yugoslavian physician Lazarevic, in 1880.[43-45]

C. Clinical significance

1. **Lumbosacral radiculopathy.** Tables 57-7 and 57-8 review the diagnostic accuracy of the bedside examination in patients with nerve pain of one leg (i.e., "sciatica"). Table 57-7 applies to all patients with sciatica. Table 57-8 applies only to patients with known lumbosacral radiculopathy and addresses how accurately findings localize the level of the lesion.

In patients with sciatica, the findings arguing *for* disc herniation and lumbosacral

TABLE 57-7 Lumbosacral radiculopathy, in patients with sciatica*

Finding[†]	Sensitivity (%)	Specificity (%)	Positive LR	Negative LR
Motor Examination				
Weak ankle dorsiflexion[34]	54	89	4.9	0.5
Ipsilateral calf wasting[34]	29	94	5.2	0.8
Sensory Examination				
Leg sensation abnormal[34]	16	86	NS	NS
Reflex Examination				
Abnormal ankle jerk[34]	48	89	4.3	0.6
Other Tests				
Straight-leg raising maneuver[31,34,46,47]	73-98	11-61	NS	0.2
Crossed straight-leg raising maneuver[34,46-48]	23-43	88-98	4.3	0.8

NS, Not significant.

Diagnostic standard: For *lumbosacral radiculopathy,* surgical finding of disc herniation compressing nerve root.

†*Definition of findings:* For *ipsilateral calf wasting,* maximum calf circumference at least 1 cm smaller than contralateral side[34]; for *straight-leg raising maneuvers,* flexion at hip of supine patient's leg, extended at the knee, causes radiating pain in affected leg (pain confined to back or hip is negative response); for *crossed straight-leg raising maneuver,* raising contralateral leg provokes pain in affected leg.

TABLE 57-8 Localizing lumbosacral radiculopathy*

Finding[†]	Sensitivity (%)	Specificity (%)	Positive LR	Negative LR
Motor Examination				
Weak hallux extension, detecting L5 radiculopathy[30,34]	12-51	72-91	1.8	NS
Weak ankle plantarflexion, detecting S1 radiculopathy[34]	26	99	26.6	0.7
Ipsilateral calf wasting, detecting S1 radiculopathy[34]	43	82	2.4	0.7
Sensory Examination				
Sensory loss L5 distribution, detecting L5 radiculopathy[30,34]	20-28	94-98	4.6	0.8
Sensory loss S1 distribution, detecting S1 radiculopathy[30,34]	32-49	86-90	3.0	NS
Reflex Examination				
Asymmetric quadriceps reflex, detecting L3 or L4 radiculopathy[30]	30	96	6.9	NS
Asymmetric Achilles reflex, detecting S1 radiculopathy[30,34]	63-91	69-94	NS	NS

NS, Not significant.

*Diagnostic standard: For level of radiculopathy, surgical findings or myelography.

†Definition of findings: For ipsilateral calf wasting, maximum calf circumference at least 1 cm smaller than contralateral side.[34]

radiculopathy[d] are calf wasting (LR = 5.2), weak ankle dorsiflexion (LR = 4.9), the absent ankle jerk (LR = 4.3), and the *crossed* straight-leg raising maneuver (LR = 4.3). A *negative* straight-leg raising maneuver argues *against* disc herniation (LR = 0.2).

In patients with sciatica and lumbosacral radiculopathy (see Table 57-8), the abnormal quadriceps reflex accurately predicts radiculopathy at the L3 or L4 level (LR = 6.9). The best test for L5 radiculopathy is an L5 sensory loss (dorsum of the foot; LR = 4.6), weak hallux extension being only a weak predictor (LR = 1.8). The best predictors for the S1 level are weak ankle plantarflexion (LR = 26.6), sensory loss in the S1 distribution (lateral heel, LR = 3.0), and ipsilateral calf wasting (LR = 2.4). The absent Achilles reflex does not reliably indicate the level of the lesion.

2. **Lumbosacral plexopathy**
   a. **Cancer patients.** In patients with known cancer and prior pelvic irradiation who present with lumbosacral plexopathy, findings confined to one leg argue for *recurrent tumor* (LR = 4.5) whereas findings in both legs argue for *radiation plexopathy* (LR = 7.5).[37]
   b. **Diabetic amyotrophy.**[49-53] Diabetic amyotrophy (or "diabetic proximal neuropathy") is a lumbosacral plexopathy of diabetic patients with presenting symptoms of weak thigh muscles and severe pain in the thighs or back, or both. The quadriceps, adductor, and iliopsoas muscles are weak 100% of the time, and the glutei and hamstrings 50% of the time (all are proximal muscles). The weakness may

---

[d] An L4-L5 disc compresses the L5 root and an L5-S1 disc compresses the S1 root.

be unilateral or bilateral, but it is always asymmetric. Sensation is normal (70% of the time) or diminished over the thigh (30% of the time). The quadriceps reflex is absent in 80% of patients.

Although patients with diabetes also develop femoral neuropathy,[54] femoral neuropathy affects only thigh flexion and knee extension and spares other proximal leg muscles.

REFERENCES

1. Haig AJ, Tzeng HM, and LeBreck D. The value of electrodiagnosis consultation for patients with upper extremity nerve complaints: a prospective comparison with the history and physical examination, *Arch Phys Med Rehabil* 80:1273-1281, 1999.

2. Kothari MJ and others. Electrodiagnostic studies: are they useful in clinical practice, *Arch Phys Med Rehabil* 79:1510-1511, 1998.

3. Wilbourn AJ and Aminoff MJ. AAEM minimonograph 32: the electrodiagnostic examination in patients with radiculopathies, *Musc Nerv* 21:1612-1631, 1998.

4. Yoss RE and others. Significance of symptoms and signs in localization of involved root in cervical disk protrusion, *Neurology* 7:673-683, 1957.

5. Nieuwenhuys R. Bolk's studies of segmental anatomy, *Acta Morphol Neerl Scand* 13:7-33, 1975.

6. Wolf JK. *Segmental neurology: a guide to the examination and interpretation of sensory and motor function,* Baltimore, 1981, University Park Press.

7. Brendler SJ. The human cervical myotomes: functional anatomy studied at operation, *J Neurosurg* 28:105-111, 1968.

8. Levin KH, Maggiano HJ, and Wilbourn AJ. Cervical radiculopathies: comparison of surgical and EMG localization of single-root lesions, *Neurology* 46:1022-1025, 1996.

9. Young JH. The revision of the dermatomes, *Aust N Z J Surg* 18:171-186, 1949.

10. Makin GJV, Brown WF, and Ebers GC. C7 radiculopathy: importance of scapular winging in clinical diagnosis, *J Neurol Neurosurg Psych* 49:640-644, 1986.

11. Medical Research Council. *Aids to the examination of the peripheral nervous system,* London, 1986, Bailliere Tindall.

12. Reid RI and Ashby MA. Ulnar nerve palsy and walking frames, *Br Med J* 285:778, 1982.

13. Maimaris C and Zadeh HG. Ulnar nerve compression in the cyclist's hand: two case reports and review of the literature, *Br J Sports Med* 24:245-246, 1990.

14. Massey EW and Pleet AB. Handcuffs and cheiralgia paresthetica, *Neurology* 28:1312-1313, 1978.

15. Spurling RG and Scoville WB. Lateral rupture of the cervical intervertebral discs: A common cause of shoulder and arm pain, *Surg Gynecol Obstet* 78:350-358, 1944.

16. Viikari-Juntura E, Porras M, and Laasonen EM. Validity of clinical tests in the diagnosis of root compression in cervical disc disease, *Spine* 14:253-257, 1989.

17. Lunsford LD and others. Anterior surgery for cervical disc disease. Part 1: Treatment of lateral cervical disc herniation in 253 cases, *J Neurosurg* 53:1-11, 1980.

18. Kori SH, Foley KM, and Posner JB. Brachial plexus lesions in patients with cancer: 100 cases, *Neurology* 31:45-50, 1981.

19. Katz JN and others. A self-administered hand symptom diagram in the diagnosis and epidemiologic study of carpal tunnel syndrome, *J Rheumatol* 17:1495-1498, 1990.

20. Gerr F and others. Sensitivity and specificity of vibrometry for detection of carpal tunnel syndrome, *J Occup Environ Med* 37:1108-1115, 1995.

21. Kuhlman KA and Hennessey WJ. Sensitivity and specificity of carpal tunnel syndrome signs, *Am J Phys Med Rehabil* 76:451-457, 1997.

22. Golding DH, Rose DM, and Selvarajah K. Clinical tests for carpal tunnel syndrome: an evaluation, *Br J Rheumatol* 25:388-390, 1986.

23. Katz JN and others. Carpal tunnel syndrome: diagnostic utility of history and physical examination findings, *Ann Intern Med* 112:321-327, 1990.

24. Buch-Jaeger N and Foucher G. Correlation of clinical signs with nerve conduction tests in the diagnosis of carpal tunnel syndrome, *J Hand Surg (Br)* 19B:720-724, 1994.

25. Heller L and others. Evaluation of Tinel's and Phalen's signs in the diagnosis of the carpal tunnel syndrome, *Eur Neurol* 25:40-42, 1986.

26. Burke DT and others. Subjective swelling: a new sign for carpal tunnel syndrome, *Am J Phys Med Rehabil* 78:504-508, 1999.

27. DeSmet L and others. Value of clinical provocative tests in carpal tunnel syndrome, *Acta Orthop Belg* 61:177-182, 1995.

28. D'Arcy C and McGee S. Does this patient have carpal tunnel syndrome? *JAMA* 283:3110-3117, 2000.

29. Lum PB and Kanaklamedala R. Conduction of the palmar cutaneous branch of the median nerve, *Arch Phys Med Rehabil* 67:805-806, 1986.

30. Kortelainen P and others. Symptoms and signs of sciatica and their relation to the localization of the lumbar disc herniation, *Spine* 10:88-92, 1985.

31. Kosteljanetz M and others. Predictive value of clinical and surgical findings in patients with lumbago-sciatica: a prospective study (Part 1), *Acta Neurochirurgica* 73:67-76, 1984.

32. Jonsson B and Stromqvist B. Symptoms and signs in degeneration of the lumbar spine: a prospective, consecutive study of 300 operated patients, *J Bone Joint Surg (Br)* 75-B:381-385, 1993.

33. Supik LF and Broom MJ. Sciatic tension signs and lumbar disc herniation, *Spine* 19:1066-1069, 1994.

34. Kerr RSC, Cadoux-Hudson TA, and Adams CBT. The value of accurate clinical assessment in the surgical management of the lumbar disc protrusion, *J Neurol Neurosurg Psych* 51:169-173, 1988.

35. Liguori R, Krarup C, and Trojaborg W. Determination of the segmental sensory and motor innervation of lumbosacral spinal nerves, *Brain* 115:915-934, 1992.

36. Thage O. The myotomes L2-S2 in man, *Acta Neurol Scand* 41(suppl 13):241-243, 1965.

37. Thomas JE, Cascino TL, and Earle JD. Differential diagnosis between radiation and tumor plexopathy of the pelvis, *Neurology* 35:1-7, 1985.

38. Pettigrew LC and others. Diagnosis and treatment of lumbosacral plexopathies in patients with cancer, *Arch Neurol* 41:1282-1285, 1984.

39. Katirji MB and Wilbourn AJ. Common peroneal mononeuropathy: a clinical and electrophysiologic study of 116 lesions, *Neurology* 38:1723-1728, 1988.

40. Yuen EC, Olney RK, and So YT. Sciatic neuropathy: clinical and prognostic features in 73 patients, *Neurology* 44:1669-1674, 1994.

41. Massey EW. Sensory mononeuropathies, *Semin Neurol* 18:177-183, 1998.

42. Goddard MD and Reid JD. Movements induced by straight leg raising in the lumbo-sacral roots, nerves and plexus, and in the intrapelvic section of the sciatic nerve, *J Neurol Neurosurg Psych* 28:12-18, 1965.

43. Pearce JMS. Lasegue's sign, *Lancet* 1:436, 1989.

44. Sugar O. Charles Lasegue and his 'considerations on sciatica,' *JAMA* 253:1767-1788, 1985.

45. Dyck P. Lumbar nerve root: the enigmatic eponyms, *Spine* 9:3-5, 1984.

46. Kosteljanetz M, Bang F, and Schmidt-Olsen S. The clinical significance of straight-leg raising (Lasegue's sign) in the diagnosis of prolapsed lumbar disc: interobserver variation and correlation with surgical findings, *Spine* 13:393-395, 1988.

47. Spangfort EV. The lumbar disc herniation: a computer-aided analysis of 2504 operations, *Acta Orthop Scand* (suppl) 142:1-95, 1972.

48. Hudgins WB. The crossed straight leg raising test: a diagnostic sign of herniated disc, *J Occup Med* 21:407-408, 1979.

49. Subramony SH and Wilbourn AJ. Diabetic proximal neuropathy: clinical and electromyographic studies, *J Neurol Sci* 53:293-304, 1982.

50. Bastron JA and Thomas JE. Diabetic polyradiculopathy: clinical and electromyographic findings in 105 patients, *Mayo Clin Proc* 56:725-732, 1981.

51. Chokroverty S and others. The syndrome of diabetic amyotrophy, *Ann Neurol* 2:181-194, 1977.

52. Asbury AK. Proximal diabetic neuropathy, *Ann Neurol* 2:179-180, 1977.

53. Sander HW and Chokroverty S. Diabetic amyotrophy: current concepts, *Semin Neurol* 16:173-178, 1996.

54. Fraser DM and others. Mononeuropathy in diabetes mellitus, *Diabetes* 28:96-101, 1979.

CHAPTER 58

Coordination and Cerebellar Testing

I. **INTRODUCTION.** In the 1920s, after closely observing patients with cerebellar tumors and World War I soldiers with gunshot wounds to the posterior fossa, the British neurologist Gordon Holmes concluded that the following four physical signs were fundamental to cerebellar disease: ataxia, nystagmus, hypotonia, and dysarthria.[1-4]

II. **THE FINDINGS**

   A. **Ataxia.** Ataxia refers to incoordinated voluntary movements that lack the speed, smoothness, and appropriate direction seen in normal persons. Because the cerebellum's role is to organize and administer movement, testing for ataxia is only possible in patients with adequate motor strength (i.e., 4 or 5 on the MRC scale; see Chapter 54). Tests of ataxia include observation of the patient's gait (see Chapter 5), the finger-nose-finger test, heel-knee-shin test, and rapid alternating movements.

      1. **Finger-nose-finger test.** In this test, the seated patient takes the index finger of his outstretched hand and alternately touches his own nose and the clinician's index finger being held a couple of feet away. The patient with cerebellar disease may misjudge the

range of movement (i.e., **dysmetria**), over-shooting the target (i.e., **hypermetria**, as in missing the nose and slapping the hand into his own face) or undershooting the target (i.e., **hypometria**, as in stopping before reaching the clinician's finger). The patient's finger also may deviate from a smooth course, especially if clinician shifts the target during the test. As the patient's finger approaches the target, an increasing side-to-side tremor may appear (i.e., **intention tremor** or "kinetic tremor").

2. **Heel-knee-shin test.** In this test, the supine patient places the heel of one leg on the opposite knee and then slides it down the shin. Like the finger-to-nose test, a positive response may reveal any combination of ataxia, dysmetria, and intention tremor.

   Decomposition of movement denotes an abnormal sequence of actions. For example, during the heel-knee-shin test, the patient may completely flex the hip before beginning to bend the knee, thus lifting the heel abnormally high in the air before lowering to complete the movement.[2]

3. **Rapid alternating movements.** Difficulty with rapid alternating movements is called **dysdiadochokinesia** (Babinski coined the original term "adiadochokinesis").[3] The usual test is rapid pronation and supination of the forearm, but other tasks such as clapping hands, tapping a table, or stamping the foot are just as adequate.[3] In all these tests, the movements of patients with cerebellar disease are slower and significantly more irregular in rhythm, range, and accuracy.

B. **Nystagmus**

1. **Definition.** Nystagmus is an involuntary to-and-fro oscillation of the eyes. Nystagmus may be congenital or acquired, and the movements may affect both eyes ("bilat-

eral") or just one ("unilateral"). Bilateral nystagmus may be "conjugate," which means both eyes have identical movements, or "dissociated," which implies separate movements. Nystagmus may be "pendular," which means the to-and-fro movements have the same velocity, or "rhythmic," which means the movement is slow in one direction and quick in the other (rhythmic nystagmus is usually called "jerk nystagmus"). Jerk nystagmus is named after the direction of the quick component (e.g., a right conjugate jerk nystagmus). Finally, the direction of the nystagmus may be horizontal, vertical, or rotatory.

2. **Patterns of nystagmus.** Although nystagmus is a complicated subject that sometimes defies general principles,[a] several well-recognized patterns are described below.

   a. **Cerebellar nystagmus.** The most common nystagmus of cerebellar disease is a conjugate horizontal jerk nystagmus on lateral gaze (see Section III-A-2-a below).

      One rare type of nystagmus, "rebound nystagmus," has been described only in patients with cerebellar disease.[6,7] To test for this nystagmus, the patient first looks to one direction (say, to the right). In patients with a positive response, a brisk nystagmus with its fast component to the right appears. If the patient continues looking in this direction for about 20 seconds, the nystagmus fatigues and disappears (sometimes even reversing direction). The patient then returns his eyes to the primary position (i.e., straight ahead), and nystagmus to the left, not present

---

[a] One famous neuro-ophthalmologist once advised his students, "Never write on nystagmus, it will lead you nowhere."[5]

initially, appears, although it fatigues over time. In these patients, the direction of the nystagmus in primary gaze can be reversed at will, depending on whether the patient looks first to the left or right.[6]

b. Nystagmus and noncerebellar disorders. Other useful patterns of nystagmus (not features of cerebellar disease) are optokinetic nystagmus (see Chapter 51), the nystagmus of internuclear ophthalmoplegia (see Chapter 52), and the nystagmus of vestibular disease (which is usually a conjugate rotatory jerk nystagmus).

3. Effect of retinal fixation. "Retinal fixation" means the patient is focusing his eyes on an object. Spontaneous nystagmus that diminishes during retinal fixation argues that the responsible lesion is located in the peripheral vestibular system; nystagmus that increases or remains unchanged during fixation argues that the lesion is in the central nervous system (i.e., brain stem or cerebellum). Neuro-ophthalmologists usually use electronystagmography to detect the effects of fixation (by comparing eye movements with eyes open with those with eyes closed), but general clinicians can accomplish the same during direct ophthalmoscopy. In a dimly lit room, the clinician examines the optic disc of one eye and compares its movements as the patient fixes the opposite eye on a distant target with those when the patient's opposite eye is covered. If rhythmic movements of the optic disc first appear or worsen when the fixating eye is occluded, a peripheral vestibular disturbance is likely.[8]

C. Hypotonia (see Chapter 54). The limbs of patients with cerebellar disease offer no resistance to passive displacement, sometimes resembling (in the words of Gordon Holmes) the

"muscles of a person deeply under an anaes-
thetic, or of a corpse recently dead."[1] Holding
the forearms vertically causes the wrist to bend
to an angle much more acute than normal.
Displacing the patient's outstretched arm downwards causes abnormally wide and prolonged
up-and-down oscillations, even when the patient is requested to resist such movements.
Striking the patellar tendon causes pendular
knee jerks, traditionally defined as three or
more swings,[9] although, as already stated in
Chapter 54, this threshold will have to be revised upward because many normal persons
also demonstrate three or more swings.[10]

D. Dysarthria. The speech of patients with cerebellar disease is slow, slurred, and irregular in
volume and rhythm, findings that are collectively referred to as "dysarthria." In contrast to
patients with aphasia, however, patients with
dysarthria can name objects, repeat words, comprehend language, and speak sentences with
words whose order makes sense.

III. CLINICAL SIGNIFICANCE
A. Individual findings

1. **Ataxia.** Ataxia of gait is the most common
finding in all cerebellar syndromes (see below), and therefore, examination of the gait
should be part of every patient with suspected cerebellar disease. Many patients
with cerebellar disease have difficulty walking despite lacking all other findings of limb
ataxia.

Simple measurements of the patient's
dysdiadochokinesia—such as how quickly
and accurately the patient can alternately
tap two buttons spaced about 12 inches
apart[b]—are accurate measures of ataxia

---

[b] Ninety percent of normal persons can accomplish at least 32 taps
within 15 seconds, whereas 90% of patients with cerebellar ataxia
cannot.[11]

that correlate well with other measures of disability.[11]

2. **Nystagmus.** Seventy-five percent of cerebellar nystagmus is a conjugate horizontal jerk nystagmus that appears on lateral gaze (15% is a rotatory nystagmus and 10% a vertical nystagmus). Nonetheless, a horizontal jerk nystagmus is not specific for cerebellar disease and also occurs in peripheral vestibular disease and other central nervous system disorders. The direction of the jerk nystagmus has less localizing value than tests of ataxia (see Section B-1-a below).

The clinical utility of rebound nystagmus is limited because it is a late finding, and all patients described with the finding have had many other obvious cerebellar signs.[6,7]

3. **Dysarthria.** Dysarthria, the least common of the fundamental cerebellar signs (see below), appears more often with lesions of the left cerebellar hemisphere than with those of the right hemisphere.[12]

B. **Cerebellar syndromes.** Most patients with cerebellar disease present with difficulty walking or headache, or both.[9,13] In adults, four cerebellar syndromes are common, each of which is characterized by a different distribution of the principal cerebellar signs.

1. **Cerebellar hemisphere syndrome**

   a. **Cerebellar findings.** Table 58-1 presents the physical findings of 444 patients with focal lesions (mostly tumors) confined to one hemisphere.[9,13] According to traditional teachings, cerebellar signs appear on the side of the body *ipsilateral* to the lesion. This teaching proved generally correct in the patients of Table 58-1, in whom signs of limb ataxia (i.e., dysmetria, intention tremor, dysdiadochokinesia) were unilateral 85% of the time, and, if unilateral, were on the side ipsilateral to the lesion 80% to 90% of the

TABLE 58-1 Unilateral cerebellar lesions*

Physical Finding†	Frequency (%)‡
Ataxia	
Gait ataxia	80-93
Limb ataxia	
Dysmetria	71-86
Intention tremor	29
Dysdiadochokinesia	47-69
Nystagmus	54-84
Hypotonia	76
Pendular knee jerks	37
Dysarthria	10-25

Data from 444 patients from references 9 and 13.

Diagnostic standard: Clinical imaging, surgical findings, or postmortem examination.

†*Definition of findings:* see text.

‡Results are overall mean frequency or, if statistically heterogenous, the range of values.

time. These patients also had more hypotonia on the side of the lesion and tended to fall toward the side of the lesion when walking.

Nystagmus has less localizing value. When present, nystagmus is unilateral in only 65% of patients, and in these, the direction of nystagmus points to the side of the lesion only 70% of the time.

b. Associated findings. Despite having a lesion confined to the cerebellum, many patients with structural cerebellar lesions also have (1) cranial nerve findings (10% to 20% of patients; usually of cranial nerves 5, 6, 7, or 8, ipsilateral to the side of the lesion 75% of the time[9,13]); (2) altered mental status (38% of patients, from compression of the brain stem or complicating hydrocephalus); (3) upper motor neuron signs such as hyperactive reflexes and Babinski's sign (28% of patients); and (4) papilledema (68% of patients).

In contrast, severe weakness and sensory disturbance are both uncommon, affecting only 4%.

2. **Anterior cerebellar degeneration (rostral vermis syndrome).**[14] In contrast to the cerebellar hemisphere syndrome, these patients have ataxia of gait (100%) and of both legs (88%) but not of the arms (only 16% of patients). Nystagmus and dysarthria also are much less frequent (9%, for both findings). This syndrome most often results from chronic alcohol ingestion.

3. **Pancerebellar syndrome.** This syndrome causes the same signs listed in Table 58-1, but instead of being on one side of the body, the cerebellar signs are symmetric. Causes include drug intoxication (e.g., phenytoin), inherited disorders, and paraneoplastic syndromes.

4. **Cerebellar infarction.** The physical signs of cerebellar infarction resemble those of the cerebellar hemisphere syndrome described above, with three exceptions: In infarction, (1) all signs appear *abruptly*, (2) there is significantly more dysarthria (44% of patients), and (3) there is significantly more weakness (22% have hemiparesis; 24% have quadriparesis).[15-18] The two main arteries supplying the cerebellum are the superior cerebellar and posterior cerebellar arteries. An associated lateral medullary syndrome (see Table 55-2 in Chapter 55) suggests an infarct in the distribution of the posterior inferior cerebellar artery.[17,19]

REFERENCES

1. Holmes G. Clinical symptoms of cerebellar disease and their interpretation: Lecture 1, *Lancet* 1:1177-1182, 1922.

2. Holmes G. Clinical symptoms of cerebellar disease and their interpretation. Lecture 2, *Lancet* 1:1231-1237, 1922.

3. Holmes G. Clinical symptoms of cerebellar disease and their interpretation. Lecture 3, *Lancet* 2:59-65, 1922.

4. Holmes G. Clinical symptoms of cerebellar disease and their interpretation. Lecture 4, *Lancet* 2:111-115, 1922.

5. Wartenberg R. *Diagnostic tests in neurology: a selection for office use,* Chicago, 1953, Year Book Publishers, Inc.

6. Hood JD, Kayan A, and Leech J. Rebound nystagmus, *Brain* 96:507-526, 1973.

7. Morales-Garcia C and others. Clinical significance of rebound nystagmus in neuro-otological diagnosis, *Ann Otol Rhinol Laryngol* 87:238-242, 1978.

8. Zee DS. Ophthalmoscopy in examination of patients with vestibular disorders, *Ann Neurol* 3:373-374, 1978.

9. Gilman S, Bloedel JR, and Lechtenberg R. Disorders of the cerebellum. In Plum F, McDowell FH, and Baringer JR, editors. *Contemporary neurology series,* Philadelphia, 1981, FA Davis, Co.

10. Bickett JB and Tatum EJ. Pendular knee reflexes: a reliable sign of hypotonia? *Lancet* 2:236-237, 1984.

11. Notermans NC and others. Measuring ataxia: quantification based on the standard neurological examination, *J Neurol Neurosurg Psych* 57:22-26, 1994.

12. Lechtenberg R and Gilman S. Speech disorders in cerebellar disease, *Ann Neurol* 3:285-290, 1978.

13. Amici R, Avanzini G, and Pacini L. Cerebellar tumors: clinical analysis and physiopathologic correlations. In Cohen MM, editor. *Monographs in neural sciences,* vol 4, Basel, 1976, S. Karger.

14. Victor M, Adams RD, and Mancall EL. A restricted form of cerebellar cortical degeneration occurring in alcoholic patients, *Arch Neurol* 1:579-688, 1959.

15. Scotti G and others. Cerebellar softening, *Ann Neurol* 8:133-140, 1980.

16. Tohgi H and others. Cerebellar infarction: clinical and neuroimaging analysis in 293 patients, *Stroke* 24:1697-1701, 1993.

17. Kase CS and others. Cerebellar infarction: clinical and anatomic observations in 66 cases, *Stroke* 24:76-83, 1993.

18. Sypert GW and Alvord EC. Cerebellar infarction: a clinicopathological study, *Arch Neurol* 32:357-363, 1975.

19. Amarenco P. The spectrum of cerebellar infarctions, *Neurology* 41:973-979, 1991.

CHAPTER 59

Examination of Hysterical Neurologic Disorders

I. **TRADITIONAL PHYSICAL FINDINGS OF HYS-TERICAL DISEASE.** Hysterical neurologic disorders (also called "nonorganic," "psychogenic," or "functional") occur commonly, accounting for 9% of admissions to a neurologic service, according to one study.[1] The traditional bedside findings that suggest functional disease are listed below:

A. **Findings whose severity fluctuates during the examination.** Examples are the patient who falls suddenly while walking but catches himself with knees and hips flexed, a position that requires considerable strength, or the patient whose stance is unstable until distracted by asking him to perform the finger-nose test.[2]

B. **Findings that defy neuroanatomic explanation,** including (1) hysterical hemianopia, as in the patient who has right hemianopia with both eyes open or just the right eye open, but normal visual fields when just the left eye is open[3,4]; (2) **wrong-way tongue deviation** (i.e., the tongue deviates away from the hemiparetic side; in cerebral hemispheric disease, the tongue deviates toward the hemiparetic side, see Chapter 53)[5]; (3) **peripheral facial palsy and ipsi-**

lateral hemiparesis (if a single lesion causes peripheral facial weakness and hemiparesis, the lesion is in the brain stem and the findings should be on opposite sides of the body).[6]

C. **Bizarre movements not normally seen in organic disease.** Examples are the patient who drags the hemiparetic leg after him as if it were an inanimate object,[2,7] or the ataxic patient who sways dramatically without falling.[4]

D. **Findings elicited during special tests** include **(1) optokinetic nystagmus** testing for functional blindness; because patients with intact vision cannot suppress this nystagmus (see Chapter 51), the presence of optokinetic nystagmus uncovers that the blindness is functional and **(2) procedures that confuse the patient of sidedness,** such as a maneuver that mixes up the fingers to uncover hysterical hemianalgesia (Figure 59-1).[8]

II. CLINICAL SIGNIFICANCE: CAVEATS TO THE DIAGNOSIS OF HYSTERICAL DISORDERS.

Despite these traditional teachings, the clinician should be very reluctant to diagnose hysterical disease, primarily because many of these "nonorganic" findings, when subjected to serious study, also appear in patients with organic disease. For example, in studies of patients with known organic causes of their findings, 8% "split" their sensory findings precisely at the midline, up to 85% feel vibration less in numb areas, 48% have sensory findings that change between examinations or make no sense neuroanatomically, and 33% have "give-away" weakness.[9,10] All of these findings, at one point in time, have been presented as reliable markers of psychogenic disease.[11]

Rare disorders also will trip up the unwary clinician. For example, patients with the medial medullary syndrome also may point their tongue to the "wrong" side, and patients with advanced Huntington's disease are often regarded as having an hysterical gait when it is viewed in isolation.[7]

FIGURE 59-1 Test for hysterical hemianalgesia. This test simply mixes up the fingers and confuses the body image. In the first step (*top row*), the patients hands are pronated so their little fingers are on top, palms are outward, and fingers are interlocked. In the second step (*bottom row*), the hands are rotated downward, inward, and upward, so the interlocked fingers are positioned in front of the chest. The clinician then repeats the sensory examination to determine if the patient is consistent in describing his sensory loss. In the final position, the fingertips end up on the same side of the body as their respective arms, and the thumbs (which are not interlocked) end up on the side opposite the fingers.

In one study, up to 40% of patients given a diagnosis of hysterical neurologic disease were subsequently found to have a neurologic disease to account for the finding.[12] The diagnosis of hysterical illness, then, is often a diagnostic snare, best left to the experts who are paid to take on such risks.

REFERENCES

1. Lempert T and others. Psychogenic disorders in neurology: frequency and clinical spectrum, *Acta Neurol Scand* 82:335-340, 1990.
2. Lempert T and others. How to identify psychogenic disorders of stance and gait, *J Neurol* 238:140-146, 1991.
3. Keane JR. Hysterical hemianopia: the 'missing half' field defect, *Arch Ophthalmol* 97:865-866, 1979.
4. Keane JR. Patterns of hysterical hemianopia, *Neurology* 51:1230-1231, 1998.
5. Keane JR. Wrong-way deviation of the tongue with hysterical hemiparesis, *Neurology* 36:1406-1407, 1986.
6. Keane JR. Hysterical hemiparesis accompanying Bell's palsy, *Neurology* 43:1619, 1993.
7. Keane JR. Hysterical gait disorders: 60 cases, *Neurology* 39:586-589, 1989.
8. Bowlus WE and Currier RD. A test for hysterical hemianalgesis, *N Engl J Med* 269:1253-1254, 1963.
9. Rolak LA. Psychogenic sensory loss, *J Nerv Ment Dis* 176:686-687, 1988.
10. Gould R and others. The validity of hysterical signs and symptoms, *J Nerv Ment Dis* 174:593-597, 1986.
11. Haerer AF. *DeJong's The neurologic examination*, Philadelphia, 1992, JB Lippincott.
12. Slater ETO and Glithero E. A follow-up of patients diagnosed as suffering from "hysteria," *J Psychosom Res* 9:9-13, 1965.

PART TWELVE

Likelihood Ratios and Their Confidence Intervals

CHAPTER 60

Likelihood Ratios and Their Confidence Intervals

Table 60-1 displays the point estimates and 95% confidence intervals for all of the likelihood ratios presented in this book. Chapter 2 presents the methods used to obtain these estimates, and individual chapters define each physical finding and further discuss its significance.

TABLE 60-1 Likelihood ratios—point estimates and 95% confidence intervals

Finding	Positive LR (95% CI)	Negative LR (95% CI)
Table 4-1 Dementia and Delirium		
Abnormal clock drawing test	9.6 (4.9, 18.6)	0.4 (0.2, 0.8)
Mini-mental status, ≤23	9.0 (5.7, 14.3)	0.2 (0.1, 0.3)
Mini-mental status, ≤20	14.5 (6.8, 31.1)	—
Mini-mental status, 21-25	2.2 (1.6, 3.0)	—
Mini-mental status, ≥26	0.1 (0.1, 0.2)	—
Confusion assessment method, detecting delirium	8.8 (3.6, 21.3)	0.2 (0, 0.8)
Chapter 5 Stance and Gait		
Stops talking when walking, predicting falls	8.8 (2.1, 36.5)	0.6 (0.4, 0.8)
Table 6-1 Hepatocellular Jaundice		
Weight loss	0.8 (0.2, 3.2)	1.3 (0.5, 3.3)
Spider angiomata	4.7 (1.1, 22.4)	0.6 (0.5, 0.9)
Palmar erythema	9.8 (1.4, 67.6)	0.5 (0.4, 0.7)
Distended abdominal veins	17.5 (1.1, 277)	0.6 (0.5, 0.8)
Ascites	4.4 (1.1, 17.1)	0.6 (0.5, 0.8)
Palpable spleen	2.9 (1.2, 6.8)	0.7 (0.6, 0.9)

Palpable gallbladder	0.04 (0, 0.7)	1.4 (1.1, 1.9)
Palpable liver	0.9 (0.8, 1.1)	1.4 (0.6, 3.4)
Liver tenderness	1.4 (0.8, 2.6)	0.8 (0.7, 1.1)
Table 6-2 Cirrhosis		
Spider angiomata	1.3 (0.9, 1.8)	0.7 (0.4, 1.2)
Palpable spleen	1.4 (1.1, 1.8)	0.5 (0.4, 0.8)
Ascites	3.9 (1.5, 10.5)	0.8 (0.6, 0.9)
Jaundice	14.2 (1.9, 104.9)	0.9 (0.8, 0.9)
Encephalopathy	17.5 (2.3, 130.2)	0.7 (0.6, 0.9)
Chapter 7 Cyanosis		
Central cyanosis, detecting arterial deoxyhemo-globin level of ≥2.38 g/dl	7.4 (1.5, 36.8)	0.2 (0.1, 0.5)
Table 8-1 Anemia		
Pallor at multiple sites	4.5 (3.1, 6.6)	0.7 (0.6, 0.8)
Facial pallor	3.8 (2.5, 5.8)	0.6 (0.5, 0.7)
Nailbed pallor	1.7 (1.4, 2.2)	0.6 (0.5, 0.8)
Palmar pallor	2.5 (1.9, 3.3)	0.5 (0.4, 0.6)
Palmar crease pallor	7.9 (1.8, 35.3)	0.9 (0.9, 1.0)
Conjunctiva rim pallor present	16.7 (2.2, 124.7)	—
Conjunctiva rim pallor borderline	2.3 (1.5, 3.5)	—
Conjunctiva rim pallor absent	0.6 (0.5, 0.8)	—

Continued

TABLE 60-1 Likelihood ratios—point estimates and 95% confidence intervals—cont'd

Finding	Positive LR (95% CI)	Negative LR (95% CI)
Table 9-1 Hypovolemia		
Dry axilla	2.8 (1.4, 5.4)	0.6 (0.4, 1.0)
Dry mucous membranes of mouth and nose	2.0 (1.0, 4.0)	0.3 (0.1, 0.6)
Longitudinal furrows on tongue	2.0 (1.0, 4.0)	0.3 (0.1, 0.6)
Sunken eyes	3.4 (1.0, 12.2)	0.5 (0.3, 0.7)
Confusion	2.1 (0.8, 5.7)	0.6 (0.4, 1.0)
Weakness	2.3 (0.6, 8.6)	0.7 (0.5, 1.0)
Speech not clear or expressive	3.1 (0.9, 11.1)	0.5 (0.3, 0.8)
Chapter 10 Protein-calorie Malnutrition and Weight Loss		
Underestimation of weight loss, predicting organic cause	5.4 (2.0, 14.5)	0.6 (0.5, 0.8)
Overestimation of weight loss, predicting nonorganic cause	3.6 (2.0, 6.5)	0.4 (0.2, 0.6)
Table 10-1 Protein-Energy Malnutrition		
Weight loss >10%	1.4 (1.1, 1.7)	1.0 (0.9, 1.0)
Low body weight	2.0 (1.4, 2.9)	0.9 (0.8, 1.0)
Upper arm circumference <85% predicted	2.5 (1.7, 3.6)	0.8 (0.7, 0.9)

Forearm circumference <85% predicted	3.2 (2.0, 5.1)	0.8 (0.6, 0.9)
Reduced grip strength	2.1 (1.6, 2.9)	0.3 (0.2, 0.6)

Chapter 12 Cushing's Syndrome

Clinically apparent osteoporosis, detecting Cushing's syndrome	17.6 (7.8, 39.4)	0.4 (0.3, 0.5)

Table 12-2 Cushing's Syndrome

Hypertension	2.3 (1.5, 3.7)	0.8 (0.6, 0.9)
Moon facies	1.6 (1.1, 2.5)	0.1 (0, 0.9)
Central obesity	3.0 (2.0, 4.4)	0.2 (0.1, 0.3)
Generalized obesity	0.1 (0, 0.2)	2.5 (2.1, 3.1)
Thin skinfold	115.6 (7.2, 1853.8)	0.2 (0.1, 0.6)
Plethora	2.7 (2.1, 3.5)	0.3 (0.1, 0.5)
Hirsutism, in women	1.7 (1.2, 2.5)	0.7 (0.5, 0.9)
Ecchymoses	4.5 (1.2, 16.4)	0.5 (0.4, 0.6)
Red or blue striae	1.9 (1.3, 2.7)	0.7 (0.6, 0.9)
Acne	2.2 (1.5, 3.2)	0.6 (0.5, 0.8)
Proximal muscle weakness	4.4 (1.0, 19.6)	0.4 (0.3, 0.6)
Edema	1.8 (1.1, 3.1)	0.7 (0.6, 0.9)

Continued

TABLE 60-1 Likelihood ratios—point estimates and 95% confidence intervals—cont'd

Finding	Positive LR (95% CI)	Negative LR (95% CI)
Chapter 13 Pulse Rate and Contour		
Pulsus paradoxus >12 mm Hg, detecting tamponade	5.9 (2.4, 14.3)	0.03 (0, 0.2)
Delayed carotid artery upstroke, detecting severe aortic stenosis	3.7 (2.5, 5.5)	0.4 (0.2, 0.9)
Hyperkinetic arterial pulse in mitral stenosis, detecting mitral regurgitation	14.2 (7.4, 27.2)	0.3 (0.2, 0.4)
Table 13-1 Tachycardia		
Predicting mortality, myocardial infarct	1.6 (1.3, 2.1)	0.8 (0.7, 0.9)
Predicting mortality, septic shock	2.0 (1.3, 3.3)	0.1 (0, 0.5)
Predicting complications, gallstone pancreatitis	6.8 (3.7, 12.5)	0.2 (0, 1.0)
Predicting mortality, pneumonia	2.1 (1.1, 3.8)	0.7 (0.5, 1.0)
Predicting mortality, pontine hemorrhage	25.4 (1.6, 395.3)	0.3 (0.2, 0.6)
Table 13-2 Pulsus Paradoxus and Asthma		
Pulsus paradoxus >10 mm Hg, predicting severe asthma	2.7 (1.7, 4.3)	0.5 (0.4, 0.7)

Finding		
Pulsus paradoxus >20 mm Hg, predicting severe asthma	8.2 (1.7, 40.3)	0.8 (0.7, 0.9)
Pulsus paradoxus >25 mm Hg, predicting severe asthma	22.6 (1.4, 363.2)	0.8 (0.8, 0.9)
Chapter 14 Abnormalities of Pulse Rhythm		
Pounding sensation in neck, detecting intranodal reentrant tachycardia	350.7 (22.0, 5594)	0.1 (0, 0.2)
Table 14-1 Atrioventricular Dissociation		
Varying arterial pulse	2.1 (1.0, 4.4)	0.5 (0.3, 1.0)
Intermittent cannon A waves	3.8 (1.8, 8.2)	0.1 (0, 0.4)
Changing intensity of S_1	24.4 (1.5, 384.5)	0.4 (0.3, 0.7)
Chapter 15 Blood Pressure		
Murmur of aortic insufficiency, detecting type A dissection	11.9 (5.0, 28.3)	0.5 (0.2, 1.3)
Absence of peripheral pulse, detecting type A dissection	3.3 (1.9, 5.9)	0.8 (0.5, 1.2)
Proportional pulse pressure <0.25, detecting low cardiac index	5.4 (1.9, 15.4)	0.1 (0, 0.3)
Large pulse pressure, moderate-to-severe aortic regurgitation	10.9 (1.5, 77.1)	0.5 (0.2, 0.8)

Continued

TABLE 60-1 Likelihood ratios—point estimates and 95% confidence intervals—cont'd

Finding	Positive LR (95% CI)	Negative LR (95% CI)
Table 15-2 Hypotension		
Predicting mortality, intensive care unit	4.0 (3.6, 4.3)	0.8 (0.8, 0.9)
Predicting mortality, pneumonia	10.0 (5.6, 17.6)	0.8 (0.7, 1.0)
Predicting mortality, myocardial infarction	15.5 (12.2, 19.6)	0.7 (0.7, 0.7)
Chapter 16 Temperature		
Shaking chills, detecting bacteremia	1.8 (1.4, 2.2)	0.8 (0.6, 1.0)
Temperature >39° C in pontine hemorrhage, predicting hospital mortality	23.7 (1.5, 371)	0.4 (0.2, 0.6)
Temperature <36.1° C in pneumonia, predicting hospital mortality	2.0 (1.1, 3.5)	0.9 (0.9, 1.0)
Table 16-1 Detection of Fever		
Patient's report of fever	4.9 (3.9, 6.1)	0.2 (0.1, 0.4)
Patient's forehead abnormally warm	2.5 (1.8, 3.5)	0.4 (0.3, 0.6)
Chapter 17 Respiratory Rate and Abnormal Breathing Patterns		
Asynchronous breathing, predicting hospital death or intubation	3.2 (1.3, 7.8)	0.5 (0.2, 1.0)
Paradoxical abdominal movements, detecting diaphragm weakness	3.3 (1.7, 6.3)	0.1 (0, 1.1)
Orthopnea, detecting low ventricular ejection fraction	2.7 (1.5, 4.9)	0.04 (0, 0.7)

Continued

Table 17-1 Tachypnea

Finding		
Predicting failure of weaning	2.9 (1.2, 7.1)	0.1 (0, 1.4)
Predicting cardiopulmonary arrest	3.0 (1.8, 5.0)	0.6 (0.4, 0.7)
Detecting pneumonia	2.0 (1.4, 2.8)	0.8 (0.7, 0.9)
Predicting mortality, pneumonia	2.0 (1.7, 2.5)	0.6 (0.4, 0.9)

Chapter 19 The Pupils

Finding		
Cocaine test, detecting Horner's syndrome	96.8 (6.1, 1527.3)	0.1 (0, 0.1)
Asymmetric facial sweating in Horner's syndrome, detecting first or second order neuron lesion	2.4 (0.9, 6.1)	0.6 (0.4, 0.9)
Anisocoria, detecting intraocular inflammation	6.5 (2.6, 16.3)	0.8 (0.8, 0.9)

Table 20-2 Diabetic Retinopathy

Finding		
Nondilated pupils	5.8 (2.5, 13.5)	0.5 (0.4, 0.8)
Dilated pupils, general providers	10.0 (5.9, 17.0)	0.4 (0.3, 0.5)
Dilated pupils, specialists	18.1 (5.6, 58.2)	0.3 (0.2, 0.5)

Table 21-2 Hearing Tests

Finding		
Abnormal whispered voice test, detecting hearing loss	6.0 (4.4, 8.2)	0.03 (0, 0.3)
Rinne test, detecting conductive hearing loss	16.8 (13.8, 20.4)	0.2 (0.1, 0.8)
Weber test lateralizes to good ear, detecting neurosensory hearing loss	2.7 (1.2, 6.4)	0.5 (0.3, 1.1)

TABLE 60-1 Likelihood ratios—point estimates and 95% confidence intervals—cont'd

FINDING	POSITIVE LR (95% CI)	NEGATIVE LR (95% CI)
Table 21-2 Hearing Tests—cont'd		
Weber test lateralizes to bad ear, detecting conductive hearing loss	6.4 (1.0, 43.3)	0.5 (0.3, 0.8)
Chapter 22 The Thyroid and Its Disorders		
Precise measurement of reflex time, hypothyroidism	18.7 (13.3, 26.3)	0.1 (0, 0.2)
Table 22-2 Goiter		
No goiter, palpation or inspection	0.4 (0.3, 0.5)	—
Goiter by palpation, visible after neck extension	0.9 (0.4, 2.1)	—
Goiter, palpation and inspection in normal position	26.3 (5.2, 131.7)	—
Table 22-3 Goiter and Carcinoma		
Vocal cord paralysis	45.2 (2.7, 762.1)	0.8 (0.6, 0.9)
Cervical adenopathy	13.4 (4.6, 39.2)	0.6 (0.4, 0.7)
Fixation to surrounding tissue	9.7 (4.5, 21.2)	0.4 (0.3, 0.6)
Goiter nodular (vs. diffuse)	1.5 (1.2, 1.9)	0.5 (0.3, 0.8)
Pyramidal lobe present	0.3 (0.1, 1.7)	1.1 (1.0, 1.2)

Table 22-3 Thyroid Nodules and Carcinoma

Vocal cord paralysis	12.0 (2.0, 70.5)
Cervical adenopathy	7.4 (2.9, 19.0)
Fixation to surrounding tissues	7.2 (1.7, 30.8)
Very firm nodule	3.3 (0.4, 30.6)

Table 22-4 Hypothyroidism

Coarse skin	5.6 (2.5, 12.6)
Cool and dry skin	4.7 (3.1, 7.1)
Cold palms	1.6 (1.0, 2.7)
Dry palms	1.5 (1.0, 2.4)
Periorbital puffiness	2.8 (1.8, 4.3)
Puffiness of wrists	2.9 (1.7, 4.9)
Hair loss of eyebrows	1.9 (1.1, 3.6)
Hypothyroid speech	5.4 (2.7, 10.7)
Pulse <70 beats/min	4.1 (3.1, 5.5)
Enlarged thyroid	2.8 (2.3, 3.4)
Billewicz score less than −15 points	0.1 (0, 0.2)
Billewicz score −15 to +29 points	0.9 (0.4, 2.1)
Billewicz score +30 points or more	18.8 (1.2, 300.5)

	0.9 (0.8, 1.0)
	0.7 (0.6, 0.9)
	0.9 (0.8, 1.0)
	1.0 (0.9, 1.0)
	0.7 (0.6, 0.9)
	0.9 (0.8, 0.9)
	0.8 (0.6, 1.1)
	0.8 (0.6, 1.1)
	0.6 (0.4, 0.8)
	0.7 (0.5, 0.9)
	0.8 (0.7, 1.0)
	0.7 (0.5, 0.9)
	0.8 (0.7, 0.8)
	0.6 (0.6, 0.7)
	—
	—
	—

Continued

TABLE 60-1 Likelihood ratios—point estimates and 95% confidence intervals—cont'd

FINDING	POSITIVE LR (95% CI)	NEGATIVE LR (95% CI)
Table 22-6 Hyperthyroidism		
Pulse ≥90 beats/min	4.4 (3.8, 5.1)	0.2 (0.2, 0.3)
Skin moist and warm	6.7 (5.0, 9.1)	0.7 (0.7, 0.7)
Enlarged thyroid	2.3 (2.1, 2.5)	0.1 (0.1, 0.2)
Eyelid retraction	31.5 (16.6, 59.7)	0.7 (0.6, 0.7)
Eyelid lag	17.6 (9.2, 33.7)	0.8 (0.8, 0.8)
Fine finger tremor	11.4 (8.7, 14.8)	0.3 (0.3, 0.4)
Wayne index <11 points	0.1 (0, 0.3)	—
Wayne index 11-19 points	1.2 (0.7, 2.0)	—
Wayne index ≥20 points	18.2 (2.9, 113.5)	—
Table 23-2 Subarachnoid Hemorrhage		
Neck stiffness	10.3 (5.2, 20.7)	0.4 (0.3, 0.7)
Neurologic findings not focal	5.9 (3.5, 9.9)	0.4 (0.2, 0.7)
Age ≤60 years	1.8 (1.4, 2.3)	0.3 (0.1, 0.8)
Seizures	2.2 (1.1, 4.5)	0.8 (0.6, 1.1)

Table 25-2 Percussion of the Chest

Conventional dullness, detecting pneumonia	3.0 (1.7, 5.2)	0.9 (0.8, 1.0)
Conventional dullness, detecting any abnormality	3.0 (1.4, 6.3)	0.9 (0.9, 1.0)
Hyperresonance, detecting chronic airflow obstruction	5.1 (1.7, 15.6)	0.7 (0.5, 1.0)
Diaphragm excursion <2 cm, detecting chronic airflow obstruction	5.3 (0.8, 35.0)	0.9 (0.7, 1.1)
Auscultatory dullness, detecting any abnormality	1.7 (1.0, 3.0)	0.8 (0.6, 1.1)
Auscultatory dullness, detecting pleural fluid	18.6 (9.8, 35.2)	0.04 (0, 0.1)

Table 26-2 Breath Sounds and Vocal Resonance

Diminished breath sounds, detecting pneumonia	2.3 (1.9, 2.8)	0.8 (0.7, 0.9)
Diminished breath sounds, detecting asthma	4.2 (1.9, 9.5)	0.3 (0.1, 0.6)
Breath sound score ≤9, detecting chronic airflow obstruction	10.2 (4.6, 22.7)	—
Breath sound score 10-12, detecting chronic airflow obstruction	3.6 (1.4, 9.5)	—
Breath sound score 13-15, detecting chronic airflow obstruction	0.7 (0.3, 1.5)	—
Breath sound score >15, detecting chronic airflow obstruction	0.1 (0, 0.3)	—
Bronchial breath sounds, detecting pneumonia	3.3 (2.0, 5.6)	0.9 (0.8, 1.0)
Egophony, detecting pneumonia	4.1 (2.1, 7.8)	0.9 (0.9, 1.0)

Continued

TABLE 60-1 Likelihood ratios—point estimates and 95% confidence intervals—cont'd

FINDING	POSITIVE LR (95% CI)	NEGATIVE LR (95% CI)
Table 26-4 Crackles and Wheezes		
Crackles, detecting pulmonary fibrosis	5.9 (2.0, 17.2)	0.2 (0.1, 0.5)
Crackles, detecting high left atrial pressure	3.4 (1.6, 7.2)	0.7 (0.6, 1.0)
Crackles, detecting pneumonia	2.0 (1.5, 2.7)	0.8 (0.7, 0.9)
Early crackles, detecting obstructive disease	14.6 (3.0, 70)	0.4 (0.1, 1.4)
Early crackles, detecting severe obstruction	20.8 (3.0, 142.2)	0.1 (0, 0.4)
Unforced wheezes, detecting obstructive disease	6.0 (2.4, 15.1)	0.7 (0.6, 1.0)
Methacholine wheezes, detecting asthma	6.0 (1.5, 24.3)	0.6 (0.4, 0.9)
Table 27-1 Ancillary Tests		
Forced expiratory time <3 sec, detecting chronic airflow obstruction	0.2 (0.1, 0.3)	—
Forced expiratory time 3-9 sec, detecting chronic airflow obstruction	1.3 (0.5, 2.9)	—
Forced expiratory time ≥9 sec, detecting chronic airflow obstruction	4.8 (1.3, 17.6)	—
Snider test, detecting FEV$_1$ ≤1.6 L	9.6 (5.5, 16.6)	0.2 (0.1, 0.8)

Table 28-1 Pneumonia

Cachexia	4.0 (1.7, 9.6)
Abnormal mental status	2.2 (1.1, 4.3)
Temperature >37.8° C	2.2 (1.6, 3.1)
Respiratory rate >28/min	2.0 (1.4, 2.8)
Heart rate >100 beats/min	1.6 (1.4, 1.8)
Percussion dullness	3.0 (1.7, 5.2)
Diminished breath sounds	2.3 (1.9, 2.8)
Bronchial breath sounds	3.3 (2.0, 5.6)
Egophony	4.1 (2.1, 7.8)
Crackles	2.0 (1.5, 2.7)
Wheezes	0.8 (0.7, 1.1)
Heckerling score, 0 or 1 finding	0.3 (0.2, 0.4)
Heckerling score, 2 or 3 findings	1.0 (0.9, 1.2)
Heckerling score, 4 or 5 findings	8.2 (5.8, 11.5)

	0.9 (0.8, 1.0)
	0.9 (0.9, 1.0)
	0.7 (0.6, 0.7)
	0.8 (0.7, 0.9)
	0.7 (0.6, 0.9)
	0.9 (0.8, 1.0)
	0.8 (0.7, 0.9)
	0.9 (0.8, 1.0)
	0.9 (0.9, 1.0)
	0.8 (0.7, 0.9)
	1.1 (1.0, 1.1)
	—
	—
	—

Table 28-2 Pneumonia and Mortality

Abnormal mental status	2.3 (1.8, 2.9)	0.6 (0.5, 0.8)
Respiratory rate >30/min	2.0 (1.7, 2.4)	0.6 (0.4, 0.9)
Systolic blood pressure <90 mm Hg	10.0 (5.6, 17.6)	0.8 (0.7, 1.0)
Heart rate >100 beats/min	2.1 (1.1, 3.8)	0.7 (0.5, 1.0)

Continued

TABLE 60-1 Likelihood ratios—point estimates and 95% confidence intervals—cont'd

Finding	Positive LR (95% CI)	Negative LR (95% CI)
Table 28-2 Pneumonia and Mortality—cont'd		
Hypothermia	3.5 (1.1, 10.9)	0.8 (0.5, 1.2)
Prognostic score (with confusion)	4.5 (2.2, 9.4)	0.7 (0.5, 0.9)
Prognostic score (with BUN)	4.2 (3.4, 5.2)	0.3 (0.1, 0.6)
Table 29-1 Chronic Obstructive Lung Disease		
Subxiphoid cardiac impulse	7.4 (2.0, 27.1)	0.9 (0.7, 1.1)
Absent cardiac dullness	11.8 (1.2, 121.4)	0.9 (0.7, 1.1)
Hyperresonance	5.1 (1.7, 15.6)	0.7 (0.5, 1.0)
Diaphragm excursion <2 cm	5.3 (0.8, 35.0)	0.9 (0.7, 1.1)
Breath sound score, ≤9	10.2 (4.6, 22.7)	—
Breath sound score 10-12	3.6 (1.4, 9.5)	—
Breath sound score 13-15	0.7 (0.3, 1.5)	—
Breath sound score, >15	0.1 (0, 0.3)	—
Early inspiratory crackles	14.6 (3.0, 70.0)	0.4 (0.1, 1.4)
Unforced wheezes	6.0 (2.4, 15.1)	0.7 (0.6, 1.10)
Forced expiratory time, <3 sec	0.2 (0.1, 0.3)	—
Forced expiratory time, 3-9 sec	1.3 (0.5, 2.9)	—

Forced expiratory time, ≥9 sec	4.8 (1.3, 17.6)	—
Combined findings, 2 of 3	25.7 (6.2, 105.5)	0.3 (0.2, 0.7)

Table 30-2 Pulmonary Embolism

Known cancer	4.1 (2.0, 8.6)	0.8 (0.7, 0.9)
Heart rate >90 beats/min	1.8 (1.3, 2.5)	0.3 (0.1, 0.8)
Heart rate increased by 20 beats/min	2.5 (1.2, 5.3)	0.7 (0.5, 1.0)
Respiratory rate >20/min	1.7 (1.3, 2.2)	0.5 (0.3, 0.8)
Pleural friction rub	1.5 (0.6, 3.8)	1.0 (0.8, 1.1)
Loud P_2	1.1 (0.4, 3.1)	1.0 (0.8, 1.2)
Calf pain or swelling	2.6 (1.4, 4.9)	0.6 (0.4, 0.9)
Hypoxemia	1.1 (1.0, 1.1)	0.8 (0.6, 1.1)
Increased A-a gradient	1.1 (1.0, 1.2)	0.3 (0, 2.4)

Table 30-3 Hoellerich Rule for Pulmonary Embolism

1-10 points	0.1 (0, 0.6)	—
11-18 points	0.7 (0.4, 1.3)	—
19-23 points	3.7 (1.5, 9.5)	—
24-31 points	17.3 (2.3, 131.5)	—

Continued

TABLE 60-1 Likelihood ratios—point estimates and 95% confidence intervals—cont'd

FINDING	POSITIVE LR (95% CI)	NEGATIVE LR (95% CI)
Table 30-4 Wells Rule for Pulmonary Embolism		
Low clinical probability	0.2 (0.1, 0.2)	—
Moderate clinical probability	1.8 (1.5, 2.1)	—
High clinical probability	17.1 (10.9, 26.8)	—
Chapter 31 Inspection of the Neck Veins		
Intermittent cannon A waves, detecting atrioventricular dissociation	3.8 (1.8, 8.2)	0.1 (0, 0.4)
Table 31-1 Inspection of Neck Veins		
Detecting measured CVP >8 cm H_2O	9.0 (3.7, 22.1)	0.2 (0, 1.5)
Detecting measured CVP >12 cm H_2O	10.4 (5.5, 19.9)	0.1 (0, 0.6)
Detecting elevated left heart diastolic pressures	3.9 (1.6, 9.4)	0.7 (0.5, 1.0)
Detecting low left ejection fraction	4.0 (0.2, 72.8)	1.0 (0.9, 1.0)
Predicting postoperative pulmonary edema	11.3 (5.0, 25.8)	0.8 (0.7, 1.0)
Predicting postoperative infarction or death	9.4 (4.0, 22.4)	0.8 (0.7, 1.0)
Abdominojugular test, detecting elevated left heart pressures	8.0 (2.1, 31.2)	0.3 (0.2, 0.6)

Table 32-1 Percussion of the Heart

Dullness >10.5 cm from midsternal line, detecting cardiothoracic ratio >0.5	2.5 (1.8, 3.4)	0.05 (0, 0.3)
Dullness >10.5 cm from midsternal line, detecting increased left ventricular volume	1.4 (1.1, 1.7)	0.2 (0, 1.3)
Dullness extending beyond midclavicular line, detecting cardiothoracic ratio >0.5	2.4 (1.1, 5.2)	0.1 (0, 0.4)

Table 33-1 Palpable Apical Impulse

Supine apical impulse lateral to midclavicular line, detecting cardiothoracic ratio >0.5	3.4 (1.6, 7.3)	0.6 (0.5, 0.8)
Supine apical impulse lateral to midclavicular line, detecting ejection fraction <50%	5.7 (1.6, 20.5)	0.8 (0.7, 0.9)
Supine apical impulse lateral to midclavicular line, detecting increased ventricular volume	8.0 (1.9, 33.0)	0.7 (0.6, 0.9)
Supine apical impulse lateral to midclavicular line, detecting wedge pressure >12 mm Hg	5.8 (1.3, 26.0)	0.6 (0.4, 1.0)
Supine apical impulse >10 cm from midsternal line, detecting cardiothoracic ratio >0.5	4.3 (0.3, 70.8)	0.5 (0.3, 0.8)
Apical beat diameter 4 cm or more in lateral decubitus position, detecting increased ventricular volume	4.7 (2.1, 10.2)	0.4 (0.2, 1.0)

Continued

TABLE 60-1 Likelihood ratios—point estimates and 95% confidence intervals—cont'd

Finding	Positive LR (95% CI)	Negative LR (95% CI)
Table 33-2 Abnormal Palpable Movements		
Hyperkinetic apical movement in mitral stenosis, detecting additional valvular lesion	11.2 (6.4, 19.5)	0.3 (0.2, 0.4)
Sustained apical movement, detecting severe aortic stenosis	4.1 (1.7, 10.1)	0.3 (0.1, 0.5)
Sustained apical movement, detecting moderate-to-severe aortic regurgitation	2.4 (1.4, 4.0)	0.1 (0, 0.9)
Sustained left lower parasternal movement, detecting right ventricular pressure >50 mm Hg	3.6 (1.4, 8.9)	0.4 (0.2, 0.7)
Palpable P_2, detecting pulmonary hypertension	3.6 (1.5, 8.8)	0.05 (0, 0.8)
Table 35-1 First and Second Heart Sounds		
Changing intensity of S_1, detecting atrioventricular dissociation	24.4 (1.5, 384.5)	0.4 (0.3, 0.7)
Fixed wide splitting of S_2, detecting atrial septal defect	2.6 (1.6, 4.3)	0.1 (0, 0.8)
Paradoxic splitting of S_2, detecting significant aortic stenosis	2.4 (0.8, 7.0)	0.6 (0.2, 1.7)
Loud P_2, detecting pulmonary hypertension	1.2 (0.9, 1.5)	0.8 (0.3, 1.9)
Palpable P_2, detecting pulmonary hypertension	3.6 (1.5, 8.8)	0.05 (0, 0.8)

Table 36-1 Third and Fourth Heart Sounds

S_3, detecting ejection fraction <0.5	3.8 (1.9, 7.7)	0.7 (0.5, 1.0)
S_3, detecting ejection fraction <0.3	4.1 (2.3, 7.3)	0.3 (0.2, 0.5)
S_3, detecting elevated filling pressures	5.7 (3.1, 10.3)	0.8 (0.7, 1.0)
S_3, predicting postoperative pulmonary edema	14.6 (5.7, 37.3)	0.8 (0.7, 1.0)
S_3, predicting postoperative infarction or death	8.0 (2.7, 23.4)	0.9 (0.8, 1.0)
S_3, detecting moderate/severe mitral regurgitation	1.8 (1.4, 2.4)	0.8 (0.7, 0.9)
S_4, predicting 5-yr mortality after infarction	3.2 (1.3, 7.8)	0.8 (0.6, 1.1)
S_4, detecting elevated filling pressures	1.4 (0.8, 2.6)	0.6 (0.3, 1.4)
S_4, detecting severe aortic stenosis	0.9 (0.5, 1.9)	1.1 (0.6, 1.9)

Table 38-2 Murmurs and Valvular Heart Disease

Abnormal heart examination, detecting valvular heart disease	38.3 (9.5, 154.1)	0.3 (0.2, 0.5)
Systolic murmur, detecting aortic stenosis	3.3 (2.8, 3.9)	0.1 (0, 0.1)
Systolic murmur, detecting mild mitral regurgitation or worse	5.4 (3.7, 8.1)	0.4 (0.2, 0.7)
Systolic murmur, detecting moderate-to-severe mitral regurgitation	3.3 (2.7, 4.1)	0.2 (0.1, 0.4)
Systolic murmur, detecting mild tricuspid regurgitation or worse	14.6 (4.5, 47.1)	0.8 (0.7, 0.9)

Continued

TABLE 60-1 Likelihood ratios—point estimates and 95% confidence intervals—cont'd

FINDING	POSITIVE LR (95% CI)	NEGATIVE LR (95% CI)
Table 38-2 Murmurs and Valvular Heart Disease—cont'd		
Systolic murmur, detecting moderate-to-severe tricuspid regurgitation	10.1 (5.8, 17.8)	0.4 (0.2, 0.7)
Diastolic murmur, detecting mild aortic regurgitation or worse	9.9 (4.9, 20.0)	0.3 (0.2, 0.4)
Diastolic murmur detecting moderate-to-severe aortic regurgitation	4.3 (2.1, 8.6)	0.1 (0.1, 0.2)
Diastolic murmur, detecting pulmonary regurgitation	17.4 (3.6, 83.2)	0.9 (0.8, 1.0)
Table 38-4 Systolic Murmurs and Maneuvers		
Louder during inspiration, detecting right-sided murmurs	7.8 (3.7, 16.7)	0.2 (0.1, 0.5)
Louder with Valsalva strain, detecting hypertrophic cardiomyopathy	14.0 (3.4, 57.4)	0.3 (0.1, 0.8)
Louder with squatting-to-standing, detecting hypertropic cardiomyopathy	6.0 (2.9, 12.3)	0.1 (0, 0.8)
Softer with standing-to-squatting, detecting hypertrophic cardiomyopathy	7.6 (2.5, 22.7)	0.1 (0, 0.4)

Softer with passive leg elevation, detecting hypertrophic cardiomyopathy	9.0 (3.5, 23.3)	0.1 (0, 0.7)
Softer with isometric hand grip, detecting hypertrophic cardiomyopathy	3.6 (2.0, 6.4)	0.1 (0, 0.9)
Louder with isometric hand grip, detecting mitral regurgitation or ventricular septal defect	5.8 (1.9, 17.3)	0.3 (0.2, 0.5)
Louder with transient arterial occlusion, detecting mitral regurgitation or ventricular septal defect	48.7 (3.1, 768.5)	0.2 (0.1, 0.5)
Softer with amyl nitrite inhalation, detecting mitral regurgitation or ventricular septal defect	10.5 (5.1, 21.5)	0.2 (0.1, 0.6)

Table 39-1 Characteristics of Severe Aortic Stenosis

Delayed carotid artery upstroke	3.7 (2.5, 5.5)	0.4 (0.2, 0.9)
Reduced carotid artery volume	2.3 (1.8, 2.9)	0.3 (0.2, 0.5)
Brachioradial delay	2.5 (1.4, 4.7)	0.04 (0, 0.7)
Sustained apical impulse	4.1 (1.7, 10.1)	0.3 (0.1, 0.5)
Apical-carotid delay	2.6 (1.4, 5.2)	0.05 (0, 0.7)
Absent A_2	4.5 (1.4, 14.1)	0.8 (0.7, 1.0)
Absent or diminished A_2	3.6 (2.6, 5.1)	0.4 (0.3, 0.6)
S_4 gallop	0.9 (0.5, 1.9)	1.1 (0.6, 1.9)
Late peaking murmur	4.4 (2.5, 7.6)	0.2 (0.1, 0.3)
Prolonged murmur	3.9 (2.1, 7.3)	0.2 (0.1, 0.5)

Continued

TABLE 60-1 Likelihood ratios—point estimates and 95% confidence intervals—cont'd

FINDING	POSITIVE LR (95% CI)	NEGATIVE LR (95% CI)
Table 39-1 Characteristics of Severe Aortic Stenosis—cont'd		
Murmur loudest over aortic area	1.8 (1.1, 2.9)	0.6 (0.4, 0.7)
Murmur transmits to neck	1.4 (1.1, 1.8)	0.1 (0, 0.8)
Table 40-1 Aortic Regurgitation		
Diastolic murmur, detecting mild aortic regurgitation or worse	9.9 (4.9, 20.0)	0.3 (0.2, 0.4)
Diastolic murmur, detecting moderate-to-severe aortic regurgitation	4.3 (2.1, 8.6)	0.1 (0.1, 0.2)
Diastolic murmur loudest at right sternum, detecting dilated aortic root or endocarditis	8.2 (5.0, 13.3)	0.7 (0.7, 0.8)
Diastolic murmur softer with amyl nitrite inhalation, detecting aortic regurgitation (vs. Graham Steell)	5.7 (0.5, 71.4)	0.1 (0, 0.3)
Table 40-2 Moderate-to-Severe Aortic Regurgitation		
Murmur grade 3 or louder	8.2 (2.2, 31.1)	0.6 (0.4, 0.9)
Diastolic blood pressure, >70 mm Hg	0.2 (0.1, 0.9)	—
Diastolic blood pressure, 51-70 mm Hg	1.1 (0.7, 1.7)	—

Finding		
Diastolic blood pressure, ≤50 mm Hg	19.3 (2.7, 140.6)	—
Pulse pressure, <60 mm Hg	0.3 (0.1, 0.9)	—
Pulse pressure, 60-79 mm Hg	0.8 (0.2, 2.9)	—
Pulse pressure, ≥80 mm Hg	10.9 (1.5, 77.1)	—
Hill's test, <40 mm Hg	0.3 (0.2, 0.8)	—
Hill's test, 40-59 mm Hg	2.4 (0.6, 9.7)	—
Hill's test, ≥60 mm Hg	17.3 (1.1, 284.3)	—
Enlarged or sustained apical impulse	2.4 (1.4, 4.0)	0.1 (0, 0.9)
Duroziez's sign, femoral pistol shot, water hammer pulse	3.4 (0.4, 31.0)	0.7 (0.5, 0.9)

Table 41-1 Severity of Mitral and Tricuspid Regurgitation

Finding		
Murmur grade 3 or louder, detecting moderate-to-severe mitral regurgitation	4.4 (2.9, 6.7)	0.2 (0.1, 0.3)
S_3, detecting moderate-to-severe mitral regurgitation	1.8 (1.4, 2.4)	0.8 (0.7, 0.9)
Pulsatile liver, detecting moderate-to-severe tricuspid regurgitation	3.9 (1.4, 11.4)	0.8 (0.6, 1.0)
Systolic regurgitant venous waveform, detecting moderate-to-severe tricuspid regurgitation	1.5 (0.9, 2.5)	0.7 (0.5, 1.1)

Continued

TABLE 60-1 Likelihood ratios—point estimates and 95% confidence intervals—cont'd

FINDING	POSITIVE LR (95% CI)	NEGATIVE LR (95% CI)
Table 41-2 Mitral Stenosis		
Graham Steell murmur, detecting pulmonary hypertension	4.2 (1.1, 15.5)	0.4 (0.2, 0.9)
Hyperkinetic apical movement, detecting mitral regurgitation or aortic valve disease	11.2 (6.4, 19.5)	0.3 (0.2, 0.4)
Hyperkinetic arterial pulse, detecting mitral regurgitation	14.2 (7.4, 27.2)	0.3 (0.2, 0.4)
Chapter 42 Disorders of the Pericardium		
Pericardial rub in cancer patient, detecting idiopathic/radiation pericarditis	5.5 (1.4, 21.9)	0.4 (0.2, 0.9)
Pulsus paradoxus >12 mm Hg, detecting tamponade	5.9 (2.4, 14.3)	0.03 (0, 0.2)
Chapter 43 Congestive Heart Failure		
Proportional pulse pressure <0.25, detecting low cardiac index	5.4 (1.9, 15.4)	0.1 (0, 0.3)
Table 43-1 Elevated Left Heart Filling Pressure		
Heart rate >100 beats/min	5.5 (1.3, 24.1)	0.9 (0.9, 1.0)
Abnormal Valsalva response	7.6 (1.7, 34.3)	0.1 (0, 0.8)
Crackles	1.6 (0.8, 2.9)	0.9 (0.9, 1.0)

Elevated jugular venous pressure	3.9 (1.6, 9.4)	0.7 (0.5, 1.0)
Positive abdominojugular test	8.0 (2.1, 31.2)	0.3 (0.2, 0.6)
Supine apical impulse lateral to MCL	5.8 (1.3, 26.0)	0.6 (0.4, 1.0)
S_3 gallop	5.7 (3.1, 10.3)	0.8 (0.7, 1.0)
S_4 gallop	1.4 (0.8, 2.6)	0.6 (0.3, 1.4)
Edema	1.4 (0.6, 3.2)	1.0 (0.9, 1.0)

Table 43-2 Low Ejection Fraction

Abnormal Valsalva response	7.6 (4.9, 11.8)	0.3 (0.2, 0.4)
Crackles	2.9 (0.3, 27.3)	0.9 (0.7, 1.1)
Elevated neck veins	4.0 (0.2, 72.8)	1.0 (0.9, 1.0)
Supine apical impulse lateral to MCL	5.7 (1.6, 20.5)	0.8 (0.7, 0.9)
S_3 gallop	3.8 (1.9, 7.7)	0.7 (0.5, 1.0)
Murmur of mitral regurgitation	2.2 (0.9, 5.7)	0.8 (0.7, 1.0)
Hepatomegaly	0.9 (0.1, 9.4)	1.0 (0.9, 1.1)
Edema	4.9 (0.3, 86.6)	0.9 (0.9, 1.0)

Chapter 45 Palpation and Percussion of the Abdomen

Palpable spleen and adenopathy, detecting liver disease	0.04 (0, 0.6)	—
Palpable spleen and liver, detecting liver disease	2.7 (1.8, 3.9)	—
Massive splenomegaly, detecting hematologic disease	2.1 (1.1, 3.8)	—

Continued

TABLE 60-1 Likelihood ratios—point estimates and 95% confidence intervals—cont'd

Finding	Positive LR (95% CI)	Negative LR (95% CI)
Table 45-1 Liver and Spleen		
Palpable liver, detecting actual liver edge	233.7 (14.6, 3737)	0.5 (0.5, 0.6)
Palpable liver, detecting hepatomegaly	1.7 (1.4, 2.1)	0.5 (0.4, 0.7)
Palpable spleen, detecting splenomegaly	9.6 (5.7, 16.3)	0.6 (0.5, 0.7)
Positive spleen percussion sign (Castell's), detecting splenomegaly	1.9 (1.2, 2.8)	0.7 (0.5, 0.9)
Positive Nixon method, detecting splenomegaly	1.8 (1.0, 3.4)	0.8 (0.6, 1.0)
Traube's space dullness, detecting splenomegaly	2.0 (1.5, 2.6)	0.8 (0.7, 1.0)
Table 45-2 Gallbladder and Aorta		
Palpable gallbladder, detecting obstructed bile ducts	26.0 (1.5, 439.9)	0.7 (0.5, 0.9)
Palpable gallbladder, detecting malignant obstruction	2.6 (1.5, 4.6)	0.7 (0.6, 0.9)
Expansile pulsation epigastrium, detecting abdominal aortic aneurysm	7.6 (3.8, 15.0)	0.6 (0.5, 0.7)
Table 45-3 Ascites		
Bulging flanks	1.9 (1.4, 2.6)	0.4 (0.2, 0.6)
Edema	3.8 (2.2, 6.6)	0.2 (0, 0.6)
Flank dullness	1.8 (0.9, 3.4)	0.3 (0.1, 0.7)

Shifting dullness	2.3 (1.5, 3.5)	0.4 (0.2, 0.6)
Fluid wave	5.0 (2.5, 9.9)	0.5 (0.3, 0.7)

Chapter 46 Abdominal Pain and Tenderness

Loin tenderness, detecting ureterolithiasis	27.7 (10.7, 71.9)	0.9 (0.8, 0.9)
Renal tenderness, detecting ureterolithiasis	3.6 (3.1, 4.1)	0.2 (0.1, 0.3)
Microscopic hematuria, detecting ureterolithiasis	73.1 (41.7, 128.1)	0.3 (0.2, 0.4)

Table 46-1 Acute Abdominal Pain, Detecting Peritonitis

Guarding	2.6 (1.7, 3.9)	0.6 (0.5, 0.8)
Rigidity	5.1 (2.1, 12.2)	0.9 (0.8, 1.0)
Rebound tenderness	2.1 (1.6, 2.7)	0.5 (0.4, 0.6)
Abnormal bowel sounds	2.2 (0.5, 9.7)	0.8 (0.7, 0.9)
Rectal tenderness	1.2 (0.9, 1.7)	0.9 (0.9, 1.0)
Positive abdominal wall tenderness test	0.1 (0, 0.7)	1.9 (0.9, 4.4)
Positive cough test	2.4 (1.1, 5.4)	0.3 (0.2, 0.5)

Table 46-2 Acute Right Lower Abdominal Pain, Detecting Appendicitis

Fever	1.8 (1.2, 2.7)	0.5 (0.3, 0.7)
Severe right lower quadrant tenderness	1.6 (0.7, 3.8)	0.2 (0.1, 0.3)
McBurney's point tenderness	3.4 (1.6, 7.2)	0.4 (0.2, 0.7)
Rovsing's sign	2.5 (1.4, 4.4)	0.7 (0.6, 0.8)

Continued

TABLE 60-1 Likelihood ratios—point estimates and 95% confidence intervals—cont'd

Finding	Positive LR (95% CI)	Negative LR (95% CI)
Table 46-2—cont'd		
Rectal tenderness	1.1 (1.0, 1.2)	0.9 (0.9, 1.0)
Psoas sign	2.3 (0.7, 7.8)	0.9 (0.8, 1.0)
Obturator sign	1.4 (0.4, 4.5)	1.0 (0.9, 1.1)
Table 46-3 Acute Right Upper Abdominal Pain, Detecting Cholecystitis		
Murphy's sign	2.0 (1.5, 2.7)	0.2 (0, 2.4)
Back tenderness	0.4 (0.3, 0.6)	2.0 (1.4, 3.0)
Right upper quadrant mass	0.8 (0.5, 1.2)	1.1 (0.9, 1.2)
Table 46-4 Acute Abdominal Pain, Detecting Bowel Obstruction		
Visible peristalsis	18.8 (4.3, 81.9)	0.9 (0.9, 1.0)
Distended abdomen	9.6 (5.0, 18.6)	0.4 (0.3, 0.5)
Guarding	1.0 (0.6, 1.7)	1.0 (0.7, 1.4)
Rigidity	1.2 (0.4, 3.6)	1.0 (0.9, 1.2)
Rebound tenderness	0.9 (0.7, 1.1)	1.1 (1.0, 1.2)
Hyperactive bowel sounds	5.0 (2.4, 10.6)	0.6 (0.5, 0.8)
Abnormal bowel sounds	3.2 (1.7, 6.1)	0.4 (0.3, 0.5)
Rectal tenderness	0.9 (0.6, 1.5)	1.0 (1.0, 1.1)

Table 46-5 Chronic Upper Abdominal Pain

Right upper quadrant tenderness, detecting cholelithiasis	1.1 (0.9, 1.4)	0.9 (0.7, 1.2)
Lower abdominal tenderness, detecting cholelithiasis	0.5 (0.3, 0.7)	1.4 (1.2, 1.6)
Epigastric tenderness, detecting positive upper endoscopy	0.9 (0.7, 1.3)	1.2 (0.6, 2.3)

Table 47-1 Auscultation of the Abdomen

Any abdominal bruit, detecting renovascular hypertension	4.8 (2.6, 9.0)	0.7 (0.7, 0.8)
Any abdominal bruit, detecting abdominal aortic aneurysm	2.0 (0.5, 8.6)	0.9 (0.8, 1.1)
Systolic/diastolic bruit, detecting renovascular hypertension	38.9 (9.5, 159.6)	0.6 (0.5, 0.7)

Chapter 48 Peripheral Vascular Disease

Abnormal femoral pulse, detecting aortoiliac disease	31.0 (1.9, 500.6)	0.6 (0.5, 0.8)
Limb bruit, detecting arterial stenosis	3.2 (1.2, 8.7)	0.3 (0.1, 0.6)

Continued

TABLE 60-1 Likelihood ratios—point estimates and 95% confidence intervals—cont'd

FINDING	POSITIVE LR (95% CI)	NEGATIVE LR (95% CI)
Table 48-2 Peripheral Vascular Disease		
Wounds or sores on foot	7.0 (3.2, 15.6)	1.0 (1.0, 1.0)
Foot color abnormally pale, red, or blue	2.8 (2.4, 3.2)	0.7 (0.7, 0.8)
Atrophic skin	1.7 (1.2, 2.3)	0.7 (0.5, 1.0)
Absent lower limb hair	1.7 (1.2, 2.3)	0.7 (0.6, 1.0)
Foot asymmetrically cooler	6.1 (4.2, 8.9)	0.9 (0.9, 0.9)
Absent femoral pulse	6.1 (3.8, 10.0)	0.9 (0.9, 1.0)
Absent posterior tibial and dorsalis pedis pulses	14.9 (3.3, 66.3)	0.3 (0.3, 0.4)
Limb bruit present	7.3 (3.6, 14.9)	0.7 (0.5, 0.9)
Capillary refill time ≥5 sec	1.9 (1.2, 3.2)	0.8 (0.7, 1.0)
Venous filling time >20 sec	3.6 (1.9, 6.8)	0.8 (0.7, 1.0)
Table 49-1 The Diabetic Foot		
Unable to sense the 5.07 monofilament, detecting subsequent ulceration	2.9 (1.1, 7.8)	0.5 (0.4, 0.6)
Positive probe test, detecting osteomyelitis	4.3 (1.7, 10.8)	0.4 (0.3, 0.6)
Ulcer area >2 cm², detecting osteomyelitis	7.2 (1.1, 48.9)	0.5 (0.3, 0.8)
Ulcer deeper than 3 mm or bone exposed, detecting osteomyelitis	3.6 (1.3, 9.7)	0.2 (0.1, 0.5)
Erythema, swelling, purulence, detecting osteomyelitis	1.5 (0.5, 4.7)	0.8 (0.6, 1.3)

Chapter 50 Edema and Deep Vein Thrombosis

Active cancer, detecting deep vein thrombosis	3.2 (1.8, 5.5)
Recent immobilization, detecting deep vein thrombosis	2.3 (1.7, 3.2)

Table 50-1 Deep Vein Thrombosis

Any calf or ankle swelling	1.2 (1.0, 1.4)
Asymmetric calf swelling, ≥2 cm difference	2.1 (1.8, 2.5)
Thigh swelling	2.5 (1.6, 3.8)
Superficial venous dilation	1.9 (1.3, 3.0)
Erythema	1.0 (0.6, 1.7)
Superficial thrombophlebitis	0.9 (0.2, 5.1)
Tenderness	1.0 (0.9, 1.1)
Asymmetric skin warmth	1.4 (1.2, 1.7)
Palpable cord	1.1 (0.7, 1.6)
Homan's sign	1.1 (0.9, 1.3)

The active cancer and immobilization values above correspond to 0.8 (0.7, 0.9) and 0.8 (0.7, 0.9) respectively; the DVT signs correspond to 0.7 (0.5, 0.9), 0.6 (0.4, 0.7), 0.6 (0.5, 0.8), 0.8 (0.7, 1.0), 1.0 (0.8, 1.2), 1.0 (0.9, 1.1), 0.9 (0.7, 1.2), 0.7 (0.5, 1.2), 1.0 (0.9, 1.1), 1.0 (0.9, 1.1).

Table 50-3 Wells Score Scheme

Low pretest probability	0.2 (0.1, 0.3)
Moderate pretest probability	1.0 (0.8, 1.3)
High pretest probability	13.2 (9.1, 19.3)

Continued

TABLE 60-1 Likelihood ratios—point estimates and 95% confidence intervals—cont'd

FINDING	POSITIVE LR (95% CI)	NEGATIVE LR (95% CI)
Table 51-1 Visual Field Defects		
Anterior detects	4.2 (2.6, 6.7)	0.7 (0.5, 0.9)
Posterior defects	6.8 (2.6, 17.8)	0.4 (0.2, 0.8)
Asymmetric optokinetic nystagmus, detecting parietal lobe disease	5.7 (3.2, 10.1)	0.1 (0, 0.3)
Associated hemiparesis or aphasia, detecting parietal lobe disease	18.3 (6.0, 56.2)	0.1 (0, 0.7)
Chapter 53 Miscellaneous Cranial Nerves		
Hutchinson's sign, detecting ocular complications	3.2 (1.4, 7.5)	0.5 (0.3, 0.8)
Table 53-2 Aspiration After Stroke		
Abnormal voluntary cough	1.9 (1.2, 2.9)	0.5 (0.4, 0.7)
Dysphonia	1.3 (1.0, 1.6)	0.4 (0.2, 0.8)
Drowsiness	2.2 (1.3, 3.6)	0.4 (0.2, 0.8)
Absent pharyngeal sensation	2.4 (1.6, 3.6)	0.03 (0, 0.5)
Abnormal gag reflex	1.8 (1.2, 2.6)	0.5 (0.4, 0.7)
Water swallow test	5.6 (2.4, 12.9)	0.2 (0.1, 0.5)

Table 54-2 Parkinson's Disease

All 3 traditional findings present	2.2 (1.2, 4.2)	0.5 (0.3, 0.7)
Asymmetric onset and no atypical features	3.0 (1.5, 6.1)	0.3 (0.2, 0.5)
Asymmetric onset, no atypical features, no alternative diagnosis	4.1 (1.7, 10.2)	0.4 (0.3, 0.6)

Table 54-8 Unilateral Cerebral Hemispheric Disease

Arm rolling test	36.3 (2.3, 562.9)	0.1 (0.1, 0.3)
Upper arm drift	33.0 (2.1, 511.9)	0.2 (0.1, 0.4)
Finger tapping test	11.0 (2.3, 51.7)	0.2 (0.1, 0.4)
Facial weakness	32.3 (2.1, 501.7)	0.2 (0.1, 0.4)
Hemiparesis	31.7 (2.0, 491.5)	0.3 (0.2, 0.4)
Wrist extensor weakness	29.0 (1.9, 450.8)	0.3 (0.2, 0.5)
Babinski response	19.0 (1.2, 297.8)	0.6 (0.4, 0.7)
Hemianopia	12.5 (0.8, 199)	0.7 (0.6, 0.9)
Hemisensory disturbance	12.3 (0.8, 195.9)	0.7 (0.6, 0.9)

Chapter 56 Examination of the Reflexes

Absent bulbocavernosus reflex, detecting S2-S4 disease, men	13.0 (5.9, 28.9)	0.3 (0.2, 0.5)
Absent bulbocavernosus reflex, detecting S2-S4 disease, women	2.7 (1.6, 4.6)	0.6 (0.5, 0.9)
Grasp reflex, detecting frontal lobe or deep brain lesions	20.2 (4.8, 84.5)	0.9 (0.8, 0.9)

Continued

TABLE 60-1 Likelihood ratios—point estimates and 95% confidence intervals—cont'd

Finding	Positive LR (95% CI)	Negative LR (95% CI)
Table 57-3 Localizing Cervical Radiculopathy		
Weak elbow flexion, detecting C5 radiculopathy	5.3 (2.7, 10.5)	0.2 (0, 2.5)
Weak wrist extension, detecting C6 radiculopathy	2.3 (1.1, 5.0)	0.8 (0.5, 1.1)
Weak elbow extension, detecting C7 radiculopathy	4.0 (1.8, 9.2)	0.4 (0.3, 0.6)
Weak finger flexion, detecting C8 radiculopathy	3.8 (1.7, 8.5)	0.6 (0.3, 1.1)
Sensory loss affecting thumb, detecting C6 radiculopathy	8.5 (2.3, 31.1)	0.7 (0.5, 1.0)
Sensory loss affecting middle finger, detecting C7 radiculopathy	3.2 (0.2, 60.1)	1.0 (0.9, 1.0)
Sensory loss affecting little finger, detecting C8 radiculopathy	41.4 (2.1, 807.3)	0.8 (0.6, 1.1)
Diminished biceps or brachioradialis reflex, detecting C6 radiculopathy	14.2 (4.3, 46.7)	0.5 (0.3, 0.8)
Diminished triceps reflex, detecting C7 or C8 radiculopathy	28.3 (1.8, 440.9)	0.4 (0.3, 0.5)

Table 57-4 Carpal Tunnel Syndrome

"Classic" or "probable" hand diagram	2.4 (1.6, 3.5)	0.5 (0.3, 0.7)
"Unlikely" hand diagram	0.2 (0, 0.7)	—
Weak thumb abduction	1.8 (1.4, 2.3)	0.5 (0.4, 0.7)
Thenar atrophy	1.6 (0.9, 2.8)	1.0 (0.9, 1.0)
Hypalgesia	3.1 (2.0, 5.1)	0.7 (0.5, 1.1)
Abnormal 2 point discrimination	1.3 (0.6, 2.7)	1.0 (0.9, 1.1)
Abnormal vibration sensation	1.6 (0.8, 3.0)	0.8 (0.4, 1.3)
Tinel's sign	1.4 (1.0, 1.9)	0.8 (0.7, 1.0)
Phalen's sign	1.3 (1.1, 1.6)	0.7 (0.6, 0.9)

Table 57-7 Lumbosacral Radiculopathy, in Patients with Sciatica

Weak ankle dorsiflexion	4.9 (1.9, 12.5)	0.5 (0.4, 0.7)
Ipsilateral calf wasting	5.2 (1.3, 20.8)	0.8 (0.6, 0.9)
Leg sensation abnormal	1.2 (0.5, 2.9)	1.0 (0.8, 1.1)
Abnormal ankle jerk	4.3 (1.7, 11.1)	0.6 (0.5, 0.7)
Straight-leg raising maneuver	1.3 (1.0, 1.7)	0.2 (0.1, 0.6)
Crossed straight-leg raising maneuver	4.3 (1.8, 10.3)	0.8 (0.7, 0.8)

Continued

TABLE 60-1 Likelihood ratios—point estimates and 95% confidence intervals—cont'd

Finding	Positive LR (95% CI)	Negative LR (95% CI)
Table 57-8 Localizing Lumbosacral Radiculopathy		
Weak hallux extension, detecting L5 radiculopathy	1.8 (1.4, 2.3)	0.8 (0.6, 1.1)
Weak ankle plantarflexion, detecting S1 radiculopathy	26.6 (1.6, 436.4)	0.7 (0.6, 0.9)
Ipsilateral calf wasting, detecting S1 radiculopathy	2.4 (1.2, 4.7)	0.7 (0.5, 0.9)
Sensory loss L5 distribution, detecting L5 radiculopathy	4.6 (1.3, 16.8)	0.8 (0.7, 0.9)
Sensory loss S1 distribution, detecting S1 radiculopathy	3.0 (1.5, 6.2)	0.7 (0.5, 1.0)
Asymmetric quadriceps reflex, detecting L3-L4 radiculopathy	6.9 (2.4, 19.9)	0.7 (0.5, 1.1)
Asymmetric Achilles reflex, detecting S1 radiculopathy	5.2 (0.7, 36.6)	0.2 (0, 1.3)

INDEX

A

Abdominal aortic aneurysm
  bruit in, 636
  κ-statistic for, 38t
  palpation of, 603t, 606,
    608-609
Abdominal auscultation,
  633-637
  bowel sounds in,
    636-637
  bruits in, 633-634,
    635t, 636
  hepatic rub in, 636
  likelihood ratios of,
    861t
Abdominal bruits, 633-634,
  635t, 636
  clinical finding of, 633
  in healthy persons, 633
  in malignancies, 634
  rare causes of, 634-635
  with renovascular hyper-
    tension, 634
Abdominal distention,
  κ-statistic for, 38t
Abdominal inspection,
  589-592
  ecchymosis of abdominal
    wall in, 589-591
  κ-statistic for, 38t
  Sister Mary Joseph's
    nodule in, 591-592

Page numbers followed by "t"
and "n" indicate tables and text
footnotes, respectively, and *italic*
page numbers indicate figures.

Abdominal movements
  and abnormal respira-
    tion, 212-215, *213*
  paradoxical, 214-215
Abdominal obesity,
  113, 114
Abdominal pain, 615-629
  acute, 615-627; *see also*
    Acute abdomen
  chronic, 627, 628t, 629
  likelihood ratios of, 859,
    861t
Abdominal palpation
  κ-statistic for, 38t
  likelihood ratios of,
    857t
  of liver, 596, 597t, 598
  of spleen, 597t,
    599-600
  technique of, 594
Abdominal percussion
  κ-statistic for, 38t
  likelihood ratios of,
    857t
  of liver; *see* Liver
    percussion
  of spleen, 597t, 600-601
Abdominal reflex, superficial, 781
Abdominal veins, dilated,
  81-82
Abdominal wall tenderness
  test, 617-618
Abdominojugular test,
  409-410
  elevated venous pressure
    and, 411
  κ-statistic for, 37t

869